Understanding Prevention for HIV Positive Gay Men

Leo Wilton

Editor

Understanding Prevention for HIV Positive Gay Men

Innovative Approaches in Addressing the AIDS Epidemic

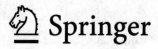 Springer

Editor
Leo Wilton
Department of Human Development
College of Community and Public Affairs (CCPA)
State University of New York at Binghamton
Binghamton, NY, USA

Faculty of Humanities
University of Johannesburg
Johannesburg, South Africa

ISBN 978-1-4939-0073-2   ISBN 978-1-4419-0203-0   (eBook)
DOI 10.1007/978-1-4419-0203-0

Library of Congress Control Number: 2017953104

Printed on acid-free paper

This Springer imprint is published by Springer Nature
The registered company is Springer Science+Business Media LLC
The registered company address is: 233 Spring Street, New York, NY 10013, USA

Contents

Contributors

Vincent C. Allen Jr Department of Psychiatry and Biobehavioral Sciences, Semel Institute for Neuroscience and Human Behavior, University of California, Los Angeles (UCLA), Los Angeles, CA, USA

Department of Psychology, University of California, Los Angeles (UCLA), Los Angeles, CA, USA

Emily A. Arnold Center for AIDS Prevention Studies, Department of Medicine, University of California, San Francisco (UCSF), San Francisco, CA, USA

Marlon M. Bailey Women and Gender Studies Program, School of Social Transformation, Arizona State University, Tempe, AZ, USA

Jason D.P. Bird Department of Social Work, School of Arts and Sciences-Newark, Rutgers University-Newark, Newark, NJ, USA

Alida M. Bouris School of Social Service Administration, Chicago Center for HIV Elimination, University of Chicago, Chicago, IL, USA

Russell A. Brewer Louisiana Public Health Institute, New Orleans, LA, USA

Ben Cabangun Asian & Pacific Islander American Health Forum, Oakland, CA, USA

Sean Cahill The Fenway Institute, Fenway Health, Boston, MA, USA

Department of Health Sciences, Bouvé College of Health Sciences, Northeastern University, Boston, MA, USA

Gabriel R. Galindo Public Health Research Services, LLC, Los Angeles, CA, USA

College of Southern Nevada, Las Vegas, NV, USA

Ja'Nina J. Garrett-Walker Department of Psychology, College of Arts and Sciences, University of San Francisco (USF), San Francisco, CA, USA

Janna R. Gordon Joint Doctoral Program in Clinical Psychology, University of California, San Diego (UCSD)/San Diego State University (SDSU), San Diego, CA, USA

Cynthia I. Grossman *FasterCures*, a center of the Milken Institute, Washington, DC, USA

Division of AIDS Research, National Institute of Mental Health (NIH/NIMH), Bethesda, MD, USA

Sabina Hirshfield Division of Research and Evaluation, Public Health Solutions, New York, NY, USA

Keith J. Horvath Division of Epidemiology & Community Health, University of Minnesota, Minneapolis, MN, USA

Kenneth T. Jones Office of Health Equity, U.S. Department of Veterans Affairs, Washington, DC, USA

Division of HIV/AIDS Prevention, National Center for HIV/AIDS, Viral Hepatitis, STD, and TB Prevention, Centers for Disease Control and Prevention (CDC), Atlanta, GA, USA

Carl A. Latkin Department of Health, Behavior and Society, Johns Hopkins Bloomberg School of Public Health, Johns Hopkins University, Baltimore, MD, USA

David J. Malebranche Department of Medicine, Morehouse School of Medicine, Atlanta, GA, USA

Kenneth H. Mayer Harvard Medical School, Boston, MA, USA

Department of Global Health and Population, Harvard T. H. Chan School of Public Health, Boston, MA, USA

Beth Israel Deaconess Medical Center, Boston, MA, USA

The Fenway Institute, Fenway Health, Boston, MA, USA

Matthew J. Mimiaga The Fenway Institute, Fenway Health, Boston, MA, USA

Departments of Epidemiology and Behavioral & Social Health Sciences, Brown School of Public Health, Providence, RI, USA

Department of Psychiatry & Human Behavior, Alpert Medical School, Brown University, Providence, RI, USA

Kevin L. Nadal Department of Psychology, John Jay College of Criminal Justice—City University of New York, New York, NY, USA

LaRon E. Nelson School of Nursing, University of Rochester, Rochester, NY, USA

Centre for Urban Health Solutions, Li Ka Shing Knowledge Institute, St. Michael's Hospital, Toronto, ON, Canada

John E. Pérez Department of Psychology, College of Arts and Sciences, University of San Francisco (USF), San Francisco, CA, USA

John A. Schneider Departments of Medicine and Public Health Sciences, Chicago Center for HIV Elimination, University of Chicago, Chicago, IL, USA

Steven Shoptaw Department of Family Medicine, David Geffen School of Medicine, University of California, Los Angeles (UCLA), Los Angeles, CA, USA

Michael J. Stirratt Division of AIDS Research, National Institute of Mental Health (NIH/NIMH), Bethesda, MD, USA

Karin E. Tobin Department of Health, Behavior and Society, Johns Hopkins Bloomberg School of Public Health, Johns Hopkins University, Baltimore, MD, USA

Dexter R. Voisin School of Social Service Administration, University of Chicago, Chicago, IL, USA

Jordan J. White Desmond M. Tutu Fellow of Public Health and Human Rights, Johns Hopkins Bloomberg School of Public Health, Johns Hopkins University, Baltimore, MD, USA

Jaclyn M. White Hughto Department of Chronic Disease Epidemiology, Yale School of Public Health, New Haven, CT, USA

The Fenway Institute, Fenway Health, Boston, MA, USA

Y. Omar Whiteside Division of HIV/AIDS Prevention, National Center for HIV/AIDS, Viral Hepatitis, STD, and TB Prevention, Centers for Disease Control and Prevention, Atlanta, GA, USA

John K. Williams Department of Psychiatry and Biobehavioral Sciences, Semel Institute for Neuroscience and Human Behavior, University of California, Los Angeles (UCLA), Los Angeles, CA, USA

Leo Wilton Department of Human Development, College of Community and Public Affairs (CCPA), State University of New York at Binghamton, Binghamton, NY, USA

Faculty of Humanities, University of Johannesburg, Johannesburg, South Africa

The chapters in this book, *Understanding Prevention for HIV Positive Gay Men: Innovative Approaches in Addressing the AIDS Epidemic*, were required to have a pre-publication double-blind peer review process in that reviewer and author identities were anonymous throughout the review process.

About the Editor

Leo Wilton is Professor in the Department of Human Development in the College of Community and Public Affairs (CCPA) at the State University of New York at Binghamton. He is affiliated with the Department of Africana Studies and Latin American and Caribbean Area Studies (LACAS) program at Binghamton University. Dr. Wilton is a Senior Research Associate in the Faculty of Humanities at the University of Johannesburg in Johannesburg, South Africa. His primary research interests include health disparities and inequities (primary and secondary HIV prevention); community-based research and evaluation; and Black psychological development and mental health. Dr. Wilton's scholarly research on the AIDS epidemic focuses on the intersectionality of race, gender, and sexuality, as situated in macro- and micro-level inequalities in Black communities, both nationally and internationally. The overall objective of his scholarly research program focuses on the impact of socio-structural/−cultural factors that influence sexual/drug risk and protective behavior and mental health for Black men who have sex with men (MSM). A key emphasis is placed on understanding how these domains influence people's development and well-being within African and African Diasporic communities for same-gender practicing men, with specific implications for addressing social justice and human rights. His research examines socio-structural/−cultural factors that provide the basis for the development of culturally congruent HIV prevention interventions for Black MSM.

Dr. Wilton was appointed to the NIH Director's Council of Public Representatives (COPR) for a four-year term. He was invited to the White House by the Office of National AIDS Policy as part of a select group of nationally recognized experts to participate in a research meeting that addressed the state of the AIDS epidemic among Black men in the USA. He was a Regional Trainer for the HOPE program with the American Psychological Association. He is a lifetime member of the Association of Black Psychologists and Association for the Study of the Worldwide African Diaspora (ASWAD). He is a founding member and immediate past Chair of the Board of Directors of the Black Gay Research Group (BGRG), an international organization of Black gay men engaged in interdisciplinary and intersectional research in the fields of public health, psychology, African Diaspora studies, gender studies, and sexuality studies.

Dr. Wilton is a recipient of the Chancellor's Award for Excellence in Teaching in the State University of New York (SUNY) and the Distinguished Contributions to Ethnic Minority Issues Award by Division 44 of the American Psychological Association. He completed a PhD degree in counseling psychology at New York University, MPH degree at the University of Massachusetts-Amherst, predoctoral clinical psychology fellowship in the Department of Psychiatry at the Yale University School of Medicine, postdoctoral research fellowship in HIV behavioral research and evaluation at New York University, and a postdoctoral summer fellowship in the Empirical Summer Program in Multi-Ethnic Research at the University of Michigan. He was a Visiting Professor at the Center for AIDS Prevention Studies (CAPS) in the Department of Medicine at the University of California, San Francisco.

Part I
Contexts

Chapter 1
Assessing the Diverse Factors that Influence the Behaviors and Experiences of Gay Men and Other Men Who Have Sex with Men (MSM) Living with HIV in the United States: Implications for Prevention and Improved Health

Russell A. Brewer and Kenneth H. Mayer

Introduction

This chapter provides an historical overview of the HIV epidemic and its impact on the health and lives of gay men and other men who have sex with men in the USA. It explores the wide range of factors that influence the behaviors and experiences of MSM living with HIV infection in the USA at the individual, interpersonal, organizational, community, and broader societal level with implications and recommendations for prevention and improved health.

Socio-historical Contexts of the HIV Epidemic in the United States

In the early 1980s, what came to be known as AIDS was first recognized in the USA as an array of atypical diseases among gay men, with associated immune dysfunction (Avert, 2017; Fenton, 2011). The report described the presence of Pneumocystis

R.A. Brewer (✉)
Louisiana Public Health Institute, New Orleans, LA, USA
e-mail: rbrewer@lphi.org

K.H. Mayer
Harvard Medical School, Boston, MA, USA

Department of Global Health and Population, Harvard T. H. Chan School of Public Health, Boston, MA, USA

Beth Israel Deaconess Medical Center, Boston, MA, USA

The Fenway Institute, Fenway Health, Boston, MA, USA

© Springer Science+Business Media LLC 2017
L. Wilton (ed.), *Understanding Prevention for HIV Positive Gay Men*,
DOI 10.1007/978-1-4419-0203-0_1

Carinii Pneumonia (PCP) among five gay men in New York and California. Almost a month after the release of this report, the *New York Times* reported that 41 gay men had been diagnosed with Kaposi's Sarcoma. By the end of 1981, 5–6 new cases of the disease were reported each week (Avert, 2017).

By early 1982, the outbreak had acquired a variety of names including gay-related immune deficiency (GRID) and gay compromise syndrome. By June 1982, 355 cases of Kaposi's Sarcoma and other serious opportunistic infections among previously healthy young individuals had been reported to the Centers for Disease Control and Prevention (CDC) by 20 states and they were not only occurring among gay men. There were a small number of cases among heterosexual men and women and more than half of the identified cases among heterosexuals were linked to shared needles for injection drug use. It was not until July 1982 that the burgeoning epidemic was called the "Acquired Immune Deficiency Syndrome" or AIDS as the disease was no longer solely affecting gay men but also heterosexual men, women, and children (Avert, 2017).

By December 1992, the CDC reported that three heterosexual hemophiliacs had died after developing PCP and other AIDS-related opportunity infections. What these three individuals shared in common was that they had all received a blood transfusion (Avert, 2017). Around the same time, the CDC also received reports of AIDS among a small number of immigrants from Haiti. Medical journals and books started to claim that AIDS originated in Haiti and that Haitians were responsible for the AIDS epidemic in the USA (Avert, 2017). By the end of 1982, based on the groups that were initially impacted by AIDS in the USA, it become known as a disease of the "4H club"—homosexuals, heroin addicts, hemophiliacs, and Haitians (Avert, 2017). From the onset, AIDS was associated with a high level of social marginalization. This form of stigma and discrimination persisted given the unknown context associated with this new and devastating disease at the time in terms of what was causing it, how it was transmitted, as well as how it was linked to gay men and injection drug users—groups that were already highly stigmatized and discriminated against in the USA. This prejudice and lack of information was also reflected in the White House's failed response to the epidemic (Avert, 2017).

By 1985, consensus had been reached that the epidemic was caused by a newly discovered retrovirus, named HIV (Human Immunodeficiency Virus). Thirty years later, HIV/AIDS has become one of the most politicized, feared, and controversial diseases (Avert, 2017) that continues to impact the health and lives of gay men and other MSM in the USA and throughout the world (Fenton, 2011).

Impact of HIV in the USA and Among MSM

Of an estimated 1.2 million people living with HIV infection in the USA, nearly 13% (one in eight individuals) do not know that they are infected (CDC, 2015). The number of individuals living with HIV infection has increased dramatically since the early 1980s as a result of advances in HIV treatment and resulting increases in life expectancy (CDC, 2013). Overall, the annual number of new HIV infections has remained stable with approximately 50,000 cases observed annually (CDC, 2015). MSM remain the group most heavily impacted by HIV in the USA. Although MSM represent approximately 4% of the male population in the USA, they accounted for more than three-fourths (78%) of new HIV infections among men and nearly two-thirds (63%) of all new HIV infections in 2010 (CDC, 2015). In addition, MSM accounted for more than half of all individuals living with HIV infection by the end of 2011 (CDC, 2015). Approximately 311,087 MSM diagnosed with AIDS have died in the USA since the beginning of the epidemic (CDC, 2015).

In terms of new HIV infections among MSM by race/ethnicity, Black MSM accounted for 11,201 or 38%, White MSM accounted for 9,008 or 31%, and Hispanic/Latino MSM accounted for 7,552 or 26% of all new HIV diagnoses among MSM in 2014 (CDC, 2016). HIV infection disproportionately impacts Black MSM, specifically young Black MSM. In 2010, young (13–24 years of age) Black MSM accounted for almost half (45%) of new HIV infections among Black MSM and 55% of new HIV infections among young MSM (CDC, 2015).

Sexual Risk Behaviors of HIV-Infected MSM in the USA

Although the annual number of newly diagnosed HIV infections has remained relatively stable since 1991 (CDC, 2009, 2011a), increases in HIV prevalence and sexually transmitted infections (STIs) among MSM in the USA (CDC, 2009, 2011a) underscore the need to fully examine and understand the individual, social, and structural factors and their impact among MSM living with HIV infection. MSM are more susceptible to HIV because of the increased efficiency of HIV transmission via condomless anal intercourse (CAI) (Khosropour et al., 2016). As a result, HIV-infected insertive partners are particularly likely to infect their uninfected receptive anal partners (Scott et al., 2014). Additionally, MSM can engage in role versatility, i.e., an HIV-uninfected MSM may be most susceptible to HIV, but once he becomes infected, he can efficiently transmit HIV to new partners if he is the insertive partner (Sullivan et al., 2012).

Two comprehensive reviews have explored the sexual risk behaviors of HIV-infected MSM in the USA (Crepaz et al., 2009; Van Kesteran, Hospers, & Kok, 2007). Crepaz et al. (2009) conducted a meta-analysis to determine the prevalence of UAI among HIV-infected MSM in the USA. Among half of the included studies, MSM of color (primarily Black and Latino) comprised the majority of the sample. The aggregate findings from the 30 studies showed that the estimated prevalence of CAI with any male partner among HIV-infected MSM was 43% (95% Confidence Interval [CI] = 37, 48). A second group of researchers conducted a literature review to identify studies describing sexual risk behaviors among HIV-infected MSM with a small number of studies occurring outside the USA from January 2000 to October 2005. The researchers found that more than half (29) of the 53 studies included in the analysis showed CAI prevalence rates among HIV-infected MSM of over 40%

(range 6–84%) (Van Kesteran et al., 2007). These results indicate that a sizeable percentage of HIV-infected MSM in the USA engage in CAI with their male partners, underscoring a major challenge for HIV prevention, although some sexual risk behaviors are with HIV seroconcordant partners (Khosropour et al., 2016).

MSM living with HIV infection have adopted several harm reduction strategies to reduce their risk of HIV transmission, including but not limited to abstinence (i.e., no sex); only engaging in oral sex; condom use; seroadaptive strategies; and withdrawal before oral and anal ejaculation with primary and non-primary sexual partners (Eaton et al., 2017; Grey, Rothenberg, Sullivan, & Rosenberg, 2015; Halkitis, Green, et al., 2005; McFarland et al., 2012; Parsons et al., 2005; Snowden, Raymond, & McFarland, 2009). Seroadaptive strategies consist of strategies that MSM use to reduce transmission risks through the selection of sexual partners based on serostatus, which may include "serosorting," or the selection of other HIV-infected partners for CAI and/or "seropositioning" (i.e., only engaging in receptive anal intercourse with HIV-uninfected partners given the relative reduced risk of HIV transmission) (Le Talec & Jablonski, 2008).

Data from 2,491 HIV-infected MSM in 16 states collected from 2000 to 2002 highlighted a variety of HIV prevention approaches utilized by HIV-infected MSM (CDC, 2004). Almost one-third (31%) of HIV-infected MSM reported that they were abstinent and 61% reported having sex in the last 12 months. Among sexually active MSM, 30% reported oral sex exclusively, 13% anal sex exclusively, and 55% reported both behaviors. CAI (insertive) at last sexual encounter was less likely to occur with HIV-uninfected partners and partners of unknown status than with HIV-infected partners. Furthermore, among men who reported insertive anal intercourse, CAI (insertive) was significantly less likely to occur with HIV-uninfected partners than with HIV-infected partners (CDC, 2004).

Several studies in California and New York have explored the sexual risk behaviors and HIV prevention strategies of HIV-infected MSM. A longitudinal study of 732 MSM in San Francisco showed that 11% of HIV-infected MSM did not engage in sex, 15% used condoms consistently, 13% were exclusive serosorters, and 20% were seropositioners (McFarland et al., 2012). A cross-sectional study of 1,211 HIV-uninfected and 251 HIV-infected MSM in San Francisco showed that approximately 18% of HIV-infected MSM did not engage in anal intercourse in the last 6 months (Snowden et al., 2009). Of those that engaged in anal intercourse, 21% used condoms all the time. Among HIV-infected MSM who had CAI, 20% were pure serosorters. Finally, among HIV-infected MSM who reported serodiscordant CAI, 14% were seropositioners (Snowden et al., 2009). A randomized controlled study specifically among 1,168 HIV-infected MSM enrolled in the Seropositive Urban Men's Intervention Trial (SUMIT) conducted in New York City and San Francisco from 1999 to 2002 also showed that HIV-infected MSM have adopted a variety of harm reduction sexual health approaches (Halkitis, Green, et al., 2005). Fifty-one percent (51%) HIV-infected MSM engaged in sexual experiences with other HIV-infected MSM and among those men, 62% engaged in CAI with their seroconcordant partner (Halkitis, Green, et al., 2005).

Studies also indicate that some HIV-infected MSM practice withdrawal before ejaculation during anal and oral sex as a harm reduction strategy (Parsons et al., 2005). The researchers found that men in New York and San Francisco reported more acts of oral sex without ejaculation than with ejaculation, and that HIV-infected MSM in San Francisco were more likely to use withdrawal before ejaculation during anal sex as a harm reduction strategy than men in New York City. A second study also explored sexual risk-taking behavior among 463 HIV-infected MSM in San Francisco and New York City. One hundred and seventy-nine (179) of the men reported that they were in primary relationships. The researchers found that seroconcordant and discordant couples engaged in unprotected insertive and receptive anal intercourse with and without ejaculation (Hoff et al., 2004).

There are limitations to seroadaptive and withdrawal before ejaculation approaches among HIV-infected MSM (Wilton et al., 2015). Seroadaptive strategies may not be effective in reducing HIV superinfection (infection with another strain of HIV in someone who is already HIV-infected) which is fortunately uncommon and the acquisition of other STIs which is unfortunately quite common (Blackard, Cohen, & Mayer, 2002; Kalichman, Rompa, & Cage, 2000; Van Kesteran et al., 2007). However, observational and mathematical modeling data support the premise that serosorting has reduced HIV transmission in some locations (Cassels, Menza, Goodreau, & Golden, 2009; Truong et al., 2006). For example, Truong et al. (2006) proposed that serosorting appeared to explain the rise in CAI and STIs yet stable HIV incidence among MSM in San Francisco. This analysis utilized an ecological approach with multiple pre-existing data sources (i.e., STI case reporting and HIV counseling and testing data) to assess whether increases in HIV serosorting among MSM may contribute to preventing the further expansion of the epidemic in San Francisco. A second group of researchers utilized mathematical modeling to estimate how serosorting may affect HIV prevalence and individual risk among MSM in Seattle, Washington (Cassels et al., 2009). Data from the 2003 random digit dial study of 400 MSM in Seattle was used to create the model. In their model based on observed levels of serosorting, the researchers predicted an HIV prevalence of 16%. In contrast, if serosorting was eliminated in the population, the predicted HIV prevalence would increase to 24.5%. The researchers concluded that under realistic scenarios of sexual behavior and testing for HIV, serosorting can be an effective harm reduction strategy for MSM in the USA (Cassels et al., 2009).

Additional limitations to seroadaptive strategies are that they rely on accurate assessment of HIV serostatus by both parties and mutual disclosure (Crepaz et al., 2009; Eaton, West, Kenny, & Kalichman, 2009; Van Kesteran et al., 2007). For HIV-infected MSM, serosorting may be "seroguessing," resulting in transmission from partners who were unaware of their HIV infection. Additionally, there may be some residual risk associated with the withdrawal before ejaculation approach because of the presence of HIV in pre-ejaculatory fluid and the possibility that the insertive partner may not withdraw before ejaculation, even if the initial intent was to do so (Parsons et al., 2005).

Several explanations have been proposed for the sizeable percentage of HIV-infected MSM in the USA who engage in CAI. One explanation points to the

availability of highly active antiretroviral therapy (HAART) and associated therapeutic optimism (i.e., treatment makes HIV infection a less serious concern) as a
direct cause of the increase in sexual risk behavior (Levy et al., 2017). A meta-
analysis of twenty-five (25) studies revealed that the likelihood of unprotected sex
was higher among HIV-infected individuals who believed that HIV transmission
would be less likely to occur if they were on HAART, have an undetectable viral
load or reported being less concerned about having unprotected sex given that
HAART was readily available (Crepaz, Hart, & Marks, 2004; Van Kesteran et al.,
2007). Another explanation is that HIV-infected MSM who are living longer as a
result of HAART have become tired of always having to monitor their sexual behavior ("prevention fatigue") (Ostrow et al., 2002; Van Kesteran et al., 2007) A cross-
sectional study among 547 HIV-infected and –uninfected MSM enrolled in the
Multicenter AIDS Cohort Study found that HIV-infected MSM with the least concern about their infectiousness due to the availability of HAART and/or safer sex
fatigue were more likely to report CAI (insertive) for HAART and safer sex fatigue
compared with other HIV-infected MSM (Ostrow et al., 2002).

   Another factor that may contribute to the increase in unprotected sex among
HIV-infected MSM relates to the behavioral phenomenon of barebacking (intentional unprotected anal sex) (Halkitis, Wilton, et al., 2005; Van Kesteran et al.,
2007). Data from 1,168 HIV-infected MSM in New York City and San Francisco
enrolled in SUMIT revealed that 27.2% of participants identified as barebackers.
Men from San Francisco were also more likely to identify as barebackers than men
from New York City (35.7% vs. 28.4%). In terms of adherence to therapy, barebackers were more likely to report having missed a medication dose in the 30 days
before the survey than non-barebackers (68.2% vs. 55.8%) (Halkitis, Wilton, et al.,
2005). Barebacking has become an important and compelling behavior for some
HIV-infected MSM who believe that it enhances intimacy, wholeness, and connectedness (Halkitis, Wilton, et al., 2005).

Psychosocial Issues Associated with Transmission Risk Behaviors Among HIV-Infected MSM

Another explanation for the high prevalence of CAI among HIV-infected MSM may
be due to the frequent presence of co-occurring psychosocial health issues among
MSM, such as depression, substance use, partner and homophobic societal violence, and childhood sexual abuse (Friedman et al., 2017; Mimiaga et al., 2015).
Stall et al. (2003) explored the associations between multiple co-occurring psychosocial conditions (i.e., polydrug use, depression, childhood sex abuse, and partner
violence), HIV status, and high-risk sexual behavior among 2,881 MSM in four
urban cities (Los Angeles, San Francisco, Chicago, and New York). Multivariable
logistic regression analyses revealed that polydrug use (Odds Ratio [OR] = 2.2;
95% CI = 1.7, 2.8) and partner violence (OR = 1.5; 95% CI = 1.2, 1.9) were significantly associated with HIV seropositivity. In addition, polydrug use (OR = 2.0; 95%

CI = 1.5, 2.7), partner violence (OR = 1.7; 95% CI = 1.3, 2.3), and childhood sexual abuse (OR = 1.4; 95% CI = 1.1–1.9) were significantly associated with high-risk sexual behavior among the cross-sectional sample of MSM enrolled from 1996 to 1998. The researchers also explored whether the interconnection or presence of multiple psychosocial health conditions increased vulnerability to HIV infection and likelihood of engaging in high-risk sexual behavior. After controlling for demographic variables, Stall et al. (2003) found that a greater number of psychosocial health conditions was associated with ascending odds ratios for having high-risk sex and ascending prevalence rates for HIV infection compared with the MSM who did not report any psychosocial health problems, suggesting that there were synergistic epidemics (syndemics) potentiating HIV risk (Stall et al., 2003).

Several structural- and environmental-level factors may also help explain the high prevalence of CAI among HIV-infected MSM (Lewnard & Berrang-Ford, 2014). Access and utilization of the Internet and commercial sex environments may facilitate the spread of HIV and other STIs among MSM in general (Van Kesteran et al., 2007). One example is the increase in early syphilis in the San Francisco City STI Clinic from 41 cases in 1998 to 495 cases in 2002 (CDC, 2003). This increase was also accompanied with an increase in the proportion of syphilis cases among MSM, from 22% in 1998 to 88% in 2002. The San Francisco Department of Public Health analyzed surveillance data from MSM to assess the association between early syphilis infection, Internet use, and other modalities among MSM to meet sexual partners. Of the more than 400 MSM with syphilis included in the analysis, almost one-third (32.6%) reported meeting their sexual partner(s) via the Internet and 31.4% reported meeting their sexual partner(s) at a commercial sex environment such as a bathhouse, sex club, and adult bookstore (CDC, 2003). These environments can facilitate HIV and STI risk by allowing MSM to have access to multiple partners in a short time interval.

Homelessness and unstable housing may also account for the sizeable percentage of HIV-infected MSM in the USA who engage in CAI. These structural-level factors have been associated with HIV risk behaviors and poorer health outcomes among HIV-infected individuals (Kidder, Wolitski, & Royal, 2007). Aidala, Cross, Stall, Harre, and Sumartojo (2005) explored the impact of housing among more than 2,000 individuals living with HIV infection receiving services at 16 medical and social service agencies. The researchers found an association between unstable housing, drug use, and sexual risk behavior. Thirty-four percent (34%) of the sample identified as an MSM living with HIV infection. Among HIV-infected MSM in the study, almost 60% were either homeless or had unstable housing. Participants whose housing status improved over time significantly reduced their risk of drug use, needle use, needle sharing, and unprotected sex by half in comparison to individuals whose housing status had not changed (Aidala et al., 2005). This study not only shows that unstable housing is associated with high rates of drug and sexual risk behaviors but it also shows that improvements in housing status is strongly associated with changes in HIV risk behaviors. Thus housing is a structural-level HIV prevention intervention (The National AIDS Housing Coalition, 2005).

Interventions to Decrease HIV Transmission Behaviors Among HIV-Infected MSM

Several individual-, group-, and community-level behavioral interventions have been developed to reduce HIV and STI risk behaviors among HIV-infected MSM and MSM in general (Herbst et al., 2017). Crepaz et al. (2006) conducted a meta-analytic review of HIV interventions for persons living with HIV infection to determine overall efficacy in reducing HIV risk behaviors. Twelve studies from 1988 to 2004 met the study criteria. Four of those studies included samples that were more than two-thirds MSM. Overall, individual- and group-level interventions significantly reduced instances of unprotected sex (OR 0.57; 95% CI = 0.40–0.82) and decreased STI acquisition (OR 0.20; 95% CI = 0.05–0.73) among persons living with HIV infection. A more recent meta-analysis was conducted to examine the effects of behavioral interventions designed to reduce HIV and STI transmission among MSM (Johnson et al., 2008). The researchers identified 44 studies evaluating 58 interventions with 18,585 participants. Twenty-six of the interventions were small group-level interventions, 21 were individual-level interventions, and 11 were community-level interventions. Sixteen of the 58 interventions focused specifically among HIV-infected MSM. Forty of the interventions that were measured against minimal to no HIV prevention intervention reduced instances of or partners for UAI by 27% (95% CI = 15%, 37%). The other 18 interventions reduced UAI by 17% (95% CI = 5%, 27%) beyond changes observed in the standard or other intervention group (Johnson et al., 2008). These meta-analyses indicate that there are effective individual-, group-, and community-level interventions in place for HIV-infected MSM and MSM in general. However, they may not be reaching the population. Data from the National HIV Behavioral Surveillance System revealed that only 18% of MSM in 21 cities have participated in either an individual- or group-level intervention in the last 12 months (CDC, 2011b).

Behavioral interventions for MSM have been designed from a deficit-based model or framework with a focus on the deficits (e.g., substance use, childhood sexual abuse, CAI) of MSM and not their assets or strengths. MSM may perceive these interventions as judgmental and may be less likely to accept, adhere, and complete these behavioral interventions (Herrick et al., 2011). These deficit models or frameworks, while important and necessary, are limited and need to be complemented with other perspectives such as an assets-based approach (Morgan & Ziglio, 2007). Health assets are defined as the resources that individuals and communities have at their disposal, which protect them from risky behaviors, negative health outcomes and/or promote health (Morgan & Ziglio, 2007). There is evidence of strength or assets among MSM (Herrick, Stall, Goldhammer, Egan, & Mayer, 2013) but they also have not been fully conceptualized and systematically measured. An example is the presence of a social support network among HIV-infected MSM. The concept of social support and its positive impact on health has been studied extensively since the 1970s (Hall, 1999). It has been examined in diverse age groups, populations, and health conditions (Hall, 1999). Hall (1999) conducted a literature review to examine the existing research on the relationship between social support and health among HIV-infected MSM. MSM living with HIV infection did report a social support network that consisted of partners, friends, family members, and other individuals. Another example documenting the assets of MSM is from Herrick et al. (2013). The researchers found from a sample of 4,066 MSM that about 75% of MSM with one or more psychosocial issues were still able to avoid high-risk sexual behaviors and to remain HIV uninfected (Herrick et al., 2013). Interventions that therefore focus on the assets or strengths of HIV-infected MSM and MSM in general need to be developed. These types of interventions may also improve intervention acceptability and efficacy (Herrick et al., 2011). MSM will also benefit substantially from structural-level interventions such as stable housing in order to reduce sexual risk behaviors that are more likely to transmit HIV and other STIs.

Antiretroviral Therapy Access and Adherence Among HIV-Infected MSM

The use of highly active antiretroviral therapy (HAART) has been shown to be effective in slowing down the progression of AIDS and in reducing HIV-related illnesses and deaths (Laffoon et al., 2015; Mayer et al., 2012; Siegfried, Uthman, & Rutherford, 2010). In addition, starting antiretroviral therapy earlier has been shown to reduce HIV transmission among serodiscordant sexual partners (Cohen et al., 2011; HIV Prevention Trials Network [HPTN], 2012) in the HPTN 052 study. Established in 2000, the HPTN is a worldwide clinical trials network funded by the National Institutes of Health (NIH) to develop and test the safety and efficacy of interventions to prevent the acquisition and transmission of HIV (HPTN, 2013). HPTN 052 study enrolled 1,763 HIV serodiscordant couples at 13 sites in Africa, Asia, and North and South America. Almost all (97%) of the couples were heterosexual. HIV-infected participants with CD4 counts between 350 and 550 cells/mm^3 and their partners were randomly assigned to one of two study arms: (1) immediate ART treatment of the HIV-infected partner at enrollment, or (2) delayed initiation of ART for the HIV-infected partner until two consecutive CD4 cell counts at or below 250 cells/mm^3 or the presence of an AIDS-defining illness. A total of 39 individuals who were HIV uninfected at enrollment became infected with HIV during the course of the study. Twenty-eight (28) of these cases were virologically linked to the infected partner with only one occurring in the early treatment group (hazard ratio, 0.04; 95% CI = 0.01–0.27). As a result, early initiation of ART led to a 96% reduction in HIV transmission to the HIV-uninfected partner (Cohen et al., 2011; HPTN, 2012).

The findings that increasing access to earlier initiation of HAART lead to reductions in HIV transmission have also been corroborated by ecological studies in British Columbia, San Francisco and KwaZulu-Natal, South Africa (Charlebois, Das, Porco, & Havlir, 2011; Eaton et al., 2012; Montaner, Lima, Barrios, Yip, & Wood, 2010; Tanser, Bärnighausen, Grapsa, Zaidi, & Newell, 2013). However, a recent study from Denmark, where the HIV epidemic is almost exclusively among

MSM, did not find a decrease in HIV incidence in conjunction with wider access to HAART. The authors found that some of the new transmissions were occurring in the setting of acute HIV infection (i.e., clusters of individuals who are most infectiousness and often aware of their new HIV infection), as well as some individuals presenting late into care (Audelin et al., 2013). It is also conceivable that since anal HIV transmission is more efficient than heterosexual transmission, that the magnitude of the benefit seen in HPTN 052 may not be as great for MSM, and observational studies of MSM discordant couples are underway in Europe and Australia to help further refine understanding of the risk of HIV transmission from an MSM partner who is on suppressive antiretroviral therapy (Muessig et al., 2012).

Combining Biomedical with Behavioral and Structural Interventions

The prevention benefits of early initiation of antiretroviral therapy resulting in viral suppression and reduced HIV transmission can be augmented with individual- or couple-level and community-level behavioral prevention interventions (Das et al., 2010). For HIV-infected MSM to fully benefit from HAART, they must first know that they have HIV (Gardner, McLees, Steiner, Del Rio, & Burman, 2011), enter care soon after diagnosis (Tinsley & Xavier, 2011), be engaged in regular HIV care, and initiate and adhere to their medications (Gardner et al., 2011). Recent data from the CDC (2012b) was used to inform the stages of engagement in HIV care for MSM in the USA (Fig. 1.1). The stages of engagement in HIV care or treatment cascade provides a visual depiction of the number of individuals living with HIV infection who are actually receiving the full benefits of medical care and treatment (Valdiserri, 2012). This cascade is being used at the national, state, and local levels to identify gaps in care and opportunities to reduce barriers to care and improve the

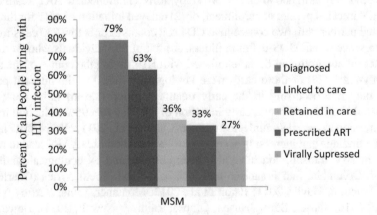

Fig. 1.1 Stages of HIV care by MSM category (CDC, 2012b)

delivery of services for persons living with HIV infection across the five stages of engagement in HIV care—from diagnosis of HIV infection and linkage in care to the initiation of ART, retention in care, and ultimate goal of viral suppression (Valdiserri, 2012). Only about one-quarter of all MSM living with HIV infection in the USA are in ongoing care and are virologically suppressed (CDC, 2012b). This points to the critical need to develop and/or expand upon effective interventions to support linkage and retention in HIV care.

Medication adherence is also necessary in order to achieve viral suppression for HIV-infected MSM engaged in care. Several studies have identified lower HIV adherence rates among HIV-infected MSM of color (Jacobson et al., 2001; Kleeberger et al., 2001, 2004; Oh et al., 2009). Four separate analyses from the Multicenter AIDS Cohort Study (MACS), a prospective study of HIV infection among 5,622 MSM in the USA, found that Black MSM living with HIV infection were more likely to report lower adherence than their White counterparts (Jacobson et al., 2001; Kleeberger et al., 2001, 2004; Oh et al., 2009). One study analyzing data from the Seropositive Urban Men's Study ($N = 456$), a formative study of HIV-infected MSM in two US cities, did not find a significant difference between adherence by race/ethnicity after controlling for confounders (Halkitis, Parsons, Wolitski, & Remien, 2003).

Several studies have also documented racial/ethnic differences in ART access among HIV-infected MSM (Halkitis et al., 2003; Jacobson et al., 2001; Stall et al., 2001). In these studies, Black MSM reported less access to ART than their White counterparts (Halkitis et al., 2003; Jacobson et al., 2001; Stall et al., 2001). Some explanations have been proposed to describe the disparity in ART access by race given that research has shown that Black MSM living with HIV infection were as likely as their White counterparts to report having health insurance (Halkitis et al., 2003; Kass, Flynn, Jacobson, Chmiel, & Bing, 1999; Millett, Peterson, Wolitski, & Stall, 2006). They may be in part due to health care provider biases, prejudices, and uncertainty when treating people of color as documented in the Institute of Medicine (IOM) report (IOM, 2002); mistrust of the health care system due to previous injustices such as the Tuskegee study (Freimuth et al., 2001); and perceived stigma about accessing care in unsympathetic clinical settings (CDC, 2011c; Eaton et al., 2015; Kinsler, Wong, Sayles, Davis, & Cunningham, 2007; Sayles, Wong, Kinsler, Martins, & Cunningham, 2009), which may discourage Black MSM living with HIV infection from engaging in needed care.

As HIV-infected MSM are engaged in the stages of HIV care, ongoing prevention counseling to reduce the likelihood of new HIV transmissions and acquisition of STIs should be a critical component of their care and treatment plan. The Medical Monitoring Project (MMP) documented a need for ongoing prevention counseling among MSM living with HIV infection (CDC, 2011d). The MMP collects clinical and behavioral data from a national representative sample of HIV-infected adults receiving medical care in outpatient facilities in the USA and Puerto Rico. Of the 1980 MSM enrolled in the MMP from 2008 to 2010, ART prescriptions were documented for 89% of MSM. Of those prescribed ART, 81% had achieved viral suppression, but only 39% of MSM had received prevention counseling (CDC, 2011d).

Identifying, Linking, and Retaining HIV-Infected MSM in Care

Several interventions have been shown to improve access to care and ultimately health outcomes for HIV-infected MSM in the USA and prevent the transmission of HIV. Two main linkage to care models have been shown to be effective in engaging newly diagnosed HIV-infected individuals in stable HIV care—the use of health system navigators and professional case managers (Bradford, Coleman, & Cunningham, 2007; Craw et al., 2008, 2010; Gardner et al., 2005). The patient health navigation model involves training community-based near peers to work with clients newly diagnosed with HIV infection. Bradford et al. (2007) explored the impact of this model in decreasing barriers to care and improving health outcomes for persons living with HIV infection. The researchers followed a cohort of 437 HIV-infected individuals over a 3-year period in four US cities (Portland, Seattle, Boston, and DC). Bradford et al. (2007) found that self-reported barriers to care (i.e., no health insurance, problem making an appointment, and worried about how to pay for care) were significantly reduced at 6 and 12 month follow-up compared to baseline measures at enrollment. In terms of health outcomes, the proportion of participants with an undetectable viral load was 50% greater at 12 months follow-up than at baseline. This study therefore showed that a patient health navigation model can reduce barriers to HIV care and enhanced linkage and engagement in HIV primary care.

In addition to the health navigation model, brief case management interventions have also been shown to improve linkage to care for persons newly diagnosed with HIV infection (Craw et al., 2008, 2010; Gardner et al., 2005). The Antiretroviral Treatment Access Study (ARTAS)-I was conducted in four US locations (Atlanta, Baltimore, Los Angeles, and Miami) among 273 persons newly diagnosed with HIV infection. Participants were randomized to a case management intervention (five sessions with a case manager over 90 days) or standard of care group (information about HIV and local care resources as well as passive referral to a local HIV medical care provider). The results indicated that a greater percentage of the case-managed participants than the standard of care participants visited an HIV clinician at least once within 6 months (78% versus 60%) and at least twice within a year (64% vs. 49%). The brief case management intervention was therefore associated with significantly higher rates of linkage to HIV care at 6 and 12 months (Gardner et al., 2005).

Given the successful results of the ARTAS-I study, CDC funded a demonstration project called ARTAS-II to evaluate the feasibility of implementing the brief case management intervention in local and state health departments and community-based organizations (CBOs) (Craw et al., 2008, 2010). Ten health departments and CBOs from across the USA were involved in the study from 2005 to 2006. Of the 626 individuals newly diagnosed with HIV infection enrolled in ARTAS-II, 497 (79%) visited an HIV clinician at least once within the first 6 months. The positive results of the ARTAS-II study indicated that the brief case management intervention is a useful model for health departments and CBOs to use in order to ensure that recently diagnosed HIV-infected persons are linked to HIV care within a reasonable period of time (Craw et al., 2008, 2010).

A variety of strategies have been documented to specifically identify, link, and engage HIV-infected MSM (specifically young MSM of color) in primary medical care (Hidalgo et al., 2011) but the effectiveness of these approaches has not been well documented. During the Health Resources and Service Administration's, Special Projects of National Significance—Young MSM of Color Initiative, part or full-time paraprofessional workers were employed by all of the funded eight demonstration sites to conduct outreach and linkage services (Hidalgo et al., 2011). These parapro-fessionals had a variety of job titles including outreach workers, connection to care specialists, peer youth advocates or specialists, supportive care managers, service linkage workers, and Disease Investigation Services (Hidalgo et al., 2011). In terms of outreach and identifying young MSM of color living with HIV infection, a major-ity of the funded sites conducted HIV outreach and education at bars, college cam-puses, gay pride events, and health fairs. Half of the sites utilized HIV mapping techniques to identify geographic areas with high HIV rates for more focused out-reach activities in these areas. Social marketing campaigns were also utilized by a few of the sites to raise awareness about the importance of HIV testing and treatment. Some sites also participated on HIV prevention planning groups to coordinate ser-vices and disseminate information. A few of the funded sites utilized drop-in centers to enhance self-efficacy to enter HIV care; conducted outreach and testing with HIV mobile vans; and recruitment and outreach using print and online advertisements and social networking sites including chat rooms and dating sites (Hidalgo et al., 2011).

Following identification of HIV-infected MSM of color, all of the eight sites uti-lized their outreach works and other paraprofessionals to enhance linkage in HIV care. These workers performed similar roles and responsibilities as ARTAS-I and –II linkage case managers and patient health navigators. This included assistance with scheduling medical appointments, arranged transportation for appointments, reminder telephone calls, and case finding for clients with missed appointments. In addition, most of the outreach workers also escorted individuals identified through outreach to their initial medical visit. As a result of these combined approaches, 87% of young MSM ($n = 291$) included in the analysis of 334 participants were linked to medical care within 3 months (Hidalgo et al., 2011). Given the dramatic increase in HIV incidence among young Black MSM (CDC, 2012a) and that younger Americans (25–34 years of age) living with HIV infection are less likely to be virally sup-pressed (CDC, 2012a) there needs to be a continued focus on engaging and retaining young MSM of color living with HIV infection in primary medical care.

Policy and Structural Approaches to HIV Prevention and Care for HIV-Infected MSM

Policy and structural-level factors including stigma, HIV confidentiality and dis-ability laws, laws banning the entry of HIV-infected persons into the USA, HIV nondisclosure laws, discrimination within the workplace, and expanded health care coverage impact the health and well-being of HIV-infected MSM in the USA. After three decades of extensive public health education efforts, voluntary HIV testing, and counseling about HIV in the USA, one would think that HIV-related prejudice and discrimination in the USA are now relics of the past. Unfortunately, this is not the case (Herek, 1999; The Body, 2003). Individuals living with HIV infection in the USA, including HIV-infected MSM, have been and continue to be the target of stigma and discrimination since the first cases of HIV infection were diagnosed.

HIV-related stigma refers to unfavorable beliefs, attitudes, policies, and related behaviors directed toward individuals perceived to be living with HIV infection as well as their loved ones, associates, social groups, and communities (Mitzel et al., 2015; The Body, 2003). A national representative survey of Americans on HIV/AIDS conducted by the Kaiser Family Foundation showed that a substantial number of Americans still continue to hold potentially stigmatizing attitudes toward individuals living with HIV infection. For example, 45% of Americans reported that they would be uncomfortable having their food prepared by someone who is HIV positive, 36% with having an HIV positive roommate, and 18% working with someone living with HIV/AIDS (Kaiser Family Foundation, 2011). Stigmatizing attitudes toward HIV-infected MSM from HIV negative MSM have also been documented in the literature (Wohl et al., 2013). According to Diaz (2003), when HIV negative Latino MSM were asked "Do you believe HIV-infected people are responsible for having gotten infected?" and "Do you believe that HIV-infected people are more sexually promiscuous?" 57 and 52% of HIV negative Latino MSM affirmed these statements.

HIV-related stigma fuels the HIV epidemic in the USA and among MSM. It discourages discussion and disclosure of HIV status with providers and sexual partners (CDC, 2011c; The Body, 2003; Center for AIDS Prevention Studies [CAPS], 2006), it deters testing and knowledge of HIV status (CAPS, 2006), and it also reduces access to HIV care and services (Kinsler et al., 2007; Sayles et al., 2009). Some MSM living with HIV infection may be less inclined to disclose their HIV status as it may lead to partner rejection, limit their sexual opportunities, or put them at increased risk for physical and sexual violence (CAPS, 2006). For example, 11.5% of MSM reported experiencing physical harm since their HIV diagnosis in the HIV Costs and Service Utilization Study of 2,864 adults living with HIV infection (Zierler et al., 2000). In terms of HIV testing, a study of 847 men and 1,126 women in seven US cities found that HIV testing behavior was related to low levels of STD-related stigma (Fortenberry, McFarlane, & Bleakley, 2002).

Stigma as a barrier to HIV care has also been documented in the literature. Sayles et al. (2009) conducted a cross-sectional study of 202 HIV-infected persons (predominantly Black) in Los Angeles County to examine the association between stigma and self-reported access to medical care. One-third of the participants reported high levels of stigma. The researchers also found that internalized HIV stigma measured using a 28-item scale was significantly associated with poor access to care (OR = 4.42; 95% CI = 1.88, 10.37) after adjusting for demographic, clinical, and other characteristics. A second prospective study also conducted in Los Angeles County explored the effect of perceived stigma on access to care among 223 low-income individuals living with HIV infection. Forty-six percent (46%) of the study population self-identified as Black and 26% of respondents reported at least one form of stigma from a health care provider using a 4-item scale. Perceived stigma was found to be associated with low access to care at baseline (OR = 3.29; 95% CI = 1.55, 7.01) and 6 months follow-up (OR = 2.85; 95% CI = 1.06, 7.65) after controlling for sociodemographic and clinical factors (Kinsler et al., 2007). A more recent study of the impact of stigma specifically among Black MSM showed that among Black MSM living with HIV, stigma from health care providers was associated with longer gaps in time since their last HIV care appointment (Eaton et al., 2015). Interventions to reduce stigma may therefore help to reduce new HIV cases and the impact of the epidemic in the USA (CDC, 2011c; The Body, 2003).

Sengupta, Banks, Jonas, Miles, and Smith (2011) conducted a systematic review of the literature to identify and determine the effectiveness of HIV-related interventions in reducing HIV-related stigma. Nineteen studies were included in the review. Nine of the studies were random clinical trials (RCTs), six were non-randomized control group studies, and four were pretest/post-test without a control group. Studies were conducted in North America, Europe, Asia, and Africa. The interventions focused on students, women, providers, persons living with HIV infection, parents, and the community. The duration of the interventions ranged from 15 min to 2 years. Fourteen of the nineteen studies demonstrated effectiveness in reducing HIV-related stigma. The authors assessed the quality of these studies and indicated that only two of the fourteen effective studies were considered "good" studies based on internal validity, the extent to which the interventions addressed stigma reduction, the stigma measures used, and the statistics reported to demonstrate effectiveness. Furthermore, the authors concluded that even with a well-designed intervention that shows a reduction in HIV-related stigma, we still know every little about how or if the change in stigma led to improvements in HIV testing, access to care, improved mental health outcomes, and enhanced policy support for people living with HIV infection. Therefore, the paucity of quality studies within the last 20 years identified in the review demonstrates the current gaps in evidenced-based interventions to reduce HIV-related stigma in the USA and the rest of the world (Sengupta et al., 2011).

Given the stigma and discrimination associated with HIV early on in the epidemic, legal protections were an essential component of the USA's response to stigma and discrimination (The Body, 2003). The recognition of the negative consequences of HIV-related stigma prompted the enactment of statutory protections for persons living with HIV infection, particularly related to the confidentiality of HIV testing results. The confidentiality of HIV test results is considered a protection under State laws and the US Constitution. These privacy laws aimed to protect individuals diagnosed with HIV infection from stigma and its consequences by keeping their health information confidential (The Body, 2003). HIV also qualifies as a disability under Federal and State laws as a result of a landmark case *Bragdon v. Abbot* (1998), the first HIV-related discrimination case that was brought to the US Supreme Court. The Supreme Court ruled that Congress intended HIV/AIDS to be included as a disability under the Americans with Disability Act of 1990. This protected persons living with HIV infection from discrimination in employment; housing; government services; and public places including schools, hotels, and medical offices (The Body, 2003).

Other laws and policies have and continue to contribute to HIV-related stigma and discrimination in the USA. As of 2010, 37 states have enacted legislation that criminalizes nondisclosure of HIV status in the USA (Lambda Legal, 2010). This may actually deter MSM from getting testing and knowing their HIV status. In some cases, the laws punish safer sex practices that are part of a risk reduction strategy. It is not known to what extent these nondisclosure laws deter high-risk behavior but it does fuel HIV-related stigma in the USA (Shriver, Everett, & Morin, 2000).

Another example of a law that was viewed by public health officials and advocates as stigmatizing and a barrier to HIV prevention was the statutory ban on immigration and travel into the USA by HIV-infected persons (Shriver et al., 2000). In 1993, Congress passed a law that prohibited HIV-infected individuals from traveling to the USA, including those wanting to live and work in the USA legally. This became known as the HIV Travel Ban (Kirberger, 2013). It was not until 2009 that the ban was lifted by President Obama (PBS, 2009).

Stigma and discrimination continue to persist for MSM in the work setting. A 2008 national probability survey found that 42% of lesbian, gay, and bisexual (LGB) respondents had experienced at least one form of sexual orientation-based discrimination (i.e., workplace harassment or lost a job) in their lifetime and 27% had experienced employment discrimination within the last 5 years prior to completing the survey. Discrimination and fear of discrimination can have negative effects on LGB employees in terms of mental and physical health, workplace productivity, job satisfaction, and job opportunities (Sears & Mallory, 2011). On April 25, 2013, the Employment Non-Discrimination Act (ENDA) prohibiting workplace discrimination based on sexual orientation and gender identity for lesbian, gay, bisexual, and transgender persons was introduced in the U.S. Senate and House for consideration (The Press-Enterprise, 2013). The passage of this Act has favorable implications for gay and bisexual men in the USA in terms of job security, satisfaction, salary, job performance, and overall health.

Health care policies or laws that expand access to HIV medical care and supportive services are important policy-level approaches with benefits for persons living with HIV infection including HIV-infected MSM. Key programs that currently provide health insurance coverage, care, and support for persons living with HIV infection in the USA include Medicaid, Medicare, and the Ryan White Program (Kaiser Family Foundation, 2012). A 2012 analysis of data from a network of high-volume HIV clinics found that 42% of persons with HIV in care were covered by Medicaid, 12% by Medicare, 24% by Ryan White, and only 13% of patients had private insurance (Fleishman & Gebo, 2012).

Health Reform and Prevention for HIV-Infected MSM

The Affordable Care Act (ACA), signed into law on March 23, 2010, by President Obama, represents one of the most significant overhauls to the US health care system since the passage of Medicaid and Medicare in 1965 (Vicini & Stempel, 2012).

The goal of the ACA is to expand access to affordable health insurance coverage and reduce the number of uninsured Americans. As such, it is expected to expand access to care for persons living with HIV infection including HIV-infected MSM (Crowley & Kates, 2012). Beginning in 2014, insurers have been no longer able to terminate or deny insurance coverage for persons living with HIV infection based on their pre-existing condition. They will also not be allowed to impose annual limits on how much the insurance company will cover over an individual's lifetime (AIDS.gov, 2012; Black AIDS Institute, 2010; Kaiser Family Foundation, 2012). The ACA also expanded Medicaid eligibility to include individuals with incomes below 133% of the Federal poverty line. As a result, persons living with HIV infection who meet this income threshold will be eligible for Medicaid in a state that is implementing Medicaid expansion. In addition, HIV-infected individuals who do not meet the eligibility criteria for Medicaid, Medicare, or Ryan White will have the option to buy coverage from the health insurance marketplace (Kaiser Family Foundation, 2012).

One of President Obama's top HIV/AIDS policy priorities was the development and implementation of a National HIV/AIDS Strategy (NHAS) for the USA. Shortly after the passage of the ACA, the NHAS was released in July 2010 to provide a roadmap with key benchmarks and greater coordination to respond to the HIV epidemic in the USA (The White House, 2010). The three primary goals of the NHAS are to reduce the number of new HIV infections; increase access to quality care for persons living with HIV infection; and reduce HIV-related health disparities among between groups (The White House, 2010). In addition to describing the disproportionate impact of HIV infection among gay and bisexual men, the NHAS also influenced the research and prevention efforts of federal agencies. For example, in order to meet the goals of the NHAS, the CDC implemented a High-Impact Prevention approach that consists of directing resources to geographic areas, interventions, and populations (i.e., MSM) that could have the greatest impact on HIV rates and health equity (CDC, 2011e).

Recommendations and Conclusions

Despite increasing evidence and awareness that earlier initiation of HIV treatment is associated with decreased HIV transmission, the numbers of new HIV infections among US MSM has continued to increase in recent years. Factors that are facilitating this increase include perceptions that HIV is not as serious as before, so that unprotected sex may be more acceptable, as well as the syndemic effects of substance use, depression, and other responses to the adversity that many MSM experience (Mimiaga et al., 2015). Social and structural factors, including unstable housing, homophobia, institutional racism, stigma, and discrimination, play an important role in potentiating the epidemic among MSM, particularly those from communities of color. Therefore, policy and structural-level changes can impact the health and well-being of HIV-infected MSM in the USA.

Evidence-based individual and group interventions have contributed to decreases in high-risk behaviors among some HIV-infected MSM. Early initiation of treatment has been associated with decreased HIV transmission, but recently, only about one-quarter of US MSM are virologically suppressed. Interventions using professional case managers and peer health system navigators have been shown to improve engagement in care and virological suppression. New modalities, such as culturally tailored behavioral interventions and those based on the existing assets of MSM (e.g., support systems), need to be combined to improve engagement in care, virological suppression, decreased instances of unprotected sex, and improved medical adherence. If many of these promising approaches can be scaled up and culturally tailored for the diverse subgroups of MSM living with HIV infection, more effective prevention of new HIV transmissions is feasible.

References

Aidala, A., Cross, J., Stall, R., Harre, D., & Sumartojo, E. (2005). Housing status and HIV risk behaviors: Implications for prevention and policy. *AIDS and Behavior, 9*, 251–265.

AIDS.gov. (2012). *The affordable Care Act helps people living with HIV/AIDS*. Retrieved from http://aids.gov/pdf/how-does-the-aca-help-plwh.pdf.

Audelin, A. M., Cowan, S. A., Obel, N., Nielsen, C., Jørgensen, L. B., & Gerstoft, J. (2013). Phylogenetic of the Danish HIV epidemic: The role of very late presenters in sustaining the epidemic. *Journal of Acquired Immune Deficiency Syndromes, 62*, 102–108.

Avert. (2017). *History of HIV & AIDS: United States of America*. Retrieved from http://www.avert. org/history-hiv-and-aids.htm.

Black AIDS Institute. (2010). *The Black AIDS Institute applauds Congress' passage of Historic health care reform bill*. Retrieved from http://www.thebody.com/content/art56015.html.

Blackard, J., Cohen, D., & Mayer, K. (2002). Human immunodeficiency virus superinfection and recombination: Current state of knowledge and potential clinical consequences. *Clinical Infectious Disease, 34*, 1108–1114.

Bradford, J., Coleman, S., & Cunningham, W. (2007). HIV system navigation: An emerging model to improve access to care. *AIDS Patient Care and STDs, 21*, S49–S58.

Cassels, S., Menza, T., Goodreau, S., & Golden, M. (2009). HIV serosorting as a harm reduction strategy: Evidence from Seattle, Washington. *AIDS, 23*, 2497–2506.

Center for AIDS Prevention Studies (CAPS). (2006). *How does stigma affect HIV prevention and treatment?* Retrieved from http://caps.ucsf.edu/uploads/pubs/FS/pdf/stigmaFS.pdf.

Centers for Disease Control and Prevention. (2003). Internet use and early syphilis infection among men who have sex with men—San Francisco, California, 1999–2003. *Mortality and Morbidity Report, 52*, 1229–1232.

Centers for Disease Control and Prevention. (2004). High-risk sexual behavior by HIV-positive men who have sex with men—16 sites, United States, 2000–2002. *Mortality and Morbidity Report, 53*, 891–894. Retrieved from http://www.cdc.gov/mmwr/preview/mmwrhtml/mm5338a1.htm.

Centers for Disease Control and Prevention. (2009). *HIV prevention in the United States. At a critical crossroads*. Atlanta, GA: National Center for HIV/AIDS, Viral Hepatitis, STD, and TB Prevention; Division of HIV/AIDS Prevention. Retrieved from http://www.cdc.gov/hiv/ resources/reports/pdf/hiv_prev_us.pdf.

Centers for Disease Control and Prevention. (2011a). *New multi-year data show annual HIV infections in U.S. relatively stable. Alarming increase among young, black gay and bisexual men requires urgent action*. Atlanta, GA: National Center for HIV/AIDS, Viral Hepatitis, STD, and

TB Prevention; Division of HIV/AIDS Prevention. Retrieved from http://www.cdc.gov/nchh-stp/newsroom/HIVIncidencePressRelease.html.

Centers for Disease Control and Prevention. (2011b). HIV risk, prevention, and testing behaviors among men who have sex with men—National HIV Behavioral Surveillance System, 21 U.S. cities, United States, 2008. *Mortality and Morbidity Report, 60*, 1–38.

Centers for Disease Control and Prevention. (2011c). *Stigma and Discrimination*. Atlanta, GA: National Center for HIV/AIDS, Viral Hepatitis, STD, and TB Prevention; Division of HIV/AIDS Prevention. Retrieved from http://www.cdc.gov/msmhealth/stigma-and-discrimination.htm.

Centers for Disease Control and Prevention. (2011d). Vital signs: HIV prevention through care and treatment-United States. *Morbidity and Mortality Weekly Report, 60*, 1618–1624.

Centers for Disease Control and Prevention. (2011e). *High-impact HIV prevention. CDC's approach to reducing HIV infections in the United States*. Atlanta, GA: National Center for HIV/AIDS, Viral Hepatitis, STD, and TB Prevention; Division of HIV/AIDS. Retrieved from http://www.cdc.gov/hiv/strategy/dhap/pdf/nhas_booklet.pdf.

Centers for Disease Control and Prevention. (2012a). *HIV among gay and bisexual men*. Atlanta, GA: National Center for HIV/AIDS, Viral Hepatitis, STD, and TB Prevention; Division of HIV/AIDS Prevention. Retrieved from http://www.cdc.gov/hiv/topics/msm/pdf/msm.pdf.

Centers for Disease Control and Prevention. (2012b). *HIV in the United States: The stages of care*. Atlanta, GA: National Center for HIV/AIDS, Viral Hepatitis, STD, and TB Prevention; Division of HIV/AIDS Prevention.

Centers for Disease Control and Prevention. (2013). *Today's HIV/AIDS Epidemic*. Retrieved from http://www.cdc.gov/nchhstp/newsroom/docs/HIVFactSheets/TodaysEpidemic-508.pdf.

Centers for Disease Control and Prevention. (2015). *HIV in the United States: At a glance*. Retrieved from https://www.cdc.gov/hiv/pdf/statistics_basics_ataglance_factsheet.pdf.

Centers for Disease Control and Prevention. (2016). *HIV among gay and bisexual men*. Retrieved from https://www.cdc.gov/hiv/pdf/group/msm/cdc-hiv-msm.pdf.

Charlebois, E. D., Das, M., Porco, T. C., & Havlir, D. (2011). The effect of expanded antiretroviral treatment strategies on the HIV epidemic among men who have sex with men in San Francisco. *Clinical Infectious Disease, 52*, 1046–1049.

Cohen, M. S., Chen, Y. Q., McCauley, M., Gamble, T., Hosseinipour, M. C., Kumarasamy, N., … HPTN 051 Study Team. (2011). Prevention of HIV-1 infection with early antiretroviral therapy. *The New England Journal of Medicine, 365*, 493–505.

Craw, J. A., Gardner, L. I., Marks, G., Rapp, R. C., Bosshart, J., Duffus, W.A., … Schmitt, K. (2008). Brief strengths-based case management promotes entry into HIV medical care: Results of the antiretroviral treatment access study-II. *Journal of Acquired Immune Deficiency Syndromes, 45*, 600–601.

Craw, J., Gardner, L., Rossman, A., Gruber, D., Noreen, O., Jordan, D., … Phillips, K. (2010). Structural factors and best practices in implementing a linkage to HIV care program using the ARTAS model. *BMC Health Services Research, 10*, 1–10.

Crepaz, N., Hart, T., & Marks, G. (2004). Highly active antiretroviral therapy and sexual risk behavior. *Journal of American Medical Association, 14*, 224–236.

Crepaz, N., Lyles, C. M., Wolitski, R. J., Passin, W. F., Rama, S. M., Herbst, J. H., … HIV/AIDS Prevention Research Synthesis (PRS) Team. (2006). Do prevention interventions reduce HIV risk behaviours among people living with HIV? A meta-analytic review of controlled trials. *AIDS, 20*, 143–157.

Crepaz, N., Marks, G., Liau, A., Mullins, M. M., Aupont, L. W., Marshall, K. J., … HIV/AIDS Prevention Research Synthesis (PRS) Team. (2009). Prevalence of unprotected anal intercourse among HIV-diagnosed MSM in the United States: a meta-analysis. *AIDS, 23*, 1617–1629.

Crowley, J., & Kates, J. (2012). *The Kaiser Family Foundation. The Affordable Care Act, The Supreme Court, and HIV: What are the implications?* Retrieved from http://kff.org/health-reform/issue-brief/the-affordable-care-act-the-supreme-court/.

Das, M., Chu, P., Santos, G. M., Scheer, S., Vittinghoff, E., McFarland, W., & Colfax, G. N. (2010). Decreases in community viral load are accompanied by reductions in new HIV infections in San Francisco. *PLoS One, 5*, 1–9.

Diaz, R. (2003). *HIV stigmatization and mental health outcomes in Latino gay men.* Paper presented at the Biennial meeting of the Society for Community Research and Action, Las Vegas, NM.

Eaton, L. A., Driffin, D. D., Kegler, C., Smith, H., Conway-Washington, C., White, D., & Cherry, C. (2015). The role of stigma and medical mistrust in the routing health care engagement of Black men who have sex with men. *American Journal of Public Health, 105*, e65–e82.

Eaton, J. W., Johnson, L. F., Salomon, J. A., Bärnighausen, T., Bendavid, E., Bershteyn, A., ... Hallett, T. B. (2012). HIV treatment as prevention: Systematic comparison of mathematical models of the potential impact of antiretroviral therapy on HIV incidence in South Africa. *PLoS Medicine, 9*, 1–20.

Eaton, L. A., Kalichman, S. C., Kalichman, M. O., Driffin, D. D., Baldwin, R., Zohren, L., & Conway-Washington, C. (2017). Randomised controlled trial of a sexual risk reduction intervention for STI prevention among men who have sex with men in the USA. *Sexually Transmitted Infections.* doi:10.1136/sextrans-2016-052835.

Eaton, L., West, T., Kenny, D., & Kalichman, S. (2009). HIV transmission risk among HIV seroconcordant and serodiscordant couples: Dyadic processes of partner selection. *AIDS Behavior, 13*, 185–195.

Fenton, K. (2011). *Addressing the HIV epidemic among gay and bisexual men.* Retrieved from http://blog.aids.gov/2011/09/addressing-the-hiv-epidemic-among-gay-and-bisexual-men.html.

Fleishman, J., & Gebo, K. (2012, March). Agency for Healthcare Research and Quality, 2012, as presented to the Institute of Medicine Committee to Review Data Systems for Monitoring HIV Care, referenced in Institute of Medicine, monitoring HIV care in the United States: Indicators and data systems. Retrieved from http://www.iom.edu/Reports/2012/Monitoring-HIV-Care-in-the-United-states.aspx.

Fortenberry, J., McFarlane, M., & Bleakley, A. (2002). Relationships of stigma and shame to gonorrhea and HIV screening. *American Journal of Public Health, 92*, 378–381.

Freimuth, V. S., Quinn, S. C., Thomas, S. B., Cole, G., Zook, E., & Duncan, T. (2001). African Americans' views on research and the Tuskegee Syphilis Study. *Social Science and Medicine, 52*, 797–808.

Friedman, M. R., Coulter, R. W., Silvestre, A. J., Stall, R., Teplin, L., Shoptaw, S., ... Plankey, M. W. (2017). Someone to count on: Social support as an effect modifier of viral load suppression in a prospective cohort study. *AIDS Care, 29*, 469–480.

Gardner, E. M., McLees, M. P., Steiner, J. F., Del Rio, C., & Burman, W. J. (2011). The spectrum of engagement in HIV care and its relevance to test-and-treat strategies for prevention of HIV infection. *Clinical Infectious Diseases, 52*, 793–800.

Gardner, L. I., Metsch, L. R., Anderson-Mahoney, P., Loughlin, A. M., del Rio, C., Strathdee, S., ... Antiretroviral Therapy and Access Study Group. (2005). Efficacy of a brief case management intervention to link recently diagnosed HIV-infected persons to care. *AIDS, 19*, 423-431.

Grey, J. A., Rothenberg, R., Sullivan, P. S., & Rosenberg, E. S. (2015). Racial differences in the accuracy of perceived partner HIV status among men who have sex with men (MSM) in Atlanta, Georgia. *Journal of the International Association of Providers in AIDS Care, 14*, 26–32.

Halkitis, P. N., Green, K. A., Remien, R. H., Stirratt, M. J., Hoff, C. C., Wolitski, R. J., & Parsons, J. T. (2005). Seroconcordant sexual partnering of HIV-seropositive men who have sex with men. *AIDS, 19*, S77–S86.

Halkitis, P., Parsons, J. T., Wolitski, R., & Remien, R. (2003). Characteristics of HIV antiretroviral treatments, access and adherence in an ethnically diverse sample of men who have sex with men. *AIDS Care, 15*, 89–102.

Halkitis, P. N., Wilton, L., Wolitski, R. J., Parsons, J. T., Hoff, C. C., & Bimbi, D. S. (2005). Barebacking identity among HIV-positive gay and bisexual men: Demographic, psychological, and behavioral correlates. *AIDS, 19*, S27–S35.

Hall, V. (1999). The relationship between social support and health in gay men with HIV/AIDS: An integrative review. *Journal of the Association of Nurses in AIDS Care, 10*, 74–86.

Herbst, J. H., Mansergh, G., Pitts, N., Denson, D., Mimiaga, M. J., & Holman J. (2017). Effects of brief messages about antiretroviral therapy and condom use benefits among Black and Latino MSM in three US cities. *Journal of Homosexuality.* doi:10.1080/00918369.2017.

Herek, G. (1999). AIDS and stigma. *American Behavioral Scientist, 42*, 1106–1116.

Herrick, A. L., Lim, S. H., Wei, C., Smith, H., Guadamuz, T., Friedman, M. S., & Stall, R. (2011). Resilience as an untapped resource in behavioral intervention design for gay men. *AIDS Behavior, 15*, S25–S29.

Herrick, A. L., Stall, R., Goldhammer, H., Egan, J. E., & Mayer, K. H. (2013). Resilience as a research framework and as a cornerstone of prevention research for gay and bisexual men: Theory and evidence. *AIDS Behavior.* Retrieved from http://link.springer.com/article/10.1007/s10461-012-0384-x/fulltext.html.

Hidalgo, J., Coombs, E., Cobbs, W. O., Green-Jones, M., Phillips, G., II, Wohl, A. R., & Young MSM of Color SPNS Initiative Study Group. (2011). Roles and challenges of outreach workers in HIV clinical and support programs serving young racial/ethnic minority men who have sex with men. *AIDS Patient Care and STDs, 25*, S15–S22.

HIV Prevention Trials Network (HPTN). (2012). *HPTN Study 052. Initiation of antiretroviral therapy (ART) prevents the sexual transmission of HIV in serodiscordant couples.* Retrieved from http://www.hptn.org/web%20documents/IndexDocs/HPTN052FactSheet19Jul2011.pdf.

HIV Prevention Trials Network (HPTN). (2013). *About the HPTN.* Retrieved from http://www.hptn.org/AboutHPTN.htm.

Hoff, C. C., Gomez, C., Faigeles, B., Purcell, D., Halkitis, P. N., Parsons, J. T., & Remien, R. H. (2004). Serostatus of primary partner impacts sexual behavior inside and outside the relationship: A description of HIV-positive MSM in primary relationships. *Journal of Psychology, 16*, 77–95.

Institute of Medicine. (2002). *Unequal treatment. What healthcare consumers need to know about racial and ethnic disparities in healthcare.* Retrieved from http://publichealthva.org/sites/default/files/What%20healthcare%20consumers%20need%20to%20know%20about%20racial%20and%20ethnic%20disparities%20in%20healthcare.pdf.

Jacobson, L. P., Gore, M. E., Strathdee, S. A., Phair, J. P., Riddler, S., Detels, R., & Multicenter AIDS Cohort Study. (2001). Therapy naivete in the era of potent antiretroviral therapy. *Journal of Clinical Epidemiology, 54*, 149–156.

Johnson, W. D., Diaz, R. M., Flanders, W. D., Goodman, M., Hill, A. N., Holtgrave, D., ... McClellan, W. M. (2008). Behavioral interventions to reduce risk for sexual transmission of HIV among men who have sex with men. *Cochran Database Systematic Review.* doi:10.1002/14651858.CD001230.pub2.

Kaiser Family Foundation. (2011). *HIV/AIDS at 30. A public opinion perspective.* Retrieved from http://www.kff.org/kaiserpolls/upload/8186.pdf.

Kaiser Family Foundation. (2012). *How the ACA changes pathways to insurance coverage for people with HIV.* Retrieved from http://kff.org/health-reform/perspective/how-the-aca-changes-pathways-to-insurance-coverage-for-people-with-hiv/.

Kalichman, S., Rompa, D., & Cage, M. (2000). Sexually transmitted infections among HIV seropositive men and women. *Sexual Transmitted Infections, 76*, 350–354.

Kass, N., Flynn, C., Jacobson, L., Chmiel, J. S., & Bing, E. G. (1999). Effect of race on insurance coverage and health service use for HIV-infected gay men. *Journal of Acquired Immune Deficiency Syndromes and Human Retroviruses, 20*, 85–92.

Khosropour, C. M., Dombrowski, J. C., Kerani, R. P., Katz, D. A., Barbee, L. A., & Golden, M. R. (2016). Changes in condomless sex and serosorting among men who have sex with men after HIV diagnosis. *Journal of Acquired Immune Deficiency Syndrome, 73*, 475–481.

Kidder, D., Wolitski, R., & Royal, S. (2007). Access to housing as a structural intervention for homeless and unstably housed people living with HIV: Rational, methods, and implementation of the housing and health study. *AIDS Behavior, 11*, 149–161.

Kinsler, J. J., Wong, M. D., Sayles, J. N., Davis, C., & Cunningham, W. E. (2007). The effect of perceived stigma from a health care provider on access to care among low-income HIV-positive population. *AIDS Patient Care and STDs, 21*, 584–592.

Kirberger, P. C. (2013). *HIV travel ban background*. Retrieved from http://immigration-lawyer.com/hiv-travel-ban-faq/.

Kleeberger, C. A., Buechner, J., Palella, F., Detels, R., Riddler, S., Godfrey, R., & Jacobson, L. P. (2004). Changes in adherence to highly active antiretroviral therapy medications in the Multicenter AIDS Cohort Study. *AIDS, 18*, 683–688.

Kleeberger, C. A., Phair, J. P., Strathdee, S. A., Detels, R., Kingsley, L., & Jacobson, L. P. (2001). Determinants of heterogeneous adherence to HIV-antiretroviral therapies in the Multicenter AIDS Cohort Study. *Journal of Acquired Immune Deficiency Syndromes, 26*, 82–92.

Laffoon, B. T., Hall, H. I., Surendera Babu, A., Benbow, N., Hsu, L. C., & Hu, Y. W. (2015). HIV infection and linkage to HIV-related medical care in large urban areas in the United States. *Journal of Acquired Immune Deficiency Syndromes, 69*(4), 487–492.

Lamda Legal. (2010). *HIV criminalization: State laws criminalizing conduct based on HIV status*. Retrieved from http://www.lambdalegal.org/sites/default/files/publications/downloads/fs_hiv-criminalization_1.pdf.

Le Talec, J., & Jablonski, O. (2008). *Seroadaptation instead of serosorting: A broader concept and more precise process model*. XVII International AIDS Conference, Mexico City, Abstract WEPE 0311.

Levy, M. E., Phillips, G., II, Magnus, M., Kuo, I., Beauchamp, G., Emel, L., ... Mayer, K. (2017). Treatment optimism is associated with HIV acquisition and transmission risk behaviors: A longitudinal analysis of Black men who have sex with men in HPTN 061. *AIDS and Behavior*. doi:10.1007/s10461-017-1756-z.

Lewnard, J. A., & Berrang-Ford, L. (2014). Internet-based partner selection and risk for unprotected anal intercourse in sexual encounters among men who have sex with men: A meta-analysis of observational studies. *Sexually Transmitted Infections, 90*, 290–296.

Mayer, K. H., Bekker, L. G., Stall, R., Grulich, A. E., Colfax, G., & Lama, R. (2012). Comprehensive clinical care for men who have sex with men: An integrated approach. *Lancet, 28*, 378–387.

McFarland, W., Chen, Y. H., Nguyen, B., Grasso, M., Levine, D., Stall, R., ... Raymond, H. F. (2012). Behavior, intention or chance? A longitudinal study of HIV seroadaptive behaviors, abstinence and condom use. *AIDS Behavior, 16*, 121–131.

Millett, G., Peterson, J., Wolitski, R., & Stall, R. (2006). Greater risk for HIV infection of Black men who have sex with men: A critical literature review. *American Journal of Public Health, 96*, 1007–1017.

Mimiaga, M. J., O'Cleirigh, C., Biello, K. B., Robertson, A. M., Safren, S. A., Coates, T. J. ... Mayer, K. H. (2015). The effect of psychosocial syndemic production on 4-year HIV incidence and risk behavior in a large cohort of sexually active men who have sex with men. *Journal of Acquired Immune Deficiency Syndromes, 68*, 329–336.

Mitzel, L. D., Vanable, P. A., Brown, J. L., Bostwick, R. A., Sweeney, S. M., & Carey, M. P. (2015). Depressive symptoms mediate the effect of HIV-related stigmatization on medication adherence among HIV-infected men who have sex with men. *AIDS and Behavior, 19*(8), 1454–1459.

Montaner, J. S., Lima, V. D., Barrios, R., Yip, B., & Wood, E. (2010). Association of highly active retroviral therapy coverage, population viral load, and yearly new HIV diagnoses in British Columbia, Canada: A population-based study. *The Lancet, 376*, 532–539.

Morgan, A., & Ziglio, E. (2007). Revitalising the evidence base for public health: An assets model. *Promotion and Education, 14*, 17–22.

Muessig, K. E., Smith, M. K., Powers, K. A., Lo, Y.-R., Burns, D. N., Grulich, A. E., ... Cohen, M. S. (2012). Does ART prevent HIV transmission among MSM? *AIDS, 26*, 2267-2273.

Oh, D. L., Sarafian, F., Silvestre, A., Brown, T., Jacobson, L., Badri, S., & Detels, R. (2009). Evaluation of adherence and factors affecting adherence to combination antiretroviral therapy among White, Hispanic, and Black men in the MACS Cohort. *Journal of Acquired Immune Deficiency Syndromes, 52*, 290–293.

Ostrow, D. E., Fox, K. J., Chmiel, J. S., Silvestre, A., Visscher, B. R., Vanable, P. A., ... Strathdee, S. A. (2002). Attitudes toward highly active antiretroviral therapy are associated with sexual risk taking among HIV-infected and uninfected homosexual men. *AIDS, 16*, 775–780.

Parsons, J. T., Schrimshaw, E. W., Wolitski, R. J., Halkitis, P. N., Purcell, D. W., Hoff, C. C., & Gomez, C. A. (2005). Sexual harm reduction practices of HIV-seropositive gay and bisexual men: Serosorting, strategic positioning, and withdrawal before ejaculation. *AIDS, 19*, S13–S25.

PBS. (2009). *Obama announces end of HIV ban*. Retrieved from http://www.pbs.org/newshour/updates/politics/july-dec09/travel_10-30.html.

Sayles, J. N., Wong, M. D., Kinsler, J., Martins, D., & Cunningham, W. E. (2009). The association of stigma with self-reported access to medical care and antiretroviral therapy adherence in persons living with HIV/AIDS. *Journal of General Internal Medicine, 24*, 1101–1108.

Scott, H. M., Vittinghoff, E., Irvin, R., Sachdev, D., Liu, A., Gurwith, M., & Buchbinder, S. P. (2014). Age, race/ethnicity, and behavioral risk factors associated with peer contact risk of HIV infection among men who have sex with men in the United States. *Journal of Acquired Immune Deficiency Syndromes, 65*, 115–1121.

Sears, B., & Mallory, C. (2011). *Documented evidence of employment discrimination and its effects on LGBT people*. The Williams Institute. Retrieved from http://williamsinstitute.law.ucla.edu/wp-content/uploads/Sears-Mallory-Discrimination-July-20111.pdf.

Sengupta, S., Banks, B., Jonas, D., Miles, M. S., & Smith, G. C. (2011). HIV interventions to reduce HIV/AIDs stigma: A systematic review. *AIDS Behavior, 15*, 1075–1087.

Shriver, M., Everett, C., & Morin, S. (2000). Structural interventions to encourage primary HIV prevention among people living with HIV. *AIDS, 14*, S57–S62.

Siegfried, N., Uthman, O., & Rutherford, G. (2010). Optimal time for initiation of antiretroviral therapy in asymptomatic, HIV-infected, treatment-naive adults (Review). *Cochrane Database of Systematic Reviews*. doi:10.1002/14651858.CD008272.pub2.

Snowden, J., Raymond, H., & McFarland, W. (2009). Prevalence of seroadaptive behaviours of men who have sex with men, San Francisco, 2004. *Sexually Transmitted Infections, 85*, 469–476.

Stall, R., Mills, T. C., Williamson, J., Hart, T., Greenwood, G., Paul, J., ... Catania, J. A. (2003). Association of co-occurring psychosocial health problems and increased vulnerability to HIV/AIDS among urban men who have sex with men. *American Journal of Public Health, 93*, 939–942.

Stall, R., Pollack, L., Mills, T. C., Martin, J. N., Osmond, D., Paul, J., ... Catania, J. A. (2001). Use of antiretroviral therapies among HIV-infected men who have sex with men: A household-based sample of 4 major American cities. *American Journal of Public Health, 91*, 767–773.

Sullivan, P. S., Carballo-Diéguez, A., Coates, T., Goodreau, S. M., McGowan, I., Sanders, E. J., ... Sanchez, J. (2012). Successes and challenges of HIV prevention in men who have sex with men. *The Lancet, 380*, 388–399.

Tanser, F., Bärnighausen, T., Grapsa, E., Zaidi, J., & Newell, M. L. (2013). High coverage of ART associated with decline in risk of HIV acquisition in rural KwaZulu-Natal, South Africa. *Science, 339*, 966–971.

The Body. (2003). *HIV/AIDS stigma*. Retrieved from http://www.thebody.com/content/art12405.html?ts=pf.

The National AIDS Housing Coalition. (2005). *Housing is the foundation of HIV prevention and treatment*. Retrieved from http://www.nationalaidshousing.org/PDF/Housing%20&%20HIVAIDS%20Policy%20Paper%2005.pdf.

The Press-Enterprise. (2013). *Gay rights: Employment discrimination still legal and common*. Retrieved from http://blog.pe.com/multicultural-beat/2013/04/25/gay-rights-employment-discrimination-still-legal-and-common/.

The White House. (2010). *The national HIV/AIDS strategy*. Retrieved from http://www.whitehouse.gov/administration/eop/onap/nhas/.

Tinsley, M., & Xavier, J. (2011). Outreach, care and prevention to engage HIV seropositive young men of color who have sex with men: A special project of national significance program initiative. *AIDS Patient Care and STDs, 25*, S1–S2.

Truong, H. M., Kellogg, T., Klausner, J. D., Katz, M. H., Dilley, J., Knapper, K., … McFarland, W. (2006). Increases in sexually transmitted infections and sexual risk behavior without a concurrent increase in HIV incidence among men who have sex with men in San Francisco: A suggestion of HIV serosorting? *Sexually Transmitted Infections, 82*, 461–466.

Valdiserri, R. (2012). *HIV/AIDS treatment cascade helps identify gaps in care, retention.* Retrieved from http://blog.aids.gov/2012/07/hivaids-treatment-cascade-helps-identify-gaps-in-care-retention.html.

Van Kesteran, N., Hospers, H., & Kok, G. (2007). Sexual risk behavior among HIV-positive men who have sex with men: A literature review. *Patient Education and Counseling, 65*, 5–20.

Vicini, J., & Stempel, J. (2012). *WRAPUP 4-US top court upholds healthcare law in Obama triumph.* Retrieved from http://www.reuters.com/article/2012/06/28/usa-healthcare-court-idUSL2E8HS4WG20120628.

Wilton, L., Koblin, B., Nandi, V., Xu, G., Latkin, C., Seal, D., … Spikes, P. (2015). Correlates of seroadaptation strategies among Black men who have sex with men (MSM) in 4 US cities. *AIDS and Behavior, 19*, 2333–2346.

Wohl, A. R., Galvan, F. H., Carlos, J. A., Myers, H. F., Garland, W., Witt, M. D., … George, S. (2013). A comparison of MSM stigma, HIV stigma and depression in HIV-positive Latino and African American men who have sex with men (MSM). *AIDS and Behavior, 17*, 1454–1464.

Zierler, S., Cunningham, W., Andersen, R., Shapiro, M. F., Nakazono, T., Morton, S., … Bozzette, S. A. (2000). Violence victimization after HIV infection in a US probability sample of adult patients in primary care. *American Journal of Public Health, 90*, 208–215.

Chapter 2
Comprehensive Primary Health Care for HIV Positive Gay Men

LaRon E. Nelson and David J. Malebranche

The Comprehensive Primary Health Care Approach

The concept of primary health care (PHC), as largely practiced within the context of the United States (USA), is understood as a person's first contact with the health care system, which is expected to be nonhospital-based preventative clinical services provided by physicians, nurse practitioners, and physician assistants (Stoeckle, 2009). Research advances in primary health care medicine and the development of evidence-based practice guidelines have provided a robust set of clinical tools to address physiological and psychological needs of patients that prevent severe acute illness events that result in lengthy, expensive, and avoidable hospital admissions (Aberg et al., 2009). Nonetheless, the concept and practice of primary health care does not sufficiently accommodate the complexity of life experiences that impact the health of individuals in the community, including gay-identified men who are living with Human Immunodeficiency Virus (HIV). The disease/illness management focus of the United States' version of primary health care has led health experts to call for it to be more precisely labeled "selective primary health care" (Cueto, 2004; Magnussen, Ehiri, & Jolly, 2004). By contrast, the comprehensive primary health care approach is one that attends to the social, cultural, and political realities of individuals and is well suited as an approach to care for HIV positive gay men who may be experiencing a multitude of social oppressions that impact their health.

L.E. Nelson (✉)
School of Nursing, University of Rochester, Rochester, NY, USA

Centre for Urban Health Solutions, Li Ka Shing Knowledge Institute, St. Michael's Hospital, Toronto, ON, Canada
e-mail: Laron_Nelson@URMC.Rochester.edu

D.J. Malebranche
Department of Medicine, Morehouse School of Medicine, Atlanta, GA, USA

© Springer Science+Business Media LLC 2017
L. Wilton (ed.), *Understanding Prevention for HIV Positive Gay Men*,
DOI 10.1007/978-1-4419-0203-0_2

Comprehensive primary health care is a concept that was commissioned by leaders in global health policy and clinical practice who understood that population advances in health could not be achieved without addressing social determinants of health and the inequitable social processes that led to disproportionately poor health outcomes in some groups compared to others (Lynam & Crowley, 2007). This is articulated in the Declaration of Alma Ata—adopted by the World Health Organization in 1978—a policy statement that advanced a holistic definition of health that included social and economic wellness and proposed structural level intervention strategies necessary to achieve "health" for all (International Conference on Primary Health Care, 1978). Initially trumpeted as a solution for resource-limited countries, the comprehensive PHC approach has also been embraced by advanced capitalist societies such as France, Brazil, and Canada—all of whom have outpaced the USA in the gains made in the prevention and management of HIV infection among gay men (Hutchison, Levesque, Strumpf, & Coyle, 2011; Rickets, Naiditch, & Bourgueil, 2012). In this chapter, we move beyond the concept of primary care towards a more serious embrace of comprehensive primary health care considerations for HIV positive gay men. Our objective in writing this chapter is for the reader to gain a core understanding of what is *comprehensive primary health care* and its applicability as an approach to clinical practice with gay-identified men living with HIV.

Principles of Comprehensive Primary Health Care

There are five principles in comprehensive primary health care. These principles are interrelated in that each is a necessary component for maximizing the degree to which an individual's life is not only disease-free (biomedical and selective primary care models), but also lived to its full potential capacity for social and economic wellness (Magnussen et al., 2004). In order for primary health care to be impactful on the health of individuals and communities there must be a sufficient number of qualified health practitioners trained with the requisite skills to appropriately care for them. The principle of (1) *health care provider capacity development* indicates that health care teams should be composed of personnel (e.g., nurses, physicians, social workers) who are prepared to work together to support individuals in the management of their physical and social wellness needs. The second principle, (2) *community participation*, stipulates that individuals and their communities must be involved in decision-making regarding policies and practices that will ultimately structure how they receive health care as well as the nature and volume of care that will be provided. This is envisioned as a collaborative process actively engaged with individuals and/or communities that lead to greater self-determination for their health and overall wellness. Recognizing that some of the life complexities that accompany an HIV diagnosis are outside the scope of what health care practitioners can address, the principle of (3) *intersectoral collaboration* is proposed as the coordinated assemblage of resources and services from an array of sectors that are relevant to the individual being able to achieve an optimal state of health and wellness. This goes beyond popular notions of interprofessional or interdisciplinary care, which are typically intrasectoral collaborations across areas such as nursing, pharmacy, social work, and psychology.

The comprehensive PHC principle of intersectoral collaboration calls for coordinating with services outside of the health care sector—for example, housing, criminal justice, employment and education sectors—to more wholly address factors that impact on an individual's health. In order to support individual health maintenance and the prevention of, and recovery from, illness events the (4) *appropriate use of technology* principle stipulates that providers should utilize clinical, social, and behavioral innovations that are not only scientifically sound but also culturally congruent and ones that can be sustained within an individual's and/or communities' economic means. Last, the principle of (5) *accessibility and equity* states that services needed to achieve and sustain optimal states of wellness should be universally accessible to all individuals in a society. Underlying the principles of accessibility is the active and deliberate disruption of institutionalized social processes (such as homophobia, racism, patriarchy) that impede an individual's ability to seek and receive the care at the time and in the quantity and quality that it is needed to achieve optimal wellness (Nelson, Walker, DuBois, & Giwa, 2014).

Evidence-Base for Comprehensive Primary Health Care

Social Determinants of Health

The literature on social determinants of health provides a foundation for grounding a discussion regarding comprehensive primary health care (Baum, 2008; Centers for Disease Control and Prevention, 2010; Rachilis et al., 2016). Research conducted over several years has established that poor health outcomes cluster together with poor social, economic, and political conditions—in particular is the position that marginalization, be it social, cultural, or political (or any combination of the three), negatively impacts the health of those who are the subject of it (Lynam & Crowley, 2007; Navarro & Muntaner, 2004; Nelson et al., 2016). This is particularly the case with HIV infection among many gay men. While there are examples of the mainstreaming of same-gender practices in the USA, gay men remain a socially marginalized group. The marginalization of HIV positive gay men's sexualities is compounded by the intersection of HIV stigma that can occur even within lesbian, gay, bisexual, and transgender communities (Smit et al., 2012). Homophobia, heteronormativity, racism, and HIV/AIDS stigma are all social processes that impact various subcommunities of HIV positive gay men and that comprehensive primary health care approaches can help to mitigate (Courtenay-Quirk, Wolitski, Parsons, & Gomez, 2006; Malebranche & Nelson, 2013; Nelson et al., 2014, 2016).

As mentioned earlier, the comprehensive primary health care approach moves beyond the biomedical management of illness but includes attention to factors that impact the overall health and well-being of HIV positive gay men. The use of comprehensive primary health care as a public health system strategy for the effective management of HIV among gay men has increased in health systems globally. Communities around the world have made great strides in delaying progression to AIDS and reducing HIV/AIDS mortality among gay men and other men who have sex with other men (Berkman, Garcia, Munoz-Laboy, Paiva, & Parker, 2005; Beyrer et al., 2011; Flowers & Davis, 2012; Galvão, 2005; Helleberg et al., 2012; Parker, 2009; van Griensven & van Wijngaarden, 2010). This is partly accomplished through addressing inequitable social processes and implementing anti-oppression strategies that facilitate engagement in medical care, and ensure equitable access to medical attention (Nelson et al., 2014; Seffner, Garcia, Muñoz-Laboy, & Parker, 2011).

Social Inequities and HIV Outcomes

A number of studies have been conducted that indicate the poor HIV outcomes are not evenly distributed across the entire population of people living with HIV. This is important because HIV positive gay men cross a multitude of socioeconomic spectra. Homophobia and HIV stigma are two important indicators of HIV outcomes (Garcia et al., 2016; Mayer, Bekker, et al., 2012). A study examining the relationship among stigma, medication adherence self-efficacy, and HIV outcomes among 202 HIV positive patients found that HIV stigma mediated the relationship between self-efficacy and quality of life (Li et al., 2011). These results are consistent with other HIV research on stigma and social marginalization (Kinsler, Wong, Sayles, Davis, & Cunningham, 2007; Mahajan et al., 2008; Nelson et al., 2016; Vanable, Carey, Blair, & Littlewood, 2006), indicating that anti-stigma and anti-oppression clinic environments optimize wellness outcomes among HIV positive gay men. Nonetheless, HIV/ AIDS stigma and other oppressions are not limited to the clinic environment. Even in the communities where they live and socialize, the degree to which HIV positive gay men experience other societal marginalization will impact on their overall quality of life including their experiences of wellness, and vulnerabilities to illness and death (Cole & Omari, 2003; Courtenay-Quirk et al., 2006).

Inequitable Distribution in HIV Care

There have been considerable advancements with the advent of HIV antiretroviral therapies. Unfortunately, these gains are not equally distributed across the entire population of HIV positive gay men and are often tempered by the intersection of social inequities that interfere with the ability of marginalized subgroups of HIV positive gay men to optimize self-management of their therapies (Rachilis et al., 2016). The U.S. Health Resources and Services Administration (HRSA) operates the Ryan White HIV/AIDS Comprehensive AIDS Resource Emergency (CARE) program that covers health care costs for people living with HIV who do not have sufficient income or insurance coverage to pay for HIV-related services (HRSA, 2010). The program has been in existence since 1990 and serves nearly 900,000 people per year (HRSA, 2010). Even with the additional HIV care capacity created by the Ryan White HIV/AIDS CARE program, inequities exist among gay men and other MSM with regard to enrollment and maintenance in HIV care (Young et al., 2016).

In a 7-city study of 610 marginalized (e.g., substance using, mental illness history, incarceration history) HIV positive people, researchers found that the uninsured, homeless, and those without access to mental health care had less access to HIV primary medical care (Cunningham et al., 2007). Results also showed that these groups were more likely to receive their HIV care in emergency situations. These and other disparities in access to HIV care have been documented in the literature for nearly two decades (Shapiro et al., 1999). Similar inequities exist with regard to young HIV positive gay males. Compared to MSM who acquire HIV infection in adulthood, MSM who sexually acquire HIV during their youth have lower rates of retention in HIV care. Numerous studies indicate that the major challenge for HIV positive adolescents is the risk of being lost-to-care between transitions from pediatric to adult care (Agwu et al., 2012; Chandwani et al., 2012; Dowshen & D'Angelo, 2011; Hussen, Chahroudi, et al., 2015). For example, in a retrospective study of 287 HIV positive youth (age 12–24) enrolled in multisite (n = 18) HIV treatment trials aimed at linking them to pediatric HIV/AIDS care between 2002 and 2008, Agwu et al. (2012) found that while two-thirds of youth initiated HAART, one-third of those transferred to adult care discontinued HAART. Researchers in this study also found that 50% of those who discontinued HAART on transition to adult clinical site were not virally suppressed. Further, the only independent predictor of HAART discontinuation identified in their regression analysis was transition to adult HIV care (adjusted hazard ratio: 1.23; 95% CI: 0.80–1.87) (Agwu et al., 2012). This phenomenon disproportionately affects MSM since they represent the majority of adolescent and pediatric cases of HIV (Centers for Disease Control and Prevention, 2015). Progression to AIDS and decreased access to quality HIV primary medical care are also more likely to occur within predominantly poor urban communities than in middle and upper class communities (Heslin, Andersen, Ettner, & Cunningham, 2005; Losina et al., 2009; Miles et al., 2013; Moore, 2011).

Inequities in HIV Outcomes and Care Quality Indicators

Advances in HIV antiretroviral therapy has helped to extend the lifespan of people living with HIV. Health science has developed more sophisticated models for treating HIV as well as managing the patients experience of treatment by such mechanisms as combination formulations which reduce the number of pills that must be taken at once and also formulations that allow for once daily dosing which makes self-management of HIV antiretroviral therapy drugs more manageable for many HIV positive gay men. Health services research in the areas of patient HIV outcomes also provides evidence of unequal distribution in the quality of HIV care and its associated outcomes (Hall, Byers, Ling, & Espinoza, 2007; Karach, Hall, Tang, Hu, & Mermin, 2015; Laffon et al., 2015; Simard, Fransua, Naishadham, & Jemal, 2012).

For example, a large population study of HIV positive gay- and non-gay-identified MSM was conducted using epidemiologic data from 33 US states on HIV/AIDS cases between 1996 and 2004 to examine inequities in HIV prevalence and progression to AIDS (Hall et al., 2007). Researchers found that, compared to White (25%) MSM, higher percentages of Blacks (33%) and Latino (32%) MSM progressed to AIDS within 3 years of their initial HIV diagnosis (Hall et al., 2007). The researchers also found among the 62,045 MSM with AIDS during 1996–2002, a significantly higher percentage of non-Hispanic Blacks (34%) had severely weakened immune systems (<50 CD4 cells/μL) at the time of their AIDS diagnosis than did Hispanics (28%) and non-Hispanic Whites (24%). Furthermore, non-Hispanic Black MSM were significantly more likely than non-Hispanic Whites or Hispanics to have died within 3 years of receiving an AIDS diagnosis (Hall et al., 2007). This specific analysis of Black MSM is important since stress, including the stress of everyday experiences of racism, is known to negatively impact on HIV outcomes such as viral load and CD4 T-cell count (Lesserman, 2008; Oramasionwu et al., 2009).

Reducing disparities in HIV outcomes require more comprehensive approach than that offered by biomedical science and practice alone (Mayer, Bekker, et al., 2012). An interdisciplinary approach to care that more fully accommodates the complexities of the lives of HIV positive gay men is needed in order to regain momentum in the reduction of new infections and increased quality of life. Here, we will specifically outline strategies within a comprehensive primary health care approach for HIV positive gay men—focusing on the five guiding principles of PHC and the ways in which they can be operationalized at the clinical encounter level as well as clinic/institutional policy level.

Applying the Comprehensive Primary Health Care Approach: Health Care Provider Capacity Development

Demonstration of HIV Clinical Excellence

As research in HIV nursing, medicine, and pharmacotherapeutics yield more clinical tools with which to support optimal physiological functioning of HIV positive gay men, health care practitioners will need to be current with regard to how to utilize these advances in the context of the patients' life situations. A number of organizations provide discipline specific continuing education offerings that allow practitioners to attain advanced levels of clinical training in HIV care. The American Academy of HIV Medicine (AAHIV) provides board certification for physicians, nurse practitioners, physician assistants, and pharmacists. Health care providers who attain this certification have an advanced level of clinical expertise as assessed by their practice experience and a national certification examination (AAHIV, 2013). Registered professional nurses are also able to attain advanced clinical preparation through the HIV/AIDS Nursing Certification Board (HANCB) that offers continuing education to registered nurses leading to the certification as AIDS Care Registered Nurse and Advanced AIDS Care Registered Nurse (HANCB, 2013). The Association of Nurses in AIDS Care (ANAC) and the HIV Medicine Association (HVMA) do not offer certifications, but have published online guidance and links to continuing education resources intended to encourage a high standard of practice for nurses and physicians providing ongoing clinical care to HIV positive gay men and others living with HIV and AIDS (ANAC, 2013; HVMA, 2010). More recently, HRSA announced its intention to invest funding to support the development of graduate education programs aimed at creating nurse practitioner and physician assistant specialists in HIV care (HRSA, 2013). The expansion of the number of health professions graduate programs that train providers to specialize in the care of HIV positive people is consistent with the U.S. National HIV/AIDS Strategy and is a crucial step in building and maintaining a competent HIV health workforce until an effective cure is found.

Multicultural Competencies

Health care practitioners can also improve their level of practice by increasing their capacity to understand patients in the patients' own sociocultural contexts (Nelson et al., 2014). These contexts are multifaceted and include LGBT culture, ethnic culture, and spiritual practice contexts (Hussen, Chahroudi, et al., 2015). Numerous studies indicate that patients rate their clinical experiences more favorably when they perceive that their differences with regard to age, ethnicities, sexualities, and spiritualties are respected and appreciated by their health care providers (Campbell, Ramsay, & Green, 2001; Trevino et al., 2010). Among HIV positive gay men, health care provider cultural competency is also associated with retention in care and self-reported quality of care (Hightow-Weidman, Smith, Valera, Matthews, & Lyons, 2011; Magnus et al., 2010). Opportunities for multicultural competency continuing education exist through HRSA funded AIDS Education & Training Centers (AETCs). The 11 AETCs across the USA routinely offer trainings for practitioners on best practices in providing care to HIV positive gay men and subpopulations (e.g., HIV positive gay men who use illicit substances; HIV positive gay men with mental illness) with unique sociocultural nuances that must be considered when working to develop plans of care (Ciesla & Roberts, 2001; Cunningham et al., 2007; Hatcher, Toldson, Godette, & Richardson, 2009; Shoptaw et al., 2012; Young, Shoptaw, Weiss, Munjas, & Gorbach, 2011; Young et al., 2016). Each AETC is responsible for providing technical assistance and continuing education to specific geographic regions of the country. Information regarding how to participate in continuing education through your regional AETC can be found by visiting their national website at www.aids-ed.org.

Life Stage-Specific Needs

HIV medical care is generally categorized into either pediatric or adult specialty practices. These life stage-specific HIV specialties are important given that there are a host of generational needs that must be attended to involving the physiology, psychology, and social context of HIV positive gay male youth compared to HIV positive adult gay men (Gayles, Kuhns, Kwon, Mustanski, & Garofalo, 2016; Hussen, Harper et al., 2015). Continued attention must be given to addressing the needs of these age groups. Nonetheless, tremendous opportunities remain for health care providers to expand their capacity to address the needs of subpopulations that are often subsumed—and many times made invisible—within the pediatric and adult HIV specialty categories (Young et al., 2016). Here, we will discuss the importance of HIV providers to develop capacities to serve adolescent (pediatric) and older adult (adult) HIV positive gay men.

Adolescents

Based on current national surveillance data, youth ages 20–24 had the highest age-specific number of new HIV infections in the United States (Centers for Disease Control and Prevention, 2015). This age group is considered to be "adolescence" since it is the time of life in which the brain has matured to a point that one has accomplished all the major pediatric developmental milestones but has not yet reached the full stage of adult development (Weinberger, Elvevag, & Giedd, 2005). Adolescents' specific developmental stage—which is heavily focused on exploration and establishing independence from authority figures—has implications for what are the best strategies to promote retention in HIV medical care, adherence to antiretroviral treatment and preventing onward transmission of HIV (Fielden, Chapman, & Cadell, 2011; Hagan, Shaw, & Duncan, 2008; Leonard, Markham, Bui, Shegog, & Paul, 2010).

There is a growing body of research focused on intervention models that support retention in care and treatment adherence for HIV positive gay adolescent males (Centers for Disease Control and Prevention, 2014; Gayles et al., 2016). Much of this research has yielded evidence regarding specific characteristics that optimize retention of HIV positive adolescent males. These include ensuring that clinic personnel exhibit multicultural competencies in their clinical practice and service delivery (Fortenberry, Martinez, Rudy, & Monte, 2012; Gilliam et al., 2011; Magnus et al., 2010) and that adolescents are provided with coordinated services to address some of their complex psychosocial needs (Bird, LaSaa, Hidalgo, Kuhns, & Garofalo, 2016; Birnbaum, Loundsbury, Eastwood, Palma, & Jo, 2013; Fortenberrry et al., 2012; Magnus et al., 2010). Other researchers are conducting research on interventions that take advantage of new technologies and capitalize on their popularity as communication mechanisms to promote treatment adherence (Hirshfield et al., 2016; Shegog, Markham, Leonard, Bul, & Paul, 2012). For example, Shegog et al. (2012) developed and tested a web-based ARV adherence support application for HIV positive adolescents and found that the intervention program was associated with increased adherence self-efficacy ($p < 0.05$) and increased understanding of the importance of maintaining a regular daily dosage schedule ($p < 0.01$). The utilization of technologies that are most compatible with the communication modes used among HIV positive gay adolescent males is a strategy that is consistent with comprehensive PHC's "*appropriate technology*" principle.

Older Adults

For older adult men, the experience of living with HIV can be complicated by declines in the expansiveness in their social networks or intersecting perceptions of decreased social significance within a LGBT community-context that has historically placed high value on the norms of youth and youthful body images (Grov, Golub, Parsons, Brennan, & Karplak, 2010; Halkitis et al., 2012; Heckman et al., 2002; Lyons, Pitts, Grierson, Thorpe, & Powell, 2010). There is significant research indicating that many HIV positive adult gay men experience depression related to experiences of loneliness, rejection, and HIV-related stigma (Grov et al., 2010). Decreases in perceived sexual desirability may create a situation where older adult HIV positive men are uncomfortable disclosing their HIV status due to the threat of rejection—that may be compounded by the ongoing (even if latent) perceived threat of rejection due to their age (Halkitis, Kapadia, Ompad, & Perez-Figueroa, 2015; Sankar, Nevedal, Neufeld, Berry, & Luborsky, 2011; van Kesteren, Hospers, van Empelen, van Breukelen, & Kok, 2007). A number of interventions have been developed to support interpersonal communication skills development among HIV positive gay men (Eaton, West, Kenny, & Kalichman, 2009; Kalichman et al., 2001). One well-known intervention is Healthy Relationships, an evidence-based group intervention program that promotes self-efficacy and relational skills development for people living with HIV (Kalichman et al., 2001; Kalichman, Rompa, & Cage, 2005). Based on social cognitive theory (Bandura, 1985), Healthy Relationships has a strong emphasis on skill development by having intervention participants first observe and then practice the target behaviors, attitudes, or expectations being modeled (Kalichman et al., 2001, 2005). Other interventions focus specifically on supporting men's decision-making skills regarding the disclosure of their HIV status in various situations (Serovich, Reed, Grafsky, & Andrist, 2009; Serovich, Reed, Grafsky, Hartwell, & Andrist, 2011). These complex life stage-specific needs require serious attention by providers working to increase their capacity to deliver quality care to HIV positive men—young and old alike.

Accessibility and Equity

With decreased access to care and mounting societal discrimination, HIV positive gay men require care that establishes access and longitudinal medical management. Treatment will be most effective only when access to care has been well established. In order to provide comprehensive primary health care for HIV positive gay men, it is not only necessary to provide a supportive care environment, but also necessary to implement a deliberate anti-racism, anti-oppression framework for practice (Mullaly, 2010; Nelson et al., 2016; Yee, 2005). Due to White supremacy, racism, heteronormativity, and homophobia, White and heterosexual men are granted explicit and implicit social privileges when compared with those who are non-white and/or self-identify as gay (Nelson et al., 2014). Practice frameworks can begin by attending to specific language that supports underlying hegemonic inequities that disenfranchise HIV positive gay men. For example, barriers to access for HIV positive gay men can come in forms as simple as the advertising of your clinic or community-based program. A deliberate anti-oppressive framework requires that health programs do more than "not discriminate" but specifically advertise that their services are inclusive of HIV positive gay men. Additionally, ensuring that program services are advertised at businesses and events that historically target and attract gay men demonstrates a willingness to be visibly associated with gay-identified activities—which is an important anti-oppression strategy (Nelson et al., 2014).

Another area where anti-oppressive practice can be exercised is in the interpersonal communication between the client and the providers. The manner in which health histories, risk assessments, and other clinical data are collected can be experienced as oppressive. For example, if an HIV positive gay man discloses that he has performed anal insertive sex with multiple partners in the past 3 months, an inquiry to him of: "Please, tell me about what motivated your sexual practices with these various partners" is consistent with anti-oppressive practice versus asking for the man to "please tell me the reasons why you were promiscuous and put other peoples lives at risk." If the patient is exhibiting signs of anxiety or distress, the practitioner may even wish to verbally acknowledge the psycho-emotional difficulties that the patient may be experiencing. In this way, the practitioner does not necessarily normalize the behavior, but makes an inquiry that avoids a moral evaluation of the behavior and reduces the risk of creating an interpersonal environment where the patient may not feel comfortable to further disclose or discuss his needs and concerns. Adopting some of these practices and identifying and incorporating other anti-oppressive practices can help generate environments where comprehensive primary health care can be more equitably accessed.

Community Participation

Health Program Integration

Including HIV positive gay men in the implementation of health programs are common mechanisms by which both clinic and community-based HIV/AIDS service programs achieve their goals for community participation. Health program integration benefits organizations by having individuals, who live the experience of being a gay man diagnosed with HIV, to help deliver services to others in this population. In addition to integrating HIV positive gay men into health programs, consumer advisory boards are sometimes utilized for generating feedback on how to improve organizational practices on working with HIV positive gay men. The consumer advisory boards can also be useful in identifying emerging social, cultural, and health trends among HIV positive gay men that may stimulate the development of new programs or treatment strategies. Consumer advisory boards are also helpful in ensuring that the clinics and programs are maximally responsive to the interests of HIV positive gay men. This can include interests related to clinic policies that affect the men. For example, a clinic that is contemplating a change in policy that reduces the number of wellness visits that are booked within a 12-month period, for patients who pay a reduced sliding scale fee for clinic services, should include full input from HIV positive gay men since such a decision will impact the care that the men can expect to receive. Consumer advisory boards could also provide input on research targeting HIV positive gay men with the aim of ensuring that the studies are as fair, relevant, and beneficial as possible to the men who will enroll. Health program integration can be achieved in numerous ways. Whichever methods are chosen, token participation should be avoided and full, serious input into program design and implementation must be the goal.

Developing a Client-Centered Treatment Plan

There is increasing attention given to the benefits of developing treatment plans that are centered on the client's sociocultural context and other situational factors that may be occurring at the time of the plan development. Numerous studies indicate that client-centered treatment plans are associated with greater treatment plan adherence by patients (Bogart et al., 2012; Church & Simon, 2010; Farrisi & Dietz, 2013; Gilman, Hidalgo, Thomas, Au, & Hargreaves, 2012). Moreover, health care providers have a moral imperative to ensure that the treatment plans for patients are based on what the patients' believe are in their own best interest (Beauchamp & Childress, 2001). HIV positive gay men who are fully informed about treatment options may decide to exercise options that the treating physician or nurse practitioner may not agree is the best course of action. It is important that the provider's understanding of the clinical situation is reconciled with the patient's understanding of what is the plan that they want for themselves. Nonetheless, it remains that the interests of the health care provider must not be prioritized over the self-expressed interests of the patient—regardless of the outcome implications. Major professional medical organizations have published statements that are consistent with the notion that treatment plans and approaches must be centered on the self-expressed interests of the patients (American Board of Internal Medicine Foundation, American College of Physicians American Society of Internal Medicine Foundation, & European Federation of Internal Medicine, 2002). Additionally, there is an abundance of evidence-based interventions for assisting providers to improve communications with patients such that the patients' needs and wishes are more likely to result in a plan of care that reflects the patients' interests (Harrington, Noble, & Newman, 2004; Kaymeg, Howard, Clochesy Mitchell, & Suresky, 2010; Rao, Anderson, Inui, & Frankel, 2007; Tennstedt, 2000). Providers can use these and other interventions to better enhance their skills in listening to HIV positive gay men's needs and incorporating them accordingly into their plans of care.

Intersectoral Collaboration

Health and Social Service Sectors

Collaboration between disciplines within health care is necessary to effectively promote physical and social wellness for HIV positive gay male patients. For example, the primary physician, nurse practitioner, or physician assistant should, whenever indicated, work in conjunction with other health providers such as pharmacists, psychologists, social workers, and registered dieticians. Notwithstanding the importance of multidisciplinary collaborations within health care, a comprehensive primary health approach stipulates that multidisciplinary efforts across sectors, outside of the health care domain, are required to fully address the complexities of patients' needs. HIV positive gay men with complex needs may require that health care providers coordinate care with a myriad of sectors for such services as job placement, employment skills training, rehabilitation services, housing, and community-reintegration supportive services for ex-offenders. Partnering with these programs can enhance health care providers' abilities to meet the needs of HIV positive gay men by ensuring that other basic needs receive appropriate attention by the appropriate professionals.

Human Rights Sector

Human rights workers engage in advocacy to increase public awareness of social injustices with their aim of reducing the de facto privileges that are withheld from groups that are marginalized and otherwise made less powerful groups, such as gay men, people of color, and people living with HIV (Oldenburg et al., 2016). Human rights workers have a broad scope of practice and have the capacity to provide advocacy for HIV positive gay men on a range of important issues from marriage equality to demanding accountability from insurance companies whose coverage policies discriminate against HIV positive applicants and enrollees (Barclay, Bernstein, & Marshall, 2009). Many immigrants and refugees, especially those from HIV-endemic countries, may arrive to the USA. Many of these individuals may learn of their HIV status only after arriving in the USA. Those who are gay-identified may find that is unsafe to return to their countries of origin either because of poor HIV/AIDS care infrastructure or because engaging in HIV/AIDS care will lead to imminent disclosure of their sexual behavioral practice, which could increase their vulnerability to violence and other homophobia-based social marginalizations (Nelson et al., 2015). In these cases, human rights workers can support newcomers to the USA in navigating asylum processes and helping them link with legal professionals who specialize in immigration cases. Human rights workers may also help individuals who are undocumented, link to health service networks that practice multicultural competence and that may provide free clinical services without requiring patient's to authenticate their identities with official government documents such as social security cards, birth certificates, or drivers licenses. Such strategies may reduce fears that engagement in health care systems place them at high-risk for apprehension by police agents and deportation.

Appropriate use of Technology

Advances in ART

Antiretroviral therapy (ART) is the cornerstone of pharmacologic management of HIV. The goals of ART include CD4 count increase, decreased HIV viral load, and delayed progression to AIDS. Studies indicate that early initiation of ART decreases progression to AIDS and HIV mortality by 50% (Marks, Gardner, Craw, & Crepaz, 2010; Mayer, 2011; Zolopa & Katz, 2012). The gold standard of care is to use at least two classes of ART, from which at least three different agents are selected (Aberg et al., 2009; Zolopa & Katz, 2012). ART classes include: nucleoside reverse transcriptase inhibitors (e.g., Retrovir, Videx, Hivid, Zerit, 3TC, Emtriva), nucleoside reverse transcriptase inhibitors (Viread), protease inhibitors (Crixivan, Invirase, Norvir, Viracept, Lexiva, Kaletra, Reyataz, Norvir), non-nucleoside reverse transcriptase inhibitors (Viramune, Rescriptor, Sustiva, Intelence), entry inhibitors (Fuzeon, Selzentry), and integrase inhibitors (Isentress). Each of the drug classes has unique actions against HIV infection. These medications carry complex pharmacokinetic and pharmacodynamic properties, and as such, they should be prescribed and monitored only by experienced HIV clinicians. Most classes of ART drugs also produce side effects that require monitoring and treatment. Patients should receive sufficient education about their medications, side effects, signs/symptoms that necessitate notification of a health provider, and the importance of strict maintenance to the medication regimen. The number of pills that a patient must consume daily ("pill burden"), the patient's ability to adhere to the regimen, costs, and comorbidities and immune status should all receive consideration when working with the patient to develop a treatment plan. All things considered, the treatment plan to which the patient is most willing to commit is the one he is most likely to follow and thus should be the one selected.

Sexual Health

Sexual health promotion is of paramount importance in primary care of HIV positive gay men (Mayer, Bush, et al., 2012). The patient's own views about his sexuality and disease process should be evaluated. Any perceived deficiencies should be addressed through health counseling and education from the appropriate professional. Patients should be educated about their disease process and receive coaching on the various ways that they can express their sexualities that minimize their chances of onward transmission of HIV. Patients should also receive education on what sources of information are reliable when researching their own disease processes and how it may impact aspects of their sexual expression that may include, for some, erection and ejaculation.

Prevention of other sexually transmitted infections (STIs) is critical for HIV positive gay men. HIV positive gay men are at increased risk for coinfection with other sexually transmitted pathogens (Bachmann et al., 2009; Pando et al., 2012; Rice et al., 2016). STIs common in gay HIV positive patients include human papilloma virus (HPV), hepatitis A, B, and C, gonorrhea, syphilis, chlamydia, and herpes 1 and 2 (Zolopa & Katz, 2012). Moreover, treatment of gonorrhea, chlamydia, and syphilis can significantly reduce the amount of HIV virus present at the urethral and anal mucosal sites—consequently decreasing the odds of onward HIV transmission to sexual partners (Modjarrad & Vermund, 2010). An HIV positive gay man should also be offered hepatitis A & B vaccinations if it is determined that he has not been previously vaccinated or if verification—either by patient recollection or chart documentation—is unavailable. The HPV vaccine is now recommended for MSM through age 26, especially for HIV positive MSM. High-intensity behavioral counseling and other evidence-based behavioral interventions should be considered for use in support of STI risk reduction. HIV positive gay men who have serodiscordant sexual partnerships should be considered for pre-exposure prophylaxis (PrEP) for the HIV negative partner along with high-frequency HIV screening for early detection and treatment in the event of seroconversion (Baeten et al., 2012; Grant et al., 2010; Thigpen et al., 2012). Sexual health care for HIV positive gay men is complex, requiring provider-patient collaborations to find strategies for achieving sexual expression and health maintenance goals (Mayer et al., 2016; Weinman, 2010).

Mental Health

Mental health and wellness is an integral and foundational aspect of HIV care for gay men (Batchelder, Safren, Mitchell, Ivardic, & O'Cleirigh, 2017). A comprehensive suicide assessment and screening should be conducted at the first clinical encounter, as HIV positive persons are two times more likely to experience depression and suicidal thoughts than HIV negative persons (Ciesla & Roberts, 2001). The health provider should be sensitive as to how the diagnosis of HIV and other STI positive results are delivered to gay men, as studies have demonstrated that the manner in which the clinician communicates these results can alter the response and coping ability of the patient (Hult, Maurer, & Moskowitz, 2009). Some HIV positive gay men may also have internalized feelings of homophobia, which may be a contributing or compounding factor to their experiences of depressive symptoms. Internalized homophobia among HIV positive gay men has been linked both to increased risk of depression and to sexual risk behaviors (Ross, Rosser, & Neumaier, 2008). Linkages to psychological counseling services and support groups should be provided, wherever possible, as these have been shown to have beneficial effects on depressive symptoms (White et al., 2012). Pharmacological agents may also be necessary to support the patients' management of depression and anxiety. Given HIV positive gay men's elevated risk for developing depressive symptoms, health care providers should conduct a psychosocial assessment, even if only a brief one, at every clinical encounter and work with patients to develop a mental health plan of care and linkage to care, as appropriate.

E-Technology

As the numbers of uninsured HIV positive gay men increase, the need to treat, monitor, and educate such patients will also increase. Qualified clinicians may not always reside in the geographic location of clinical need. In such situations, clinicians may be able to conduct limited evaluations over the phone, through video conferencing, and through email (Hirshfield et al., 2016). This type of technology is best suited for follow-up evaluations, counseling, needs assessment, triage, prescription refills, and education. E-technology should not serve as an initial point of entry for physical examinations. E-technology may increase, as the numbers of insured may reach historic proportions within the context of the Affordable Health Care Act in the USA. Legal and ethical considerations must be evaluated and resolved as this emerging form of patient evaluation and treatment continues to evolve. E-technology may provide considerable relief for current gaps in access to care for HIV positive gay men across the country.

Directions for Future Research

With the passing of the Affordable Care Act (ACA) and the implementation of the National HIV/AIDS Strategy and HIV Care Continuum Initiative, the USA has begun a new chapter in the organization of health care practice approaches. This reorganization presents an optimal window for the emergence of comprehensive primary health care as an approach to HIV/AIDS care (Beyrer et al., 2012). The utilization of a comprehensive PHC approach will require research and innovation regarding how health care costs are managed (Basinga et al., 2010; Mayer et al.,

2016; Schoen et al., 2009), how health care teams are organized under ACA (Rittenhouse, Shortell, & Fisher, 2009), and the implications of multidisciplinary health care teams on HIV care quality outcomes (Mayer et al., 2016; Poulton and West, 1993; Sherer et al., 2002; Zaller, Gilliani, & Rich, 2007). Additional research should also explore how emerging solutions in data (e.g., electronic charts, local/regional patient information exchanges) and communication (telemedicine) systems can be harnessed to support more time-efficient, cost-effective, accessible, and client-centered health care services and expand access points into HIV care (Hirshfield et al., 2016; Schoen et al., 2012).

Test and treat interventions focus on reducing risk of onward transmission by suppressing the HIV viral load of HIV-infected individuals (Castel et al., 2016; Kalichman et al., 2010; Modjarrad & Vermund, 2010). Additionally, interventions that promote early linkage to and retention in care are needed to support quality outcomes for HIV positive gay men (Marks et al. 2010; Mayer, 2011; Gwadz et al., 2015; Mugavero, Norton, & Saag, 2011; Rachilis et al., 2016). It will also be important for future research to extend beyond clinical and behavioral factors that impact screening, medical care linkage and treatment towards investigating policies that interfere with the effective and efficient linkage to care (Mugavero et al. 2011; Riley et al., 2012). Although gay men generally reduce HIV transmission risk behaviors after receiving an HIV diagnosis, a substantial percentage of HIV positive gay men remain at increased risk for the onward transmission of HIV (Crepaz et al., 2009; Mayer, Bush, et al., 2012). This highlights the need for continued research evaluating innovative strategies for preventing the onward transmission of HIV to others (Safren et al., 2011; Serovich et al., 2009).

Conclusions

The comprehensive primary health care approach is a relevant practice model for working with HIV positive gay men. Within the comprehensive PHC approach, a more holistic engagement with the needs of HIV positive gay men can be accomplished (Beyrer et al., 2012; Bhatia & Rifkin, 2010). Public health practice has a long tradition of advocating for social justice reforms as interventions to improve health and wellness of vulnerable and marginalized populations (Nelson & Morrison-Beedy, 2012); however, increased attention must be given to educating nurses, physicians, and other members of the clinical team to adopt anti-racism, anti-oppression frameworks in their clinical practice (Nelson et al., 2014, 2016). The United States, through the National HIV/AIDS Strategy, has an opportunity to more fully adopt principles of comprehensive primary health care. Many of the priorities in the National HIV/AIDS Strategy are congruent with the comprehensive primary health care approach. These include expanding access to HIV primary care, maximizing the application of technological innovation in the primary and secondary prevention of HIV and the development of community-informed plans for the manner in which HIV prevention and care are organized and delivered within local communities across the USA. Implementing the principles of comprehensive PHC will require that health care professionals push the boundaries and commit to social justice aims within their clinical practice (Dean & Fenton, 2010; Easley & Allen, 2007; Eliason, Dibble, & DeJoseph, 2010; Nelson et al., 2016) and work with partners outside of the health sector to help HIV positive gay men attain their wellness goals.

References

Aberg, J. A., Kaplan, J. E., Libman, H., Emmanuel, P., Anderson, J. R., Stone, V. E., … Gallant, J. E. (2009). Primary care guidelines for the management of persons infected with human immunodeficiency virus: 2009 update by the HIV medicine association of the Infectious Diseases Society of America. Clinical Infectious Diseases, 49, 651–681.

Agwu, A. L., Siberry, G. K., Ellen, J. M., Fleishman, J. A., Rutstein, R., Gaur, A. H., … Gebo, K. A. (2012). Predictors of highly active antiretroviral therapy utilization for behaviorally HIV-1-infected youth: Impact of adult versus pediatric clinical care site. Journal of Adolescent Health, 50, 471–477.

American Academy of HIV Medicine. (2013). American Academy of HIV Medicine credentialing information. Retrieved from http://www.aahivm.org/about.

American Board of Internal Medicine Foundation, American College of Physicians, American Society of Internal Medicine Foundation, & European Federation of Internal Medicine. (2002). Medical professionalism in the new millennium: A physician charter. Annals of Internal Medicine, 136, 243–246.

Association of Nurses in AIDS Care. (2013). Professional development. Retrieved from http://www.nursesinaidscare.org/i4a/pages/index.cfm?pageid=3289.

Bachmann, L. H., Grimley, D. M., Chen, H., Aban, I., Hu, J., Zhang, S., … Hook, E. W., III. (2009). Risk behaviors in HIV positive men who have sex with men participating in an intervention in a primary care setting. International Journal of STD and AIDS, 20, 607–612.

Baeten, J. M., Donnell, D., Ndase, P., Mugo, N. R., Campbell, J. D., Wangisi, J., … Celum, C. (2012). Antiretroviral prophylaxis for HIV prevention in heterosexual men and women. New England Journal of Medicine, 367, 399–410.

Bandura, A. (1985). Social foundations of thought and action. Prentice-Hall, NJ: Englewood Cliffs.

Barclay, S., Bernstein, M., & Marshall, A. (2009). Queer mobilizations: LGBT activists confront the law. New York, New York University Press.

Basinga, P., Gertler, P. J., Binagwaho, A., Soucat, A. L. B., Sturdy, J. R., & Vermeersch, C. (2010). Paying primary health care centers for performance in Rwanda (World Bank Policy Research Working Paper No. 5190). Geneva: World Bank.

Batchelder, A. W., Safren, S., Mitchell, A. D., Ivardic, I., & O'Cleirigh, C. (2017). Mental health in 2020 for men who have sex with men in the United States. Sexual Health. doi:10.1071/SH16083, 14, 59.

Baum, F. (2008). The commission on the social determinants of health: Reinventing health promotion for the twenty-first century. Critical Public Health, 18, 457–466.

Beauchamp, T. L., & Childress, J. F. (2001). Principles of biomedical ethics (5th ed.). New York: Oxford University Press.

Berkman, A., Garcia, J., Muñoz-Laboy, M., Paiva, V., & Parker, R. (2005). A critical analysis of the Brazilian response to HIV/AIDS: Lessons learned for controlling and mitigating the epidemic in developing countries. American Journal of Public Health, 95, 1162–1172.

Beyrer, C., Sullivan, P. S., Sanchez, J., Dowdy, D., Altman, D., Trapence, G., … Sidibe, M. (2012). A call to action for comprehensive HIV services for men who have sex with men. Lancet, 380, 424–438.

Beyrer, C., Wirtz, A. L., Valker, D., Johns, B., Sifakis, F., & Baral, S. D. (2011). The global HIV epidemics among men who have sex with men. Washington, DC: The World Bank.

Bhatia, M., & Rifkin, S. (2010). A renewed focus on primary health care: Revitalize or reframe. *Globalization and Health, 6*. doi:10.1186/1744-8603-6-13, 6.

Bird, J. D., LaSaa, M. C., Hidalgo, M. A., Kuhns, L. M., & Garofalo, R. (2016). "I had to go to the streets to get love": Pathways from parental rejection to HIV risk among young gay and bisexual men. *Journal of Homosexuality, 19*, 1–22.

Birnbaum, J. M., Loundsbury, D. W., Eastwood, E., Palma, A., & Jo, G. Y. (2013). 128. Use of system dynamics modeling as a tool for evaluation and intervention planning for HIV+ adolescents and their retention in care in an urban adolescent HIV clinic. *Journal of Adolescent Health, 52*, S82–S83.

Bogart, L. M., Wagner, G. J., Mutchler, M. G., Risley, B., McDavitt, B. W., McKay, T., & Klein, D. J. (2012). Community HIV treatment advocacy programs may support treatment adherence. *AIDS Education and Prevention, 24*, 1–14.

Campbell, J. L., Ramsay, J., & Green, J. (2001). Age, gender, socioeconomic, and ethnic differences in patients' assessment of primary health care. *Quality Health Care, 10*, 90–95.

Castel, A. D., Kalmin, M. M., Hart, R. L., Young, H. A., Hays, H., Benator, D., ... Greenberg, A. E. (2016). Disparities in achieving and sustaining viral suppression among a large cohort of HIV-infected persons in care—Washington, DC. *AIDS Care, 28*, 1355–1364.

Centers for Disease Control and Prevention. (2010). *Establishing a holistic framework to reduce inequities in HIV, viral hepatitis, and tuberculosis in the United States*. Atlanta, GA: U.S. Department of Health and Human Services—Centers for Disease Control and Prevention.

Centers for Disease Control and Prevention. (2014). Men living with diagnosed HIV who have sex with men: Progress along the continuum of HIC care—United States, 2010. *Morbidity and Mortality Weekly Report, 63*, 829–833.

Centers for Disease Control and Prevention. (2015). *HIV/AIDS surveillance report: Diagnoses of HIV infection in the United States and dependent areas, 2011*. Retrieved from http://www.cdc.gov/hiv/topics/surveillance/resources/reports/.

Chandwani, S., Koenig, L. J., Sill, A. M., Abramowitz, S., Conner, L. C., & D'Angelo, L. (2012). Predictors of antiretroviral medication adherence among a diverse cohort of adolescents with HIV. *Journal of Adolescent Health, 51*, 242–251.

Church, K., & Simon, L. (2010). Delivering integrated services: Time for a client-centered approach to meet the sexual and reproductive health needs of people living with HIV. *AIDS, 24*, 189–193.

Ciesla, J. A., & Roberts, J. E. (2001). A meta-analysis of the relationship between HIV infection and risk for depressive disorders. *American Journal of Psychiatry, 158*, 725–730.

Cole, E. R., & Omari, S. R. (2003). Race, class and the dilemmas of upward mobility for African Americans. *Journal of Social Issues, 59*, 785–802.

Courtenay-Quirk, C., Wolitski, R. J., Parsons, J. T., & Gomez, C. A. (2006). Is HIV/AIDS stigma dividing the gay community? Perceptions of HIV-positive men who have sex with men. *AIDS Education and Prevention, 18*, 56–67.

Crepaz, N., Marks, G., Liau, A., Mullins, M. M., Aupont, L. W., Marshall, K. J., ... HIV/AIDS Prevention Research Synthesis Team. (2009). Prevalence of unprotected anal intercourse among HIV-diagnosed MSM in the United States: A meta-analysis. *AIDS, 23*, 1617–1629.

Cueto, M. (2004). The origins of primary health care and selective primary health care. *American Journal of Public Health, 94*, 1864–1874.

Cunningham, C. O., Sohler, N. L., Wong, M. D., Relf, M., Cunningham, W. E., Drainoni, M., ... Cabral, H. D. (2007). Utilization of health care services in hard-to-reach marginalized HIV-infected individuals. *AIDS Patient Care and STDs, 21*, 177–186.

Dean, H. D., & Fenton, K. A. (2010). Addressing social determinants of health in the prevention and control of HIV/AIDS, viral hepatitis, sexually transmitted infections, and tuberculosis. *Public Health Reports, 125*, 1–5.

Dowshen, N., & D'Angelo, L. (2011). Health care transition for youth living with HIV/AIDS. *Pediatrics, 128*, 762–771.

Easley, C. E., & Allen, C. E. (2007). A critical intersection: Human rights, public health nursing, and nursing ethics. *Advances in Nursing Science, 30*, 367–382.

Eaton, L. A., West, T. V., Kenny, D. A., & Kalichman, S. C. (2009). HIV transmission risk among HIV seroconcordant and serodiscordant couples: Dyadic processes of partner selection. *AIDS and Behavior, 13*, 185–195.

Eliason, M. J., Dibble, S., & DeJoseph, J. (2010). Nursing's silence on lesbian, gay, bisexual, and transgender issues: The need for emancipatory efforts. *Advances in Nursing Science, 33*, 206–218.

Farrisi, D., & Dietz, N. (2013). Patient navigation is a client-centered approach that helps to engage people in HIV care. *HIV Clinician, 25*, 1–3.

Fielden, S. J., Chapman, G. E., & Cadell, S. (2011). Managing stigma in adolescent HIV: Silence, secrets and sanctioned spaces. *Culture, Health and Sexuality, 13*, 267–281.

Flowers, P., & Davis, M. M. (2012). Understanding the biopsychosocial aspects of HIV disclosure amongst HIV-positive gay men in Scotland. *Journal of Health Psychology*. doi:10.1177/1359105312454037, 18, 711.

Fortenberry, J. D., Martinez, J., Rudy, B. J., & Monte, D. (2012). Linkage to care for HIV-positive adolescents: A multisite study of the adolescent medicine trials units of the adolescent trials network. *Journal of Adolescent Health, 51*, 551–556.

Galvão, J. (2005). Brazil and access to HIV/AIDS drugs: A question of human rights and public health. *American Journal of Public Health, 95*, 1110–1116.

Garcia, J., Parker, C., Parker, R. G., Wilson, P. A., Philbin, M., & Hirsch, J. S. (2016). Psychosocial implications of homophobia and HIV stigma in social support networks: Insight for high-impact HIV prevention among black men who have sex with men. *Health Education and Behavior, 43*, 217–225.

Gayles, T. A., Kuhns, L. M., Kwon, S., Mustanski, B., & Garofalo, R. (2016). Socioeconomic disconnection as a risk factor for increased HIV infection in young men who have sex with men. *LGBT Health, 3*, 219–224.

Gilliam, P. P., Ellen, J. M., Leonard, L., Kinsman, S., Jevitt, C. M., & Straub, D. M. (2011). Transition of adolescents with HIV to adult care: Characteristics and current practices of the adolescent trials network for HIV/AIDS interventions. *Journal of the Association of Nurses in AIDS Care, 22*, 283–294.

Gilman, B., Hidalgo, J., Thomas, C., Au, M., & Hargreaves, M. (2012). Linkages to care for newly diagnosed individuals who test HIV positive in nonprimary care settings. *AIDS Patient Care and STDs, 26*, 132–140.

Grant, R. M., Lama, J. R., Anderson, P. L., MacMahan, V., Liu, A. Y., Vargas, L., … Glidden, D. V. (2010). Preexposure chemprophylaxis for HIV prevention in men who have sex with men. *The New England Journal of Medicine, 363*, 2587–2599.

Grov, C., Golub, S. A., Parsons, J. T., Brennan, M., & Karplak, S. E. (2010). Loneliness and HIV-related stigma explain depression among older HIV-positive adults. *AIDS Care, 22*, 630–639.

Gwadz, M., Cleland, C. M., Applegate, E., Belkin, M., Gandhi, M., Salomon, N., … Heart to Heart Collaborative Research Team. (2015). Behavioral intervention improves treatment outcomes among HIV-infected individuals who have delayed, declined, or discontinued antiretroviral therapy: A randomized controlled trail of a novel intervention. AIDS and Behavior, 19, 1801–1817.

Hagan, J. F., Shaw, J. S., & Duncan, P. M. (2008). *Bright futures: Guidelines for health supervision of infants, children, and adolescents* (3rd ed.). Elk Grove Village, IL: American Academy of Pediatrics.

Halkitis, P. N., Kapadia, F., Ompad, D. C., & Perez-Figueroa, R. (2015). Moving toward a holistic conceptual framework for understanding healthy aging among gay men. *Journal of Homosexuality, 62*, 571–587.

Halkitis, P. N., Kupprat, S. A., Hampton, M. B., Perez-Figueroa, R., Kingdon, M., Eddy, J. A., Ompad, D. C. (2012). Evidence for a syndemic in aging HIV-positive gay, bisexual, and other MSM: Implications for a holistic approach to prevention and healthcare. *National Resource Model, 36*. doi:10.1111/napa.12009, 365.

Hall, H. I., Byers, R. H., Ling, Q., & Espinoza, L. (2007). Racial/ethnic and age disparities in HIV prevalence and disease progression among men who have sex with men in the United States. *American Journal of Public Health, 97*, 1060–1066.

Harrington, J., Noble, L. M., & Newman, S. P. (2004). Improving patients' communication with doctors: A systematic review of intervention studies. *Patient Education and Counseling, 52,* 7–16.

Hatcher, S. S., Toldson, I. A., Godette, D. C., & Richardson, J. B. (2009). Mental health, substance abuse, and HIV disparities in correctional settings: Practice and policy implications for African Americans. *Journal of Health Care for the Poor and Underserved, 20,* 6–16.

Health Resources & Services Administration. (2010). *Going the distance: The Ryan white HIV/ AIDS program, 20 years of leadership, a legacy of care.* Rockville, MD: Author.

Health Resources & Services Administration. (2013). *AETC education for nurse practitioners and physician assistants.* Grant announcement. Retrieved February 28, 2015, from http://www. hrsa.gov/grants/index.html.

Heckman, T. G., Heckman, B. D., Kochman, A., Sikkema, K. J., Suhr, J., & Goodkin, K. (2002). Psychological symptoms among persons 50 years of age and older living with HIV disease. *Aging and Mental Health, 6,* 121–128.

Helleberg, M., Engsig, F. N., Kronborg, G., Larsen, C. S., Pedersen, G., Pedersen, C., … Obel, N. (2012). Retention in a public healthcare system with free access to treatment: A Danish nationwide HIV cohort study. *AIDS, 26,* 741–748.

Heslin, K. C., Andersen, R. M., Ettner, S. L., & Cunningham, W. E. (2005). Racial and ethnic disparities in access to physicians with HIV-related expertise. *Journal of General Internal Medicine, 20,* 283–289.

Hightow-Weidman, L. B., Smith, J. C., Valera, E., Matthews, D., & Lyons, P. (2011). Keeping them in "STYLE": Finding, linking, and retaining young HIV-positive black and Latino men who sex with men in care. *AIDS Patient Care and STDs, 25,* 37–45.

Hirshfield, S., Downing, M. J., Jr., Parsons, J. T., Grov, C., Gordon, R. J., Houang, S. T., … Chiasson, M. A. (2016). Developing a video-based ehealth intervention for HIV-positive gay, bisexual, and other men who have sex with men: Study protocol for a randomized controlled trial. JMIR Research Protocol, 5, e125. doi:10.2196/resprot.5554.

HIV Medicine Association. (2010). *Qualifications for physicians who manage the longitudinal HIV treatment of patients with HIV.* Arlington, VA: Author.

HIV/AIDS Nursing Certification Board. (2013). *Certification information.* Retrieved February 1, 2013, from http://www.hancb.org/certification.htm.

Hult, J. R., Maurer, S. A., & Moskowitz, J. T. (2009). "I'm sorry, you're positive": A qualitative study of individual experiences of testing positive for HIV. *AIDS Care, 21,* 185–188.

Hussen, S. A., Chahroudi, A., Boylan, A., Camacho-Gonzalez, A. F., Hackett, S., & Chakraborty, R. (2015). Transition of youth living with HIV infection pediatric to adult-centered healthcare: A review of the literature. *Future Virology, 9,* 921–929.

Hussen, S. A., Harper, G. W., Bauermeister, J. A., Hightow-Weidman, L. B., & Adolescent Medicine Trials Network for HIV/AIDS Interventions. (2015). Psychosocial influences on engagement in care among HIV-positive young black gay/bisexual and other men who have sex with men. *AIDS Patient Care and STDs, 29,* 77–85.

Hutchison, B., Levesque, J. F., Strumpf, E., & Coyle, N. (2011). Primary health care in Canada: Systems in motion. *Milbank Quarterly, 89,* 256–288.

International Conference on Primary Health Care. (1978). *Declaration of Alma Ata, USSR, September 6–12, 1978.* Published online by World Health Organization. Retrieved February 8, 2015 from http://www.who.int/publications/almaata_declaration_en.pdf.

Kalichman, S. C., Cherry, C., Amaral, C. M., Swerzes, C., Eaton, L., Macy, R., … Kalichman, M. O. (2010). Adherence to antiretroviral therapy and HIV transmission risks: Implications for test-and-treat approaches to HIV prevention. AIDS Patient Care and STDs, 24, 271–277.

Kalichman, S. C., Rompa, D., & Cage, M. (2005). Group intervention to reduce HIV transmission risk behavior among persons living with HIV/AIDS. *Behavior Modification, 29,* 256–285.

Kalichman, S., Rompa, D., Cage, M., DiFonzo, K., Simpson, D., Austin, J., … Graham, J. (2001). Effectiveness of an intervention to reduce HIV transmission risks in HIV-positive people. American Journal of Preventive Medicine, 21, 84–92.

Karach, D. L., Hall, H. I., Tang, T., Hu, X., & Mermin, J. (2015). Comparative mortality among people diagnosed with HIV infection or AIDS in the U.S., 2001–2010. *Public Health Reports, 130*, 253–260.

Kaymeg, K., Howard, V. M., Clochesy, J. M., Mitchell, A. M., & Suresky, J. M. (2010). The impact of high fidelity human simulation on self-efficacy of communication skills. *Issues on Mental Health Nursing, 31*, 315–323.

Kinsler, J. J., Wong, M. D., Sayles, J. N., Davis, C., & Cunningham, W. E. (2007). The effect of perceived stigma from a health care provider on access to care among a low-income HIV-positive population. *AIDS Patient Care and STDs, 21*, 584–592.

Laffon, B. T., Hall, H. I., Surendera, B. A., Benbow, N., Hu, Y. W., & Urban Areas HIV Surveillance Workgroup. (2015). HIV infection and linkage to HIV-related medical care in large urban areas in the United States, 2009. *Journal of Acquired Immune Deficiency Syndromes, 69*(4), 487–92.

Leonard, A. D., Markham, C. M., Bui, T., Shegog, R., & Paul, M. E. (2010). Lowering the risk for secondary transmission: Insights from HIV-positive youth and health care providers. *Perspectives on Sexual and Reproductive Health, 42*, 100–116.

Lesserman, J. (2008). Role of depression, stress, and trauma in HIV disease progression. *Psychosomatic Medicine, 70*, 539–545.

Li, X., Huang, L., Wang, H., Fennie, K. P., He, G., & Williams, A. B. (2011). Stigma mediates the relationship between self-efficacy, medication adherence, and quality of life among people living with HIV/AIDS in China. *AIDS Patient Care and STDs, 25*, 665–671.

Losina, E., Schackman, B. R., Sadownik, S. N., Gebo, K. A., Walensky, R. P., Chiosi, J. J., … Freedberg, K. A. (2009). Racial and sex disparities in life expectancy losses among HIV-infected persons in the United States: Impact of risk behavior, late initiation, and early discontinuation of antiretroviral therapy. Clinical Infectious Diseases, 49, 1570–1578.

Lynam, M. J., & Cowley, S. (2007). Understanding marginalization as a social determinant of health. *Critical Public Health, 17*, 137–149.

Lyons, A., Pitts, M., Grierson, J., Thorpe, R., & Powell, J. (2010). Ageing with HIV: Health and psychosocial well-being of older gay men. *AIDS Care, 22*, 1236–1244.

Magnus, M., Jones, K., Phillips, G., Binson, D., Hightow-Weidman, L. B., Richards-Clarke, C., … Hidalgo, J. (2010). Characteristics associated with retention among African American and Latino adolescent HIV-positive MSM: Results from the outreach, care and prevention to engage HIV-seropositive young MSM of color special project of national significance. Journal of Acquired Immune Deficiency Syndrome, 53, 529–536.

Magnussen, L., Ehiri, J., & Jolly, P. (2004). Comprehensive versus selective primary health care: Lessons for global health policy. *Health Affairs, 23*, 167–176.

Mahajan, A. P., Sayles, J. N., Patel, V. A., Remien, R. H., Ortiz, D., Szekeres, G., & Coates, T. J. (2008). Stigma in the HIV/AIDS epidemic: A review of the literature and recommendations for the way forward. *AIDS, 22*, S67–S79.

Malebranche, D. J., & Nelson, L. E. (2013). Intersections of race, culture, and sexuality. In J. Schneider & V. Silenzio (Eds.), *The gay and lesbian medical association handbook of LGBT health*. Washington, DC: Gay and Lesbian Medical Association.

Marks, G., Gardner, L. I., Craw, J., & Crepaz, N. (2010). Entry and retention in medical care among HIV-diagnosed persons: A meta-analysis. *AIDS, 24*, 2665–2678.

Mayer, K. H. (2011). Linkage, engagement, and retention in HIV care: Essential for optimal individual- and community-level outcomes in the era of highly active antiretroviral therapy. *Clinical Infectious Diseases, 52*, S205–S207.

Mayer, K. H., Bekker, L. G., Stall, R., Grulich, A. E., Colfax, G., & Lama, J. R. (2012). Comprehensive clinical care for men who have sex with men: An integrated approach. *Lancet, 380*, 378–387.

Mayer, K. H., Bush, T., Henry, K., Overton, E. T., Hammer, J., Richardson, J., … The SUN Investigators. (2012). Ongoing sexually transmitted disease acquisition and risk-taking behavior among US HIV-infected patients in primary care: Implications for prevention interventions. *Sexually Transmitted Diseases, 39*, 1–7.

Mayer, K. H., Vanderwarker, R., Grasso, C., & Boswell, S. L. (2016). Emerging models of clinical services for men who have sex with men: Focused versus comprehensive approaches. *Sexual Health*. doi:10.1071/SH16119, 14, 133.

Miles, I. J., Le, B. C., Wejnert, C., Oster, A., DiNenno, E., & Paz-Bailey, G. (2013). HIV infection among heterosexuals at increased risk—United States, 2010. *MMWR, 62*, 183–188.

Modjarrad, K., & Vermund, S. H. (2010). Effect of treating co-infections on HIV-1 viral load: A systematic review. *The Lancet, 10*, 455–463.

Moore, R. (2011). Epidemiology of HIV infection in the United States: Implications for linkage to care. *Clinical Infectious Diseases, 52*, S208–S213.

Mugavero, M. J., Norton, W. E., & Saag, M. S. (2011). Health care system and policy factors influencing engagement in HIV medical care: Piecing together the fragments of a fractured health care delivery system. *Clinical Infectious Diseases, 52*, S238–S246.

Mullaly, B. (2010). Oppression: An overview. In B. Mullaly (Ed.), Challenging oppression and confronting privilege: A critical social work approach (2ndnd ed., pp. 34–65). Toronto: Oxford University Press.

Navarro, V., & Muntaner, C. (2004). Towards an integrated political, economic, and cultural understanding of health inequalities. In V. Navarro & C. Muntaner (Eds.), *Political and economic determinants of population health and well being: Controversies and developments* (pp. 1–6). Amityville, NY: Baywood Publishers.

Nelson, L. E., & Morrison-Beedy, D. (2012). Conducting intervention research in public health settings. In B. M. Melnyk & D. Morrison-Beedy (Eds.), *Designing, conducting, analyzing and funding intervention research: A practical guide for success* (pp. 247–254). New York: Springer.

Nelson, L. E., Walker, J. J., DuBois, S. N., & Giwa, S. (2014). Your blues ain't like mine: Considering integrative antiracism in HIV prevention research with black men who have sex with men in Canada and the United States. *Nursing Inquiry, 21*, 270–282.

Nelson, L. E., Wilton, L., Agyarko-Poku, T., Zhang, N., Alucoh, M., Thach, C. T., … Adu-Sarkodie, Y. (2015). The association of HIV stigma and HIV/STD knowledge with sexual risk behaviors among adolescent and adult men who have sex with men in Ghana, West Africa. Research in Nursing and Health, 38, 194–206.

Nelson, L. E., Wilton, L., Moineddin, R., Zhang, N., Siddiqi, A., Sa, T., … HPTN 061 Study Team. (2016). Economic, legal and social hardships associated with HIV risk among black men who have sex with men in six US cities. Journal of Urban Health, 93, 170–188.

Oldenburg, C. E., Perez-Brumer, A. G., Reisner, S. L., Mayer, K. H., Mimiaga, M. J., Hatzenbuehler, M. L., & Bärnighausen, T. (2016). Human rights protections and HIV prevalence among MSM who sell sex: Cross-country comparisons from a systematic review and meta-analysis. *Global Public Health, 15*, 1–12.

Oramasionwu, C. U., Hunter, J. M., Skinner, J., Ryan, L., Lawson, K. A., Brown, C. M., … Frei, C. R. (2009). Black race as a predictor of poor health outcomes among a national cohort of HIV/AIDS patients admitted to US hospitals: A cohort study. *BMC Infectious Diseases, 9*. doi:10.1186/1471-2334-9-127, 9.

Pando, M. A., Balan, I. C., Marone, R., Dolezal, C., Leu, C., Squiquera, L., … Avila, M. M. (2012). HIV and other sexually transmitted infections among men who have sex with men recruited by RDS in Buenos Aires, Argentina: High HIV and HPV infection. PloS One, 7(6). http://dx.doi.org/10.1371/journal.pone.0039834, e39834

Parker, R. G. (2009). Civil society, political mobilization, and the impact of HIV scale-up on health systems in Brazil. *Journal of Acquired Immune Deficiency Syndrome, 52*, S49–S51.

Poulton, B. C., & West, M. A. (1993). Effective multidisciplinary teamwork in primary health care. *Journal of Advanced Nursing, 18*, 918–925.

Rachilis, S., Burchell, A. N., Gardner, S., Light, L., Raboud, J., Antoniou, T., … Ontario HIV Treatment Network Cohort Study. (2016). Social determinants of health and retention in HIV care in a clinical cohort in Ontario, Canada. *AIDS Care, 27*, 1–10.

Rao, J., Anderson, L., Thomas, I., & Frankel, R. (2007). Communication interventions make a difference in conversations between physicians and patients: A systematic review of the evidence. *Medical Care, 45*, 340–349.

Rice, C. E., Maierhofer, C., Fields, K. S., Ervin, M., Lanza, S. T., & Turner, A. N. (2016). Beyond anal sex: Sexual practices of men who have sex with men and associations with HIV and other sexually transmitted infections. *Journal of Sexual Medicine, 13*, 374–382.

Rickets, T., Naiditch, M., & Bourgueil, Y. (2012). Advancing primary care in France and the United States. *Journal of Primary Care and Community Health, 3*, 221–225.

Riley, E. D., Neilands, T. B., Moore, K., Cohen, J., Bangsberg, D. R., & Havlir, D. (2012). Social, structural and behavioral determinants of overall health status in a cohort of homeless and unstably housed HIV-infected men. PloS One, 7, e35207. doi:10.1371/journal.pone.0035207.

Rittenhouse, D. R., Shortell, S. M., & Fisher, E. S. (2009). Primary care and accountable care—Two essential elements of delivery-system reform. *New England Journal of Medicine, 361*, 2301–2303.

Ross, M. W., Rosser, B. R., & Neumaier, E. R. (2008). The relationship of internalized homonegativity to unsafe sexual behavior in HIV-seropositive men who have sex with men. *AIDS Education and Prevention, 20*(6), 547–557.

Safren, S. A., O'Cleirigh, C., Skeer, M. R., Driskell, J., Goshe, B. M., Covahey, C., & Mayer, K. H. (2011). Demonstration and evaluation of a peer-delivered, individually-tailored, HIV prevention intervention for HIV-infected MSM in their primary care setting. *AIDS and Behavior, 15*, 949–958.

Sankar, A., Nevedal, A., Neufeld, S., Berry, R., & Luborsky, M. (2011). What do we know about older adults and HIV? A review of social and behavioral literature. *AIDS Care, 23*, 1187–1207.

Schoen, C., Osborn, R., Doty, M. M., Squires, D., Peugh, J. P., & Applebaum, S. (2009). A survey of primary care physicians in eleven countries, 2009: Perspectives on care, costs, and experiences. *Health Affairs, 28*, 1171–1183.

Schoen, C., Osborn, R., Squires, D., Doty, M., Rasmussen, P., Pierson, R., & Applebaum, S. (2012). A survey of primary care doctors in ten countries shows progress in use of health information technology, less in other areas. *Health Affairs, 31*, 2805–2816.

Seffner, F., Garcia, J., Muñoz-Laboy, M., & Parker, R. (2011). A time for dogma, a time for the bible, a time for condoms: Building a Catholic theology of prevention in the face of public health policies at casa Fonte Colombo in Porto Alegre, Brazil. *Global Public Health, 6*, S271–S283.

Serovich, J. M., Reed, S. J., Grafsky, E. L., & Andrist, D. (2009). An intervention to assist men who have sex with men disclose their serostatus to casual sex partners. *AIDS Education and Prevention, 21*, 207–219.

Serovich, J. M., Reed, S. J., Grafsky, E. L., Hartwell, E. E., & Andrist, D. W. (2011). An intervention to assist men who have sex with men disclose their serostatus to family members: Results from a pilot study. *AIDS and Behavior, 15*, 1647–1653.

Shapiro, M. F., Morton, S. C., McCaffrey, D. F., Senterfitt, J. W., Fleishman, J. A., Perlman, J. F., … Bozzette, M. A. (1999). Variations in the care of HIV-infected adults in the United States: Results from the HIV costs and services utilization study. JAMA, 281, 2305–2315.

Shegog, R., Markham, C. M., Leonard, A. D., Bul, T. C., & Paul, M. E. (2012). "+ CLICK": Pilot of a web-based training program to enhance ART adherence among HIV-positive youth. *AIDS Care, 24*, 310–318.

Sherer, R., Stieglitz, K., Narra, J., Jasek, J., Green, L., Moore, B., … Cohen, M. (2002). HIV multidisciplinary teams work: Support services improve access to and retention in HIV primary care. AIDS Care, 14, 31–44.

Shoptaw, S., Stall, R., Bordon, J., Kao, U., Cox, C., Li, X., … Plankey, M. W. (2012). Cumulative exposure to stimulants and immune function outcomes among HIV-positive and HIV-negative men in the multicenter AIDS cohort study. International Journal of STD and AIDS, 23, 576–580.

Simard, E. P., Fransua, M., Naishadham, D., & Jemal, A. (2012). The influence of sex, race/ethnicity, and educational attainment on human immunodeficiency virus death rates among adults, 1993–2007. *Archives of Internal Medicine, 172,* 1591–1598.

Smit, P. J., Brady, M., Carter, M., Fernandes, R., Lamore, L., Meulbroek, M., … Thompson, M. (2012). HIV-related stigma within communities of gay men: A literature review. AIDS Care, 24, 405–412.

Stoeckle, J. D. (2009). The practice of primary care. In A. H. Goroll & A. G. Mulley's (Eds.), *Primary care medicine: Office evaluation and management of the adult patients* (6th ed., pp. 1–9). Philadelphia, PA: Lippincott, Williams, and Wilkins.

Tennstedt, S. L. (2000). Empowering older patients to communicate more effectively in the medical encounter. *Clinical Geriatric Medicine, 16,* 61–70.

Thigpen, M. C., Kebaabetswe, P. M., Paxton, L. A., Smith, D. K., Rose, C. E., Segolodi, T. M., Henderson, F. L., … Brooks, J. T. (2012). Antiretroviral preexposure prophylaxis for heterosexual HIV transmission in Botswana. New England Journal of Medicine, 367, 423–434.

Trevino, K. M., Pargament, K. I., Cotton, S., Leonard, A. C., Hahn, J., Caprini-Faigin, C. A., & Tsevat, J. (2010). Religious coping and physiological, psychological, social, and spiritual outcomes in patient with HIV/AIDS: Cross-sectional and longitudinal findings. *AIDS and Behavior, 14,* 379–389.

van Griensven, F., & van Wijngaarden, D. L. V. (2010). A review of the epidemiology of HIV infection and prevention responses among MSM in AIDS. *AIDS, 24,* S30–S40.

van Kesteren, N. M., Hospers, H. J., van Empelen, P., van Breukelen, G., & Kok, G. (2007). Sexual decision-making in HIV positive men who have sex with men: How moral concerns and sexual motives guide intended condom use with steady and casual partners. *Sexual Behavior, 36,* 437–449.

Vanable, P. A., Carey, M. P., Blair, D. C., & Littlewood, R. A. (2006). Impact of HIV-related stigma on health behaviors and psychological adjustment among HIV-positive men and women. *AIDS and Behavior, 10,* 473–482.

Weinberger, D. R., Elvevag, B., & Giedd, J. N. (2005). *The adolescent brain: A work in progress.* Washington, DC: The National Campaign to Prevent Teen Pregnancy.

Weinman, M. (2010). Living well and sexual self-determination: Expanding human rights discourse about sex and sexuality. *Law, Culture and the Humanities, 7,* 101–120.

White, W., Grant, J., Pryor, E. R., Keltner, N. L., Vance, D. E., & Raper, J. L. (2012). Do social support, stigma, and social problem-solving skills predict depressive symptoms in people living with HIV: A mediation analysis. *Research and Theory for Nursing Practice, 26,* 182–204.

Yee, J. (2005). Critical anti-racism praxis in social work: The concept of whiteness implicated. In S. Hick, R. Pozzuto, & J. Fook (Eds.), *Social work: A critical turn* (pp. 87–104). Toronto: Thompson Educational Publishing.

Young, L. E., Jonas, A. B., Michaels, S., Jackson, J. D., Pierce, M. L., Schneider, J. A., & uConnect Study Team. (2016). Social-structural properties and HIV prevention among young men who have sex with men in the ballroom house and independent gay family communities. *Social Science and Medicine, 174,* 26–34.

Young, S. D., Shoptaw, S., Weiss, R. E., Munjas, B., & Gorbach, P. M. (2011). Predictors of unrecognized HIV infection among poor and ethnic men who have sex with men in Los Angeles. *AIDS and Behavior, 15,* 643–649.

Zaller, N., Gilliani, F. S., & Rich, J. D. (2007). A model of integrated primary care for HIV-positive patients with underlying substance use and mental illness. *AIDS Care, 19,* 1128–1133.

Zolopa, A. R., & Katz, M. H. (2012). HIV infection and AIDS. In S. J. McPhee, M. A. Papadakis, & M. W. Rabow (Eds.), *Current medical diagnosis and treatment, CMDT 2012* (Vol. 31, 51st ed.). New York: McGraw Hill, Lange.

Chapter 3
From Pathology to Resiliency: Understanding the Mental Health of HIV Positive Gay Men

Ja'Nina J. Garrett-Walker and Gabriel R. Galindo

Introduction

Research suggests that stress, stigma, and synergistic coupling of disease conditions have resulted in health-related disparities among sexual minority men, including gay men and other men who have sex with men (MSM[1]) (Batchelder et al., 2017). Sexual minority men experience unique oppression due to structural injustices in relation to their sexual orientation (White Hughto et al., 2017). For gay men living with HIV, their HIV status adds an additional level of stigma that impacts their mental health (Rendina et al., 2017). Social oppression and marginalization have continuously been shown to have a negative effect on the mental health and well-being of gay men and individuals living with HIV (Bostwick et al., 2014; Choi, Paul, Ayala, Boylan, & Gregorich, 2013; Cochran & Mays, 2015; Díaz, Ayala, & Bein, 2004; Hays, Turner, & Coates, 1992; Mays, Cochran, & Barnes, 2007; Meyer, 1995; Meyer, Dietrich, & Schwartz, 2008; Meyer, Schwartz, & Frost, 2008; Siegel, Lune, & Meyer, 1998; Mimiaga et al., 2015; Wheeler, 2005; Wilson, Stadler, Boone & Bolger, 2014; Wong, Schrager, Holloway, Meyer, & Kipke, 2014). In this chapter, we examine existing literature related to mental health concerns for HIV positive gay men in the USA. The chapter seeks to better understand and conceptualize: (1) current research related to the mental health of gay men and HIV positive gay men; (2) psychological distress

---

[1] "MSM" is a public health term used by academics and surveillance specialists, but it does not capture the complex meanings that men ascribe to their sexual identities, communities, and networks. In this chapter, the term "gay" is preferred; however, where appropriate, MSM is used to stay consistent with previous study data.

J.J. Garrett-Walker (✉)
Department of Psychology, College of Arts and Sciences, University of San Francisco (USF), San Francisco, CA, USA
e-mail: jgarrettwalker@usfca.edu

G.R. Galindo
Public Health Research Services, LLC, Los Angeles, CA, USA

College of Southern Nevada, Las Vegas, NV, USA

© Springer Science+Business Media LLC 2017
L. Wilton (ed.), *Understanding Prevention for HIV Positive Gay Men*,
DOI 10.1007/978-1-4419-0203-0_3

and resiliency among HIV positive gay men, including the role of stigma, shame, and silence regarding sexual behavior and HIV status; and (3) public health considerations and implications for HIV prevention strategies.

Mental Health for Gay Men and HIV Positive Gay Men

Minority Stress Theory

Meyer (1995) proposed the notion that negative societal perceptions of same-sex behavior directly impacted the mental health of gay men. Meyer (1995) found that internalized homophobia, stigma, and prejudice events each independently predicted psychological distress (i.e., demoralization [e.g., anxiety, sadness, helplessness, hopelessness], guilt, sex problems, and suicide) in a sample of gay men. These findings provided an empirical basis to correlate the negative impact of sexual minority stress on mental health outcomes. Minority stress theory posits that experiences of social discrimination based on gender, sexual and/or ethnoracial[2] minority status work to reduce the overall health profile of minority individuals. This process occurs over time as individuals with minority status are exposed to both explicit (i.e., "proximal") and implicit (i.e., "distal") experiences of discrimination and social marginalization. Combined, these experiences may cause chronic stress to an individual, which in turn lowers self-esteem and increases negative mental health outcomes. This process of minority stress renders the individual more vulnerable to serious psychosocial health problems (Meyer, 2003). In effect, minority stress is an additive stress (i.e., a stress in addition to stressors encountered by non-stigmatized counterparts) faced by those who experience distal and proximal stressful events based on their minority status(es).

Among sexual minority men, including gay men, evidence suggests that minority stress increases their risk for salient health issues, including depression, anxiety, substance use, and sexual risk behaviors (Lelutiu-Weinberger et al., 2013; Meyer, Dietrich, et al., 2008; Meyer, Schwartz, et al., 2008; Rendina et al., 2017). The model describes stress processes, including experiences of prejudice, expectations of rejection, hiding, concealing, internalized homophobia, and impaired positive coping processes such as social support systems (Meyer, 1995, 2003). Based on the minority stress model, Meyer (1995, 2003, 2016) contends that macro-contextual factors, such as homophobia and sexual stigma, may arise from the environment. These societal factors require an individual to not only adapt, but may also cause significant stress, which can ultimately affect the health and well-being of an individual. The underlying concepts held within the model indicate that minority stressors (both proximal and distal) are unique (i.e., not experienced by non-stigmatized

---

[2] Building from Omi & Winant's (1986) classical work surrounding racial formation in the USA, the term ethnoracial (as opposed to "race" or "ethnicity") is used to describe encompassing categories of associated heritage and cultural group affiliations.

counterparts), chronic (i.e., occurring over time), and socially based (i.e., constructed via social processes, institutions, and structures) (Meyer, Dietrich, et al., 2008; Meyer, Schwartz, et al., 2008). Minority stress has consistently been shown to impact the mental health and sexual risk behavior for gay men, which supports Meyer's claim that attention must be provided to the ways in which societal marginalization impacts health outcomes of gay men (Hamilton & Mahalik, 2009; Han et al. 2015; Hequembourg & Brallier, 2009; Kimmel & Mahalik, 2005; Rendina et al., 2017).

Mental Health for Gay Men

Research has indicated that, due to social oppression, gay men experience increased prevalence of mental health disorders compared to their heterosexual counterparts (Bränström, 2017; Choi et al., 2013; Cochran & Mays, 2003; Greene, 1994; Herek & Garnets, 2007; Meyer, 2003). Using data from the National Health and Nutrition Examination Survey III, Cochran and Mays (2000, 2003) found that men reporting any male partners in their lifetime were significantly more likely than their exclusively heterosexual counterparts to report lifetime prevalence of recurring depression. Findings showed that 15% of men who had any male partner in their lifetime met diagnostic criteria for depression (Cochran & Mays, 2000, 2003). Using data from the Midlife in the United States (MIDUS) survey, the first national survey of middle life adulthood, findings demonstrated that the sample of self-identified MSM showed a higher prevalence of depression than their male heterosexual counterparts (Cochran, Sullivan, & Mays, 2003). Recent findings (Blosnich et al., 2016) from the California Quality of Life Surveys ($n = 1478$ sexual minority and 3465 heterosexual individuals) showed that homosexually experienced men, as compared to heterosexual men, reported about 7 times higher risk of a history of suicide attempts.

However, other research has suggested that gay and heterosexual men do not differ on mental health outcomes. For example, Bybee et al. (2009) found no significant differences on psychological well-being based on sexual orientation. This may be due to the small size of the sample ($n = 81$ gay men, $n = 86$ heterosexual men) (Bybee, Sullivan, Zielonka, & Moes, 2009) or due to other demographic differences, such as socioeconomic status or affiliation to sexual minority communities. Based on a sample of 2605 MSM from the Urban Men's Health Study (UMHS), Barrett and Pollack (2005) noted that as levels of education and income decreased, MSM were more likely to report sexual intercourse with women, and less likely to report involvement with gay communities or to endorse gay community affiliation (Barrett & Pollack, 2005).

Demographic differences have been found among gay men in regard to their mental health (Moeller, Halkitis, Pollack, Siconolfi, & Barton, 2013). Using a diverse sample of 388 New York City residents, Meyer and colleagues (2008) found that ethnoracial differences existed within sexual minority populations.

The findings indicated that Black participants tended to report fewer mental health concerns than their Latino and White counterparts. However, Latino participants reported significantly more suicide attempts than their Black and White counterparts. In regard to age, younger LGB participants (18–44 years old) reported significantly lower mood disorder prevalence than older participants (Meyer, Dietrich, et al., 2008).

Bybee et al. (2009) found that gay men under the age of 25 reported more depression, suicidality, anger, negative self-esteem, emotional instability, emotional non-responsiveness, shame, and guilt when compared to gay men over the age of 25. These age findings may be due to the developmental period younger participants are experiencing. For example, McDermott, Roen, and Scourfield (2008) contend that due to societal level homophobia, sexual minority youth incorporate shame-avoidance coping strategies to manage homophobia. Without expectation of support from family, this may in turn make sexual minority youth more vulnerable to self-destructive behaviors (McDermott, Roen, & Scourfield, 2008). Given that these younger participants are still developing and solidifying their identities, they may experience instability in their psychological well-being as they experience the process of merging their multiple identities (Arnett, 2000; Walker et al., 2015). In addition to these demographic differences, impaired mental health has been shown to influence HIV sexual risk behavior (Batchelder et al., 2017; O'Cleirigh, Skeer, Mayer, & Safren, 2009; Safren, Blashill, & O'Cleirigh, 2011). For HIV negative gay men, anxiety has been related to increases in condomless anal intercourse, sex under the influence of substances as well as number of days in which substances were utilized in the last 30 days (Lelutiu-Weinberger et al., 2013).

Mental Health for HIV Positive Gay Men

While the experiences of ethnoracial, gender, and sexual minorities have been explored using the minority stress model as a conceptual framework, a major limitation is the role of minority status in relation to HIV positive serostatus (Rendina et al., 2017). Gay men living with HIV experience discrimination from society because of their sexual orientation in addition to marginalization based on their HIV status (Batchelder et al., 2017). There exists a growing body of literature that substantiates evidence that psychosocial factors, such as stressful life events and passive coping strategies (e.g., denial), may affect disease progression in those infected with HIV (Friedman et al., 2017; Leserman et al., 2002). It has been well demonstrated that HIV positive gay men experience psychosocial health problems, such as substance use, depression, anxiety, victimization, and participation in high-risk sexual behaviors (Safren et al., 2010; Safren et al., 2013) in different contexts than their HIV negative serostatus counterparts (Leserman et al. 2002). Much of the research in this area has provided a core foundation for studying HIV-specific cognitive behavioral therapies in an effort to better understand the role of stressors on the immune systems of HIV positive individuals (Batchelder et al., 2017).

Stress-management interventions, including bereavement support groups, have been shown to reduce distress and have a salutary effect on immune and other physical health-related measures in individuals living with HIV (Leserman et al. 2002).

While the research on mental health provides innovative directions for the management and care of HIV, particularly among gay men and MSM, there is a paucity of psychological clinical trials (Batchelder et al., 2017). Specifically, a majority of the peer-reviewed studies on psychosocial moderators of HIV infection have been conducted on MSM and were primarily initiated before the advent of highly active antiretroviral medications, such as protease inhibitors (Safren et al., 2013). Still, advances in research on social stress and biomedical health outcomes indicate that stress and passive coping are related to immune change and HIV disease progression (Friedman et al., 2017; Leserman, 2003). Despite the usefulness in using the minority stress model to explain psychological mental health outcomes among sexual minority populations, limited research has used this model to link social stressors to physical health outcomes (Rendina et al., 2017). In addition to understanding the additive role of minority stress among individuals, for those living with HIV, it may be equally important to recognize the ways in which cognitive behavioral treatments may ameliorate the negative effects of stress and passive coping, and as such, have a beneficial impact on the course of HIV infection, particularly among sexual minority men who are subject to increased social stressors (Mimiaga et al., 2015; Safren et al., 2013).

Psychological Distress and Resiliency Among HIV Positive Gay Men

Understanding potential barriers and facilitators to impaired mental health for HIV positive gay men, including a consideration of resiliency, is of great importance as: (1) individuals are living longer with HIV and (2) younger populations are continuing to see increased HIV prevalence rates (CDC, 2015; Halkitis, Kapadia, et al., 2013; Herrick, Stall, Goldhammer, Egan, & Mayer, 2013, Kingdon et al., 2013; Moeller et al., 2013; Peterson, Miner, Brennan, & Rosser, 2012; Walker & Longmire-Avital, 2013). In order to provide individuals with adequate care, we must examine the social structures that contribute to impaired mental health and the resources that increase positive mental health outcomes (Batchelder et al., 2017). For example, recent innovative work surrounding sexual minority populations has revealed that negative social environments for sexual minority youth can increase suicidal attempts (Hatzenbuehler, 2011), and that institutional discriminatory policies can create harmful consequences for the mental health of sexual minority populations (Hatzenbuehler, McLaughlin, Keyes, & Hasin, 2010). However, Cramer, Burks, Plöderl and Durgampudi (2017) has posited that positive social environments can influence the mental health and quality of life for sexual minority individuals, which impact health inequities. For example, engagement in community centers has been shown to buffer poor mental health outcomes (Ramirez-Valles, 2002), and recent research has suggested the utilization of student health organizations as a strategy in reducing health-related disparities in "underserved" communities (Mays, Ly, Allen, & Young, 2009).

Theory of Syndemic Production

Psychosocial health problems such as substance use, depression, and intimate partner violence have been found to interact in such a way that their impact on the overall health of an individual is greater than one would expect the additive effect to be (Friedman et al., 2017; Halkitis, Moeller et al., 2013; Herrick, et al., 2014; Parsons, Grov, & Golub, 2012; Safren et al., 2010; Stall et al., 2003). Building from the literature surrounding HIV and sexual minority health, the Theory of Syndemic Production posits that the combination of one or more negative psychosocial health outcomes are thought to interact to form a syndemic (i.e., co-occurring health conditions that together can lower an individual's overall health), thereby making them more susceptible to disease (Stall et al. 2003). Beyond comorbidity research, which tends to focus on the boundaries and overlap of diagnoses, syndemic research focuses on communities experiencing multiple epidemics that additively increase negative health outcomes (Stall, Friedman, & Catania, 2007). Within this model, it is possible for two disorders to be comorbid but not represent a syndemic (e.g., the disorders are not epidemic in the studied population or their co-occurrence is not accompanied by additional adverse health consequences). The Theory of Syndemic Production is pioneering insofar as it implies not only a focus on health disparities but also on the social conditions that perpetrate these health disparities (Herrick, Lim, et al., 2013; Stall et al., 2003; Stall et al., 2007). Within syndemic productions of health disparities, there may be ethnoracial differences among gay male populations. Dyer et al. (2012) used data from a large prospective cohort study to confirm that syndemic theory assists in explaining complexities which sustain HIV-related sexual transmission behaviors among Black gay men (Dyer et al., 2012).

Recent studies have demonstrated that as the number of psychosocial conditions endorsed by an individual increase, their likelihood of engagement in HIV sexual risk behaviors increased, as did their likelihood of HIV infection (Mustanski, Garofalo, Herrick, & Donenberg, 2007). It has been suggested that this set of co-occurring psychosocial health problems (i.e., the presence of a syndemic condition) may actually be driving the HIV epidemic among MSM and may similarly reinforce other health disparities (e.g., depression and anxiety). While the Theory of Syndemic Production advances public health considerations, it is limited in its consideration of socio-structural factors that may also influence health outcomes of sexual minority men. In particular, social oppression (defined as racism, homophobia, and poverty) has been shown to impact the lives of sexual minority men, in ways that go beyond synergistic syndemic productions of disease (Ayala, Bingham, Kim, Wheeler, & Millett, 2012; Bogart et al., 2011; Choi et al., 2013). For example, the research of Díaz et al. (2001, 2006) focused on ethnoracial sexual minority men has shown that multiple minority identities can increase experiences of distal and proximal stressors, through racism, homophobia, and poverty (Díaz, Ayala, Bein, Henne, & Martin, 2001; Díaz, Bein, & Ayala, 2006).

These multileveled stressors can be even more pronounced for HIV positive sexual and ethnoracial minority men (Friedman et al., 2017). In a study of HIV positive gay men, depression (58.1%), anxiety (38.2%), and HIV-related issues (21.8%) were the main concerns that brought participants in for treatment. Participants in this study had an average CD4 count of 508 (SD = 255; Range = 99–1200), 41.5% reported a detectable viral load, and 64.3% reported currently being on HAART medications (Berg, Mimiaga, & Safren, 2004). In a sample of older (44–75 years old) gay men (37.62% HIV positive), gay stigma, excessive HIV bereavements, and concerns regarding independence significantly predicted depression (Wight, LeBlanc, de Vries, & Detels, 2012). Stigma and mental health concerns are of increased importance for HIV positive gay men due to the ways in which impaired psychological well-being impacts the physical health of these men.

Sources of Psychological Distress

As previously discussed, social oppression is a painful reality for HIV positive gay men that affects their mental health. In the USA, society has historically marginalized gay communities as well as other stigmatized groups, such as individuals living with HIV (Drescher, 2010; Han et al., 2015; White Hughto et al., 2017; Szymanski & Gupta, 2009). It is often assumed that HIV positive gay men have acquired HIV through sexual contact with another man. This assumption has framed much of the discourse about HIV, for gay men, involving a cycle of sexual shame, stigma, and silence (Jeffries et al., 2015). Shame fuels hatred, mistrust, violence and often forces individuals to hide critical parts of themselves. The internalization of societal shaming, along with the distress that shaming causes, often leads to depression, other mental health concerns, and risk behavior (Kaufman & Raphael, 1996). Stigma, associated with same-sex behavior, has been associated with increased high-risk sexual acts (condomless anal sex with an unknown status or HIV positive partner) for HIV negative gay men (Lelutiu-Weinberger et al., 2013). This sexual shaming has been derived through society and is often passed through cultures, families, and generations (Kaufman and Raphel, 1996).

Internalized Homonegativity

Internalized homonegativity is a concept that greatly affects individuals within gay and sexual minority communities (Herrick, Stall, Chmiel et al., 2013). Internalized homonegativity is defined as "negative attitudes and affects toward homosexuality in other persons and toward homosexual features in oneself'" (Shidlo, 1994, p. 178). Internalized homonegativity has been shown to increase psychological distress, depression, social isolation, and lower self-esteem (Boone, Cook, & Wilson, 2016; Díaz et al., 2001; Mayfield, 2001; Rosser, Bockting, Ross, Miner, & Colemen, 2008). For gay men living with HIV, marginalization does not come solely from the larger society, but also from subgroups of the population such as families, religious communities, and even gay communities. Due to social expectations regarding sexual orientation, families of gay men may reject them because of their same-sex behaviors. This rejection, and internalization of negative rhetoric and societal values, particularly for youth, can lead to depression, substance use, sexual risk behavior, and suicidal ideation and attempts (Ryan, Huebner, Díaz, & Sanchez, 2009).

Substance Use

Individuals often partake in substance use (e.g., alcohol, crystal methamphetamine, cocaine, poppers) (Buttram & Kurtz, 2015; Halkitis et al., 2011; Mimiaga et al., 2012) as a form of escapism to relieve the heightened mental distress associated with marginalization (Jerome, Halkitis, & Siconolfi, 2009; McKirnan, Ostrow, & Hope, 1996; Semple, Strathdee, Zians, & Patterson, 2012; Shoptaw et al., 2009). McCabe et al. (2010) found that LGB participants were two times more likely than their heterosexual counterparts to have had a substance use disorder in the last year. McCabe et al. also found that for LGB individuals who reported gender, racial, *and* sexual orientation discrimination, in the past year, were four times as likely to have reported a substance use disorder in the past year compared to those reporting no discrimination (McCabe, Bostwick, Hughes, West, & Boyd, 2010). Taken together, these studies help to provide focus to the growing body of research examining the multiple, co-occurring epidemics of health among sexual minority male populations. Additionally, interventions specific to exploring substance use among gay male populations have indicated that gay-specific, culturally tailored cognitive behavioral therapy can produce reliable, significant, and sustained reductions in stimulant use, particularly methamphetamine, and sexual risk behaviors (Shoptaw et al., 2008). A review by Carrico (2011) highlighted the role of increased substance use patterns on HIV progression and the resulting physical health consequences.

HIV-Related Stigma

HIV stigma has been defined as prejudice, negative attitudes, abuse, and maltreatment directed at people living with HIV and AIDS and has a multitude of consequences for an individual (UNAIDS, 2011). These include, but are not limited to, being ostracized by family, peers, and the wider community, poor treatment in healthcare and education settings, a dismantling of rights, psychological damage, and a negative effect on the success of HIV testing and treatment (UNAIDS, 2011). For gay men, HIV-related stigma becomes more salient as there is often a sexuality-based "moral component" attached to same-sex behavior and HIV infection (Jeffries, Sutton, and Eke, 2017; Valdiserri, 2002). Given local norms and values, those who do not adhere to socially constructed moral behaviors within a population may be perceived as "deviants," and therefore further subjected to stigmatization processes. Moreover, even within sexual minority populations, community members may stigmatize their peers in order to enhance their personal standing within their local world (Galindo, 2013). To avoid rejection from their family, or other members of the gay community, some individuals living with HIV may not disclose their HIV status (Bird, Fingerhut, and McKirnan, 2011). A recent review on HIV-related stigma within gay communities noted a growing division between HIV positive and HIV negative gay men, as well as fragmentation of gay communities along lines of HIV status (Boone et al., 2016; Smit et al., 2012). Research has suggested that this fragmentation of gay men, based on HIV serostatus, has underpinning roots with respect to disclosure and intentional high-risk sexual practices, such as condomless anal intercourse (Sheon & Crosby, 2004). The concept that individuals have to hide parts of their core identities, for fear of retribution, fuels the cycle of shame, stigma and silence around sexual orientation and serostatus for sexual minority populations. In essence, by reducing the meaning and value that these men ascribe to their respecting identities, their ability to cope and adapt to proximal and distal stressors is thereby reduced as well. This, in turn, may further exacerbate psychological distress for these men.

Additionally, psychological distress and HIV-related stigma have had a profound effect on the course of the HIV epidemic. Globally, the World Health Organization (WHO) notes that fears of stigma and discrimination constitute a core reason why individuals are reticent to have HIV testing, to disclose their HIV status, and engage in HIV treatment and care (WHO, 2014). For example, one review of studies investigating antiretroviral adherence among HIV-infected youth in the USA noted that HIV-related stigma increased reported depression and anxiety, and was consistently associated with poorer adherence across studies (Reisner et al., 2009). Additionally, research, including a review of interventions, to reduce HIV/AIDS stigma, highlighted that stigma remains an obstacle in HIV testing rates (Brown, Macintyre, and Trujillo, 2003; Dowson, Kober, Perry, Fisher, and Richardson, 2012). Because stigma serves as a barrier for an individual to take a HIV test, more individuals are diagnosed late (i.e., when the virus has already progressed to AIDS), which can make treatment options less optimal. In order to effectively confront the negative impact of HIV-related stigma on public health efforts, it is imperative to continue to support research in the domains of intervention, program operations, and policy formulation. Such endeavors will add to our understanding of how stigma hampers society from effectively responding to HIV/AIDS, particularly among MSM populations.

Sources of Resiliency

While there is clear evidence to support facilitators to psychological distress, there are some barriers to many of the mental health concerns that impact HIV positive gay men (Friedman et al., 2017). As indicated by Herrick et al. (2011), natural sources of strength, or "resilience," from gay male populations remain a largely untapped reserve in the design of behavioral interventions for gay men (Herrick et al., 2011). Social Support has continuously been shown to contribute to positive psychological well-being (Frost, Meyer, & Schwartz, 2016; Hays et al., 1992; Kalichman et al., 2003; Serovich et al., 2001). Among HIV positive gay men specifically, satisfaction with emotional, informational, and practical social support all decreased depression among participants. Early work with HIV positive gay men noted that informational support has been shown to buffer the stress associated with symptoms associated with HIV (Friedman et al., 2017; Hays, Turner, and Coates, 1992).

Due to societal thoughts on same-sex behavior and HIV infection, some men lose their main source of social support, family. Given familial rejection in reaction to sexual behavior, sexual identities, and HIV status, many gay men have sought social support outside of their traditional families and within *fictive kinships*. Fictive kinships are best understood as familial-like relationships among individuals without genetic or marital ties (Stewart, 2007). These relationships allow people to define "family" for themselves allowing them to include individuals who may, or may not, be part of the gay or HIV positive communities. The ability to define family for oneself, especially when ones native family has contributed to mental distress through stigma and discrimination, has been shown to contribute to positive mental health outcomes (Oswald, 2002; Stewart, 2007).

In addition to familial support, religious faith has also been shown to serve as a source of resiliency for many populations (see Hood, Hill, and Spilka, 2009; Lassiter et al., 2017). However, negative religious rhetoric, regarding sexual behavior, has been shown to be a source of distress for gay men, particularly ethnoracial minority gay men (Miller, 2007; Garrett-Walker & Torres, 2016; Nelson et al., 2016). Wilson et al. (2011), in their qualitative investigation of Black churches and the role of religiosity in the lives of Black MSM, noted the ways in which religious ideologies may both impede and facilitate church dialogue involving sexuality through heightened responses to the domestic HIV crisis (Wilson et al., 2011). However, much of the previous work around religious rhetoric, sexuality, and HIV has not addressed the stigma often imposed by religious institutions (Nelson et al., 2016). Other innovative work exploring the positive impact of spirituality in the lives of individuals with HIV has discussed the positive role that a relationship with a Higher Power (not a particular religious institution) has on their ability to stay adherent to their HIV medications. It was expressed that a connection to a High Power promoted physical health by decreasing mental distress associated with HIV symptomology (Foster, Arnold, Rebchook, and Kegeles, 2011). Given the complex interplay between religious faith, internalized homonegativity, and resiliency, researchers and clinicians must further explore the ways in which organized religion may be a source of distress for some individuals, while the individualized connection to one's spiritual self may serve as a source of resiliency (Walker & Longmire-Avital, 2013; Garrett-Walker & Torres, 2016).

Health, Policy, and Research

In order to understand best practices in intervention design for HIV positive sexual minority men, it is imperative to examine the current sociopolitical landscape. In this section, we highlight an evolving public health field, put into context the role of policy in advancing the health of the population, and put forth research considerations to meet the healthcare needs of HIV positive sexual minority men.

Emerging Biomedical Interventions

The success of biomedical interventions such as male circumcision, the use of pre-exposure prophylaxis (PrEP) to prevent HIV transmission and the reduction of HIV infectiousness through the use of antiretroviral medications, has spurred new paradigms in approaches to HIV prevention (Buchbinder & Liu, 2015; Koblin et al., 2011; Padian, Buve, Balkus, Serwadda, and Cates, 2008; Grant et al., 2010). While initial approaches in the HIV epidemic have emphasized behavioral interventions to reduce risk behavior, the use of advanced biomedical technologies is evolving the HIV public health field. In particular, the HPTN 052 study involving 1763 HIV serodiscordant couples was completed in 2011. Findings indicated that those who began antiretroviral therapy as soon as they were diagnosed with HIV significantly lowered the risk of HIV transmission to their sexual partners, compared to those starting treatment later, when their CD4 count had fallen below 250 cells/mm^3 (HPTN, 2011). Of those who took part in the study and were infected from their partner, only one person became infected from the early treatment group, versus 27 from the later treatment group—a 96% reduction in risk of transmission (Cohen et al., 2011). Still, in light of these recent medical advances in HIV "treatment as prevention," a successful biomedical strategy has to be scaled up in ways that affect both behavioral components and structural institutions, such as the healthcare system. This is a particularly important point for gay men with little to no access to the healthcare industry, such as Black and Latino sexual minority men. In recognizing this concern, the HPTN 073 trial is the first of the HIV Prevention Treatment Network's studies to specifically focus on PrEP uptake and adherence among Black MSM in three US cities (HPTN, 2013). Ultimately in order for biomedical interventions to truly be efficacious, an integrated approach will inevitably be needed.

Integrating Social Dimensions of Health with Medical Advances

Despite impressive scientific gains, biomedical interventions cannot be sustained on their own in nonclinical study settings. A critique of institutional barriers will be needed to fill gaps in our understanding of healthcare access and delivery. An accumulated body of empirical findings has clearly demonstrated that social and cultural factors influence health by affecting factors such as exposure and vulnerability to disease, risk-taking behaviors, the effectiveness of health promotion efforts, and access to, availability of, and quality of healthcare (Malebranche et al., 2004; Matthews & Adams, 2009; Mayer et al., 2012; Millett et al., 2012; Sullivan et al., 2012). All components have a critical role in shaping individuals' responses to health concerns and the impact of poor health on individuals' lives and well-being. Social dimensions of health are also essential to understanding current and changing population rates of morbidity, survival, mortality, and use of health services (Safren et al., 2013). This requires that we take into account the various demographic, social, economic, cultural structures, and dynamics of the population. For example, intersectionality as a unifying public health framework addresses multiple interlocking systems of privilege and oppression such as racism, sexism, and heterosexism, that many ethnoracial and sexual minority HIV positive men face (Bowleg, 2012; Nelson et al., 2016). With the advent of medical advances in the HIV field, the operational issues of the sustained cost, the target population, methods of distribution, and long-term side effects, remain paramount (Galindo et al., 2012). Emerging biomedical strategies will still necessitate both behavioral dimensions and structural components.

Role of the Affordable Care Act in Linking HIV Positive Gay Men to Healthcare

Historically, individuals living with HIV/AIDS have experienced significant challenges obtaining private health insurance and have been particularly vulnerable to insurance industry protocols. However, consistent with the goals of the National HIV/AIDS Strategy (ONAP, 2010), the Affordable Care Act (ACA, 2010) set into place an effort that helps to ensure that Americans, including those living with HIV/AIDS, have secure, stable, affordable health insurance and the relief they need from ever-increasing healthcare costs. With the leadership of President Barack Obama, beginning with its implementation in 2014, the ACA prohibits insurers from cancelling or rescinding coverage based on "pre-existing conditions," including HIV/AIDS. Insurers can no longer impose lifetime limits on insurance benefits. These changes will dramatically begin to improve access to care for those impacted by HIV/AIDS and other chronic conditions as well as help people retain the coverage they have. Furthermore, individuals with low and middle incomes will be eligible for tax subsidies that will help them buy coverage from new state health insurance Exchanges (ACA, 2010).

Additionally, the ACA broadens Medicaid eligibility to generally include individuals with income below 133% of the Federal poverty line (FPL; $14,400 for an individual and $29,300 for a family of 4), including single adults who have not traditionally been eligible for Medicaid benefits. As a result, a person living with

HIV who meets this income threshold no longer has to wait for a clinical AIDS diagnosis in order to receive services from Medicaid. In particular, for sexual minority men living with HIV/AIDS, the ACA phases out the *Medicare Part D* prescription drug benefit requirement (also known as the "donut hole"), thereby giving Medicare enrollees living with HIV/AIDS the ability to better afford their medications. However, even when implemented, social dimensions of HIV infection, including HIV-related stigma, will still impact the ways in which individuals access care and treatment. This is particularly true for HIV positive ethnoracial sexual minority men who face various stressors related to their multiple intersecting identities. Thus, the health of those impacted by HIV/AIDS is influenced not only by their ability to obtain coverage but also by economic, social, and physical factors. While the ACA expands and increases vital funding for community health centers (an important safety-net for low-income individuals and families), it is unknown if these facilities will be competent in addressing the sociocultural concerns of a population that has not historically accessed their services. Still, the ACA will lead to significant new investments to support critical healthcare workforce expansions to better serve vulnerable populations.

Maintaining and Sustaining Funding Mechanisms

Currently, fewer than one in five (17%) people living with HIV has some form of private health insurance and nearly 30% do not have any access to care (ACA, 2010). *Medicaid*, the Federal-state program that provides healthcare benefits to low-income people and those living with disabilities, is a major source of coverage for people living with HIV/AIDS. *Medicare*, the Federal program for seniors and people with disabilities also plays a role in sustaining care for those affected by HIV/AIDS. The Ryan White CARE HIV/AIDS Treatment Extension Act of 2009 is another key source of funding for health and social services for this highly vulnerable population (HRSA, 2009). Even with full implementation of the ACA, it is acknowledged that there will still be gaps in care and Ryan White services are sure to be needed. For example, while health benefit packages are still determined at the state level (i.e., through the Exchanges), we know that these benefits will not cover all nonmedical care services (including vision and dental services). In the post-ACA era, we will be reliant on Ryan White funding to provide wrap-around support services to cover essential gaps in care and treatment, such as case management, nutrition, transportation, mental health, substance use services, peer support, and/or premium co-payment assistance. While the ACA call for subsidized private insurance, for those with incomes between 133% and 400% FPL, the subsidies may leave many with premiums and co-pays they cannot afford. Additionally, in considering funding mechanisms for care and treatment, it is also important to note the significance of maintaining funding streams for research and intervention development for HIV positive sexual minority men. For example, both the National HIV/AIDS Strategy (ONAP, 2010) and the Institute of Medicine report on the health of

LGBT individuals (IOM, 2011) while underscoring the importance of providing empirical research that focuses on the prevention needs of HIV positive sexual minority individuals.

Enhancing Resilience of HIV Positive Gay Men

Historically, research regarding the health of HIV positive sexual minority men has come from a pathologized viewpoint. However, it is necessary to acknowledge that not all sexual minorities who have experienced adversity develop detrimental physical or psychological health conditions, and not all of those who develop negative health conditions become HIV infected. In fact, the original investigation of syndemic production among MSM found that, of the men who experienced three or more psychosocial health problems, 23% had recently engaged in high-risk sex and 22% were HIV positive (Stall, et al., 2007). While these numbers certainly bear concern, it is equally important to call attention to the fact that 77% of these men were able to avoid engaging in high-risk sexual behaviors and 78% had remained HIV negative in light of the fact that they were managing a plethora of associated psychosocial health tribulations. Recognizing that these men were able to withstand persistent sociocultural marginalization, despite the multitude of stressors associated with those experiences, indicates considerable resilience among the population. While the peer-reviewed literature on resilience is still emerging among sexual minority populations, and has yet to receive much focus, there appears to be great potential in considering asset-based approaches to the health promotion of MSM, including HIV positive gay men (Herrick et al., 2011). For example, innovative work exploring protective factors among Latino gay men has shown that community involvement moderates sexual risk behaviors and that volunteering with HIV/AIDS organizations can decrease psychological stressors (Ramirez-Valles, 2002; Trapence et al., 2012).

Integration of Mental Health and Substance Use

In light of evidence that suggests that interventions geared towards HIV positive sexual minority men would benefit from the inclusion of harm reduction strategies for alcohol and recreational drug use, and an understanding of comorbid mental health issues, there are few interventions that integrate mental health and substance use with sexual health information (Naar-King, Parsons, & Johnson, 2012; Safren et al., 2013; Wechsberg, Golin, El-Bassel, Hopkins, & Zule, 2012). This is a critical point of consideration as "almost all models of sexual risk-taking behavior are based on social psychological theories that may not fully consider the impact of comorbid psychiatric disorders" (Safren et al., 2011, p. S32). That is, while most HIV prevention strategies are grounded in psychological theories, the individuals who may benefit most from these strategies may be psychologically and physically impaired. That is, individuals experiencing mental health distress may not have the same cognitive capacity to enact or understand the importance of needed interventions within their lives as those with higher functioning cognitive abilities. For example, the Theory of Reasoned Action (Ajzen & Fishbein, 1980) assumes that one is capable of reasoned actions, when in actuality, a mental disorder may prevent the success of such an intervention that utilizes this theoretical approach. Revisiting the Theory of Syndemic Production, one can gain insight into strategies to enhance HIV prevention effectiveness. According to the theory, increasing levels of health across any or all psychosocial health conditions will have a positive impact on the levels of HIV risk and HIV prevalence, as well as other components that constitute the set of syndemic conditions. If syndemic conditions work together to *increase* vulnerability to HIV, then mitigation of one or more of these conditions should work to *decrease* HIV vulnerability. Thus, prevention interventions for HIV positive sexual minorities that successfully address psychosocial health conditions will likely improve HIV prevention behaviors even if there is not a direct focus on HIV prevention. Likewise, interventions that reduce substance use issues will most likely also improve HIV prevention behaviors among the population.

System Approaches to Prevention, Care, and Treatment

Beyond the sole consideration of HIV, a comprehensive multipath model that considers depression, substance use, poor social support, homelessness, medication nonadherence, and risky sexual behavior is needed to best understand HIV progression, and to explain how psychological distress may lead to accelerated progression to AIDS (Friedman et al., 2017). For example, the model proposed by Díaz et al. (2001) considers the importance of social oppression (i.e., poverty, racism, and homophobia) related to HIV transmission and sexual risk factors. In light of these phenomena, research has called for a holistic (i.e., system approach) to HIV prevention, care, and treatment (Díaz et al., 2001). For example, with respect to food insecurity, a recent study reported that 56% of HIV positive patients who were homeless or living in substandard housing were also food insecure (regular inability to obtain enough healthy food; Weiser et al., 2013). The researchers examined the case history of 347 HIV patients, all of whom resided in San Francisco, CA. Weiser et al. (2013) indicated that the food-insecure patients were roughly twice as likely to have visited the emergency room or been hospitalized over a given 3-month period, compared with patients who had enough to eat (Weiser, et al., 2013). Thus, food insecurity was more likely than homelessness, drug abuse, or depression to lead to emergency room visits for these HIV positive individuals.

Earlier studies, both in the USA and abroad, have found that food insecurity is also associated with missed doctors' appointments, less suppression of the HIV virus, and greater risk of death. Thus, strength-based approaches to HIV prevention will be aided greatly by the further development of a holistic theory of resilience that is specifically tailored to HIV positive sexual minority men. This can be accomplished through further investigation of naturally occurring strengths and protective factors that exist within both individuals and communities. Investigations into substance-using MSM often focus on the correlates of problematic substance use behaviors; however, studies that focus on the correlates of abstinence, non-problematic use, or spontaneous remission from use may be more informative for prevention and intervention programs. Similarly, studying how men with multiple syndemic conditions remain sexually safe and HIV negative over time, or how community mobilization can strengthen community interactions and support, will likely improve health promotion efforts among HIV positive gay men. Without sufficient information about what strengths exist among HIV positive gay men, and how these strengths contribute to resilience, it is difficult to envision an empirically supported theory of cultural resilience.

Conclusions

In sum, it is imperative to understand the ways in which social marginalization impacts the mental health of HIV positive gay men. Stigma and marginalization are complex phenomenon that are deeply embedded in the sociocultural domains of gender, ethnoracial identity, class, sexuality, and politics. Stigma has long been understood as an attribute that links a person to an undesirable stereotype, leading other people to reduce the individual from a whole person to a tainted and discounted one (Goffman, 1963). In recent years, this notion of stigma has been reconceptualized in terms of power dynamics relating to "status loss and discrimination." A more encompassing approach to viewing stigma lies in confronting the power relations that sustain differences of individuals, and highlighting that stigmatization functions at the intersection between culture, power, and difference (Link & Phelan, 2006; Parker & Aggleton, 2003). In this respect, stigma and discrimination exist as social processes that enable power dynamics within societies to maintain oppressive mechanisms between the stigmatized and the stigmatizers.

Given that stigma has the potential to be both a proximal and distal stressor for individuals, a systems approach to understanding the mental health of HIV positive gay men is needed. Future directions in prevention, care, and treatment should strongly consider: extensive research with HIV positive gay men; appropriate interventions focused on gay and MSM communities; resilience and protective factors; housing and food security; the role of employment and poverty; distal and proximal experiences of social stressors; HIV-related stigma and discrimination; and syndemic notions of disease prevention by addressing substance use and mental health comorbidities. In order to adequately serve HIV positive gay men, we must utilize holistic approaches and enhance research that seeks to understand the ways in which social injustice, *and* resiliency, impact mental health and access to care.

References

Ajzen, I., & Fishbein, M. (1980). *Understanding attitudes and predicting social behavior.* Englewood Cliffs, NJ: Prentice-Hall.

Arnett, J. (2000). Emerging adulthood: A theory of development from the late teens through the twenties. *American Psychologist, 55*(5), 469–480.

Ayala, G., Bingham, T., Kim, J., Wheeler, D. P., & Millett, G. A. (2012). Modeling the impact of social discrimination and financial hardship on the sexual risk of HIV among Latino and Black men who have sex with men. *American Journal of Public Health, S2,* S242–S249.

Barrett, D. C., & Pollack, L. M. (2005). Whose gay community? Social class, sexual self-expression, and gay community involvement. *The Sociological Quarterly, 46*(3), 437–456.

Batchelder, A. W., Ehlinger, P. P., Boroughs, M. S., Shipherd, J. C., Safren, S. A., Ironson, G. H., & O'Cleirigh, C. (2017). Psychological and behavioral moderators of the relationship between trauma severity and HIV transmission risk behavior among MSM with a history of childhood sexual abuse. *Journal of Behavioral Medicine.* doi:10.1007/s10865-017-9848-9

Blosnich, J. R., Hanmer, J., Yu, L., Matthews, D. D., & Kavalieratos, D. (2016). Health care use, health behaviors, and medical conditions among individuals in same-sex and opposite-sex partnerships: A cross-sectional observational analysis of the Medical Expenditures Panel Survey (MEPS), 2003–2011. *Medical Care, 54,* 547–554.

Berg, M. B., Mimiaga, M. J., & Safren, S. A. (2004). Mental health concerns of HIV-infected gay and bisexual men seeking mental health services: An observational study. *AIDS Patient Care and STDs, 18*(11), 635–643.

Bird, J. D. P., Fingerhut, D. D., & McKirnan, D. J. (2011). Ethnic differences in HIV-disclosure and sexual risk. *AIDS Care, 23*(4), 444–448.

Bogart, L. M., Wagner, G. J., Galvan, F. H., Landrine, H., Klein, D. J., & Sticklor, L. A. (2011). Perceived discrimination and mental health symptoms among Black men with HIV. *Cultural Diversity & Ethnic Minority Psychology, 17,* 295–302.

Boone, M. R., Cook, S. H., & Wilson, P. A. (2016). Sexual identity and HIV status influence the relationship between internalized stigma and psychological distress in Black gay and bisexual men. *AIDS Care, 28,* 764–770. doi:10.1080/09540121.2016.1164801

Bostwick, W. B., Meyer, I., Aranda, F., Russell, S., Hughes, T., Birkett, M., & Mustakni, B. (2014). Mental health and suicidality among racially/ethnically diverse sexual minority youths. *American Journal of Public Health, 104,* 1129–1136.

Bowleg, L. (2012). The problem with the phrase women and minorities: Intersectionality—An important theoretical framework for public health. *American Journal of Public Health, 102,* 1267–1273.

Bränström, R. (2017). Minority stress factors as mediators of sexual orientation disparities in mental health treatment: A longitudinal population-based study. *Journal of Epidemiology and Community Health, 71,* 446–452.

Brown, L., Macintyre, K., & Trujillo, L. (2003). Interventions to reduce HIV/AIDS stigma: What have we learned? *AIDS Education and Prevention, 15*(1), 49–69.

Buchbinder, S. P., & Liu, A. Y. (2015). CROI 2015: Advances in HIV testing and prevention strategies. *Topics in Antiviral Medicine, 23,* 8–27.

Buttram, M. E., & Kurtz, S. P. (2015). A mixed methods study of health and social disparities among substance-using African American/Black men who have sex with men. *Journal of Racial and Ethnic Health Disparities, 2,* 1–10.

Bybee, J. A., Sullivan, E. L., Zielonka, E., & Moes, E. (2009). Are gay men in worse mental health than heterosexual men? The role of age, shame and guilt, and coming out. *Journal of Adult Development, 16,* 144–154.

Carrico, A. W. (2011). Substance use and HIV disease progression in the HAART era: Implications for the primary prevention of HIV. *Life Sciences, 88*(21-22), 940–947.

Center for Disease Control. (2015). *HIV and AIDS among gay and bisexual men.* Retrieved from http://www.cdc.gov/nchhstp/newsroom/docs/fastfacts-msm-final508comp.pdf.

Choi, K. H., Paul, J., Ayala, G., Boylan, R., & Gregorich, S. E. (2013). Experiences of discrimination and their impact on the mental health among African American, Asian and Pacific Islander, and Latino men who have sex with men. *American Journal of Public Health, 103,* 868–874.

Cochran, S. D., & Mays, V. M. (2000). Lifetime prevalence of suicide symptoms and affective disorders among men reporting same-sex sexual partners: Results from NHANES III. *American Journal of Public Health, 90*(4), 573–578.

Cochran, S. D., & Mays, V. M. (2003). Estimating prevalence of mental and substance-using disorders among lesbians and gay men from existing national health data. In A. Omoto & H. Kurtzman (Eds.), *Sexual orientation and mental health: Examining identity and development in lesbian, gay, and bisexual people. Contemporary perspectives on lesbian, gay, and bisexual psychology* (pp. 143–165). Washington, DC: American Psychological Association.

Cochran, S. D., & Mays, V. M. (2015). Mortality risks among persons reporting same-sex sexual partners: Evidence from the 2008 General Social Survey-National Death Index data set. *American Journal of Public Health, 105,* 358–364.

Cochran, S. D., Sullivan, J. G., & Mays, V. M. (2003). Prevalence of mental disorders, psychological distress, and mental health services use among lesbian, gay, and bisexual adults in the United States. *Journal of Consulting and Clinical Psychology, 71,* 53–61.

Cohen, M.S., Chen, Y.Q., McCauley, M., Gamble, T. Hosseinipour, M.C. Kumarasamy, N., … Fleming, T.F. (2011). Prevention of HIV-1 infection with early antiretroviral therapy. New England Journal of Medicine, 365, 493–505.

Cramer, R. J., Burks, A. C., Plöderl, M., & Durgampudi, P. (2017). Minority stress model components and affective well-being in a sample of sexual orientation minority adults living with HIV/AIDS. *AIDS Care, 13,* 1–7.

Díaz, R. M., Ayala, G., & Bein, E. (2004). Sexual risk as an outcome of social oppression: Data from a probability sample of Latino gay men in three US cities. *Cultural Diversity and Ethnic Minority Psychology, 10*(3), 255–267.

Díaz, R. M., Ayala, G., Bein, E., Henne, J., & Marin, B. V. (2001). The impact of homophobia, poverty and racism on the mental health of Latino gay men. *American Journal of Public Health, 91,* 927–932.

Díaz, R. M., Bein, E., & Ayala, G. (2006). Homophobia, poverty, and racism: Triple oppression and mental health outcomes in Latino gay men. In A. M. Omoto & H. S. Kurtzman (Eds.), *Sexual orientation and mental health* (pp. 207–224). Washington, DC: American Psychological Association.

Dowson, L., Kober, C., Perry, N., Fisher, M., & Richardson, D. (2012). Why some MSM present late for HIV testing: A qualitative analysis. *AIDS Care, 24,* 204–209.

Drescher, J. (2010). Queer diagnoses: Parallels and contrasts in the history of homosexuality, gender variance, and the diagnostic and statistical manual. *Archives of Sexual Behavior, 39,* 427–460.

Dyer, T. P., Shoptaw, S., Guadamuz, T. E., Plankey, M., Kao, U., Ostrow, D., … Stall, R. (2012). Application of syndemic theory to black men who have sex with men in the Multicenter AIDS Cohort Study. *Journal of Urban Health, 89*(4), 697–708.

Foster, M. L., Arnold, E., Rebchook, G., & Kegeles, S. M. (2011). 'It's My Inner Strength': Spirituality, religion, and HIV in the lives of young African American men who have sex with men. *Culture, Health & Sexuality, 13*(9), 1103.

Friedman, M. R., Coulter, R. W., Silvestre, A. J., Stall, R., Teplin, L., Shoptaw, S., … Plankey, M. W. (2017). Someone to count on: Social support as an effect modifier of viral load suppression in a prospective cohort study. *AIDS Care, 29,* 469–480.

Frost, D. M., Meyer, I. H., & Schwartz, S. (2016). Social support networks among diverse sexual minority populations. *American Journal of Orthopsychiatry, 86,* 91–102.

Galindo, G. R. (2013). A loss of moral experience: Understanding HIV-related stigma in the New York City House and Ball Community. *American Journal of Public Health, 103*(2), 293–299.

Galindo, G. R., Walker, J. J., Hazelton, P., Lane, T., Steward, W. T., Morin, S. F., & Arnold, E. A. (2012). Community member perspectives from transgender women and men who have sex with men on pre-exposure prophylaxis as an HIV prevention strategy: Implications for implementation. *Implementation Science, 7*(116), 1–13.

Garrett-Walker, J. J. & Torres, V. (2016). Negative religious rhetoric in the lives of Black cisgender queer emerging adult men: A qualitative analysis. *Journal of Homosexuality*. doi:10.1080/009 18369.2016.1267465.

Goffman, E. (1963). *Stigma: Notes on the management of spoiled identity.* New York: Simon and Schuster.

Grant, R.M., Lama, J.R., Anderson, P.L., McMahan, V., Liu, A.Y., Vargas, L., ... iPrEx Study Team. (2010). Preexposure chemoprophylaxis for HIV prevention in men who have sex with men. *New England Journal of Medicine, 363*(27), 2587–2599.

Greene, B. (1994). Ethnic-minority lesbians and gay men: Mental health and treatment issues. *Journal of Consulting and Clinical Psychology, 62,* 243–251.

Halkitis, P. N., Kapadia, F., Siconolfi, D. E., Moeller, R. W., Figueroa, R. P., Barton, S. C., & Blachman-Forshay, J. (2013). Individual, psychosocial, and social correlates of unprotected anal intercourse in a new generation of young men who have sex with men in New York City. *American Journal of Public Health, 103,* 889–895.

Halkitis, P. N., Moeller, R. W., Siconolfi, D. E., Storholm, E. D., Solomon, T. M., & Bub, K. L. (2013). Measurement model exploring a syndemic in emerging adult gay and bisexual men. *AIDS and Behavior, 17,* 662–673.

Halkitis, P. N., Pollock, J. A., Pappas, M. K., Dayton, A., Moeller, R. W., Siconolfi, D., & Solomon, T. (2011). Substance use in the MSM population of New York City during the era of HIV/ AIDS. *Substance Use & Misuse, 46,* 264–273.

Hamilton, C. J., & Mahalik, J. R. (2009). Minority stress, masculinity, and social norms predicting gay men's health risk behaviors. *Journal of Counseling Psychology, 56*(1), 132–141.

Han, C. S., Ayala, G., Paul, J. P., Boylan, R., Gregorich, S. E., & Choi, K. H. (2015). Stress and coping with racism and their role in sexual risk for HIV among African American, Asian/ Pacific Islander, and Latino men who have sex with men. *Archives of Sexual Behavior, 44,* 411–420.

Hatzenbuehler, M. L., McLaughlin, K. A., Keyes, K. M., & Hasin, D. S. (2010). The impact of institutional discrimination on psychiatric disorders in lesbian, gay, and bisexual populations: A prospective study. *American Journal of Public Health, 100*(3), 452–459.

Hatzenbuehler, M. L. (2011). The social environment and suicide attempts in lesbian, gay, and bisexual youth. *Pediatrics, 127*(5), 896–903.

Hays, R. B., Turner, H., & Coates, T. J. (1992). Social support, AIDS-related symptoms, and depression among gay men. *Journal of Consulting and Clinical Psychology, 60*(3), 463–469.

Hequembourg, A. L., & Brallier, S. A. (2009). An exploration of sexual minority stress across the lines of gender and sexual identity. *Journal of Homosexuality, 56*(3), 273–298.

Herek, G. M., & Garnets, L. D. (2007). Sexual orientation and mental health. *Annual Review of Clinical Psychology, 3,* 353–375.

Herrick, A. L., Lim, S. H., Wei, C., Smith, H., Guadamuz, T., Friedman, M. S., & Stall, R. (2011). Resilience as an untapped resource in behavioral intervention design for gay men. *AIDS and Behavior, 15*(S1), S25–S29.

Herrick, A. L., Lim, S. H., Plankey, M. W., Chmiel, J. S., Guadamuz, T. E., Kao, U., ... Stall, R. (2013). Adversity and syndemic production among men participating in the multicenter AIDS cohort study: A life-course approach. *American Journal of Public Health, 103*(1), 79–85.

Herrick, A.L., Stall, R., Chmiel, J.S., Guadamuz, T.E., Penniman, T., Shoptaw, S., ... Plankey, M.W. (2013). It gets better: Resolution of internalized homophobia over time and associations with positive health outcomes among MSM. AIDS and Behavior, 17, 1423–1430.

Herrick, A. L., Stall, R., Goldhammer, H., Egan, J. E., & Mayer, K. H. (2013). Resilience as a research framework and as a cornerstone of prevention research for gay and bisexual men: Theory and evidence. *AIDS and Behavior, 15,* S25–S29.

Herrick, A., Stall, R., Egan, J., Schrager, S., & Kipke, M. (2014). Pathways towards risk: Syndemic conditions mediate the effect of adversity on HIV risk behaviors among young men who have sex with men (MSM). *Journal of Urban Health, 91*, 969–982.

HIV Prevention Trials Network. (2011). *Initiation of antiretroviral treatment protects uninfected sexual partners from HIV infection (HPTN study 052)*. Retrieved from http://www.hptn.org/web%20documents/IndexDocs/HPTN052FactSheet22July12.pdf.

HIV Prevention Trials Network. (2013). *Pre-exposure prophylaxis (PrEP) initiation and adherence among Black men who have sex with men (BMSM) in three US cities (HPTN study 073)*. Retrieved from http://www.hptn.org/research_studies/hptn073.asp.

Hood, R. W., Hill, P. C., & Spilka, B. (2009). Religion, health, psychopathology, and coping. In *The psychology of religion* (pp. 435–476). New York: Guilford.

Institute of Medicine (IOM). (2011) *The health of lesbian, gay, bisexual, and transgender people.* Retrieved from http://www.iom.edu/lgbthealth.

Jeffries, W. L., 4th, Townsend, E. S., Gelaude, D. J., Torrone, E. A., Gasiorowicz, M., & Bertoli, J. (2015). HIV stigma experienced by young men who have sex with men (MSM) living with HIV infection. *AIDS Education and Prevention, 27*, 58–71.

Jeffries, W. L., IV, Sutton, M. Y., & Eke, A. N. (2017). On the battlefield: The Black church, public health, and the fight against HIV among African American gay and bisexual men. *Journal of Urban Health, 94*(3), 384–398.

Jerome, R. C., Halkitis, P. N., & Siconolfi, D. E. (2009). Club drug use, sexual behavior, and HIV seroconversion: A qualitative study of motivations. *Substance Use and Misuse, 44*(3), 431–447.

Kaufman, G., & Raphel, L. (1996). *Coming out of shame: Transforming gay and lesbians lives.* New York: Doubleday.

Kalichman, S. C., DiMarco, M., Austin, J., Luke, W., & DiFonzo, K. (2003). Stress, social support, and HIV-status disclosure to family and friends among HIV positive men and women. *Journal of Behavioral Medicine, 26*(4), 315–332.

Kimmel, S. B., & Mahalik, J. R. (2005). Body image concerns of gay men: The roles of minority stress and conformity to masculine norms. *Journal of Consulting and Clinical Psychology, 73*(6), 1185–1190.

Kingdon, M. J., Storholm, E. D., Halkitis, P. N., Jones, D. C., Moeller, R. W., Siconolfi, D., & Solomon, T. M. (2013). Targeting HIV prevention messaging to a new generation of gay, bisexual, and other young men who have sex with men. *Journal of Health Communication, 18*, 325–342.

Koblin, B. A., Mansergh, G., Frye, V., Tieu, H. V., Hoover, D. R., Bonner, S., … Colfax, G. N. (2011). Condom-use decision making in the context of hypothetical pre-exposure prophylaxis efficacy among substance-using men who have sex with men: Project MIX. *Journal of Acquired Immune Deficiency Syndromes, 58*, 319–327.

Lassiter, J. M., Saleh, L., Starks, T., Grov, C., Ventuneac, A., & Parsons, J. T. (2017). Race, ethnicity, religious affiliation, and education are associated with gay and bisexual men's religious and spiritual participation and beliefs: Results from the One Thousand Strong cohort. *Cultural Diversity and Ethnic Minority Psychology*. doi:10.1037/cdp0000143.

Lelutiu-Weinberger, C., Pachankis, J. E., Golub, S. A., Walker, J. J., Bamonte, A. J., & Parsons, J. T. (2013). Age cohort differences in the effects of gay-related stigma, anxiety and identification with the gay community on sexual risk and substance use. *AIDS and Behavior, 17*, 340–349.

Leserman, J., Petitto, J.M., Gu, H., Gaynes, B.N., Barroso, J., Golden, R.N., … Evans, D.L. (2002). Progression to AIDS, a clinical AIDS condition, and mortality: Psychosocial and physiological predictors. Psychological Medicine, 32, 1059–1073

Leserman, J. (2003). The effects of stressful life events, coping, and cortisol on HIV infection. *CNS Spectrums, 8*(01), 25–30.

Link, B. G., & Phelan, J. C. (2006). Stigma and its public health implications. *Lancet, 367*, 528–529.

Malebranche, D. J., Peterson, J. L., Fullilove, R. E., & Stackhouse, R. W. (2004). Race and sexual identity: Perceptions about medic al culture and healthcare among Black men who have sex with men. *Journal of the National Medical Association, 96*, 97–107.

Matthews, C. R., & Adams, E. M. (2009). Using a social justice approach to prevent the mental health consequences of heterosexism. *The Journal of Primary Prevention, 30*(1), 11–26.

Mayer, K. H., Bekker, L. G., Stall, R., Grulich, A. E., Colfax, G., & Lama, J. R. (2012). Comprehensive clinical care for men who have sex with men: An integrated approach. *Lancet, 380*, 378–387.

Mayfield, W. (2001). The development of an internalized homonegativity inventory for gay men. *Journal of Homosexuality, 41*(2), 53–76.

Mays, V. M., Cochran, S. D., & Barnes, N. W. (2007). Race, race-based discrimination, and health outcomes among African Americans. *Annual Review of Psychology, 58*, 201–225.

Mays, V. M., Ly, L., Allen, E., & Young, S. (2009). Engaging student health organizations in reducing health disparities in underserved communities through volunteerism: Developing a student health corps. *Journal of Health Care for the Poor and Underserved, 20*, 914–928.

McCabe, S. E., Bostwick, W. B., Hughes, T. L., West, B. T., & Boyd, C. J. (2010). The relationship between discrimination and substance use disorders among lesbian, gay, and bisexual adults in the United States. *American Journal of Public Health, 100*(10), 1946–1952.

McDermott, E., Roen, K., & Scourfield, J. (2008). Avoiding shame: Young LGBT people, homophobia and self-destructive behaviours. *Culture, Health & Sexuality, 10*(8), 815–829.

McKirnan, D. J., Ostrow, D. G., & Hope, B. (1996). Sex, drugs and escape: A psychological model of HIV-risk sexual behaviours. *AIDS Care, 8*(6), 655–670.

Meyer, I. H. (1995). Minority stress and mental health in gay men. *Journal of Health and Social Behavior, 36*(1), 38–56.

Meyer, I. H. (2003). Prejudice, social stress, and mental health in lesbian, gay and bisexual populations: Conceptual issues and research evidence. *Psychological Bulletin, 129*, 674–697.

Meyer, I. H. (2016). Does an improved social environment for sexual and gender minorities have implications for a new minority stress research agenda? *Psychology of Sexualities Review, 7*, 81–90.

Meyer, I. H., Dietrich, J., & Schwartz, S. (2008). Lifetime prevalence of mental disorders and suicide attempts in diverse lesbian, gay, and bisexual populations. *American Journal of Public Health, 9*(6), 1004–1006.

Meyer, I. H., Schwartz, S., & Frost, D. M. (2008). Social patterning of stress and coping: Does disadvantaged social statuses confer more stress and fewer coping resources? *Social Science & Medicine, 67*, 368–379.

Miller, R. L. (2007). Legacy denied: African American gay men, AIDS and the Black church. *Social Work, 52*(1), 51–61.

Millett, G. A., Peterson, J. L., Flores, S. A., Hart, T. A., Jeffries, W. L., Wilson, P. A., … Remis, R. S. (2012). Comparisons of disparities and risks of HIV infection in Black and other men who have sex with men in Canada, UK, and USA: A meta-analysis. *Lancet, 380*, 341–348.

Mimiaga, M. J., O'Cleirigh, C., Biello, K. B., Robertson, A. M., Safren, S. A., Coates, T. J., … Mayer, K. H. (2015). The effect of psychosocial syndemic production on 4-year HIV incidence and risk behavior in a large cohort of sexually active men who have sex with men. *Journal of Acquired Immune Deficiency Syndromes, 68*, 329–336.

Mimiaga, M., Reisner, S., Pantalone, D., O'Cleirigh, C., Mayer, K., & Safren, S. (2012). A pilot trial of integrated behavioral activation and sexual risk reduction counseling for HIV-uninfected men who have sex with men abusing crystal methamphetamine. *AIDS Patient Care and STDs, 26*, 683–693.

Moeller, R. W., Halkitis, P. N., Pollock, J. A., 4th, Siconolfi, D. E., & Barton, S. (2013). When emotions really started kicking in, which ended up being a problem: Sex, HIV, and emotions among young gay and bisexual men. *Journal of Homosexuality, 60*, 773–795.

Mustanski, B., Garofalo, R., Herrick, A., & Donenberg, G. (2007). Psychosocial health problems increase risk for HIV among urban young men who have sex with men: Preliminary evidence of a syndemic in need of attention. *Annuals of Behavioral Medicine, 34*(1), 37–45.

Naar-King, S., Parsons, J. T., & Johnson, A. (2012). Motivational interviewing targeting risk reduction for people with HIV: A systematic review. *Current HIV/AIDS Reports, 9*(4), 335–343.

Nelson, L. E., Wilton, L., Zhang, N., Regan, R., Thach, C. T., Dyer, T. V., ... HPTN 061 Study Team. (2016). Childhood exposure to religions with high prevalence of members who discourage homosexuality is associated with adult HIV risk behaviors and HIV infection in Black men who have sex with men. *American Journal of Men's Health*. doi:10.1177/1557988315626264.

O'Cleirigh, C., Skeer, M., Mayer, K., & Safren, S. (2009). Functional impairment and health care utilization among HIV-infected men who have sex with men: The relationship with depression and post-traumatic stress. *Journal of Behavioral Medicine, 32*(5), 466–477.

Office of National AIDS Policy (ONAP). (2010). *National HIV/AIDS strategy for the United States*. Retrieved from http://www.whitehouse.gov/administration/eop/onap/nhas.

Omi, M., & Winant, H. (1986). *Racial formation in the United States: From the 1960s to the 1990s*. New York: Routledge.

Oswald, R. F. (2002). Resilience within the family networks of lesbians and gay men: Intentionality and redefinition. *Journal of Marriage and Family, 64*(2), 374–383.

Padian, N. S., Buve, A., Balkus, J., Serwadda, D., & Cates, W. (2008). Biomedical interventions to prevent HIV infection: Evidence, challenges and way forward. *Lancet, 372*, 585–599.

Parker, R., & Aggleton, P. (2003). HIV and AIDS-related stigma and discrimination: A conceptual framework and implications for action. *Social Science & Medicine, 57*, 13–24.

Parsons, J. T., Grov, C., & Golub, S. A. (2012). Sexual compulsivity, co-occurring psychosocial health problems, and HIV risk among gay and bisexual men: Further evidence of a syndemic. *American Journal of Public Health, 102*, 156–162.

Peterson, J. L., Miner, M. H., Brennan, D. J., & Rosser, B. R. (2012). HIV treatment optimism and sexual risk behaviors among HIV positive African American men who have sex with men. *AIDS Education and Prevention, 24*, 91–101.

Ramirez-Valles, J. (2002). The proactive effects of community involvement for HIV risk behavior: A conceptual framework. *Health Education Research, 17*(4), 389–403.

Rendina, H. J., Gamarel, K. E., Pachankis, J. E., Ventuneac, A., Grov, C., & Parsons, J. T. (2017). Extending the minority stress model to incorporate HIV-positive gay and bisexual men's experiences: A longitudinal examination of mental health and sexual risk behavior. *Annals of Behavioral Medicine, 51*, 147–158.

Reisner, S. L., Mimiaga, M. J., Skeer, M., Perkovich, B., Johnson, C. V., & Safren, S. A. (2009). A review of HIV antiretroviral adherence and intervention studies among HIV-infected youth. *Topics in HIV Medicine, 17*(1), 14–25.

Rosser, B. R., Bockting, W. O., Ross, M. W., Miner, M. H., & Coleman, E. (2008). The relationship between homosexuality, internalized homo-negativity, and mental health in men who have sex with men. *Journal of Homosexuality, 55*(1), 150–168.

Ryan, C., Huebner, D., Díaz, R., & Sanchez, J. (2009). Family rejection as a predictor of negative health outcomes in White and Latino lesbian, gay and bisexual young adults. *Pediatrics, 123*(1), 346–352.

Safren, S. A., Blashill, A. F., & O'Cleirigh, C. M. (2011). Promoting the sexual health of MSM in the context of co-morbid mental health problems. *AIDS and Behavior, 15 Suppl 1*, S30–S34.

Safren, S. A., O'Cleirigh, C. M., Skeer, M., Elsesser, S. A., & Mayer, K. H. (2013). Project enhance: A randomized controlled trial of an individualized HIV prevention intervention for HIV-infected men who have sex with men conducted in a primary care setting. *Health Psychology, 32*, 171–179.

Safren, S. A., Reisner, S. L., Herrick, A., Mimiaga, M. J., & Stall, R. D. (2010). Patterns of substance use among a large cohort of HIV-infected men who have sex with men in primary care. *Journal of Acquired Immune Deficiency Syndromes, 55*(Suppl 2), S74–S77.

Semple, S. J., Strathdee, S. A., Zians, J., & Patterson, T. L. (2012). Factors associated with experiences of stigma in a sample of HIV-positive methamphetamine-suing men who have sex with men. *Drug and Alcohol Dependence, 125*, 154–159.

Sheon, N., & Crosby, M. G. (2004). Ambivalent tales of HIV disclosure in San Francisco. *Social Science & Medicine, 58*(11), 2105–2118.

Shidlo, A. (1994). Internalized homophobia: Conceptual and empirical issues in measurement. In B. Greene & G. M. Herek (Eds.), *Lesbian and gay psychology: Theory, research and clinical applications* (pp. 176–205). Thousand Oaks, CA: Sage.

Shoptaw, S., Reback, C. J., Larkins, S., Wang, P. C., Rotheram-Fuller, E., Dang, J., & Yang, X. (2008). Outcomes using two tailored behavioral treatments for substance abuse in urban gay and bisexual men. *Journal of Substance Abuse Treatment, 35*(3), 285–293.

Shoptaw, S., Weiss, R.E., Munjas, B., Hucks-Ortiz, C., Young, S. D., Larkins, S., ... Gorbach, P. M. (2009). Homonegativity, substance use, sexual risk behaviors, and HIV status in poor and ethnic men who have sex with men in Los Angeles. Journal of Urban Health, 86 (S1), 77–92.

Serovich, J. M., Kimberly, J. A., Mosack, K. E., & Lewis, T. L. (2001). The role of family and friend social support in reducing emotional distress among HIV positive women. *AIDS Care, 13*(3), 335–341.

Siegel, K., Lune, H., & Meyer, I. H. (1998). Stigma management among gay/bisexual men with HIV/AIDS. *Qualitative Sociology, 21*(1), 3–24.

Smit, P.J., Brady, M., Carter, M., Fernandes, R., Lamore, L., Meulbroek, M., ... Thompson, M. (2012). HIV-related stigma within communities of gay men: A literature review. AIDS Care, 24 (4), 405–412.

Stall, R., Friedman, M., & Catania, J. (2007). Interacting epidemics and gay men's health: A theory of syndemic production among urban gay men. In R. J. Wolitski, R. Stall, & R. O. Valdiserri (Eds.), *Unequal opportunity: Health disparities affecting gay and bisexual men in the United States* (pp. 251–274). New York: Oxford.

Stall, R., Mills, T. C., Williamson, J., Hart, T., Greenwood, G., Paul, J., ... Catania, J. A. (2003). Association of co-occurring psychosocial health problems and increased vulnerability to HIV/ AIDS among urban men who have sex with men. *American Journal of Public Health, 93,* 939–942.

Stewart, P. (2007). Who is kin? Family definition and African American families. *Journal of Human Behavior in the Social Environment, 15*(2-3), 163–181.

Sullivan, P.S., Carballo-Dieguez, A., Coates, T., Goodreau, S.M., McGowan, I., Sanders, E.J., ... Sanchez, J. (2012). Successes and challenges of HIV prevention in men who have sex with men. Lancet, 380, 388–399.

Szymanski, D. M., & Gupta, A. (2009). Examining the relationship between multiple internalized oppressions and African American lesbian, gay, bisexual, and questioning persons' self-esteem and psychological distress. *Journal of Counseling Psychology, 56*(1), 110–118.

The Affordable Care and Patient Protection Act (ACA) of the United States. (2010). Retrieved from http://www.healthcare.gov/law/.

Trapence, G., Collins, C., Avrett, S., Carr, R., Sanchez, H., Ayala, G., ... Baral, S.D. (2012). From personal survival to public health: Community leadership by men who have ex with men in the response to HIV. Lancet, 380, 400–410.

United Nations Programme on HIV/AIDS (UNAIDS). (2011). *UNAIDS strategy 2011–2015: Getting to Zero.* Retrieved from http://www.unaids.org/en/media/unaids/contentassets/ documents/unaidspublication/2010/jc2034_unaids_strategy_en.pdf.

U.S Department of Health and Human Services, National Institutes of Health, Health Resources and Services Administration (HRSA). (2009). *About the Ryan White HIV/AIDS Program.* Retrieved from http://hab.hrsa.gov/abouthab/aboutprogram.html.

Valdiserri, R. O. (2002). HIV/AIDS stigma: An impediment to public health. *American Journal of Public Health, 92*(3), 341–342.

Walker, J. J., & Longmire-Avital, B. (2013). The impact of religious faith and internalized homo-negativity on resiliency for Black lesbian, gay, and bisexual emerging adults. *Developmental Psychology, 49,* 1723–1731.

Walker, J. J., Longmire-Avital, B., & Golub, S. (2015). Racial and sexual identities as potential buffers to risky sexual behavior for Black gay and bisexual emerging adult men. *Health Psychology, 34,* 841–846.

Wechsberg, W. M., Golin, C., El-Bassel, N., Hopkins, J., & Zule, W. (2012). Current interventions to reduce sexual risk behaviors and crack cocaine use among HIV-infected individuals. *Current HIV/AIDS Reports, 9*(4), 385–393.

Weiser, S. D., Hatcher, A., Frongillo, E. A., Guzman, D., Riley, E. D., Bangsberg, D. R., & Kushel, M. B. (2013). Food insecurity is associated with greater acute care utilization among HIV-infected homeless and marginally housed individuals in San Francisco. *Journal of General Internal Medicine, 28,* 91–98.

Wheeler, D. P. (2005). Working with positive men: HIV prevention with Black men who have sex with men. *AIDS Education and Prevention, 17,* 102–115.

White Hughto, J. M., Pachankis, J. E., Eldahan, A. I., & Keene, D. E. (2017). "You can't just walk down the street and meet someone": The intersection of social-sexual networking technology, stigma, and health among gay and bisexual men in a small city. *American Journal of Men's Health, 11,* 726–736.

Wight, R. G., LeBlanc, A. J., de Vries, B., & Detels, R. (2012). Stress and mental health among midlife and older gay-identified men. *American Journal of Public Health, 102*(3), 503–510.

Wilson, P. A., Stadler, G., Boone, M. R., & Bolger, N. (2014). Fluctuations in depression and well-being are associated with sexual risk episodes among HIV-positive gay men. *Health Psychology, 33,* 681–685.

Wilson, P. A., Wittlin, N. M., Muñoz-Laboy, M., & Parker, R. (2011). Ideologies of Black churches in New York City and the public health crisis of HIV among Black men who have sex with men. *Global Public Health, 6*(sup2), S227–S242.

Wong, C. F., Schrager, S. M., Holloway, I. W., Meyer, I. H., & Kipke, M. D. (2014). Minority stress experiences and psychological well-being: The impact of support from and connection to social networks within the Los Angeles House and Ball communities. *Prevention Science, 15,* 44–55.

World Health Organization (WHO). (2014). *Global update on the health sector response to HIV, 2014.* Geneva, Switzerland: WHO. Retrieved from http://www.who.int/hiv/pub/global-update.pdf.

Chapter 4
HIV Positive Gay Men, MSM, and Substance Use: Perspectives on HIV Prevention

Steven Shoptaw

Case Example: Mark

Mark is a 21-year-old African American man who has sex with other men (MSM) who has been living with HIV for about 2 years. Mark comes from a stable, family oriented, middle-class home in Los Angeles with both parents and a younger brother. Mark's parents love both their sons, but things got complicated when Mark was 17 and his father discovered Mark was having sex with other men. (Mark had stepped away briefly from the computer while reading his email without closing his account and his father read several of Mark's messages from a man he was arranging to meet.) Mark's parents were torn by this new understanding about their son, but made it clear that he would not be welcome to live at home if he was having sex with men. There were fights and arguments for a couple of weeks, but eventually Mark's parents asked him to be abstinent sexually or to have sex with women as a condition of living in the house after he turned 18.

Mark went on to graduate high school while living at home, but decided to move out soon thereafter. Mark found it impossible to find work that paid him enough to live on his own even with a full-time job at a fast food restaurant and part-time work on weekends at a retail store. Eventually Mark could not pay his rent and found himself without a regular place to sleep. His friends helped him out for a while by letting him sleep on their couches, but Mark felt terrible about himself and his situation. Mark began spending more of his time near the gay community in Los Angeles and 1 day was standing near the curb on Santa Monica Blvd. when a car pulled up and rolled down the window. His every impulse was to walk away, but Mark looked in the window. An older man said he had some bad weed he'd be willing to share and unlocked the doors. Mark got into the car and the man drove to a

S. Shoptaw (✉)
Department of Family Medicine, David Geffen School of Medicine, University of California, Los Angeles (UCLA), Los Angeles, CA, USA
e-mail: SShoptaw@mednet.ucla.edu

© Springer Science+Business Media LLC 2017
L. Wilton (ed.), *Understanding Prevention for HIV Positive Gay Men*, DOI 10.1007/978-1-4419-0203-0_4

secluded parking lot nearby and Mark had his first sexual experience in exchange for money. Mark promised himself that he would use this type of sex only to help make ends meet or to buy things he needed, but couldn't afford otherwise. Mark was good about keeping his promise, but found that weed didn't quite cut it the same way as if he smoked a little crack cocaine. Getting that high made exchange sex easier for him to tolerate, especially if he was asked for special favors, like having receptive condomless anal sex.

One day an HIV prevention outreach worker asked Mark to get tested. At 20 years old, Mark learned that he was HIV positive. Mark cried with the counselor who delivered the news. The counselor made an appointment for HIV medical care, but Mark never appeared for the visit for a variety of reasons, including lack of health insurance. Feeling scared, mad, alone, and newly HIV positive, Mark never told his family he lived close to the streets when between jobs for the next year. He often used unhealthy coping mechanisms, including smoking crack cocaine and marijuana to dull his psychological pain, to avoid his family and friends, and to stay away from doctors, medications, and all of that. Mark knew he did not want to move back home. But, he also did not stress about using condoms during sex anymore, as he believed someone had been careless with his health and he felt no responsibility to protect the health of anyone else.

Recently, Mark was talking with a different HIV prevention worker who convinced him to start medical care for his HIV. The worker referred him to a doctor at a nearby clinic who takes uninsured patients and called a case manager there who can relate to the concerns of young Black men to talk with Mark and help with transitioning into care. Mark kept his appointment this time and agreed to take antiretroviral medications and to reduce his substance use. Mark remains in HIV medical care for now and his viral load levels are undetectable most of the time. He is doing better accessing his supports. He no longer has condomless sex, and he is not using crack cocaine or having exchange sex. He still occasionally smokes marijuana and struggles with how to find his way, particularly as he feels rejected by his family and he is not sure whether he trusts anyone in the gay communities.

Introduction

Many aspects of the current situation of HIV/AIDS in the USA are highlighted in the case of Mark. Changes in the epidemiology of the disease in the USA have occurred over the past three decades, shifting the burden of disease from involving primarily White gay men and injection drug users (IDUs) to young men who have sex with men (MSM) and men who have sex with men and women (MSMW), primarily people of color (Carrico et al., 2016; Shoptaw, Landovitz, & Reback, 2017). The case also illustrates some of the structural, cultural, interpersonal, and individual factors that can link to HIV infection and also that can influence potential HIV transmission from personal health behaviors, including substance use, among MSM living with HIV/AIDS. In this chapter, MSM and MSMW are admittedly limited terms, but are used to encompass the populations of men in the USA who have sex with other men, independent of whether they adopt any of a range of terms (or no terms) that would represent their sexual behaviors with men (e.g., gay, bisexual, same gender loving). The chapter opens with a presentation of the current epidemiology of HIV transmission in MSM, focusing on the unique role of substance use, particularly use of stimulants, club drugs, and inhalants. A brief discussion on prevention approaches among MSM who use injection drugs follows, but the majority of the chapter focuses on non-injection substance use, the stigma and discrimination this brings to an already stigmatized group (MSM living with HIV/AIDS), and approaches to address HIV prevention that focuses on substance use.

Epidemiology of HIV in MSM and the Influence of Substance Use

In the USA and worldwide, HIV/AIDS is increasingly a disease that affects MSM, with MSM accounting for more cases of HIV than any other behavioral risk group (Centers for Disease Control and Prevention [CDC], 2015). In the USA between 2007 and 2010, the number of new diagnoses of HIV cases decreased for IDUs, for MSM who also are IDUs, and for heterosexuals. At the same time, new diagnoses of HIV cases increased for MSM (CDC, 2015). Increases in new cases of HIV did not distribute equally across US citizens and more so for American MSM. In 2010, 25,297 new HIV cases were reported, and of these cases, 46% were Black/African American males and females. This is despite the fact that Black men and women represent 13.6% of the US population (Rastogi, Johnson, Hoeffel, & Drewery, 2011). The greatest absolute number of these new HIV cases is accounted for by Black/African American MSM, who bear fully one-third (34.3%) of new cases reported among males nationally. In 2010, young Black MSM have been disproportionately affected by HIV disease burden with more than twice the number of new HIV infections when compared to other racial/ethnic groups (CDC, 2015). These findings clearly show that while MSM of all race/ethnicities experience increases in rates of new HIV cases, the disproportionate burden continues to affect Black/African American MSM.

What is concerning about this situation is that while incidence of HIV is increasing among MSM, the response by policymakers to this situation is underwhelming. In one report, HIV prevention scientists noted that HIV/AIDS is a forgotten epidemic in America (El-Sadr, Mayer, & Hodder, 2010), recognizing that the epidemic has shifted to be driven largely by MSM, a group that faces substantial stigma in the USA. Adding to the problem, a significant proportion of new infections among MSM are due directly to substance use (between 16% (Koblin et al., 2006) and 36% (Ostrow et al., 2009)), particularly stimulant drugs like methamphetamine, amphetamine, and cocaine. Other drugs used with these stimulants by MSM, like volatile nitrites ("poppers") and amphetamine analogues (MDMA/Ecstasy), also are linked to new infections due to drug-related sexual risk behaviors (Hall, Shoptaw, & Reback, 2014). Among HIV positive MSM, linkages between substance use and sexual risk behaviors have been noted for many years (Benotsch, Kalichman, & Kellly, 1999). This situation calls for a rational response to addressing the role of substance use in MSM, yet an organized response is lacking so far. While use of stimulant and other drugs influence HIV incidence in MSM, it is vital that interventionists and policymakers understand reasons that might explain these effects (Reback, Fletcher, Shoptaw, & Grella, 2013). Ron Stall and colleagues have applied the theory of syndemics (Singer, 2009) to gay and bisexual men and noted intertwining epidemics of substance use, HIV/AIDS and other STIs, psychological problems (e.g., depression, child sexual abuse) and low SES produce that consistently correspond with poor health outcomes (Greenwood et al., 2001; Herrick et al., 2013; Hirshfield et al., 2015; Stall, Friedman, & Catania, 2008; Stall et al., 2003). Effects of syndemic conditions may be greatest among sexual minorities who are persons of color, so-called "double minorities" (Dyer et al., 2012; Williams, Wyatt, Resell, Peterson, & Asuan-O'Brien, 2004), with those effects exacerbated by minority stress that can arise from the impact of stigma, prejudice, and discrimination (Meyer, Ouellette, Haile, & McFarlane, 2011). From the perspective of syndemics, HIV prevention approaches that focus solely on one aspect of the syndemics experienced by MSM living with HIV/AIDS and who use substances, would likely to be insufficient, as the impacts of the related conditions would continue to threaten health (Hirshfield et al., 2015). For example, substance using MSM living with HIV/AIDS who engage one or more sessions of HIV prevention may also continue to face challenges in adopting sustained behavior changes due to one or more other syndemic conditions, including mental illness, childhood abuse, and discrimination/victimization (Mimiaga et al., 2015).

HIV Prevention Among MSM Who Inject Drugs

Only a minority (~4%) of MSM use injection drugs and acquire HIV/AIDS (CDC, 2015). Even so, there exists effective means for preventing HIV transmission for individuals who inject drugs, meaning no drug-related, new infections should occur among substance-using MSM who inject drugs. These effective means include a combination of methods that increase access to using opioid substitution therapy to treat opioid addiction, that ensure access to needle and syringe programs to reduce harm for those who use injection methods to administer their drugs, and that facilitate consistent access to HIV medical care and to antiretroviral medications so that viral load levels remain at or near undetectable levels (Degenhardt et al., 2010; Strathdee et al., 2010). Still, many who inject drugs, including MSM, encounter barriers to accessing these effective methods for reducing drug-related transmissions. Some have called for action to address the needs of IDUs in reducing barriers to prevention that are mostly based on "addictophobia," apathy, and inaction (Strathdee et al., 2012). In the sections that follow, evidence for improving access to combination HIV prevention and to programs that reduce sexual related behaviors in substance using MSM is presented.

Combination Prevention Approaches to Reduce HIV Transmissions: A Strategy for Substance Using MSM?

Exciting new gains in HIV prevention science are offering new strategies that may guide prevention approaches to segments of the population that face exaggerated risks for HIV transmission, such as MSM living with HIV/AIDS and who use substances. The most impressive set of findings comes from the HIV Prevention Trials Network 052 study (Cohen et al., 2011), which showed a 96% decrease in HIV transmissions among HIV-serodiscordant (primarily heterosexual) couples that resulted simply by starting antiretroviral therapy early for the HIV positive partner. This dramatic decrease in HIV transmissions showed for the first time that treating the HIV positive partner early is protective as HIV prevention. For this study, treating early meant starting antiretroviral therapy when the HIV positive partners' CD-4 counts were between 350 and 550 cells per mm³. This compared to the standard at the time for deciding when to start antiretroviral therapy, which was when the HIV positive partner showed a drop in CD-4 cells or an onset of HIV symptoms. More importantly, data from this study showed that providing antiretroviral therapy early to HIV positive individuals improved that individual's health significantly, resulting in a 41% reduction in the rate of reported health complications. The success in this "proof-of-concept" study has been termed "Treatment as Prevention (or TasP) and is gaining recognition as an HIV prevention strategy in its own right. The scientific finding supporting use of TasP had such impact on the field that the prestigious journal, *Science,* named this finding as the "scientific breakthrough of the year in 2011" (J. Cohen, 2011).

HIV Positive Substance Users Have Reduced Access to ART

There exist limits to implementing combination HIV prevention strategies, such as TasP for substance-using MSM living with HIV/AIDS. Chief among these is resolving problems in ensuring access to antiretroviral medications for *all* individuals who need the medication, regardless of their status of membership in being a member of sexual and/or racial minorities, of being of lower socioeconomic class, and of being a substance user. This issue is vital, as evidence shows that HIV-infected people who start antiretroviral treatment early live longer than if they delay treatment (Kitahata et al., 2009). Moreover, these benefits become more pronounced for individuals who begin their initial treatment at progressively lower initial CD-4 counts (Ray et al., 2010), who likely are individuals carrying some form of discrimination or stigma, such as substance users. Indeed, cohort studies show convincing evidence that HIV positive individuals who either inject drugs (IDUs) or who use non-injection routes to administer their drugs (NIDUs) are *both* less likely to access antiretroviral treatments (OR = 0.47, 95% CI: 0.33, 0.67; OR = 0.62, 95% CI: 0.47, 0.81, respectively) compared to nondrug users (McGowan et al., 2011). Findings from these cohorts further document that IDUs and NIDUs who start antiretroviral therapies are significantly less likely to have consistent access to them (≥ 95% of the time under study). The first step to seriously ensuring fair and equitable access to consistent HIV medical care and HIV medications for substance using MSM who are living with HIV/AIDS will involve implementing coherent strategies that address stigma and discrimination in healthcare settings.

The Importance of Ensuring Access to Antiretroviral Therapies for HIV Positive Substance Users

There may be biological factors that emphasize unique benefits to HIV positive MSM who use substances from antiretroviral medications that are in counterpoint to the biology of HIV positive women who use substances. In the Women's Interagency HIV Study (WIHS), a cohort study of 2058 HIV positive women, crack cocaine use reported over the past 6 months associated significantly with an increase of plasma viral load levels, decrease of CD4 cell counts, and increased levels of morbidity and mortality as compared to nondrug users, even after controlling for adherence to antiretroviral therapies (Cook et al., 2008). These findings are in stark contrast in efforts to detect measurable negative health effects of substances of abuse for HIV positive men. In data collected every 6 months between October 1996 and March 2007, findings from the Multisite AIDS Cohort Study (a cohort study of MSM living with HIV/AIDS) showed that significant, but minor decrements could be measured to CD4+/CD8+ ratios per 10 cumulative use-years for methamphetamine (0.93, 95% CI: 0.88, 0.98) and cocaine (0.93, 95% CI: 0.89, 0.96). Cumulative effects of adherent antiretroviral use (≥ 95% adherence per 10 years of adherent antiretroviral use), however, produced more than four times multiplicative increases in CD4+/CD8+ ratios (4.07, 95% CI: 3.52, 4.71). Findings showing adherence to antiretroviral medications with positive immune function independent of stimulant use in HIV positive MSM provides additional evidence for ensuring access to antiretroviral medications for these men.

The evidence shows that the quality of the evidence supporting use of antiretroviral medications in HIV positive MSM who use substances is strong: antiretroviral treatments are shown consistently to reduce viral load, morbidity, and mortality, with substance using individuals demonstrating benefits to immune function when adhering to these treatments. Future domestic HIV prevention research designed to evaluate how HIV positive MSM who use substances (and their sexual and drug-using partners) can benefit from HIV treatment as prevention strategies have priority. This is particularly true among substance using MSM as all proof of concept studies that demonstrate efficacy of HIV treatment as prevention systematically excluded substance users from enrollment due to concerns over perceived inability for HIV positive substance users to adhere to HIV medication regimens sufficiently to observe the TasP effect. Such information is vital to guiding cost-benefit analyses that might determine whether HIV positive MSM who use substances may warrant the costs inherent to the approach.

Biomedical HIV Prevention in HIV Negative MSM: PrEP

Some brief mention on the use of combination HIV strategies for substance-using HIV negative MSM seems appropriate. While the size of the effect for protection against HIV transmission is about one-half that observed in HPTN 052, findings (Grant et al., 2010) showed that HIV negative MSM randomly assigned to take anti-retroviral medications in the form of a daily combination tablet of emtricitabine and tenofovir (pre-exposure prophylaxis or PrEP) and in the context of sexual HIV risk reduction strategies (i.e., using condoms) decreased HIV infections by 44% compared to those assigned to receive placebo tablets and sexual risk reduction strategies. These findings demonstrate that combination HIV prevention is efficacious (i.e., demonstrates a statistically significant effect against a control condition), but expensive. Starting HIV positive individuals early onto antiretroviral therapy adds costs for medications and medical visits compared to delaying treatment. Providing daily antiretroviral medications to individuals who are HIV negative introduces wholly new costs to HIV prevention plans. Cost-benefit analyses may ultimately identify specific groups of MSM who benefit sufficiently to warrant the costs (e.g., HIV positive MSM who use substances), but there are no data to suggest substance users are unable to engage in the kinds of consistent medication adherence behaviors (or consistent enough adherence behaviors) to gain the HIV prevention benefits of PrEP. There are, however, data from MSM who use stimulants and alcohol that show low uptake of PrEP even when the men are aware of its potential utility as an HIV prevention strategy (Oldenburg et al., 2016). Until recently, with the possible exception of opioid substitution therapies, HIV prevention services have been delivered in nonmedical settings, which may introduce a ramp-up period for providers to be able to deliver these new prevention services with cultural competence. As noted earlier, ethical concerns arise for health jurisdictions where antiretroviral medications are not available to all HIV positive individuals who need them.

Behavioral Interventions for HIV Positive Substance Using MSM

There exists an array of behavioral interventions, some with evidence showing that they have effects over a standard control condition, that they have effects over a wait-list control, or that they have effects over baseline measures in terms of reducing HIV-related risk behaviors, primarily sexual risk behaviors, in MSM. While this has been the primary focus of HIV prevention science over the past 30 years, no studies of behavioral interventions to date have demonstrated the ability to reduce HIV transmission, i.e., shown program efficacy in reducing HIV incidence. This problem likely diminished the importance placed on behavioral risk reduction programs in President Obama's National HIV/AIDS Strategy (*National HIV/AIDS Strategy for the United States*, 2010). In spite of this, there are two federal agencies that review and award recognition to behavioral risk reduction interventions with demonstrated evidence of efficacy. One is the Compendium of Evidence-Based HIV Prevention Interventions (CDC), a catalog of prevention programs with several geared toward helping people who inject drugs to reduce injection behaviors. The other is the National Registry of Evidence-Based Programs and Practices (NREPP), which is part of the Substance Abuse and Mental Health Services Administration (SAMHSA). Unfortunately, there are no interventions recommended with evidence for HIV prevention with HIV positive MSM who use substances.

Although linkages between HIV transmission and drug-related sexual behaviors for HIV positive MSM are indirect, the HIV prevention literature is replete with efforts to develop and describe interventions that reduce these correlated sex transmission behaviors. Indeed, the compendium of Evidence-Based Interventions (EBIs) has long been the backbone of HIV prevention. The CDC's new strategy for high impact prevention involves prioritizing and implementing a combination of cost-effective, scalable interventions based on the current state of the science, including biomedical interventions. In Table 4.1, a comprehensive presentation is provided for EBIs and interventions that have evidence to support their use (randomized controlled comparison conditions or wait list control conditions) and that address the needs of HIV positive MSM who use substances. As can be seen, there are few prevention programs with evidence that address the specific needs of HIV positive MSM who use substances, leave aside the subgroups of these men who may be from racial and ethnic subgroups. Interventions in Table 4.1 are listed in order of the comprehensiveness with which they address the intersection of the factors of: (1) MSM; (2) HIV Positive Specific; and (3) Substance Use Focus.

Methamphetamine Dependent MSM

The first three entries in Table 4.1 are programs that have evidence of efficacy for use with MSM who misuse methamphetamine. Each of these programs is unique in important ways, but all are intended to decrease methamphetamine-related HIV transmission behaviors, reflecting the key observation nearly 6 years ago that HIV prevalence among methamphetamine-using MSM increased concomitant with the level of use of the drug (i.e., from occasional, to regular, to addiction) (Shoptaw & Reback, 2006). In the first of these interventions (and the only one of all interventions in Table 4.1 that has evidence for use with MSM who are HIV positive and who use substances), *EDGE* was shown to be efficacious for improving both safer sex behaviors and self-efficacy regarding safer sex compared to a control condition. Moreover, these effects were shown in HIV positive MSM who were not treatment seeking. In the second, *Friends Getting Off* describes outcomes when tailoring a mainstream (Matrix Model) cognitive behavioral treatment for methamphetamine dependence for use with gay and bisexual men and combining this intervention with contingency management. The third, *Mirtazapine,* describes outcomes of a randomized, placebo-controlled trial of 30 mg of the antidepressant mirtazapine in the

Table 4.1 HIV Prevention for HIV positive substance using MSM: evidence-based interventions and results

HIV Risk-reduction program	Target population characteristics	Approach methods	Results
EDGE Mausbach, Semple, Strathdee, Zians, and Patterson (2010)	MSM ☒ yes ☐ no HIV positive specific ☒ yes ☐ no Substance use focus ☐ yes ☐ no ☒ other: Methamphetamine using HIV positive MSM only	• 8 individual sessions (5 weekly 90-min each to start and 3 booster sessions) over 4 months • Increase knowledge, self-efficacy and positive outcome expectancies for safer sex, disclosure of serostatus, and enhancing social support • Mechanisms include observation, role modeling, skill performance, positive feedback, reinforcement for implementing safer sex behaviors in the context of active substance use	Compared to an individual session control condition, EDGE participants: • ↑Protected sex acts at 8- and 12-months follow-up • ↑Ratio of protected-to-total sex acts at 12-months follow-up • ↑Self-efficacy for using condoms over the 12-month period
Friends getting off Reback and Shoptaw (2011)	MSM ☒ yes ☐ no HIV positive specific ☐ yes ☒ no ☒ other: all MSM are ok Substance use focus ☒ yes ☐ no	• 8-weeks of thrice weekly group meetings followed by 8 optional once-weekly support groups and one follow-up interview • The program combines cognitive behavioral therapy with group counseling skills that teach skills to cease methamphetamine use, prevent relapse, and reduce drug-related sexual risk behaviors • Contingency management is part of first 8-weeks of program (i.e., participants receive vouchers for drug-negative urine samples that are exchanged for gift cards	Compared to control condition at end of treatment: • ↓ Unprotected anal intercourse • ↓ Methamphetamine use Compared to baseline at 12 months: • ↓ Unprotected anal intercourse • ↓ Methamphetamine use Recent adaptation compared to former version, adapted version: • ↑ Consecutive weeks of abstinence • ↓ Past 30 days of methamphetamine use • ↓ Number of sex partners

(continued)

Table 4.1 (continued)

HIV Risk-reduction program	Target population characteristics	Approach methods	Results
Mirtazapine (30 mg) Colfax et al. (2011)	MSM ☒ yes ☐ no HIV positive specific ☐ yes ☒ no ☒ other: all MSM are ok Substance use focus ☒ yes ☐ no ☒ other: Treatment seeking methamphetamine dependent only	• Double-blind, 12-week, randomized, placebo-controlled trial of mirtazapine (30 mg)—an antidepressant medication • MSM who reported sex under the influence of methamphetamine ≥ once, 3 months prior to baseline • 30 mirtazapine; 30 placebo MSM attended clinic weekly, received study medications, provided self-report and biological data, and received once-weekly 30 min individual sessions of cognitive behavioral and motivational interviewing for drug cessation	52% of MSM were HIV positive Compared to placebo condition, MSM randomized to mirtazapine: • Fewer drug-positive urine samples (RR=0.57, 95% CI, 0.35, 0.93) • ↓ Number of male partners with whom methamphetamine was used • ↓ Number of male partners, • ↓ Number of episodes of unprotected anal sex with serodiscordant partners • No differences in adverse events
Healthy relationships Kalichman (2005) and Kalichman et al. (2001)	MSM ☒ yes ☐ no ☒ NOTE: Heterosexual Men and Women OK HIV positive specific ☒ yes ☐ no Substance use focus ☐ yes ☒ no	• In five, 120-min interactive sessions, groups focus on problem-solving and decision-making skills to address stress related to safer sex practices and revealing serostatus to others • Group members observe leaders model skills through role play • Participants respond by practicing interactions and receiving feedback from facilitators • Groups are separated by sex and sexual orientation • Each group is made up of 5–12 HIV-infected individuals • Groups are closed to new members and are led by two individuals: one male, one female • One leader is a licensed counselor and the other is a peer (who may be HIV positive)	Relative to a comparison health maintenance intervention group: ↓ Unprotected sexual behaviors • Greatest ↓ in HIV transmission behaviors with HIV-uninfected sex partners

Many Men, Many Voices (3MV) Wilton et al. (2009	MSM ☒ yes ☐ no ☒ other: Black MSM HIV positive specific ☐ yes ☒ no ☒ other: HIV-unknown status ok Substance use focus ☐ yes ☒ no	• Group-level intervention that consists of 6 consecutive 2- to 3-h sessions • Each session focuses on a different topic (e.g., The Culture of Black MSM, STI/HIV Prevention, Relationship issues, Social Support & Problem Solving to Maintain Change) • Some sessions involve role-playing communication	As compared to a wait-list control group: ↓ Unprotected anal intercourse with casual male partners ↑ Consistency in condom use in receptive anal intercourse with casual partners ↓ Number of sex partners ↑ HIV testing
d-up—Defend yourself! Jones et al. (2009)	MSM ☒ yes ☐ no ☒ other: Black MSM HIV positive specific ☐ yes ☒ no Substance use focus ☐ yes ☒ no	• Promotes an interdependent social network where each individual's behavior impacts another's • Opinion leaders, who are members of the Black MSM community, are trained to work among friends and acquaintances to deliver messages that encourage safer sex practices and to counteract homophobic and racial biases directed toward Black MSM in society	As compared to baseline levels: ↓ Unprotected receptive anal intercourse ↓ Mean number of partners for unprotected receptive anal intercourse at 12 months

(continued)

Table 4.1 (continued)

HIV Risk-reduction program	Target population characteristics	Approach methods	Results
Mpowerment Kegeles, Hays, and Coates (1996)	MSM ☒ yes ☐ no HIV positive specific ☐ yes ☒ no Substance use focus ☐ yes ☒ no	• Peer-led, 2–3 h one-time discussion groups of 8–10 young gay men • Groups discuss factors contributing to unsafe sex among men, including misconceptions about safer sex and poor communication skills • Skills-building exercises practice safer sex negotiation and correct condom use	As compared to baseline levels and relative to a similar community comparison group receiving no specific intervention: ↓ Rates of unprotected anal intercourse
Popular Opinion Leader (POL) Kelly et al. (1991)	MSM ☒ yes ☐ no HIV positive specific ☐ yes ☒ no Substance use focus ☐ yes ☐ no ☒ other: held in bars, so presumes active substance use	• A group of trusted, well-liked men who frequent gay bars are trained to interact with their peers to promote safer sex and HIV prevention and to correct misconceptions about either or both topics • Such men are given the title of "Popular Opinion Leaders (POL)". A "POL" will interact with peers in gay bars and other settings by engaging in casual, one-on-one conversations in which safer sex practices and HIV prevention is discussed (e.g., keeping condoms on hand, avoiding sex while intoxicated, resisting pressure for unsafe sex)	↓ Unprotected anal intercourse from baseline levels

context of once-weekly cognitive behavioral and motivational interviewing approaches for instilling drug abstinence. This intervention is innovative in that it integrates use of a putative pharmacotherapy for reducing methamphetamine use in MSM. Findings are among the first to describe reductions of drug-related sexual risk behaviors that can be attributed to a medication for stimulant dependence. While this type of approach is novel and exciting, it requires that participants are MSM living with HIV/AIDS and are seeking treatment for substance dependence, which may limit the ultimate reach of the strategy.

General Health Interventions

The four remaining interventions in Table 4.1 all have evidence for use with MSM, but may not have an HIV positive specific focus and none have a specific focus on substance use. *Healthy Relationships* is a broad, health intervention that has evidence of efficacy for use with HIV positive MSM and heterosexual men and women, but groups are separated both by sex and sexual orientation. The remaining interventions are developed specifically for use with Black MSM who are either HIV negative or serostatus unknown. In *Many Men, Many Voices (3MV)*, Black MSM participate in seven sessions focusing on the health and culture of Black MSM. *D-up—Defend Yourself!* also is developed for use with Black MSM and has the goal of increasing condom use and recognition of homophobic and racial biases directed toward Black MSM in society. In *MPowerment,* young gay and bisexual men (especially men of color) interact in one-time discussion groups to discuss unsafe sex and to build commitment to future safer sex behaviors. It is being adapted specifically for use with young African American gay men. No discussion of behavioral approaches for HIV prevention among MSM can be complete without recognition of the *Popular Opinion Leader* approach. This approach, which tacitly acknowledges substance use as it is implemented in gay bars, is imbued with cultural values toward substance use and sexual risk behaviors, and has been implemented worldwide.

In addition to the interventions described in Table 4.1, two interventions require mention. The *Healthy Living* project is a group-based intervention designed to be implemented in HIV care and primary care settings and to be accessed by HIV positive people. The program requires 15 sessions, 90 min each and requires implementers to be college educated. *Healthy Living* is a broad intervention that does not specifically address the concerns or needs of HIV positive MSM who use substances. An evaluation of the program along self-reported drug and sexual behaviors for participants assigned to the *Healthy Living* condition compared to a wait-list control showed that the subgroup of gay men assigned to the intervention reported fewer days of use of hard drugs than gay men who received the control group at long-term follow-up; gay men also reported more days of use of hard drugs than heterosexual men in either condition (Healthy Living Project Team, 2007). There was no evidence the intervention reduced sexual risk behaviors for gay men over the control condition, however.

A second "honorable mention" to the list is *Safety Counts* (Hershberger, Wood, & Fisher, 2003). *Safety Counts* was designed to help nontreatment seeking IDUs and crack cocaine users to develop a personalized risk reduction plan. The intervention helps participants discuss personal goals that encourage peer support and that increase self-efficacy for reducing HIV risks. Although the program was not developed for either MSM or HIV positive people specifically, outcomes showed a significant reduction in sharing of injection equipment compared to a standard, two-session counseling and testing intervention.

Techniques with Promise for New Interventions: HIV Positive MSM Who Use Substances

In addition to the literature describing behavioral interventions with efficacy, there are innovations that deserve mention for future intervention development. One especially promising technique that merits attention in the next round of intervention development involves manipulation of behavioral economics (contingent cash transfers), which is the same concept as operant conditioning (contingency management). This set of behavioral interventions seeks to help individuals institute and sustain behavior change, particularly regarding drug abstinence. Especially with drug dependent groups, contingency management (CM) is highly efficacious in producing short- and longer-term reductions of substance use (Shoptaw et al., 2005). The technique of CM involves delivering increasingly valuable reinforcements in exchange for consecutive biomarkers documenting substance abstinence. Consistent support for its use is strongest with treatment-seeking methamphetamine dependent MSM, though the evidence is mixed when using CM in settings of STI clinics and there is no motivations for reductions in substance use (Menza et al., 2010). To present, interventions using CM have only focused on reducing substance use. Other outcomes that would have significance in working with HIV positive MSM who use substances would include implementing contingencies to reinforce reductions in viral load levels and consistency in accessing HIV primary care. In reinforcing behaviors and biomarkers linked to HIV disease, however, substance use becomes a mediating behavior and those seeking to achieve the reinforcer would have to manage their substance use in relation to their antiretroviral adherence and appointment consistency.

Another set of techniques that have promise in nontreatment seeking, HIV positive substance using MSM involves text messaging. In a recent pilot study, self-reported drug use and corresponding HIV risk behaviors were reduced in MSM who were actively using methamphetamine following repeated texts that delivered health messages (Reback & Shoptaw, 2011). As development of technology advances, text messaging, social media, and online program methods likely will become stale by the time the current wave of intervention studies can accrue data that comments on the efficacy of these approaches. Still opportunities quickly appear for leveraging electronic communication technologies to improve health and are worthy of integration into new HIV prevention strategies.

Conclusions

The case example that begins and the data presented throughout this chapter demonstrate the key importance to attending to the syndemics that affect MSM living with HIV/AIDS and who use substances. This very experience requires the developer of HIV prevention interventions to think broader than designing programs that focus on altering outcomes for a single health threat. Evidence of this exhortation is that despite investment in over 30 years of HIV prevention programs, the incidence of new HIV infections has not been slowed or stopped among MSM. This contrasts with the stunning HIV prevention successes in nearly stopping incidence among IDUs and among mother to child transmissions in the USA. These successes highlight the lackluster enthusiasm that exists for addressing HIV infections among MSM who use substances. It is time to invest time and resources in slowing HIV incidence in this group, similar to what was done to accomplish the successes with IDUs and with mother-to-child transmission.

While there is no indication that incidence is slowing, there are no data that might describe the situation regarding what the situation might be regarding HIV incidence for substance using MSM in the absence of the few existing HIV prevention programs. What seems clear is that for incidence rates among MSM to begin to slow or to stop, new and/or more impactful HIV prevention approaches are necessary—not simply funding more of the same. President Obama's National HIV/AIDS Strategy outlines many of those new approaches. At the same time, the information presented describes HIV transmission as the resultant of more than a set of sexual behaviors that happen in the context of HIV—there are important correlated syndemics that encourage and support the eventual occurrence of a potential risk event. The representational case and the data presented in this chapter on the current state of HIV prevention among substance using HIV positive MSM are intended to awaken new commitments to addressing this significant health problem and to provide some suggestions to guide a strategy for a new way forward in HIV prevention.

Acknowledgements The author would like to acknowledge the support by a grant from the National Institute of Mental Health (P30 MH58107) awarded to Mary Jane Rotheram-Borus, Ph.D.

References

Benotsch, E. G., Kalichman, S. C., & Kellly, K. A. (1999). HIV positive men who have sex with men: Prevalence and predictors of high-risk behaviors. *Addictive Behaviors, 24*(6), 857–868.

Carrico, A. W., Jain, J., Discepola, M. V., Olem, D., Andrews, R., Woods, W. J., et al. (2016). A community-engaged randomized controlled trial of an integrative intervention with HIV-positive, methamphetamine-using men who have sex with men. *BMC Public Health, 16*, 673. doi:10.1186/s12889-016-3325-1

Centers for Disease Control and Prevention. (2015). Estimated HIV incidence among adults and adolescents in the United States, 2007–2010. *HIV Surveillance Supplemental Report, 2012, 17*(No. 4), 1–26. Retrieved January 4, 2015.

Cohen, J. (2011). Breakthrough of the year. HIV treatment as prevention. *Science*, *334*(6063), 1628.

Cohen, M. S., Chen, Y.Q., McCauley, M., Gamble, T., Hosseinipour, M.C., Kumarasamy, N., ... HPTN 052 Study Team. (2011). Prevention of HIV-1 infection with early antiretroviral therapy. *New England Journal of Medicine, 365*(6), 493–505.

Colfax, G. N., Santos, G.-M., Das, M., Santos, D. M., Matheson, T., Gasper, J., ... Vittinghoff, E. (2011). Mirtazapine to reduce methamphetamine use: A randomized controlled trial. *Archives of General Psychiatry, 68*(11), 1168–1175. doi:10.1001/archgenpsychiatry.2011.124

Cook, J. A., Burke-Miller, J. K., Cohen, M. H., Cook, R. L., Vlahov, D., Wilson, T. E., ... Grey, D. D. (2008). Crack cocaine, disease progression, and mortality in a multicenter cohort of HIV-1 positive women. *AIDS, 22*, 1355–1363.

Degenhardt, L., Mathers, B., Vickerman, P., Rhodes, T., Latkin, C., & Hickman, M. (2010). Prevention of HIV infection for people who inject drugs: Why individual, structural, and combination approaches are needed. *Lancet, 376*(9737), 285–301.

Dyer, T. P., Shoptaw, S., Guadamuz, T.E., Plankey, M., Kao, U., Ostrow, D., ... Stall, R. (2012). Application of syndemic theory to black men who have sex with men in the Multicenter AIDS Cohort Study. *Journal of Urban Health, 89*(4), 697–708.

El-Sadr, W. M., Mayer, K. H., & Hodder, S. L. (2010). AIDS in America—Forgotten but not gone. *New England Journal of Medicine, 362*(11), 967–970.

Grant, R. M., Lama, J.R., Anderson, P.L., McMahan, V., Liu, A.Y., Vargas, L., ... iPrEx Study Team. (2010). Preexposure chemoprophylaxis for HIV prevention in men who have sex with men. *New England Journal of Medicine, 363*(27), 2587–2599.

Greenwood, G. L., White, E. W., Page-Shafer, K., Bein, E., Osmond, D. H., Paul, J., & Stall, R. D. (2001). Correlates of heavy substance use among young gay and bisexual men: The San Francisco Young Men's Health Study. *Drug and Alcohol Dependence, 61*(2), 105–112.

Hall, T. M., Shoptaw, S., & Reback, C. J. (2014). Sometimes poppers are not poppers: Huffing as an emergent health concern among MSM substance users. *Journal of Gay and Lesbian Mental Health, 23*, 118–121.

Healthy Living Project Team. (2007). Effects of a behavioral intervention to reduce risk of transmission among people living with HIV: The healthy living project randomized controlled study. *Journal of Acquired Immune Deficiency Syndromes, 44*(2), 213–221.

Herrick, A. L., Lim, S. H., Plankey, M. W., Chmiel, J. S., Guadamuz, T. E., Kao, U., ... Stall, R. (2013). Adversity and syndemic production among men participating in the multicenter AIDS cohort study: A life-course approach. *American Journal of Public Health, 103*(1), 79–85.

Hershberger, S. L., Wood, M. M., & Fisher, D. G. (2003). A cognitive-behavioral intervention to reduce HIV risk behaviors in crack and injection drug users. *AIDS and Behavior, 7*(3), 229–243.

Hirshfield, S., Schrimshaw, E. W., Stall, R. D., Margolis, A. D., Downing, M. J., Jr., & Chiasson, M. A. (2015). Drug use, sexual risk, and syndemic production among men who have sex with men in group sexual encounters. *American Journal of Public Health, 25*, e1–e10.

Jones, K. T., Gray, P., Whiteside, Y. O., Wang, T., Bost, D., Dunbar, E., ... Johnson, W. D. (2009). Evaluation of an HIV prevention intervention adapted for Black men who have sex with men. *American Journal of Public Health, 98*(6), 1043–1050.

Kalichman, S. C. (2005). *Positive prevention: A sourcebook for HIV transmission risk reduction among people living with HIV-AIDS*. New York, NY: Springer.

Kalichman, S. C., Rompa, D., Cage, M., DiFonzo, K., Simpson, D., Austin, J., ... Graham, J. (2001). Effectiveness of an intervention to reduce HIV transmission risks in HIV-positive people. *American Journal of Preventive Medicine, 21*(2), 84–92.

Kegeles, S. M., Hays, R. B., & Coates, T. J. (1996). The Mpowerment Project: A community-level HIV prevention intervention for young gay men. *American Journal of Public Health, 86*(8(Pt 1)), 1129–1136.

Kelly, J. A., St. Lawrence, J. S., Diaz, Y. E., Stevenson, L. Y., Hauth, A. C., Brasfield, T. L., ... Andrew, M. E. (1991). HIV risk behavior reduction following intervention with key opinion leaders of a population: An experimental community level analysis. *American Journal of Public Health, 81*, 168–171.

Kitahata, M. M., Gange, S.J., Abraham, A.G., Merriman, B., Saag, M.S., Justice, A. C., ... NA-ACCORD Investigators. (2009). Effect of early versus deferred antiretroviral therapy for HIV on survival. *New England Journal of Medicine, 360*(18), 1815–1826.

Koblin, B. A., Husnik, M. J., Colfax, G., Huang, Y., Madison, M., Mayer, K., ... Buchbinder, S. (2006). Risk factors for HIV infection among men who have sex with men. *AIDS, 20*, 731–739.

Mausbach, B. T., Semple, S. J., Strathdee, S. A., Zians, J., & Patterson, T. L. (2010). Efficacy of a behavioral intervention for increasing safer sex behaviors in HIV-positive MSM methamphetamine users: Results from the EDGE study. *Drug and Alcohol Dependence, 87*(2–3), 249–257.

McGowan, C. C., Weinstein, D.D., Samenow, C.P., Stinnette, S.E., Barkanic, G., Rebeiro, P.F., ..., Hulgan, T. (2011). Drug use and receipt of highly active antiretroviral therapy among HIV-infected persons in two U.S. clinic cohorts. PloS One, 6(4), e18462.

Menza, T. W., Jameson, D. R., Hughes, J. P., Colfax, G. N., Shoptaw, S., & Golden, M. R. (2010). Contingency management to reduce methamphetamine use and sexual risk among men who have sex with men: A randomized controlled trial. *BMC Public Health, 10*, 774.

Meyer, I. H., Ouellette, S. C., Haile, R., & McFarlane, T. A. (2011). "We'd Be Free": Narratives of life without homophobia, racism, or sexism. *Sexuality Research & Social Policy, 8*(3), 204–214.

Mimiaga, M. J., O'Cleirigh, C., Biello, K. B., Robertson, A. M., Saffren, S. A., Coates, T. J., ... Mayer, K. H. (2015). The effect of psychosocial syndemic production on 4-year HIV incidence and risk behavior in a large cohort of sexually active men who have sex with men. *Journal of Acquired Immune Deficiency Syndromes, 68*, 329–336.

National HIV/AIDS Strategy for the United States. (2010). Washington DC: Retrieved from http://www.whitehouse.gov/sites/default/files/uploads/NHAS.pdf.

Oldenburg, C. E., Mitty, J. A., Biello, K. B., Closson, E. F., Safren, S. A., Mayer, K. H., & Mimiaga, M. J. (2016). Differences in attitudes about HIV pre-exposure prophylaxis use among stimulant versus alcohol using men who have sex with men. *AIDS and Behavior, 20*(7), 1451–1460.

Ostrow, D. G., Plankey, M. W., Cox, C., Li, X., Shoptaw, S., Jacobson, L. P., & Stall, R. C. (2009). Specific sex drug combinations contribute to the majority of recent HIV seroconversions among MSM in the MACS. *Journal of Acquired Immune Deficiency Syndromes, 51*(3), 349–355.

Rastogi, S., Johnson, T.D., Hoeffel, E.M., Drewery Jr., M.P. (2011). The Black Population: 2010 *Census Briefs.* https://www.census.gov/prod/cen2010/briefs/c2010br-06.pdf. Accessed 8 Apr 2017.

Ray, M., Logan, R., Stern, J. A. C., Hernandez-Diaz, S., Robins, J. M., Sabin, C., & HIV-CAUSAL Collaboration. (2010). The effect of combined antiretroviral therapy on the overall mortality of HIV-infected individuals. *AIDS, 24*, 123–137.

Reback, C. J., & Shoptaw, S. (2011). Development of an evidence-based, gay-specific cognitive behavioral therapy intervention for methamphetamine-abusing gay and bisexual men. *Addictive Behaviors, 39*(8), 1286–1291.

Reback, C. J., Fletcher, J. B., Shoptaw, S., & Grella, C. E. (2013). Methamphetamine and other substance use trends among street-recruited men who have sex with men, from 2008–2011. *Drug and Alcohol Dependence, 133*, 262–265.

Shoptaw, S., & Reback, C. J. (2006). Associations between methamphetamine use and HIV among men who have sex with men: A model for guiding public policy. *Journal of Urban Health, 83*(6), 1151–1157.

Shoptaw, S., Reback, C.J., Peck, J.A., Yang, X., Rotheram-Fuller, E., Larkins, S., ... Hucks-Ortiz, C. (2005). Behavioral treatment approaches for methamphetamine dependence and HIV-related sexual risk behaviors among urban gay and bisexual men. Drug and Alcohol Dependence, 78(2), 125–134.

Shoptaw, S., Landovitz, R. J., & Reback, C. J. (2017). Contingent vs. non-contingent rewards:Time-based intervention response patterns among stimulant-using men who have sex with men. *Journal of Substance Abuse Treatment, 72*, 19–24.

Singer, M. (2009). *Introducing syndemics: A critical systems approach to public and community health.* New York, NY: Wiley.

Stall, R., Mills, T., Williamson, J., Hart, T., Greenwood, G., Paul, J., ... Catania, J. (2003). Co-occurring psychosocial health problems among urban men who have sex with men are associated with increased vulnerability to the HIV/AIDS epidemic. American Journal of Public Health, 93(6), 939–942.

Stall, R., Friedman, M., & Catania, J. A. (2008). Intersecting epidemics and gay men's health: A theory of syndemic production among urban gay men. In R. J. Wolitski, R. Stall, & R. O. Valdeserri (Eds.), *Unequal opportunity: Health disparities affecting gay and bisexual men in the United States* (pp. 251–274). New York, NY: Oxford.

Strathdee, S. A., Hallett, T. B., Bobrova, N., Rhodes, T., Booth, R., Abdool, R., & Hankins, C. A. (2010). HIV and risk environment for injecting drug users: The past, present, and future. *Lancet, 376*(9737), 268–284.

Strathdee, S. A., Shoptaw, S., Dyer, T. P., Quan, V. M., Aramrattana, A., & Substance Use Scientific Committee of the HIV Prevention Trials Network. (2012). Towards combination HIV prevention for injection drug users: Addressing addictophobia, apathy and inattention. *Current Opinion in HIV and AIDS, 7*(4), 320–325.

Williams, J. K., Wyatt, G. E., Resell, J., Peterson, J., & Asuan-O'Brien, A. (2004). Psychosychosocial issues among gay-and non-gay-identifying HIV-seropositive African American and Latino MSM. *Cultural Diversity and Ethnic Minority Psychology, 10*(3), 268.

Wilton, L., Herbst, J.H., Coury-Doniger, P., Painter, T.M., English, G., Alvarez, M.E., … Carey, J.W. (2009). Efficacy of an HIV/STI prevention intervention for black men who have sex with men: Findings from the Many Men, Many Voices (3MV) project. AIDS and Behavior, 13(3), 532–544.

Chapter 5
Childhood Sexual Abuse and Revictimization Among Gay Men: Implications for Those Who Are HIV Positive

John K. Williams and Vincent C. Allen, Jr.

Since the beginning of the HIV/AIDS epidemic in the USA, gay and bisexual men have experienced disproportionate rates of HIV morbidity and mortality. The Centers for Disease Control and Prevention (CDC) reported that in 2013, gay, bisexual, and other men who have sex with men (MSM) accounted for 55% of people living with HIV in the USA despite comprising approximately 2% of the US population (CDC, 2016a). Among MSM, people of color and young MSM appear to be disproportionately impacted. African American and Latino MSM account for 38% (estimated 11,201) and 26% (estimated 7552) of new infections, respectively, while White MSM represent 31% (estimated 9008) of new infections among MSM (CDC, 2016b). Among the African American gay and bisexual men diagnosed with HIV, an estimated 39% (4321) were aged 13–24 (CDC, 2016b). Trauma histories, including childhood sexual abuse (CSA) and adult sexual abuse (ASA) especially in the form of intimate partner violence (IPV), are rarely examined among MSM despite being associated with increased mortality and morbidity. In this chapter, we: a) review the existing literature on child and adult sexual abuse among MSM in general, while emphasizing what research has been conducted with HIV positive gay men; b) explore the research and clinical challenges associated with the lack of operationalized abuse definitions and how it may impact the needs of HIV positive gay men; c) discuss sexual, mental, and physical health sequelae associated with trauma histories for MSM and specifically, for HIV positive gay men; and d) discuss

J.K. Williams (✉)
Department of Psychiatry and Biobehavioral Sciences, Semel Institute for Neuroscience and Human Behavior, University of California, Los Angeles (UCLA), Los Angeles, CA, USA
e-mail: keoniwmd@aol.com

V.C. Allen, Jr.
Department of Psychiatry and Biobehavioral Sciences, Semel Institute for Neuroscience and Human Behavior, University of California, Los Angeles (UCLA), Los Angeles, CA, USA

Department of Psychology, University of California, Los Angeles (UCLA),
Los Angeles, CA, USA

© Springer Science+Business Media LLC 2017
L. Wilton (ed.), *Understanding Prevention for HIV Positive Gay Men*,
DOI 10.1007/978-1-4419-0203-0_5

implications for sexual risk reduction among HIV positive gay men with histories of CSA, ASA, and IPV. Since the literature is sparse in respect to trauma histories specifically among HIV positive gay men, we distinguish the research that has been conducted with MSM versus gay men.

Framing Risk Factors for HIV

There are several commonly identified risk factors that may contribute to HIV infection rates among gay and bisexual men. Utilizing Bronfenbrenner's (1979) ecological theory of development, Mustanski, Newcomb, Du Bois, Garcia, and Grov (2011) framed their review of HIV correlates and predictors for young MSM. The ecological theory of development places the individual at the center of a model comprised of multiple environmental systems with expanding relationships moving from the individual level to interpersonal and interrelational community levels, and enveloping all of these is the broadest level which incorporates cultural, structural, and societal norms. This model also examines these relationships over time, and thus has a developmental framework that can be applied across the lifespan.

At the individual or person level, factors such as alcohol and drug use, personality characteristics, and mental health were associated with sexual risk-taking among MSM (Mustanski et al., 2011). Relationships, in which individuals have direct contact with others such as family, friends, and sexual partners, would be examined at the microsystem level. The correlates specifically for HIV risk include such factors as characteristics of intimate partner relationships, experiences of sexual abuse, and the presence, type, and quality of social and emotional support. The mesosystem level includes the environment or context in which an individual exists and the ways in which these settings influence their behaviors. In regard to sexual risk-taking, social settings such as bars and clubs commonly provide the opportunity for alcohol and drug use behaviors to intersect with sexual partner seeking behaviors. Other examples of where the sociocultural context can be associated with sexual risk-taking among MSM include the degree to which men feel connected to the gay community, the prevalence and engagement in sex work and/or attending commercial sex venues (i.e., bath houses, sex clubs), and even the availability and access of sexual partners via the Internet (Binson et al., 2001; Halkitis et al., 2013; Halkitis & Parson, 2003; Van Beneden et al., 2002; Williams et al., 2003).

At the broadest level of Bronfenbrenner's (1979) theory is the macrosystem which is comprised of societal norms and ideological values. One example of an HIV correlate at this level may include the concept of minority stress, which entails the cumulative effect of stigma, internalized homophobia, and discrimination (Brofenbrenner, 1979; Meyer, 1995; Mustanski et al., 2011). The minority stress model was developed as a way to understand the unique experiences associated with being a member of a sexual minority group (Meyer, 1995, 2003). Perceptions of these experiences as stressful were based on the contrasting differences between the minority person's culture, beliefs, and norms as compared to those of the larger society. While minority stress has been associated with increased psychological distress (Meyer, 1995), research has only recently begun to explore the effects of minority stress and other structural and institutional variables on sexual risk behaviors.

Bronfenbrenner's (1979) ecological theory of development helps to conceptualize these diverse systems and explore their relationships with health outcomes. However, these systems are multifaceted, overlapping, and dynamic. Thus, the level of complexity provides challenges to identifying key correlates of HIV risk behaviors. This is highly evident among Black MSM where racial/ethnic disparities in HIV continue to persist and where risk factors commonly associated with HIV fail or inadequately help to explain such disparities. A meta-analysis by Millett et al. (2012) found that Black MSM were more likely than other MSM to report the use of any preventive behavior against HIV infection, more likely to report HIV testing in the past year, and demonstrated no significant difference in substance use compared to other MSM. Black MSM were more likely to experience structural factors such as low education, unemployment, low income, and prior incarceration which may better explain racial disparities in HIV prevalence (Millett et al., 2012). Millett, Flores, Peterson, and Bakerman (2007) also found that sexually transmitted infections (STIs) were greater among Black MSM than White MSM. However, higher rates of HIV infections among Black MSM were not attributable to differences in substance use, sexual risk behaviors, nongay identity, or sexual disclosure (Millet, Peterson, Wolitski, & Stall, 2006; Millett et al., 2007). The challenge of addressing the HIV epidemic among Black MSM demonstrates the difficulty of identifying HIV correlates and predictors. Importantly, it supports the need to explore other factors that may be contributing to the HIV epidemic, such as past and present experiences of sexual abuse (Feldman, 2010; Glover, Williams, & Kisler, 2012; Mustanski et al., 2011). Moreover, it raises the issue of conceptualizing models of HIV risk for diverse populations, accounting for differences on variables such as race/ethnicity and HIV serostatus.

Child Sexual Abuse as a Risk Factor for HIV

In discussing the sexual behaviors of gay men as it relates to HIV risk, much emphasis is often placed on current behaviors with a focus on sexual risk reduction and condom use and sexual decision-making (Williams, Wyatt, & Wingood, 2010). However, the understanding of current sexual behaviors necessitates inquiry into the role that early experiences with sex and the exploration of one's sexuality had in shaping adult behaviors (Williams et al., 2008). This is particularly important for men whose initial and/or early sexual experiences could be defined as being sexual abuse. Understanding the relationship between childhood sexual experiences and adult sexual behaviors may have implications in the overall well-being of gay men. Providing credence to this idea is research that supports the association between CSA and poor psychological, physical, and sexual health outcomes (Bartholow et al., 1994; Brennan, Hellerstedt, Ross, & Wells, 2007; Catania et al., 2008; Holmes & Slap, 1998; Jinich et al., 1998; Lloyd & Operario, 2012; Mimiaga et al., 2009;

O'Leary, Purcell, Remien, & Gomez, 2003; Paul, Catania, Pollack, & Stall, 2001; Welles et al., 2009). While there is a paucity of research on CSA specifically among gay and bisexually identified men, there is increasing recognition that CSA may be an additional risk factor for HIV infection and transmission and that there are psychological and physical health implications among MSM (Metzger & Plankey, 2012). Research on CSA supports that abused men, as compared to nonabused men, were more likely to engage in high-risk sexual behaviors, have more lifetime sexual partners, use condoms less frequently, have higher rates of STIs and exchange sex, and have up to a twofold increase in the rate of HIV (Holmes & Slap, 1998; Lloyd & Operario, 2012) as well as higher depression symptomatology, and alcohol and illicit substance use (Brennan et al., 2007; Catania et al., 2008; Jinich et al., 1998; Mimiaga et al., 2009; O'Leary et al., 2003; Paul et al., 2001; Welles et al., 2009).

In this chapter, we review the current literature on CSA among gay men, focusing on those who are living with HIV and the associated health implications. We also examine ASA and intimate partner violence (IPV), as research supports that individuals who were abused as children are often revictimized as adults (Classen, Palesh, & Aggarwal, 2005). While the chapter's intent is to focus on the experiences of gay men, there are limitations in the literature involving research conducted with this population. Research since the early 1990s has more commonly used the "MSM" term to identify men at increased HIV transmission risk due to behaviors. Thus, the use of the MSM terminology often prevents the distinction of CSA research specifically with gay identified men.

Prevalence of Sexual Abuse

Sexual assault within the USA, which includes child and adult sexual abuse and intimate sexual partner violence, is a significant public health concern (Hornor, 2010; Rothman, Exner, & Baughman, 2011). The US Department of Health and Human Services estimates that of the 695,000 children who experienced maltreatment in 2010, 9% of them were sexually abused (US Department of Health and Human Serivces, 2011). However, a limitation of this information is that much of the literature on CSA tends to focus on the experiences of women and girls. There continues to be inadequate attention on the sexual experiences of men and boys, who may also experience CSA (Bartholow et al., 1994; Homma, Wang, Saewyc, & Kisnor, 2012). For example, an early study conducted by Finkelhor (1987) found that 3–31% of men experienced sexual abuse before the age of 18. Additional studies reported similar CSA prevalence rates among men ranging from 3% (Lodico & DiClemente, 1994) to 29% (Zierler et al., 1991). A review by Rothman et al. (2011) found variable rates of sexual assault among men and reported prevalence rates ranging from 4.1% to 59.2% for CSA, 10.8% to 44.7% for ASA, 11.8% to 54% for lifetime sexual assault, 9.5% to 57% for intimate partner sexual violence, and 3% to 19% for hate-crime-related sexual assault.

The prevalence of CSA among gay and bisexual men has been reported to be significantly greater than that of their heterosexual counterparts. In a nonclinical sample of 329 men, 49% of homosexual men reported histories of molestation, compared to 24% of heterosexual men (Tomeo, Temple, Anderson, & Kotler, 2001). Also, histories of same-sex perpetrators were significantly greater among gay men (46%) than heterosexual men (7%). A study examining histories of sexual abuse among male college students found that lifetime prevalence of sexual abuse was significantly greater among students who identified as gay (12%) than those that identified as heterosexual (4%) (Duncan, 1990). The implications of these findings are not clear as patterns of male sexual assault have not been adequately examined (Stermac, Sheridan, Davidson, & Dunn, 1996). Importantly, challenges with disclosure which include stigma regarding male sexual assault and sexual orientation may influence reporting. While additional research among all men is needed, it is particularly necessary among gay men where associations between sexual abuse and negative health outcomes have been repeatedly supported (Williams, Kisler, Glover, & Sciolla, 2011).

Variability in CSA Prevalence Rates and Its Implications

CSA prevalence rates are highly variable among men. Reasons for this variability may be due to a lack of consistency in the definition of CSA and to underreporting as a consequence of CSA stigma and issues related to masculinity (Senn, Carey, & Vanable, 2008; Stoltenborgh, van IJzendoorn, Euser, & Bakermans-Kranenburg, 2011). As a result, it is likely that reported prevalence rates underestimate the true occurrence of CSA among men and boys.

The diverse ways in which CSA is defined across studies result in sexual experiences being defined as sexual abuse in some studies but not in others (Relf, 2001). Rates of CSA prevalence among gay men may differ, in part, due to this lack of consistency, as well as the difficulties inherent in assessing CSA among men (Kisler & Williams, 2012; Williams et al., 2011; Williams et al., 2008). While it is largely understood that sexual abuse involves the sexual conduct of an adult or a significantly older child with another child, there is a large range in the ways in which histories are obtained and the specific details which constitute an experience as abusive (Hornor, 2010). Holmes and Slap (1998) examined and identified the various ways in which information about CSA was collected across studies involving men with histories of sexual abuse. Three types of questioning methods were identified: none, subjective, and objective. In cases where histories of sexual abuse were not asked directly, investigators often relied on previously collected information (i.e., child sexual abuse registries), or failed all together to report how such information was collected. Subjective methods involved asking subjects whether they had been sexually abused, assaulted, or victimized. However, these terms were not defined, leaving the interpretation of past sexual experiences up to the individual. Objective methods asked about histories of sexual abuse while offering definitions and, in some cases, providing descriptions through the use of vignettes. The method in which information is collected is important as it is directly related to the ability to reliably assess CSA prevalence rates. For example, computerized and written questionnaires completed by a sample of 200 male undergraduate students yielded rates of 14% and 8%, respectively, with 90% of subjects reporting more honestly when using computerized methods (Bagley & Genuis, 1991). Given the sensitivity of discussing CSA histories, particularly for men, the assessment of CSA may be especially sensitive to collection methodologies.

In addition to the manner in which histories of sexual abuse were obtained, Holmes and Slap (1998) identified other criteria that were used to determine if a sexual experience was abuse. The age differential between the perpetrator and the victim, which could be fixed, graded, or unspecified, was often assessed. A fixed age differential existed when the age difference between the perpetrator and the victim, typically 5 years, remained the same regardless of the age of the victim. For example, the same 5 year age differential would be used with an 8-year-old individual as it would be for a 13-year-old individual. In contrast, the graded differential takes the ages of the individuals involved into account such that for boys under 13 years of age, the perpetrator had to be at least 5 years older in order for a situation to be designated as abuse. For boys between 13 and 16, a minimum of a 10-year age difference was needed. Studies that employed an unspecified age differential simply asked the participant if, as a child, he ever had a sexual experience with an adult. Under such criterion, a 17-year-old boy could be victimized by an 18-year-old based upon the age difference.

Other criteria used to define CSA included: (1) the appraisal of the experience as "negative"; (2) the presence of force/coercion or the perception of the perpetrator as more powerful; (3) the sexual activity occurring with an authority figure; (4) the presence of physical contact; and (5) the presence of anal penetration of the child or anal or vaginal penetration of the perpetrator by the child. In total, more than 30 combinations of CSA criteria were identified. Such varied definitions and inconsistency in what constitutes CSA and the manner in which CSA histories are assessed have implications for CSA prevalence estimates and relatedly for the need of health interventions (Fromuth & Burkhart, 1987; Holmes & Slap, 1998; Senn et al., 2008; Stoltenborgh et al., 2011). As an example, in a study of 200 male college students, the requirement of physical contact yielded a CSA prevalence of 8%, the use of a graded age differential and presence of coercion yielded 10%, the use of a graded age differential alone yielded 14%, and having either a graded age differential or the presence of coercion yielded 22% (Fromuth & Burkhart, 1987). The large degree of diversity in operationalized definitions has the potential to result in an over- or underestimation of early experiences of sexual abuse and creates a significant challenge to understanding the true prevalence of CSA among gay and bisexual men.

CSA Among Gay Men

The presence of CSA histories among gay men has been consistently demonstrated at significant levels in several large-scale studies. Among nearly 3000 gay men participating in a study in an urban area, the CSA prevalence was 20% (Paul et al., 2001). Similarly, in a study of nearly 2000 gay and bisexual men recruited at gay bars and through household telephone surveys, 28% reported histories of CSA (Jinich et al., 1998). In an ethnically diverse sample of 1001 homosexual and bisexual men recruited from STI clinics in three major cities, 37% (*n* = 369) reported sexual contact with an older or more powerful individual before the age of 19 years (Doll et al., 1992). Comparable prevalence rates have also been revealed in smaller community samples of gay and bisexual men. Among a sample of 327 well educated, middle aged, predominately White gay men, 36% reported at least one experience of CSA (Lenderking et al., 1997). Rothman et al. (2011) found that overall, the prevalence of CSA reported by gay and bisexual men in the current literature ranged from 4.1 to 59.2% (median, 22.7%).

Research has also attempted to identify whether men were sexually abused more commonly by male versus female perpetrators. There has been some data suggesting that gay male CSA survivors were more commonly abused by men than women. This was demonstrated in studies by both Lenderking et al. (1997) and Jinich et al. (1998), in which 96% of the perpetrators in both studies were men. In addition, the majority of the perpetrators in those studies, 63% and 70%, respectively, were men that were unrelated to the victim (i.e., extrafamilial abuse). In the study conducted by Jinich et al. (1998), only 15.7% of the extrafamilial perpetrators were strangers, challenging the notion that most abusers are unknown to the victim.

Data has also supported that men abused as children largely report being victimized during early adolescence prior to their teenage years, when they may be particularly vulnerable. Lenderking et al. (1997) found that 63% of men experienced abuse prior to age 13, with 37% experiencing abuse between 13 and 16. Similarly, 71% of the men in Jinich et al.' (1998) study reported abuse prior to the age of 12, while 29% reported being sexually abused between 13 and 15 years of age. Consistent with these findings, the median age at time of first contact among the men who reported being abused as children in a study conducted by Doll et al. (1992) was 10, with ages ranging from 2 to 17 years of age. The median age difference between the victim and the perpetrator was 11 years (range: 0–55), with the age differential being significantly higher for those boys younger than 6 and those older than 15 years of age. Similarly, among a sample of 137 HIV positive African American and Latino MSM and men who have sex with men and women (MSMW) with histories of CSA and who identified with various gay and bisexual identity labels, the mean age of first CSA incident was 10.6 years (Williams et al., 2008).

The type and severity of abuse reported by gay men varies. Among the sample of 1001 gay and bisexual men in the study conducted by Doll et al. (1992), oral to genital (39%) and anal to genital (33%) contact were the most prevalent forms of sexual abuse reported compared to kissing (2%), exposing genitals (2%), and touching genitals (21%) (Doll et al., 1992). Other studies have found that sexual abuse without bodily contact was the most frequent (65.5%), and most commonly involved indecent exposure (Lenderking et al., 1997). Among the experiences involving bodily contact, the most frequent were being masturbated (60%) and sexualized nongenital contact (56%) (Lenderking et al., 1997). Among a sample of HIV positive African American and Latino MSM and MSMW, 12.4% reported CSA that included touching, fondling, or frottage, while 87.6% reported CSA that included performing and/or receiving oral or anal sex, digital penetration or penetration with objects (Williams et al., 2008). Among this latter group which reported more severe CSA, 53% reported anal penetration, 37% reported performing or receiving oral sex against their will, and 10% reported both. Taken together, these findings suggest that gay and bisexual men with histories of CSA may be exposed to a spectrum of sexual abuse experiences, from non-bodily to bodily contact with severe forms including penetration.

While these studies have focused on CSA experiences among gay and bisexual samples, several additional studies reported associations between CSA and being HIV positive. Arreola, Neilands, Pollack, Paul, and Catania (2008) conducted a study with gay and bisexual men which included three categories of childhood sexual experiences, those who reported no sex before age 18, consensual only (sex before age 18 that was not forced), and forced sex (having been "forced or frightened by someone into doing something sexually" before the age of 18). The prevalence of being HIV positive was higher among the forced and consensual groups as compared to the no sex group. The forced and consensual groups also had higher rates of substance use and transmission risk than the no sex group. The forced sex group had significantly higher rates of frequent drug use and high-risk sex as compared to the consensual group (Arreola et al., 2008). In another study, men who were recruited from a gay pride venue and who reported histories of CSA were more likely to report unprotected receptive anal intercourse, engage in exchange sex for drugs or money, experience nonsexual relationship violence, and report being HIV positive (Kalichman, Gore-Felton, Benotsch, Cage, & Rompa, 2004).

Consistent with these findings, gay and bisexual men who reported having "regular" CSA experiences were more likely to be HIV positive, engage in exchange sex, and be a regular user of sex-related drugs (Brennan et al., 2007). Similarly, in a study conducted by Jinich et al. (1998), gay and bisexual men with CSA histories were more likely to engage in high-risk sexual behaviors such as unprotected anal intercourse with non-primary partners. Also, perceptions of being coerced were associated with increased sexual risk behaviors and the degree of coercion was positively associated with self-reported HIV serostatus. That is, 16% of nonabused men reported being HIV positive, while 19% of men who reported no/mild coercion and 22% of men who reported strong coercion/physical force reported being HIV positive.

CSA Among Gay Men of Color

Examination of gay men by race/ethnicity reveals that gay men of color typically report higher rates of CSA and other forms of trauma (Feldman, 2010; Mimiaga et al., 2009). In the study by Doll et al. (1992), Black (52%) and Hispanic (50%) men were significantly more likely than White men (32%) to report sexual contact with an older or more powerful partner. In a study of 569 young MSM in New York, Black (28%) and Latino (49%) MSM were more likely than White (13%) MSM to report experiencing childhood victimization, including both physical and sexual abuse (Gwadz et al., 2006). However, the literature regarding racial/ethnic differences of CSA prevalence rates is not entirely consistent. Siegel, Sorenson, Golding, Burnam, and Stein (1987) found that non-Hispanic Whites (6.5%) had a higher rate of sexual abuse than Hispanics (3.2%). Nevertheless, given the findings of significant prevalence of CSA among Black and Latino gay and bisexual men, as well as the association between histories of CSA and risky behaviors, it is likely that CSA among gay men of color may contribute to racial disparities in HIV prevalence and needs further examination (Feldman, 2010).

The Sequelae of CSA

Herman (1992) states, "Repeated trauma in adult life erodes the structure of the personality already formed, but repeated trauma in childhood forms and deforms the personality." CSA has implications on the health of gay and bisexual men. Having a history of CSA has been associated with engaging in high-risk sexual behaviors, externalizing sexual decision-making to partners, and experiencing difficulties in the ability to form healthy intimate relationships, as some of the most damaging effects of CSA are intrapsychic (Burns-Loeb et al., 2002; Herman, 1992). Consequently, CSA is a risk factor for a wide range of sexual, psychological, and physical health issues in both childhood and adulthood (Burns-Loeb et al., 2002; Kendall-Tackett, 2004).

CSA and Sexual Health

There is a well-documented association between early adverse experiences, including CSA and high-risk sexual behaviors in adulthood (Paul et al., 2001; Relf, 2001; Rosario, Schrimshaw, & Hunter, 2006; Stevenson, 2000; Wilson, 2010; Zierler et al., 1991). In comparison to their nonabused peers, gay and bisexual men who experience CSA are more likely to engage in unprotected sex (Bartholow et al., 1994; Carballo-Dieguez & Dolezal, 1995; Dolezal, 2002; Feldman, 2010; Jinich et al., 1998; Strathdee et al., 1998), have more sexual partners (Dolezal, 2002; Jinich et al., 1998; Rosario et al., 2006), have more sexual episodes under the influence of recreational drugs (Jinich et al., 1998), have multiple anonymous sex partners (Zierler et al., 1991), and engage in commercial sex work/exchange sex (Bartholow et al., 1994; Zierler et al., 1991).

The relationship between CSA and high-risk sexual behaviors has also been found to be mediated by substance use during sex, engaging in anonymous sex, and intimate partner violence (Paul et al., 2001). Importantly, in one study that examined the relationship between a history of CSA and unsafe sexual behaviors, CSA was found to be the only significant predictor of unprotected receptive anal intercourse (Lenderking et al., 1997). Engaging in high-risk sexual behavior can be particularly costly for gay men by placing them at increased risk for HIV/AIDS and other STIs and influencing overall well-being across the lifespan. Research supports that being coerced sexually as a child is associated with high incidence rates of adult HIV infection (Jinich et al., 1998), and sexually abused men are twice as likely to be HIV positive as their nonabused peers (Zierler et al., 1991). It is also possible that CSA has an indirect effect on HIV risk behaviors by promoting more sexual partners, more sexual encounters, and a greater likelihood of engaging in HIV sexual risk behaviors (Rosario et al., 2006).

For the individual who experiences CSA, its impact may be experienced over their lifespan. In particular, early experiences of sexual trauma may influence an individual's sexual decision-making as an adult. Male survivors of CSA may have difficulties negotiating sexual activities and may externalize control of sexual behaviors to their sexual partners (Burns-Loeb et al., 2002; Williams et al., 2008). Relf (2001) suggests that the significant role of engaging in casual one-night stands as a mediator between CSA and risky sexual behavior for gay men is likely an indication of a lack of interpersonal regulatory ability, as well as poor risk appraisal skills. Wright (2001) describes gay men with histories of CSA as engaging in a "spiral of risk," in which men engage in high-risk sexual behaviors out of a need to feel that they belong and to avoid feelings of abandonment. While understanding the processes that drive decision-making and actions are important, there is also a critical need to recognize sexual behaviors as being potentially deleterious with long-term health implications. Despite most studies of sexual abuse being limited in examining causal effects, there is significant data that supports the relationships between CSA and the overall health of gay and bisexual men. It has been suggested that the consequences of CSA on men's self-esteem and health, both physical and mental, and the repeated engagement in unhealthy, high-risk sexual behaviors may be exacerbating the history of trauma which the men are actually trying to ameliorate (Wright, 2001). The relationship between CSA and health outcomes is important to understand especially among HIV positive gay men whose sexual behaviors may place them at increased risk for HIV reinfection, acquiring other STIs, or transmission to sexual partners.

CSA and Mental Health

Generally, CSA has been found to be associated with psychological health issues including fear, anxiety, depression, insomnia, self-destructive behaviors, headaches, aggression, anger, hostility, poor self-esteem, substance abuse, suicidal ideations and attempts, sexual maladjustment, and problems with obesity (Wilson, 2010). Gay men with histories of CSA are twice as likely as their nonabused peers to suffer from a mental health disorder (George, 1996) and have an elevated risk of substance abuse, attempted suicide, and anxiety and mood disorders (Brady, 2008; Chen et al., 2010). In a study conducted with young MSM ages 18–30 years of age, men with histories of nonconsensual sex had a higher depression score (OR = 2.08; 95% CI,

1.34–3.22), lower social support (OR = 1.94; 95% CI, 1.24–3.00), and were more likely to use recreational drugs than men who were not abuse (Strathdee et al., 1998). Also, borderline personality disorder, dissociate identity disorder, and bulimia nervosa have all been linked with CSA (Putman, 2003). While research is not able to support a causal relationship between CSA and sexual identity development, a review of the literature does suggest the need to examine the context of sexual exploration and sexual identity development and experiences of sexual abuse as these past experiences may impact psychological well-being (Relf, 2001).

Post-traumatic Stress Disorder (PTSD). While a direct causal link is difficult to establish, individuals with histories of CSA have an increased likelihood for the development of post-traumatic stress disorder (PTSD) (Rodriguez, Ryan, Rowan, & Foy, 1999; Spies et al., 2012). Psychopathology among HIV-infected individuals who have histories of CSA is highly prevalent. For example, among a sample of 247 people living with HIV, 117 of whom were gay and bisexual men, and who had histories of CSA, 40% met diagnostic criteria for PTSD (Sikkema et al., 2008).

Contributing to the complication of establishing a causal link between CSA and mental health outcomes is the presentation of sequelae not occurring in close temporal proximity to the sexual abuse. That is, symptoms such as those of PTSD may be delayed for months or possibly, for years. Also, the triggers of PTSD may be diverse. For example, among children and adolescents, triggers may include developmental milestones such as their first sexual intercourse, also known as sexual debut (Hornor, 2010). For gay men abused by other men, it is possible that engaging in sex with other men in adulthood acts as a trigger for traumatic memories associated with early abuse. Therefore, it is plausible that substance use before and during sex may act as a way for such men to numb the emergence of the traumatic feelings associated with sex. It may also explain, in part, why CSA is associated with drinking before sex (Lodico & DiClemente, 1994). Intimacy with other men in adulthood may trigger traumatic memories of early abusive experiences and possibly explain some of the challenges that gay men with CSA histories face in developing healthy intimate relationships.

Depression. CSA has been found to be strongly associated with the onset of depression in adulthood (DiLillo & Long, 1999; Paolucci, Genuis, & Violato, 2001), especially among gay men (Relf, 2001). In addition to being angry with their abuser, gay men with histories of CSA may be frustrated with society's lack of attention to sexual abuse among gay men, as well as the gay community's perceived insensitivity to survivors of CSA (Anderson, 1982). Such feelings can have negative consequences for gay men, including depression (Anderson, 1982).

Among a sample of 439 young gay and bisexual men, aged 18–30, those classified as risk-takers as compared to non-risk-takers, were significantly more likely to have a history of nonconsensual sex, greater depressive symptoms, and report using recreational drugs during the previous year (Strathdee et al., 1998). Similarly, gay and bisexual men who experienced CSA involving either strong coercion or physical force had significantly higher depressive symptoms than did men who reported no coercion or mild coercion and the nonabused men (Jinich et al., 1998). In comparison to their nonabused peers, gay men with histories of CSA are more likely to be hospitalized for depression, suggesting an elevated risk for depression overall, as well as for more severe depression (Bartholow et al., 1994; Relf, 2001).

The recognition of depression among individuals with histories of CSA is challenging as experiences of sexual abuse have the potential to change the clinical presentation of depression. That is, the neurovegetative symptoms characteristic of the typical presentation of depression may be reversed for those with histories of CSA, resulting in increased appetite, weight gain, and hypersomnia when compared to individuals with depression that lack CSA histories (Putman, 2003). Furthermore, a history of sexual abuse is often associated with an earlier onset of depressive episodes, as well as an altered response to standard treatments for depression (Hornor, 2010). The nature of the sexual abuse (i.e., penetrative vs. non-penetrative) and the relationship between the victim and the perpetrator, may also affect the development and severity of depression (Trickett, Noll, Reiffman, & Putman, 2001). While it has been suggested that emotional abuse appears to pose a greater risk for depression than sexual or physical abuse (Chapman et al., 2004), multiple forms of abuse tend to co-occur with CSA (Dong, Anda, Dube, Giles, & Felitti, 2003). Thus, it is likely that men will have experienced emotional abuse along with sexual abuse, and possibly, physical abuse or threat of abuse as well, further compounding their risk for adulthood depression.

The impact of CSA and its association with depression may also have physical health implications. One of the health consequences of depression is its ability to affect immune functioning (Irwin & Miller, 2007; Kiecolt-Glaser & Glaser, 2002; Raison & Miller, 2003). This may be of particular importance to the health of gay male survivors of CSA who are living with HIV. Such impairment in the already compromised immune system of individuals living with HIV has implications for disease progression, development of opportunistic infections, and general ability to remain healthy. Therefore, the effects of CSA, HIV, and depression may interact in ways that significantly affect men's mental and physical well-being. This complex relationship illustrates the need for interventions to address sexual health and in particular, the sexual risk behaviors of gay men, and mental and physical health, without ignoring past experiences of CSA (Gore-Felton et al., 2006).

CSA and Physical Health

CSA is often co-occurring with physical and emotional abuse (Dong et al., 2003). Survivors of such concurrent experiences may have an increased vulnerability to stress and to deleterious acute and chronic health consequences (Wilson, 2010). The stress and trauma of the experience, combined with the shame and pressure to not disclose the abuse, may be linked to immune functioning which predisposes or exacerbates health problems among survivors of CSA (Wilson, 2010). Consequently, CSA is frequently associated with negative health outcomes in adulthood with the odds of having poor health being 1.63 times greater when a history of CSA is present (Golding, 1999). Examples of health issues correlated with CSA histories include complications with gastrointestinal functioning, sexual dysfunction, psychogenic seizures, and nonspecific chronic pain (Paras et al., 2009).

Consistent with having increased physical illness, adults with histories of CSA also report more health symptoms and doctor visits than their nonabused peers (Newman et al., 2000). Those with CSA histories report more somatic symptoms including headaches, sinus pain, muscle pain, migraines, cough, fever, abdominal pain, and other gastrointestinal symptoms (Newman et al., 2000). While the association between CSA and physical health has been established, somatization must be considered as a potential explanation of poor health. Anecdotal evidence such as that reported by Brady (2008) supports a relationship between CSA and somatization. Brady (2008) explored this issue in a case study with a gay male client who had chronic health issues which healthcare providers were unable to adequately treat given their inability to identify the source of the client's pain. Treatment explored the relationship between the client's history of CSA and his experiences of psychosomatic complaints. Though the symptoms did not completely dissipate, they were significantly reduced after the client was able to recognize the link between his experience of sexual trauma and the somatic symptoms (Brady, 2008). It is important to note that the limitation in examining the effects of CSA using experimental design weakens the ability to definitively suggest that physical or psychiatric health issues are the direct result of early experiences of sexual trauma. However, the strong correlations between CSA and poor health outcomes indicate a significant association between the two, although the relationship may not be causal (Wilson, 2010).

Coping Strategies

Gay men with histories of early sexual trauma may engage in various coping strategies. High levels of substance use among gay men in sexual situations may serve to manage negative emotions and the potential re-emergence of traumatic memories related to the experiences of CSA (Relf, 2001). Relf (2001) also suggested that casual sexual encounters such as one-night stands among gay male survivors of CSA may act as a mediator between CSA and HIV.

Among adolescent males with experiences of sexual abuse, an association between CSA and externalizing behaviors such as violence, delinquency, substance use, and heavy drinking has been identified (Dube et al., 2003; Hornor, 2010; Mullers & Dowling, 2008). Externalizing behaviors may serve as a way for adolescent males to exert control when they otherwise feel helpless. Dube et al. (2003) suggested that substance use may serve as a form of coping, through avoidance/escape or dissociation, to deal with the feelings of helplessness and instability that are often characteristic of CSA. Furthermore, if the perpetrator of the abuse was male, externalizing behaviors may be a way to assert and reclaim the sense of masculinity that men and boys may feel is lost due to the male-male sexual abuse.

Developing healthy coping strategies to deal with past experiences of sexual abuse is beset with difficulty. However, being a sexual minority and being HIV positive may pose additional challenges for a man who has experienced sexual abuse. Research needs to explore the impact of CSA among HIV positive gay men and assess whether these stressors are additive and contribute to worsening health outcomes.

Adult Sexual Abuse (ASA) Among Gay Men

In addition to CSA, Rothman et al.' (2011) review of the literature on sexual assault among gay, lesbian, and bisexual individuals indicated that gay and bisexual men are at risk for experiencing diverse forms of sexual victimization throughout their lifetime. Among gay and bisexual men, adult sexual abuse (ASA) ranged from 10.8 to 44.7% (median, 14.7%) and lifetime sexual assault ranged from 11.8 to 54% (median, 30.4%). Additionally, intimate partner sexual assault ranged from 9.5 to 57% (median, 12.1%), and hate-crime related sexual assault ranged in prevalence from 3 to 19.8% (median, 14%) (Rothman et al., 2011). These findings suggest that gay and bisexual men are not only at increased risk for CSA, but that they also have an increased risk for a lifetime of sexual violence victimization. It is possible that sexual revictimization is related directly and indirectly to sequelae of early sexual trauma (Anderson, 1982; Classen et al., 2005; Fillipas & Ullman, 2006). Additional research needs to examine sexual revictimization specifically among HIV positive gay men, as being HIV-infected may increase their vulnerability to trauma exposure.

Intimate Partner Relationships Among Gay Men with CSA

Similar to their heterosexual peers, the majority of gay and bisexual men with histories of CSA were abused by other men (Brady, 2008). However, unlike their heterosexual peers who primarily have intimate partner relationships with women, gay and bisexual men must be able to establish healthy intimate relationships with other men. Histories of CSA by male perpetrators pose potential problems with many gay men in developing the ability to be intimate with other men (Brady, 2008). Furthermore, given the high incidence of CSA among gay men, evidence suggests that abused men are likely to choose abused partners (King, 2001). The intra- and interpersonal difficulties that are often the result of CSA, combined with the lack of support for gay male survivors to manage these issues, can make sex, love, and intimacy particularly difficult to manage in gay male relationships (King, 2001).

Survivors of CSA report less relationship satisfaction, poorer communication and interpersonal skills, and lower levels of trust in relationships (Wilson, 2010). Gay male survivors of CSA may be challenged in establishing healthy intimate and sexual relationships with other men due to the fact that their initial sexual experiences with men may have involved coercion, physical assault, and distrust. This could potentially lead gay men to generalize their early traumatic experiences to all their relationships with men, and potentially alter their understanding of what it means to be in a healthy relationship with another man. As a result, gay men with histories of CSA may experience intimate partner victimization, both sexual and physical, and may themselves perpetrate sexual abuse toward their partners (Brady, 2008).

Revictimization Among Gay Men of Color

Gay men of color, particularly Black and Latino men, tend to have higher rates of CSA than their White peers (Feldman, 2010; Kalichman et al., 2004; Mimiaga et al., 2009). However, an area that appears to be underexplored is the unique ways in which gay men of color manage the experience of early sexual trauma, particularly when the perpetrator is also a person of color. It is possible that racial/ethnic minority gay men who were abused by minority perpetrators experience difficulty establishing relationships with men of their same racial/ethnic group. That is, racial/ethnic concordance between the perpetrator and victim may further complicate the ability for sexually abused gay men to develop healthy intimate relationships with other men.

Racial concordance between the perpetrator and victim was explored by Brady (2008) in a case study of a HIV positive Black gay man with a history of CSA. While the patient did not have an issue reconciling his sexuality with his history of abuse, psychotherapy with the patient explored his aversion to dating other Black men, as well as his preference for White partners. Through the course of therapy the patient realized that, for him, Black men represented the Black perpetrator who had sexually abused him. As a result, the patient found himself conflicted, simultaneously being attracted to and fearing Black men. These feelings led him to perceiving White men as safe and to him only engaging in high-risk substance use and sexual behavior with other Black men anonymously (Brady, 2008).

The exploration of this issue is in no way intended to suggest that interracial relationships are a manifestation of internalized racism among minority gay male survivors of CSA with histories of racially concordant perpetrators. However, in a society where men of color, particularly Black and Latino, are stereotyped as being hypersexual and aggressive (Bush, 1999; Kisler & Williams, 2012; Majors & Billson, 1992; O'Neil, 1990; Pitt, 2010; Rasheed & Rasheed, 1999; Reese, 2004), it may be important to consider how such social heuristics interact with the experience of sexual trauma. When men of color are sexually abused by men of their racial/ethnic group, the experience may be interpreted as confirming negative racial stereotypes and generalized to the entire group. Such an experience likely differs for White gay men who are sexually abused by other White men, given the absence of a social narrative of White men as hypersexual, aggressive, or even predatory. As a result, the experience of CSA between White men and boys may be interpreted much more individually, whereas the experience between racial/ethnic minority men and boys may be seen as confirming negative stereotypes regarding racial/ethnic minority men's sexual prowess, promiscuity, violence, and aggression. As seen in Brady's (2008) case study, such early experiences of sexual abuse between men of color may have implications for men's partner selection in adulthood. For gay men of color, the relationships between early sexual abuse, internalized racism, appraisal of the trauma experience, and later partner selection are complex. These issues warrant greater examination if the potentially unique experiences of these men, including those who are HIV positive, are to be fully understood.

Sexual Abuse, Masculinity, Gender Roles, and Sexual Identity Development

One proposed theory for the increased incidence of sexual abuse among gay men is related to the idea that gay men, as children, were more likely to display "gender atypical behavior" (Brady, 2008). It has been suggested that boys who behave in a gender atypical or feminine manner are at an increased risk for being stigmatized and ostracized, and potentially to be at an increased risk for sexual, physical, and emotional abuse (Brooks, 2001). It has also been suggested that gender non-conforming behavior in childhood may be associated with homosexuality later in life (Bailey & Zucker, 1995) and that this behavior contributes to these children being targeted and susceptible to being abused (Balsam, Rothblum, & Beauchaine, 2005; Corliss, Cochran, & Mays, 2002). This idea of being stigmatized for not exhibiting masculine attributes is not only seen with boys, but also exists among men (Kisler & Williams, 2012; Reese, 2004; Robertson, 1997). Unfortunately, masculine attributes and sexuality are commonly erroneously linked together and perceived as being the same. That is, those who do not demonstrate "traditional" male gender roles and characteristics are believed to be gay.

Gay men with histories of CSA experience abuse within a larger cultural context that stigmatizes, devalues, and punishes homosexuality (King, 2001). Early experiences of being mistreated due to gender atypical behavior, early sexual trauma, and adulthood experiences of stigma associated with being a sexual minority interact in complex ways in the lives of gay men (King, 2001). Add to this the stigma and maltreatment commonly associated with being HIV positive, and such experiences can make it particularly challenging for gay male survivors of CSA living with HIV to develop an affirmative identity (Brady, 2008).

The experience of being abused by a man potentially creates difficulties for men who may struggle with the implications of the abuse for themselves as men (Brady, 2008). This can include issues around self-identity, sexuality, and concerns about becoming a perpetrator (Brady, 2008). Men may also externalize such feelings, which can manifest as homophobia. In a review of the literature, Relf (2001) found that gay and heterosexual men abused by men were: (1) "intensely" homophobic; (2) fearful of homosexuals; (3) expressing disdain of homosexuality and homosexual behavior; and (4) hostile toward homosexuality. Relf (2001) stressed that these results were from clinical samples, possibly exaggerating the intensity of homophobia and limiting the generalizability. Nevertheless, it will be important to consider the ways in which gay men, including those who are HIV positive, appraise and understand their sexual experiences, sexuality, and sexual behaviors.

Sexual identity development is a normal part of growth. However, it is not clear how trauma experiences such as sexual abuse impacts sexual identity development. It has been hypothesized that having a history of CSA impacts gender and sexual identity (Relf, 2001). For example, a qualitative study of 26 men with CSA histories identified issues surrounding sexuality and homosexuality as common themes among the participants (Lisak, 1994). Other research has also documented higher rates of gender role confusion and fears regarding intimate relationships with both men and women among men with histories of CSA (Holmes & Slap, 1998; Hunter, 1991; Jacobson & Herald, 1990; Janus, Burgess, & McCormack, 1987; McCormack, Janus, & Burgess, 1986; Sansonnet-Hayden, Haley, Marriage, & Fine, 1987). Among a sample of sexually abused adolescent boys, diverse gender roles were defined and identified as undifferentiated (52%), masculine (23%), androgynous (19%), and feminine (6%) (Richardson, Meredith, & Abbot, 1993). Abused boys, especially those who were victimized by males, were up to seven times more likely to self-identify as gay or bisexual than their nonabused counterparts (Johnson & Shrier, 1985, 1987). Among men, those with histories of CSA were more likely than those with histories of childhood physical abuse and/or childhood neglect to report having had same-sex sexual partners in their lifetime (Wilson & Widom, 2010). Unfortunately, it is difficult to identify a causal link between sexual abuse and sexual identity due to the lack of longitudinal studies. To further complicate the issue is that gender role confusion preceding experiences of sexual abuse makes it difficult to establish a linear pathway to a defined sexual identity. That is, the process of identity development for men with histories of sexual abuse may largely be affected by the chronology of the abuse and the individual's stage of identity development. Men who have engaged in sexual behaviors prior to experiencing sexual abuse may have a different experience with sexual identity development than those whose first sexual experience was within the context of CSA (Bartholow et al., 1994). For gay men whose first sexual experience was within the context of abuse, the process of questioning gay identity occurred at an earlier age and proceeded differently than for nonabused men (Bartholow et al., 1994).

The impact of CSA on sexual identity continues to pose many questions and remains poorly understood. Some adolescent males who are exploring and questioning their sexual identities may seek out and engage in sexual relationships with older men. While these encounters have the potential to be coercive in nature, for many adolescent males, there are limited avenues in which to safely engage in sexual exploration. For adolescent boys exploring their same-sex attraction, efforts to initiate contacts with other boys in their peer groups and social circles (i.e., schools, church, neighborhood) could lead to violence and harassment (Relf, 2001). Consequently, such boys who seek relationships with older men in an effort to explore their sexuality may be putting themselves at risk for sexually abusive relationships, even if they do not realize the true nature of these relationships.

Men as Victims and Social Norms

Historically, the sexual abuse of male children and adolescents has been minimized, ignored, and even denied (Anderson, 1982). As a result, clinicians, advocates, and policy makers have often neglected the needs of male survivors of sexual abuse. Societal gender role expectations pose a significant hindrance in acknowledging, identifying, and addressing CSA among male children (Bartholow et al., 1994). Such social norms dictate that males are to be dominant, strong, and even aggressive (Bush, 1999; Kisler & Williams, 2012; Majors & Billson, 1992; O'Neil, 1990; Pitt, 2010; Rasheed & Rasheed, 1999; Reese, 2004), and experiencing sexual abuse falls outside of the realm of expected social behaviors. This is particularly true when the perpetrator is a man, often causing the male victim to question his manhood and ability to live up to gender expectations. However, when the perpetrator is female, male victims are often expected to normalize the experience as nonabusive and desirable (Kisler & Williams, 2012). As a result, male survivors of CSA often experience self-blame, guilt, shame, and humiliation (Lisak, 1994).

Adult Sexual Abuse (ASA) and Intimate Partner Violence (IPV)

Victims of CSA are more likely to be sexually revictimized later in adolescence as well as in adulthood (Hornor, 2010; Roche, Runtz, & Hunter, 1999; Rumstein-McKean & Hunsley, 2001; Whiffen & MacIntosh, 2005). Adult sexual abuse (ASA) is four times more likely among those with a history of CSA (Fillipas & Ullman, 2006). Adults with histories of CSA have been found to have difficulties with romantic interpersonal adult relationships, possibly due to insecure attachments established through abusive relationships in childhood (Alexander, 1992). It is possible that victims of CSA are less able to negotiate sexual activities as adults due to these previous experiences. These findings suggest that CSA may increase the likelihood of experiencing ASA because it leads to an inability to negotiate sexual activities and the likelihood of engaging in high-risk sexual behavior. Sexual trauma must therefore be explored within the context of HIV. In particular, attention must be placed on addressing the needs of HIV-infected individuals who have histories of sexual abuse as they may be vulnerable to reinfection and for transmitting HIV to sexual partners.

Implications of Sexual Trauma Histories: Developing Sexual Risk Reduction Interventions

Effective sexual risk reduction interventions for HIV positive gay men must address the psychosocial and cultural issues that are relevant to sexual decision-making (Williams et al., 2008). This includes CSA and ASA, which are sensitive issues that are often neglected in discussions of current sexual risk behaviors (Williams et al., 2008). However, to adequately address HIV risk behavior among gay men, interventions are needed that address mental health and focus on reconciling issues related to sexual abuse (Gore-Felton et al., 2006). Furthermore, interventions aimed at sexual risk reduction should consider addressing issues beyond the scope of sexual behavior that may not seem relevant, but that are pertinent to risk behaviors and HIV (Relf, 2001). Specifically, early adverse life experiences involving childhood sexual, physical, and emotional abuse as well as abuse within a family and community context may influence sexual risk behaviors and should be addressed in interventions for gay men (Relf, 2001).

In addition to being correlated with sexual risk behavior, CSA influences stress and immune responses, as well as physical and mental health. Therefore, the sequelae of CSA may be best conceptualized using a holistic paradigm. Understanding the broader context in which abuse and adverse events occur, while assessing for resiliency factors such as personal assets and resources, will better inform the overall health needs of gay men (Arreola, Ayala, Díaz, & Kral, 2013). For many gay men, particularly those who are HIV positive, their immune status becomes the focus of their health. Unfortunately, sexual abuse survivors make up a sizeable percentage of primary care practices, accounting for roughly 13–26% (Kogan, 2004; Priebe & Swedin, 2008). However, only 5% of sexual abuse survivors report their history of abuse to their physicians (Walker, Katon, Roy-Byrne, Jemelka, & Russo, 1993). While patients consider it appropriate for physicians to ask questions regarding sexual abuse history, such questions are not routinely asked (Wendt et al., 2007). The healthcare system can be an important avenue to provide screenings for, and interventions with males who have previously experienced or who are currently experiencing sexual abuse (Chen et al., 2010). Pediatric and primary care physicians who provide healthcare to adolescent boys need to be trained on assessing for sexual abuse and for anticipating their physical and mental health needs (Hornor, 2010). Importantly, attention to these health issues must also be contextualized for the lives of HIV positive gay men and boys.

Wilson (2010) asserts that holistic perspectives that permit a greater understanding of the health consequences of CSA are essential to the healing process. Familial support, especially parental belief in the abuse allegation, acts as a significant buffer against the development of the negative sequelae often associated with CSA (Tremblay, Hebert, & Piche, 1999). Interventions which utilize resiliency factors, including support from intimate sexual partners, family, friends and community, and appropriately trained healthcare professionals, need to be developed to address the holistic health needs of HIV positive gay men with sexual abuse histories. Importantly, strategies to routinely implement these interventions into diverse venues, such as primary care settings and service agencies, are essential. Community based organizations that offer HIV testing and health programs must be prepared to address sexual health that includes experiences of sexual abuse. By contextualizing the meaning of past experiences, HIV positive gay men will be better able to assess what influences their sexual decision-making.

In conclusion, sexual abuse has been associated with negative sexual as well as mental and physical health outcomes. Addressing the health needs of gay men and specifically those who are HIV positive must include the assessment of histories of CSA and ASA. Programs that offer HIV interventions are ideal opportunities for screenings, assessments, and appropriate referrals and treatment. HIV risk reduction interventions administered in community settings and through health maintenance visits with primary care providers are excellent opportunities to explore sexual health within the context of overall health. For HIV positive gay men, this holistic paradigm ensures that health needs, such as the sequelae of sexual abuse, are not ignored.

Acknowledgements Funding to support this research and to write this manuscript was provided in part from the National Institute of Mental Health (The ES-HIM Project [1 R34 MH077550] and the Center for Culture, Trauma, and Mental Health Disparities [5P50MH073453]).

References

Alexander, P. C. (1992). Application of attachment theory to the study of sexual abuse. *Journal of Counseling and Clinical Psychology, 60*, 185–195.

Anderson, C. L. (1982). Males as sexual assault victims: Multiple levels of trauma. *Journal of Homosexuality, 7*, 145–162.

Arreola, S. G., Ayala, G., Díaz, R. M., & Kral, A. H. (2013). Structure, agency, and sexual development of Latino gay men. *Journal of Sex Research, 50*, 392–400.

Arreola, S., Neilands, T., Pollack, L., Paul, J., & Catania, J. (2008). Childhood sexual experiences and adult health sequelae among gay and bisexual men: Defining childhood sexual abuse. *Journal of Sex Research, 45*, 246–252.

Bagley, C., & Genuis, M. (1991). Psychology of computer use: XX. Sexual abuse recalled: Evaluation of a computerized questionnaire in a population of young adult males. *Perceptual and Motor Skills, 72*, 287–288.

Bailey, J. M., & Zucker, K. J. (1995). Childhood sex-typed behavior and sexual orientation: A conceptual analysis and quantitative review. *Developmental Psychology, 31*, 43–55.

Balsam, K. F., Rothblum, E. D., & Beauchaine, T. P. (2005). Victimization over the life span: Comparison of lesbian, gay, bisexual, and heterosexual siblings. *Journal of Counseling and Clinical Psychology, 73*, 477–487.

Bartholow, B. N., Dolls, L. S., Joy, D., Douglas, J. M., Bolan, G., Harrison, J. S., … McKirnan, D. (1994). Emotional, behavioral and HIV risks associated with sexual abuse among adult homosexual and bisexual men. *Child Abuse and Neglect, 18*, 747–761.

Binson, D., Woods, W. J., Pollack, L., Paul, J., Stall, R., & Catania, J. (2001). Differential HIV risk in bathhouses and public cruising areas. *American Journal of Public Health, 91*(9), 1482–1486.

Brady, S. (2008). The impact of sexual abuse on sexual identity formation in gay men. *Journal of Child Sexual Abuse, 17*(3–4), 359–376.

Brennan, D. J., Hellerstedt, W. L., Ross, M. W., & Wells, S. L. (2007). History of childhood sexual abuse and HIV risk behaviors in homosexual and bisexual men. *American Journal of Public Health, 97*, 1107–1112.

Brofenbrenner, U. (1979). *The ecology of human development: Experiments by nature and design.* Cambridge, MA: Harvard University Press.

Brooks, F. (2001). *Beneath contempt: The mistreatment of non-traditional/gender atypical boys.* Binghamton, NY: The Haworth Press.

Burns-Loeb, T., Williams, J. K., Rivkin, I., Vargas Carmona, J., Wyatt, G., Chin, D., & Asuan-O'Brien, A. (2002). Child sexual abuse: Associations with the sexual functioning of adolescents and adults. *Annual Review of Sex Research, 13*, 307–345.

Bush, L. V. (1999). Am I a man? A literature review engaging the sociohistorical dynamics of black manhood in the United States. *The Western Journal of Black Studies, 23*, 49–50.

Carballo-Dieguez, A., & Dolezal, C. (1995). Association between history of childhood sexual abuse and adult HIV-risk behavior in Puerto Rican men who have sex with men. *Child Abuse and Neglect, 19*, 595–605.

Catania, J. A., Paul, J., Osmond, D., Folkman, S., Pollack, L., Canchola, J., ... Neilands, T. (2008). Mediators of childhood sexual abuse and high-risk sex among men-who-have-sex-with-men. *Child Abuse and Neglect, 32*(10), 925–940.

Centers for Disease Control and Prevention. (2016a). *HIV Among Gay and Bisexual Men.* Retrieved December 23, 2016, from https://www.cdc.gov/hiv/group/msm/.

Centers for Disease Control and Prevention. (2016b). *HIV among African AmericanGay and Bisexual Men.* Retrieved December 23, 2016, from https://www.cdc.gov/hiv/group/msm/bmsm.html.

Chapman, D. P., Whitfield, C. L., Felitti, V. J., Dube, S. R., Edwards, V. J., & Anda, R. F. (2004). Adverse childhood experiences and the risk of depressive disorders in adulthood. *Journal of Affective Disorders, 82*, 217–225.

Chen, L. P., Murad, H., Paras, M. L., Colbenson, K. M., Sattler, A. L., Goranson, E. N., ... Zirakzadeh, A. (2010). Sexual abuse and lifetime diagnosis of psychiatric diagnosis: Systematic review and meta-analysis. *Mayo Clinic Proceedings, 85*(7), 618–629.

Classen, C., Palesh, O., & Aggarwal, R. (2005). Sexual revictimization: A review of the empirical literature. *Trauma, Violence, and Abuse, 6*(2), 103–129.

Corliss, H. L., Cochran, S. D., & Mays, V. M. (2002). Reports of parental maltreatment during childhood in the United States population based survey of homosexual, bisexual, and heterosexual adults. *Child Abuse and Neglect, 26*, 1165–1178.

DiLillo, D., & Long, P. J. (1999). Perceptions of couple functioning among female survivors and child sexual abuse. *Journal of Child Sexual Abuse, 7*(4), 59–76.

Dolezal, C. (2002). Childhood sexual experiences and the perception of abuse among Latino men who have sex with men. *Journal of Sex Research, 39*, 165–173.

Doll, L. S., Joy, D., Bartholow, B. N., Harrison, J. S., Bolan, G., Douglas, J. M., ... Delgado, W. (1992). Self-reported childhood and adolescent sexual abuse among adult homosexual and bisexual men. *Child Abuse and Neglect, 16*, 855–864.

Dong, M., Anda, R. F., Dube, S. R., Giles, W. H., & Felitti, V. J. (2003). The relationship of exposure to childhood sexual abuse to other forms of abuse, neglect, and household dysfunction during childhood. *Child Abuse and Neglect, 27*, 625–639.

Dube, S. R., Felitti, V. J., Dong, M., Chapman, D. P., Giles, W. H., & Anda, R. F. (2003). Childhood abuse, neglect, and household dysfunction and the risk of illicit drug use: The adverse childhood experiences study. *Pediatrics, 111*, 564–572.

Duncan, D. F. (1990). Prevalence of sexual assault victimization among heterosexual and gay/lesbian university students. *Psychological Reports, 66*, 65–66.

Feldman, M. B. (2010). A critical literature review to identify possible causes of higher rates of HIV infection among young black and Latino men who have sex with men. *Journal of the National Medical Association, 102*(12), 1206–1221.

Fillipas, H., & Ullman, S. E. (2006). Child sexual abuse, coping responses, self-blame, post-traumatic stress disorder and adult sexual revictimization. *Journal of Interpersonal Violence, 21*, 652–672.

Finkelhor, D. (1987). The trauma of child sexual abuse: Two models. *Journal of Interpersonal Violence, 2*, 348–366.

Fromuth, M. E., & Burkhart, B. R. (1987). Childhood sexual victimization among college men: Definitional and methodological issues. *Violence and Victims, 2*, 241–253.

George, M. (1996). Listening and hearing: Child sex abuse. *Nursing Standard, 10*(30), 22–23.

Glover, D. A., Williams, J. K., & Kisler, K. A. (2012). Using novel methods to examine stress among HIV positive African American men who have sex with men and women. *Journal of Behavioral Medicine, 36*(3), 10. doi:10.1007/s10865-012-9421-5

Golding, J. M. (1999). Sexual-assault history and long-term physical health problems: Evidence from clinical and population epidemiology. *Current Directions in Psychological Science, 8*(6), 191–194.

Gore-Felton, C., Kalichman, S. C., Brondino, M. J., Benotsch, E. G., Cage, M., & DiFonzo, K. (2006). Childhood sexual abuse and HIV risk among men who have sex with men: Initial test of a conceptual model. *Journal of Family Violence, 21*, 263–270.

Gwadz, M. V., Clatts, M. C., Yi, H., Leonard, N. R., Goldsamt, L., & Lankenau, S. (2006). Resilience among young men who have sex with men in New York City. *Sexuality Research and Social Policy, 3*(1), 13–21.

Halkitis, P. N., Kapadia, F., Siconolfi, D. E., Moeller, R. W., Figueroa, R. P., Barton, S. C., & Blachman-Forshay, J. (2013). Individual, psychosocial, and social correlates of unprotected anal intercourse in a new generation of young men who have sex with men in New York City. *American Journal of Public Health, 103*(5), 889–895. doi:10.2105/AJPH.2012.300963

Halkitis, P. N., & Parson, J. T. (2003). Intentional unsafe sex (barebacking) among HIV positive gay men who seek sexual partners on the Internet. *AIDS Care: Psychological and Sociomedical Aspects of AIDS/HIV, 15*(3), 367–378.

Herman, J. (1992). *Trauma and recovery*. New York: Basic Books.

Holmes, W. C., & Slap, G. B. (1998). Sexual abuse of boys: Definition, prevalence, correlate, sequelae, and management. *Journal of the American Medical Association, 280*(21), 1855–1862.

Homma, Y., Wang, N., Saewyc, E., & Kisnor, N. (2012). The relationship between sexual abuse and risky sexual behaviors among adolescent boys: A meta-analysis. *Journal of Adolescent Health, 51*, 18–24.

Hornor, G. (2010). Child sexual abuse: Consequences and implications. *Journal of Pediatric Health Care, 24*(6), 358–364.

Hunter, J. A. (1991). A comparison of the psychosocial maladjustment of adult males and females sexually molested as children. *Journal of Interpersonal Violence, 6*, 205–217.

Irwin, M. R., & Miller, A. H. (2007). Depressive disorders and immunity: 20 years of progress and discovery. *Brain, Behavior and Immunity, 21*, 374–383.

Jacobson, A., & Herald, C. (1990). The relevance of childhood sexual abuse to adult psychiatric inpatient care. *Hospital and Community Psychiatry, 41*, 154–158.

Janus, M., Burgess, A. W., & McCormack, A. (1987). Histories of sexual abuse in adolescent male runaways. *Adolescence, 22*, 405–417.

Jinich, S., Paul, J. P., Stall, R., Acree, M., Kegeles, S., Hoff, C., & Coates, T. J. (1998). Childhood sexual abuse and HIV risk-taking behavior among gay and bisexual men. *AIDS and Behavior, 2*(1), 41–51.

Johnson, R. L., & Shrier, D. K. (1985). Sexual victimization of boys: Experience at an adolescent medicine clinic. *Journal of Adolescent Health Care, 6*, 372–376.

Johnson, R. L., & Shrier, D. K. (1987). Past sexual victimization by females of male patients in an adolescent medicine clinic population. *American Journal of Psychiatry, 144*, 650–652.

Kalichman, S., Gore-Felton, C., Benotsch, E. G., Cage, M., & Rompa, D. (2004). Trauma symptoms, sexual behaviors, and substance abuse: Correlates of childhood sexual abuse and HIV risk among men who have sex with men. *Journal of Child Sexual Abuse, 13*(1), 1–15.

Kendall-Tackett, K. A. (2004). *Health consequences of abuse in the family: A clinical guide for evidence-based practice*. Washington, DC: American Psychological Association.

Kiecolt-Glaser, J. K., & Glaser, R. (2002). Depression and immune functioning: Central pathways to morbidity and mortality. *Journal of Psychosomatic Research, 53*, 873–876.

King, N. (2001). *Childhood sexual trauma in gay men: Social context and the imprinted arousal pattern*. Binghamton, NY: The Haworth Press.

Kisler, K. A., & Williams, J. K. (2012). Image over risk reduction: Perceptions of masculinity as HIV risk factors among nongay-identifying HIV positive black MSMW. *Journal of AIDS and Clinical Research*. Retrieved from http://dx.doi.org/10.4172/2155-6113.S1-008.

Kogan, S. M. (2004). Disclosing unwanted sexual experiences: Results from a national sample of adolescent women. *Child Abuse and Neglect, 28*, 147–165.

Lenderking, W. R., Wold, C., Mayer, K. H., Goldstein, R., Losina, E., & Seage, G. R. (1997). Childhood sexual abuse among homosexual men: Prevalence and association with unsafe sex. *Journal of General Internal Medicine, 12*, 250–253.

Lisak, D. (1994). The psychological impact of sexual abuse: Content analysis of interviews with male survivors. *Journal of Traumatic Stress, 7*, 525–548.

Lloyd, S., & Operario, D. (2012). HIV risk among men who have sex with men who have experienced childhood sexual abuse: Systematic review and meta-analysis. *AIDS Education and Prevention, 24*(3), 228–241.

Lodico, M. A., & DiClemente, R. J. (1994). The association between childhood sexual abuse and prevalence of HIV-related risk behaviors. *Clinical Pediatrics, 33*, 498–502.

Majors, R., & Billson, J. M. (1992). *Cool pose*. New York, NY: Lexington Books.

McCormack, A., Janus, M., & Burgess, A. W. (1986). Runaway youths and sexual victimization: Gender differences in an adolescent runaway population. *Child Abuse and Neglect, 10*, 387–395.

Metzger, P., & Plankey, M. (2012). Child sexual abuse and determinants of risky sexual behavior in men who have sex with men. *The Georgetown Undergraduate Journal of Health Sciences, 6*(1), 2–14.

Meyer, I. H. (1995). Minority stress and mental health in gay men. *Journal of Health and Social Behavior, 36*, 38–56.

Meyer, I. H. (2003). Prejudice, social stress, and mental health in lesbian, gay, and bisexual populations: Conceptual issues and research evidence. *Psychological Bulletin, 129*(5), 674–697.

Millet, G. A., Peterson, J. L., Wolitski, R. J., & Stall, R. (2006). Greater risk for HIV infection of black men who have sex with men: A critical literature review. *American Journal of Public Health, 96*, 1007–1019.

Millett, G. A., Flores, S. A., Peterson, J. L., & Bakerman, R. (2007). Explaining disparities in HIV infection among black and white men who have sex with men: A meta-analysis of HIV risk behaviors. *AIDS, 21*(5), 2083–2091.

Millett, G. A., Peterson, J. L., Flores, S. A., Hart, T. A., Jeffries, W. L., Wilson, P. A., … Remis, R. S. (2012). Comparisons of disparities and risks of HIV infection in black and other men who have sex with men in Canada, UK, and USA: A meta-analysis. *The Lancet, 380*(9839), 341–348.

Mimiaga, M. J., Noonan, E., Donnell, D., Safren, S. A., Koenen, K. C., Gortmaker, S., … Mayer, K. H. (2009). Childhood sexual abuse is highly associated with HIV risk-taking behavior and infection among MSM in the EXPLORE study. *Journal of Acquired Immune Deficiency Syndromes and Human Retrovirology, 51*, 340–348.

Mullers, E. S., & Dowling, M. (2008). Mental health consequences of child sexual abuse. *British Journal of Nursing, 17*, 1428–1433.

Mustanski, B. S., Newcomb, M. E., Du Bois, S. N., Garcia, S. C., & Grov, C. (2011). HIV in young men who have sex with men: A review of epidemiology, risk and protective factors, and interventions. *Journal of Sex Research, 48*(2–3), 218–253.

Newman, M. G., Clayton, L., Zuellig, A., Cashman, L., Arnow, B., & Dea, R. (2000). The relationships of childhood sexual abuse and depression with somatic symptoms and medical utilization. *Psychological Medicine, 30*, 1063–1077.

O'Leary, A., Purcell, D., Remien, R. H., & Gomez, C. (2003). Childhood sexual abuse and sexual transmission risk behavior among HIV positive men who have sex with men. *AIDS Care, 15*(1), 17–26.

O'Neil, J. M. (1990). *Assessing men's gender role conflict*. Alexandria, VA: American Association for Counseling.

Paolucci, E., Genuis, M., & Violato, C. (2001). A meta-analysis of the published research on the effects of child sexual abuse. *Journal of Psychology, 187*, 17–36.

Paras, M. L., Murad, H., Chen, L. P., Goranson, E. N., Sattler, A. L., Colbenson, K. M., … Zirakzadeh, A. (2009). Sexual abuse and lifetime diagnosis of somatic disorders: A systematic review and meta-analysis. *Journal of the American Medical Association, 85*(7), 618–629.

Paul, J., Catania, J., Pollack, L., & Stall, R. (2001). Understanding childhood sexual abuse as a predictor of sexual risk taking among men who have sex with men: The urban men's health study. *Child Abuse and Neglect, 25*, 557–584.

Pitt, R. N. (2010). "Still looking for my Jonathan": Gay black men's management of religious and sexual identity conflicts. *Journal of Homosexuality, 57*, 39–53.

Priebe, G., & Swedin, C. G. (2008). Child abuse is largely hidden from the adult society: An epidemiological study of adolescents' disclosures. *Child Abuse and Neglect, 28*, 1095–1108.

Putman, F. W. (2003). Ten-year research update review: Child sexual abuse. *Journal of the American Academy of Child and Adolescent Psychiatry, 42*, 269–278.

Raison, C. L., & Miller, A. H. (2003). When not enough is too much: The role of insufficient glucocorticoid signaling in the pathophysiology of stress-related disorders. *American Journal of Psychiatry, 160*(9), 1554–1565.

Rasheed, J. M., & Rasheed, M. N. (1999). *Social work practice with African American men: The invisible presence.* Thousand Oaks, CA: Sage.

Reese, R. (2004). *American paradox: Young black men.* Durham, NC: Carolina Academic Press.

Relf, M. V. (2001). Childhood sexual abuse in men who have sex with men: The current state of the science. *Journal of the Association of Nurses in AIDS Care, 12*(5), 20–29.

Richardson, M. F., Meredith, W., & Abbot, D. A. (1993). Sex-typed role in the male adolescent sexual abuse survivors. *Journal of Family Violence, 8*, 89–100.

Robertson, T. (1997). Gay male development: Hermeneutic and self psychological perspectives. *Dissertation Abstracts International, 57*(10-B), 6589.

Roche, D. N., Runtz, M. G., & Hunter, M. A. (1999). Adult attachment: A mediator between childhood sexual abuse and later psychological adjustment. *Journal of Interpersonal Violence, 14*, 184–207.

Rodriguez, N., Ryan, S., Rowan, A. B., & Foy, D. W. (1999). Posttraumatic stress disorder in a clinical sample of adult survivors of childhood sexual abuse. *Child Abuse and Neglect, 20*(10), 943–952.

Rosario, M., Schrimshaw, E. W., & Hunter, J. (2006). A model of sexual risk behaviors among young gay and bisexual men: Longitudinal associations of mental health, substance abuse, and the coming-out process. *AIDS Education and Prevention, 18*, 444–460.

Rothman, E. F., Exner, D., & Baughman, A. (2011). The prevalence of sexual assault against people who identify as gay, lesbian, or bisexual in the United States: A systematic review. *Trauma, Violence, and Abuse, 12*(2), 55–66.

Rumstein-McKean, O., & Hunsley, J. (2001). Interpersonal and family functioning of female survivors of childhood sexual abuse. *Clinical Psychology Review, 21*, 471–490.

Sansonnet-Hayden, H., Haley, G., Marriage, K., & Fine, S. (1987). Sexual abuse and psychopathology in hospitalized adolescents. *Journal of the American Academy of Child and Adolescent Psychiatry, 26*, 753–757.

Senn, T. E., Carey, M. P., & Vanable, P. A. (2008). Child and adolescent sexual abuse and subsequent sexual risk behavior: Evidence from controlled studies, methodological critique, and suggestions for research. *Clinical Psychology Review, 28*, 711–735.

Siegel, J. M., Sorenson, S. B., Golding, J. M., Burnam, M. A., & Stein, J. A. (1987). The prevalence of childhood sexual assault: The Los Angeles epidemiologic catchment area project. *American Journal of Epidemiology, 126*, 1141–1153.

Sikkema, K. J., Wilson, P. A., Hansen, N. B., Kochman, A., Neufel, S., Ghebremichael, M. S., & Kershaw, T. (2008). Effects of a coping intervention on transmission risk behavior among people living with HIV/AIDS and a history of childhood sexual abuse. *Journal of Acquired Immune Deficiency Syndromes and Human Retrovirology, 47*, 506–513.

Spies, G., Afifi, T. O., Archibald, S. L., Fennema-Notestine, C., Sareen, J., & Seedat, S. (2012). Mental health outcomes in HIV and childhood maltreatment: A systematic review. *Systematic Reviews, 1*, 30. doi:10.1186/2046-4053-1-30

Stermac, L., Sheridan, P. M., Davidson, A., & Dunn, S. (1996). Sexual assault of adult males. *Journal of Interpersonal Violence, 11*(1), 52–64.

Stevenson, M. (2000). Public policy, homosexuality and the sexual coercion of children. *Journal of Psychology and Human Sexuality, 12*(4), 1–19.

Stoltenborgh, M., van IJzendoorn, M. H., Euser, E. M., & Bakermans-Kranenburg, M. J. (2011). A global perspective on child sexual abuse: Meta-analysis of prevalence around the world. *Child Maltreatment, 16*, 79–101.

Strathdee, S. A., Hogg, R. S., Martindale, S. L., Cornelisse, P. G. A., Craib, K. J. P., Montaner, J. S. G., ... Schecter, M. T. (1998). Determinants of sexual risk-taking among young HIV-negative gay and bisexual men. *Journal of Acquired Immune Deficiency Syndromes and Human Retrovirology, 19*, 61–66.

Tomeo, M., Temple, D., Anderson, S., & Kotler, D. (2001). Comparative data of childhood and adolescence molestation in heterosexual and homosexual persons. *Archives of Sexual Behavior, 30*, 535–541.

Tremblay, C., Hebert, M., & Piche, C. (1999). Coping strategies and social support as mediators of consequences in child sexual abuse victims. *Child Abuse and Neglect, 23*, 929–945.

Trickett, P. K., Noll, J. G., Reiffman, A., & Putman, F. W. (2001). Variants of intrafamilial sexual abuse experience: Implications for short- and long-term development. *Development and Psychopathology, 13*, 1001–1019.

US Department of Health and Human Serivces. (2011). *Child Maltreatment*, 2010.

Van Beneden, C. A., O'Brien, K., Modesitt, S., Yusem, S., Rose, A., & Fleming, D. (2002). Sexual behaviors in an urban bathhouse 15 years into the HIV epidemic. *Journal of Acquired Immune Deficiency Syndromes and Human Retrovirology, 30*(5), 522–526.

Walker, E. A., Katon, W. J., Roy-Byrne, P. P., Jemelka, R. P., & Russo, J. (1993). Histories of sexual victimization in patients with irritable bowel syndrome or inflammatory bowel disease. *American Journal of Psychiatry, 150*, 1502–1506.

Welles, S. L., Baker, A. C., Miner, M. H., Brennan, D. J., Jacoby, S., & Rosser, B. R. (2009). History of childhood sexual abuse and unsafe anal intercourse in a 6-city study of HIV positive men who have sex with men. *American Journal of Public Health, 99*(6), 1079–1086.

Wendt, E., Hildingh, C., Lidell, E., Westerstahl, A., Baigi, A., & Marklund, B. (2007). Young women's sexual health and their views on dialogue with health professionals. *Acta Obstetricia et Gynecologica Scandinavica, 86*, 590–595.

Whiffen, V. E., & MacIntosh, H. B. (2005). Interpersonal and family functioning of female survivors of childhood sexual abuse. *Clinical Psychology Review, 21*, 471–490.

Williams, J. K., Kisler, K., Glover, D., & Sciolla, A. (2011). Exploring childhood sexual experiences and vulnerability to intimate partner violence among African American MSMW: Was that abuse or love? In L. E. Hynes (Ed.), *Sexual abuse: Types, signs and treatments*. Hauppauge, NY: Nova Science Publishers.

Williams, J. K., Wyatt, G. E., Rivkin, I., Ramamurthi, H. C., Li, X., & Liu, H. (2008). Risk reduction for HIV positive African American and Latino men with histories of childhood sexual abuse. *Archives of Sexual Behavior, 37*, 763–772.

Williams, J. K., Wyatt, G. E., & Wingood, G. (2010). The Four Cs of HIV prevention with African Americans: Crisis, condoms, culture and community. *Current Report, 7*, 185–193.

Williams, M. L., Timpson, S., Klovdahl, A., Bowen, A. M., Ross, M. W., & Keel, K. B. (2003). HIV risk among a sample of drug using male sex workers. *AIDS, 17*(9), 1402–1404.

Wilson, D. (2010). Health consequences of childhood sexual abuse. *Perspectives in Psychiatric Care, 46*(1), 56–64.

Wilson, H., & Widom, C. (2010). Does physical abuse, sexual abuse, or neglect in childhood increase the likelihood of same-sex sexual relationships and cohabitation? A prospective 30-year follow-up. *Archives of Sexual Behavior, 39*, 63–74.

Wright, D. (2001). *Illusions of intimacy*. Binghamton, NY: Haworth Press.

Zierler, S., Feingold, L., Laufer, D., Velentgas, P., Kantrowitz-Gordon, I., & Mayer, K. (1991). Adult survivors of childhood sexual abuse and subsequent risk of HIV infection. *American Journal of Public Health, 81*, 572–575.

Part II
Prevention

Chapter 6
Comprehensive Prevention with HIV Positive Gay Men

Michael J. Stirratt and Cynthia I. Grossman

Gay men have always been leaders in HIV prevention and care. Gay men were among the first to recognize and respond to the US HIV epidemic in the early 1980s, as it became clear that an ever-growing number of gay friends, neighbors, and sexual and romantic partners were dying of a mysterious, acute illness (Weissman & Weber, 2011). Even before the identification of HIV, gay men were already conducting grassroots community organizing in response to the illness, providing care and support to individuals who were ill, and alerting others to this grave and growing concern (Trapence et al., 2012; Weissman & Weber, 2011). After the identification of HIV and its mode of sexual transmission, the subsequent wide-scale adoption of condom-protected sexual behavior by gay men in response to the HIV/AIDS epidemic represented one of the most rapid and dramatic changes in health behavior ever documented in public health research (Ekstrand & Coates, 1990; Stall, Coates, & Hoff, 1988).

HIV positive gay men have long played a particularly important role in responding to the epidemic. The Denver Principles, articulated in 1983 by a group of HIV positive gay men living with HIV, established the conceptual foundation for the civil rights of HIV positive individuals and their active engagement in HIV care and prevention ("The Denver Principles," 1983; Wright, 2013). Early in the epidemic, HIV positive gay men helped to lead and conduct vigorous advocacy for HIV treatment, helping to catalyze changes in NIH research funding and the FDA drug

M.J. Stirratt (✉)
Division of AIDS Research, National Institute of Mental Health (NIH/NIMH),
Bethesda, MD, USA
e-mail: stirrattm@mail.nih.gov

C.I. Grossman
FasterCures, a center of the Milken Institute, Washington, DC, USA

Division of AIDS Research, National Institute of Mental Health (NIH/NIMH),
Bethesda, MD, USA

© Springer Science+Business Media LLC 2017   121
L. Wilton (ed.), *Understanding Prevention for HIV Positive Gay Men*,
DOI 10.1007/978-1-4419-0203-0_6

regulatory approval process (FasterCures & HCM Strategies, 2011; France, 2016). It has been argued that "development of and access to highly active antiretroviral therapy might not have arisen at all, or at least it would have been much slower and many millions more people would have died, without the advocacy of huge numbers of gay men in the USA and Europe" (Trapence et al., 2012). HIV positive gay men have also contributed important leadership and innovations to HIV prevention research. Research studies indicate that most HIV positive gay men consider HIV prevention as a high priority in their lives (Courtenay-Quirk, Wolitski, Hoff, Parsons, & Seropositive Urban Mens Study, 2003) and adopt reduced-risk practices following HIV diagnosis (Marks, Crepaz, & Janssen, 2006). Concepts such as HIV transmission risk reduction through viral suppression from antiretroviral therapy (ART) surfaced among HIV positive gay men long before receiving validation through controlled scientific research (Cox, Beauchemin, & Allard, 2004; McConnell, Bragg, Shiboski, & Grant, 2010; Remien & Borkowski, 2005).

These achievements have occurred despite the many burdens and challenges faced by gay men in general and HIV positive gay men in particular. Across the developmental spectrum, gay men must navigate their sexual experiences and identities in a context that is, at best, not fully inclusive of their identities and, at worst, hostile and stigmatizing. There is a growing appreciation that significant health disparities exist among the gay community including higher rates of depression, trauma, childhood sexual abuse, discrimination, and physical abuse when compared to their heterosexual counterparts (Mustanski, Newcomb, Du Bois, Garcia, & Grov, 2011; Parsons, Grov, & Golub, 2012; Williams et al., 2008). For HIV positive gay men, other life challenges include homophobia, HIV stigma from other men, intimate partner violence, homelessness, and social isolation (Parsons et al., 2012). It should therefore come as no surprise that men who identify as gay and the wider group of men who have sex with men (MSM) have long borne a disproportionate burden of the US HIV epidemic.

Turning the tide on HIV among US gay men and MSM will require further effort. MSM accounted for 83% of new HIV infections among men and 67% of new infections overall in 2014 (Centers for Disease Control & Prevention, 2015). MSM are between 38 and 75 times more likely to have HIV infection than other groups of men and women (Purcell et al., 2012). The number of HIV positive gay men in the USA has been growing over time, since new men continue to become HIV infected, and ART extends the life expectancies of individuals with access to medical care. Early decreases in HIV incidence among US gay men foundered in the 1990s. HIV incidence among MSM grew 6% between 2005 and 2014 and showed strong racial/ethnic and age disparities, with an 87% increase in new HIV diagnoses among young African American MSM (Centers for Disease Control & Prevention, 2015). A large study which followed nearly 2500 Black MSM for 1 year (the HIV Prevention Trials Network Protocol 061) found an annual HIV incidence rate of 2.8% among study participants, and the incidence rate was double (5.9%) among Black MSM under age 30 (Koblin et al., 2013). These data indicate that there is a large and growing group of HIV positive gay men in the USA, and that this group is characterized by racial/ethnic disparities.

Decades into the epidemic, it is clear that HIV prevention and care for gay men stands as a paramount public health priority, and that any comprehensive approach to HIV prevention must include a focus on HIV positive individuals (Millett et al., 2010). This chapter will describe a comprehensive prevention package for HIV positive gay men in the USA, as informed by scientific research with gay men, MSM, and HIV positive individuals more generally. To guide our approach, we identify and describe two concepts—combination prevention and sexual health—from which a comprehensive prevention package must be derived. A comprehensive prevention package for HIV positive gay men should encompass integrated efforts to encourage and advance: (a) the identification of men living with undiagnosed HIV infection, to facilitate access and uptake of quality medical care; (b) HIV treatment engagement, adherence, and retention to improve clinical outcomes and reduce HIV transmission through "treatment as prevention;" (c) behavioral risk reduction, as supported by counseling and peer-based programs grounded in a holistic sexual health framework; (d) efforts to address syndemic factors such as sexually transmitted infections (STIs), mental health, and substance abuse; (e) partner-related strategies, including use of pre-exposure prophylaxis (PrEP) by serodiscordant relationship partners where appropriate; and (f) community mobilization and empowerment strategies, including efforts to address large-scale social, structural, and legal/policy determinants, such as HIV stigma, homophobia, racism, and civil rights. While ambitious and broad-reaching, our hope is that prevention interventions can be developed, implemented, and sustained at every level, from the individual to the wider community, in order to address the sexual health needs and advance the HIV prevention interests of HIV positive gay men. We conclude that substantial gaps in the evidence base for such an approach remain, and must be addressed through further research and advocacy conducted in partnership with HIV positive gay men.

Setting a Historical Context: Toward Comprehensive HIV Prevention

HIV prevention activities with HIV positive gay men represent an important component of a comprehensive approach to HIV prevention more broadly, but this was not always the case. The involvement of HIV positive gay men in prevention initiatives has greatly shifted over time, and "prevention with positives" has moved from being unthinkable, in the absence of effective treatment, to a key component of a larger, comprehensive HIV prevention agenda. Early in the epidemic, there was scant attention to involving HIV positive gay men in prevention because individuals living with HIV were acutely ill and in dire need of effective treatment. Prevention messages were largely directed at generic audiences of gay men and generally exhorted condom use without consideration or attention to HIV serostatus. Further, there were concerns about developing prevention programs that targeted HIV positive gay men, for fear that these efforts would further stigmatize and shame these men.

The development of combination ART represented an important turning point for advancing prevention activities directed specifically to HIV positive gay men. With the availability of effective HIV treatment, HIV positive gay men began to live longer and had improved quality of life. This brought increased attention to their sexual and romantic lives, but the evidence base of effective prevention strategies was lacking. The 1996 International AIDS conference in Vancouver, British Columbia, marked a shift among the scientific community toward a greater emphasis on helping people living with HIV access medical care and prevention. The US Centers for Disease Control and Prevention (CDC) later launched the Serostatus Approach to Fighting the HIV Epidemic (SAFE), an approach that involves voluntary HIV testing, medical evaluation, treatment according to guidelines, and prevention services (Janssen et al., 2001). Today, there are ever-growing efforts to target prevention to meet the needs of people living with HIV and, importantly, address the epidemic among gay men. The development of the first US National HIV/AIDS Strategy (NHAS) was a historic milestone (Millett et al., 2010; White House Office of National AIDS Policy, 2010). This landmark policy document and its subsequent update (White House Office of National AIDS Policy, 2015) explicitly encompass prevention with positives and the needs of communities most impacted by HIV, including specific mention of gay men. In addition, the CDC guidance on HIV Prevention with Persons Living with HIV, first released in 2003, was updated and expanded in 2014 (Centers for Disease Control and Prevention, 2014). These developments and documents reflect how HIV positive individuals have moved from a position of silence to a position of salience in US HIV prevention initiatives over the course of the epidemic.

While a prevention approach tailored to the needs of people living with HIV is important, there is general appreciation that a comprehensive prevention approach must be just that—comprehensive—by including efforts to work with all people affected by HIV, and not just people infected with HIV. Including gay men with and without HIV infection in comprehensive HIV prevention should be more effective from a combination prevention standpoint, and recognizes that many drivers of transmission risk are common to both groups. A comprehensive approach involving those at risk for HIV as well as those living with HIV may also importantly help to unite, rather than divide, communities in addressing the HIV/AIDS epidemic, by signaling that these groups share a common interest and responsibility for such action. Developing all-inclusive combination prevention may additionally help to lessen stigma associated with HIV, as the comprehensive approach underscores the importance of having all gay men to recognize, discuss, and address the ongoing HIV epidemic in this wider community.

Touchstones for Prevention with HIV Positive Gay Men: Combination Prevention and Sexual Health

Two critical overarching concepts for current and future prevention initiatives with HIV positive gay men are combination prevention and sexual health. The concept of combination prevention maintains that multiple, multi-modal approaches across every level of intervention must be undertaken to effectively address the HIV epidemic (Bekker, Beyrer, & Quinn, 2012; Coates, Richter, & Caceres, 2008; Kurth, Celum, Baeten, Vermund, & Wasserheit, 2011). The concept is rooted in an analogy to combination ART. Just as combination therapy employs multiple drugs to intercept HIV at various junctures in its replication life cycle, combination prevention employs multiple modalities to interrupt HIV transmission at various junctures (Coates et al., 2008; Kurth et al., 2011). A combination prevention approach would therefore seek to deploy a constellation of integrated behavioral, biomedical, and structural approaches to address the HIV epidemic.

A combination prevention approach accomplishes several aims. First, it recognizes that the HIV epidemic is sustained by many complex and interlocking factors that require a multifactorial response (Coates et al., 2008). Second, it recognizes that many prevention strategies are only partially effective, and that their use in combination may be required for maximal impact (Bekker et al., 2012). Combination prevention can also encompass prevention strategies for which the evidence base is limited. As noted by Coates et al. (2008), "failure to show that a specific strategy reduces HIV infection does not render it useless in a comprehensive programme or a multilevel behavioural strategy for HIV prevention. The combination of strategies might be relevant to the end result" (pp. 672–673). Finally, combination prevention brings attention to the behavioral and social processes that are integral to the effective uptake and use for biomedical prevention strategies.

A different but complementary touchstone to combination prevention is that of sexual health promotion. In the context of a strong and sustained public health focus on HIV prevention among gay men, sexual behavior has seemingly become synonymous with sexual risk behavior. There is a growing appreciation of the need for clinicians, providers, and researchers to recognize the entirety of men's sexual health needs, and not exclusively those focused on disease prevention (Beyrer et al., 2012; Mayer et al., 2012; Rausch, Dieffenbach, Cheever, & Fenton, 2011; Sandfort & Ehrhardt, 2004). The sexual health concept recognizes that sex and sexual relationships can play a variety of meaningful roles in the lives of gay men (Halkitis & Wilton, 2005). It therefore encompasses constructive elements of sexuality such as pleasure, desire, and intimacy (Coleman, 2011; Goldhammer & Mayer, 2011; Sandfort & Ehrhardt, 2004). By seeking to acknowledge and integrate the physical, emotional, behavioral, social, and cultural aspects of men's sexual lives (Coleman, 2011; Wolitski & Fenton, 2011), sexual health promotion represents a holistic approach that encompasses not only freedom from the ill effects of disease but also freedom from fear, shame, and discrimination from others (Coleman, 2011; Wolitski & Fenton, 2011). Such an approach will not only address men's physical health in terms of HIV or other STIs, but also their mental health and healthy social relationships with other individuals and society.

By implicating the wider context of sexual and emotional relationships, including those with families, community, and society, the sexual health concept suggests that we must also work to address the advancement of civil and human rights when working with gay men (Coleman, 2011; Sandfort & Ehrhardt, 2004). This includes efforts to address the cultural stigma associated with gay identity and behavior

(Goldhammer & Mayer, 2011), as well as broad-scale social forces and policy structures that drive social marginalization and health inequities among gay men, such as racism and prejudice (Ayala, Bingham, Kim, Wheeler, & Millett, 2012; Choi, Paul, Ayala, Boylan, & Gregorich, 2013; Wilton, 2009; Wolitski & Fenton, 2011). Advancements in these wider contexts will help to sustain and reinforce sexual health, and in turn, healthy sexual practices.

Combination prevention and sexual health approaches share important connections. Both concepts harken to the need for multilevel and multicomponent strategies that attend to social relationships and cultural contexts. Combination prevention approaches recognize that there is no singular tool that will eliminate HIV transmission at present, and a sexual health framework encourages efforts to address multiple needs beyond disease prevention. These two touchstones therefore suggest that prevention with HIV positive gay men should promote physical and mental health as a foundational effort, and then extend beyond individuals and relationships to address wider community and social/legal environments designed to facilitate and sustain healthy practices and outcomes. Such an understanding also corresponds to current understandings about HIV risk, which increasingly underscore the concept of HIV risk at the community level (Das et al., 2010). HIV transmission is not strictly the product of particular sexual practices, but is importantly informed by complex contextual determinants that increase or decrease risk, including biologic susceptibility, STIs other than HIV, social and sexual mixing patterns, and community level HIV prevalence, incidence, and viral load.

A Comprehensive Prevention Package with HIV Positive Gay Men

We have sought to distill the many approaches that may be brought to bear on HIV prevention with HIV positive gay men into four primary elements: Timely diagnosis of HIV infection paired with strong HIV treatment engagement and adherence; the promotion of individual-level risk reduction through counseling interventions, STI treatment, and efforts to address psychosocial comorbidities; partner-related prevention strategies including PrEP; and enhanced community empowerment and structural approaches. Following from the combination prevention principle and sexual health concept, these interrelated approaches would aim to provide comprehensive prevention with HIV positive MSM across multiple levels of intervention, and may synergize in a manner that simultaneously strengthens sexual health and prevention outcomes. The idea is that no single approach is sufficient to stem the tide of HIV infection, and that any efforts to address the HIV prevention and sexual health needs of an individual will be better sustained and if appropriate social and structural supports are in place.

Identifying HIV Infections and Strengthening the HIV Care Continuum

A comprehensive prevention strategy should encompass efforts to identify gay men with undiagnosed infection and to strengthen participation of HIV positive gay men in the HIV care continuum. In the current era of ART treatment, individuals who receive timely HIV diagnosis and appropriate medical care are projected to maintain life expectancies that approach those of individuals without infection (Nakagawa, May, & Phillips, 2012). This is a profound advance, when contrasted with the prognosis for individuals in the earliest days of the HIV/AIDS epidemic. The lifesaving benefits of ART fully justify the need for HIV testing and treatment initiatives among gay men. The fundamental importance of HIV treatment in extending and improving quality of life among infected individuals is only reinforced by the recognition that treatment can additionally confer benefits for HIV prevention.

Evidence that HIV treatment can confer a preventive effect is now definitive, at least in the context of heterosexual transmission. Early observational studies of heterosexual HIV serodiscordant couples indicated that lower viral loads in blood plasma correspond to reduced HIV transmission (Quinn et al., 2000). Researchers in San Francisco and British Columbia subsequently linked population-level increases in ART and decreases in viral load to reductions in local HIV incidence (Das et al., 2010; Montaner et al., 2010). The landmark HPTN 052 trial has now provided direct evidence that viral suppression through ART can produce a strong preventive effect (Cohen et al., 2011, 2016). The trial was conducted with HIV serodiscordant couples in nine countries, and the vast majority of participants (97%) were heterosexual couples. HIV positive partners in these relationships were randomized to either start ART immediately or delay ART until indicated by concurrent treatment guidelines (CD4 count below 250 or development of an AIDS-related illness). All participants received intensive behavioral risk reduction counseling, free condoms, treatment for STIs, and monitoring of treatment complications and viral load. Rates of ART adherence and viral suppression in the trial were high. The final analysis of the trial determined that provision of early ART treatment reduced the risk of HIV transmission within the couple by 93% when compared to delayed treatment (Cohen et al., 2016). This landmark finding has been widely hailed as an exceptional breakthrough in HIV prevention science, and it has importantly catalyzed interest in implementing ART not only for the sake of treatment but also for prevention.

The available evidence supports the "treatment as prevention" concept in gay men, as well. The PARTNER Study is following an observational cohort of heterosexual and gay male HIV serodiscordant couples who have condomless sex and in which the HIV+ partner maintains viral suppression through ART. No within-couple HIV transmissions have been observed to date (Rodger et al., 2016). The PARTNER

Study and HPTN 052 make a compelling case for furthering prevention goals by improving HIV care outcomes. We further note that comprehensive HIV care can extend beyond ART treatment to include STI diagnosis and treatment, mental health and substance abuse treatment, and sexual risk reduction counseling—all of which can contribute to HIV prevention. These considerations join the treatment-as-prevention concept to collectively underscore the importance of facilitating participation of HIV positive MSM in primary medical care to advance prevention.

The achievement of sustained viral suppression requires most HIV positive individuals to successfully negotiate the HIV care continuum, and this presents multiple challenges that can compromise treatment outcomes and attendant prevention efforts. The HIV care continuum flows across the key junctures of HIV diagnosis, linkage to primary HIV medical care, retention in medical care, voluntary ART initiation, and adherence to ART regimens. Unfortunately, notable percentages of HIV positive individuals are lost at each point, creating an HIV treatment "cascade" (Centers for Disease Control & Prevention, 2011a; Gardner, McLees, Steiner, del Rio, & Burman, 2011; Marks, Gardner, Craw, & Crepaz, 2010). Put another way, not all individuals with HIV infection are diagnosed, not all diagnosed individuals are linked to care, not all individuals linked to care are retained, not all retained individuals initiate ART, and not all ART initiators are adherent. As a result of these gaps in the treatment cascade, it has been estimated that only 25% of HIV positive individuals living in the USA maintain viral suppression (Hall et al., 2013; Skarbinski et al., 2015). Additionally, the vast majority of HIV transmissions (91.5%) have been attributed to individuals with undiagnosed HIV infection or those who have been HIV diagnosed but not retained in care (Skarbinski et al., 2015). These challenges associated with the HIV care continuum are evident among HIV positive gay men, and they require us to address each point in the treatment cascade in order to optimize the contribution of treatment to prevention in this important population.

HIV Testing and Diagnosis

Diagnosis of HIV infection represents the first essential step toward engaging HIV positive gay men in lifesaving treatment and preventive programs. Despite increases in HIV testing among MSM in recent years (Centers for Disease Control and Prevention, 2016), undiagnosed HIV infection remains a problem. Surveillance data from 20 US metropolitan areas indicate that 34% of HIV positive MSM are unaware of their infection, and these percentages are notably higher among MSM of color and young MSM (Wejnert et al., 2013) The barriers to HIV testing and timely HIV diagnosis among MSM are complex and varied. Fear and denial about possible seropositivity is a central concern, as well as lack of perceived risk or gay identification, and concerns about potential sexual identity disclosure (Millett et al., 2011; Nelson et al., 2010). Nonetheless, one study found that Black MSM who identified as gay and who had disclosed their sexuality to their health care provider were actually more likely to have undiagnosed HIV infection than those who had not, highlighting a failure on the part of clinicians to offer HIV testing to this high-risk group (Millett et al., 2011).

These collective considerations have led the CDC to recommend at least biannual HIV and STI testing for sexually active gay men (Centers for Disease Control & Prevention, 2011b), and the updated NHAS specifies the goal of improving the proportion of people living with HIV who know their serostatus to at least 90% (White House Office of National AIDS Policy, 2015). Some strategies have shown promise for improving HIV testing uptake and identification of undiagnosed infections among MSM, including opt-out HIV testing in STI clinics and providing HIV testing in community venues (Lorenc et al., 2011). New innovations in HIV tests may also help reduce undiagnosed infections. The US FDA approved a rapid home-based HIV antibody test in 2012, which may offer increased testing convenience and privacy to those who can afford the cost. Research with MSM has found strong interest in rapid home tests for personal use and even for screening of sexual partners (Carballo-Dieguez, Frasca, Dolezal, & Balan, 2012). Until we can make further progress in the timely diagnosis of HIV infections among MSM, combination prevention efforts focused on HIV positive MSM will be substantially hindered.

Engagement and Retention in HIV Care

Rapid linkage to HIV primary medical care and sustained retention in care by HIV positive gay men should improve individual treatment outcomes as well as community-level prevention. Failure to adequately engage HIV positive gay men in care interrupts the HIV care continuum and compromises the preventive effects that treatment may confer (Gardner et al., 2011). Poor engagement in HIV primary care also reduces the access of HIV positive gay men to comprehensive care including screening and treatment for STIs, mental health disorders, and risk reduction counseling (Christopoulos, Das, & Colfax, 2011). Rates of linkage to care and retention in care among US HIV positive individuals are generally suboptimal (Gardner et al., 2011; Hall et al., 2012; Marks et al., 2010). The limited data available suggests that HIV positive MSM may have slightly favorable rates of linkage and retention relative to other US HIV-infected populations (Christopoulos et al., 2011). Nonetheless, an observational study of all known HIV patients in South Carolina over a 3-year period found significantly greater delays in entering care among MSM relative to heterosexuals (Tripathi et al., 2011). Important age and racial/ethnic disparities in care engagement and retention among US HIV positive MSM are also evident in that younger men and people of color are less likely to engage and persist in HIV medical care than older or White MSM (Hall et al., 2012). Determinants of care engagement and retention include individual factors (e.g., mental health, substance abuse, and sexual identity development), enabling factors (e.g., housing, income, and insurance), and structural factors (e.g., clinic location, hours, and support services) (Christopoulos et al., 2011).

The NHAS specifies goals for improving rapid linkage to HIV care among newly diagnosed individuals (White House Office of National AIDS Policy, 2015), but relatively few proven interventions exist to address this goal among HIV patient populations or gay men in particular (Higa, Marks, Crepaz, Liau, & Lyles, 2012). A randomized controlled trial testing the efficacy of a case management approach among newly diagnosed individuals (titled "ARTAS") demonstrated modest improvements in HIV care linkage and early care retention (Craw et al., 2008; Gardner et al., 2005). A clinic-based intervention that reinforced the importance of regular medical appointment attendance through posters, brochures, and brief messages delivered by clinicians and staff showed small but significant improvements in retention (Gardner et al., 2012). In terms of efforts directly focused on HIV positive gay men or MSM, the Health Research and Services Administration (HRSA) supported the "YMSM of Color Initiative" to address the importance of linking, engaging, and retaining young HIV positive gay men of color in HIV care (Hightow-Weidman, Jones, Wohl, et al., 2011; Magnus et al., 2010). The initiative developed age and culturally tailored demonstration projects at eight sites to link and engage newly diagnosed young MSM of color ages 16–24, and to reengage those lost to follow-up. Sites employed a variety of approaches, including intensive case management, support groups and educational programs, and youth-directed community-based outreach. High rates of care linkage and retention were reported across the programs (Hightow-Weidman, Jones, Wohl, et al., 2011; Magnus et al., 2010), indicating that young MSM of color can be successfully engaged and sustained in care through culturally competent programs.

ART Initiation and Adherence

ART use and adherence could further optimize treatment and prevention outcomes among HIV positive gay men. While treatment guidelines now recommend ART upon HIV diagnosis (Labarga, 2012), the timing of ART initiation remains a voluntary choice that must be made by the patient in consultation with a medical provider. Research indicates that not all patients who qualify for ART are receiving it. In a cohort study funded by HRSA which enrolled young MSM of color at eight sites across the USA, nearly half of the men who were eligible for ART had not initiated ART (Hightow-Weidman, Jones, Phillips, et al., 2011). A large-scale cross-sectional survey conducted through the CDC-funded National HIV Behavioral Surveillance System also found that, among MSM diagnosed with HIV, Black MSM were less likely than other MSM to be on ART (Oster et al., 2011). In light of the preventive effects of ART, such disparities in ART use may be contributing to disparities in new HIV infections (Oster et al., 2011).

ART adherence is essential to achieving viral load suppression, and viral suppression represents both the goal of HIV treatment and the fundamental driver of the strong preventive effect observed in the HPTN 052 trial. Poor ART adherence remains an important determinant of mortality among patients taking current regimens (Lima et al., 2009) and can additionally undermine the preventive benefits of treatment. Meta-analyses have found that ARV adherence is suboptimal among large proportions of US and North American HIV patients (Mills et al., 2006; Ortego et al., 2011). Population-level data indicate that more than one-third (38%) of US patients in HIV care lack durable viral suppression over a 2-year period, and that many spend substantial time at high viral load levels that could increase the risk of HIV transmission (Crepaz et al., 2016). There is some evidence indicating that average ARV adherence levels may be superior among HIV positive MSM as a whole in comparison to other populations (Ortego et al., 2011). Research has nonetheless identified racial and ethnic disparities in ARV adherence among HIV positive gay men and among patient populations more generally (Oh et al., 2009; Osborn, Paasche-Orlow, Davis, & Wolf, 2007; Simoni et al., 2012), indicating lower adherence among African Americans and Latinos relative to Whites. The reasons for these findings remain unclear, but research has linked reduced levels of ART adherence to greater experiences of racial prejudice and discrimination among African American HIV positive MSM (Bogart, Wagner, Galvan, & Klein, 2010), as well as to treatment conspiracy beliefs and treatment distrust (Bogart, Galvan, Wagner, & Klein, 2011; Bogart, Wagner, Galvan, & Banks, 2010) among African American HIV positive men, and to reduced health literacy (Osborn et al., 2007) among African American HIV positive individuals more generally.

Numerous programs to support and improve ARV adherence have been found efficacious and can help achieve viral load suppression (Amico, Harman, & Johnson, 2006; Simoni et al., 2006; Thompson et al., 2012). One of the first ARV adherence interventions to be proven effective was tested with a sample of HIV positive gay men attending an outpatient clinic specializing in HIV care for this population. The program, entitled "Life Steps," comprised a single session of cognitive-behavioral adherence counseling, self-monitoring of adherence, and brief telephone follow-up (Safren et al., 2001). Other ART adherence support programs have been tested in general US HIV clinic populations, where gay HIV positive men frequently form large components of the research samples. Examples of effective ART adherence programs include peer support and electronic reminders to encourage adherence (Simoni et al., 2009; Yard, Huh, King, & Simoni, 2011), and counseling HIV serodiscordant couples to encourage mutual care-taking and ARV adherence in the HIV positive relationship partner (Remien et al., 2005; Remien et al., 2006). More recently, ARV adherence support programs specifically tailored to HIV positive gay men are emerging, and efforts to leverage technology and incorporate peer support appear promising. Pilot trials conducted with US HIV positive gay men found that tailored SMS text messaging improved self-reported adherence and clinical outcomes (Lewis et al., 2012), and online social networking sites for HIV positive gay men can foster social support and improved adherence (Horvath et al., 2013). Programs to encourage and sustain ARV adherence among HIV positive gay men should be integrated with wider efforts to enhance HIV positive gay men's participation across the entire HIV treatment cascade—in the name of optimizing both treatment and prevention outcomes.

Addressing Individual Risk Reduction, STIs, and Comorbidities

In addition to the prevention benefits of ART that can be achieved by strengthening the HIV treatment cascade, a second important aspect of combination prevention with HIV positive gay men includes addressing those individual risk factors that impact risk behavior and health outcomes. Many HIV positive gay men could benefit from risk reduction counseling that addresses risk behavior, as well as screening and treatment for STIs and comorbidities such as mental illness and substance use (Cohen et al., 1997; Marks et al., 2006; Safren, Blashill, & O'Cleirigh, 2011). Most incident infections arise from cases where individuals are undiagnosed or poorly engaged in HIV care (Skarbinski et al., 2015), so efforts to address sexual risk reduction may help prevent HIV transmission in cases where HIV care engagement and viral suppression are lacking. Decreasing STI acquisition and addressing mental illness and substance use concerns through adequate screening and treatment would additionally improve the overall health of HIV positive gay men, thereby facilitating and supporting risk reduction. As previously mentioned, gay men have been at the forefront of behavior change in response to the HIV epidemic, and most HIV positive persons change their sexual risk behavior upon learning their diagnosis (Marks et al., 2006). However, HIV prevention requires sustained behavior change over the course of one's lifetime and not all behaviors confer equal risk for HIV transmission (Baggaley, White, & Boily, 2010; Nakagawa, Lodwick, et al., 2012; Royce, Sena, Cates, & Cohen, 1997). The development of effective behavior change interventions, particularly for HIV positive gay men, has been challenging and arguably raises more questions than answers (Grossman et al., 2011). What behaviors should interventions target for HIV positive gay men, e.g., increased condom use, serosorting, and/or medication adherence? If condoms are not used, how much of a concern should STIs be for HIV positive gay men and their partners? What is the best way to address mental illness and substance use, especially among HIV positive gay men?

Despite these challenges, meta-analyses of behavioral interventions have clearly demonstrated that individual and group based counseling can effectively reduce risk behavior, defined as increased condom use and decreased condomless anal intercourse with a serostatus negative or unknown partner (Crepaz et al., 2006; Holtgrave & Curran, 2006; Johnson et al., 2008). A meta-analysis also demonstrated that behavioral prevention interventions with HIV positive individuals significantly reduce condomless sex (OR 0.057, 95% CI, 0.40–0.82) and acquisition of STIs (OR, 0.20; 95% CI, 0.05–0.73) (Crepaz et al., 2006). The observed impact of prevention counseling on STIs is particularly important, given the disproportionate rates of STIs among gay men and MSM (Purcell et al., 2012) and the potential for STIs to facilitate HIV transmission. While the Crepaz meta-analysis included 12 studies of prevention interventions with HIV positive individuals, only five of the studies showed significant effects on transmission risk outcomes (Crepaz et al., 2006). There may be several reasons some prevention interventions for HIV positive persons have failed to demonstrate efficacy. Randomized trials of prevention interventions that employ a robust attention control comparison arm often demonstrate significant behavioral changes in the control group, compromising the ability to find a preventive effect associated with the intervention. Trials lacking a robust and meaningful control condition, however, can have problems with retention. Furthermore, few prevention interventions with HIV positive individuals have demonstrated lasting behavior change, with effects rarely seen beyond a 6-month follow-up time point. The problem of creating sustained behavioral change represents a challenge for all forms of behavioral intervention, more generally.

Research suggests that another challenge to evaluating the effectiveness of prevention interventions for HIV positive gay men and MSM is the fact that many behavioral interventions address knowledge, attitudes, and motivations associated with HIV risk behavior while either screening out participants with mental health and substance use problems or referring participants for treatment outside of the intervention (Safren, Blashill, et al., 2011). Studies show that there is a synergistic negative effect of psychosocial and substance use problems on sexual risk behavior among MSM (Mimiaga et al., 2015; Stall et al., 2003) and also specifically among HIV positive MSM (O'Cleirigh, Mimiaga, Safren, Stall, & Mayer, 2010). In addition, depression and post-traumatic stress negatively impacts health care utilization among HIV positive gay men (O'Cleirigh, Skeer, Mayer, & Safren, 2009). Safren and colleagues tried to remedy some of the previous limitations to behavioral interventions by designing a multi-session (5 sessions) intervention that included modules on substance use and mental health delivered by a medical social worker (Safren, O'Cleirigh, et al., 2011). The randomized study showed a decrease in transmission risk behavior among study participants in both the intervention arm and the comparison arm (treatment as usual with assessment). While there was not a significant difference by treatment arm, there was a significant difference among those who screened in for depression at baseline. Among those who reported depressive symptoms as baseline, those assigned to the intervention condition significantly reduced their transmission risk compared to those assigned to the control condition. This result was not found for those who did not report depression at baseline or among those who reported substance use at baseline. This finding suggests that addressing multiple factors, such as depression, is critical to demonstrating reductions in risk in a behavioral trial.

The Healthy Living Project, an intensive behaviorally based intervention for HIV positive men and women with 15 counseling sessions, demonstrated a 36% reduction in sexual risk behavior at 20 months and sustained significant reduction in sexual risk at 25 months (Healthy Living Project Team, 2007). This intervention paid significant attention to psychosocial factors that participants identified as impacting their behavior, such as addressing stress and coping, sexual and drug decision making. While attention to these factors is important in its own right, the research picture is complicated by the fact that the intervention did not significantly impact psychosocial adjustment, with no effect found among individuals presenting with mild to moderate depressive symptoms (Carrico et al., 2009). In addition, subsequent analysis demonstrated that the intervention impact on sexual risk behavior was largely explained by an increase in serosorting practices, in which the HIV positive study participants sought other HIV positive individuals as sex partners (Morin et al., 2008).

Emphasizing the need to understand sexual behavior in a context beyond condom use, one study examined a tailored video using a sexual health framework specific to the needs of HIV positive MSM (Rosser et al., 2010). The study found that sexual risk behavior with seronegative or unknown status decreased across all study arms, and it was therefore unable to demonstrate the superiority of a tailored approach for this particular group of men. A related methodological challenge was that individuals who engaged in serodiscordant condomless anal intercourse were more likely to leave the study (Rosser et al., 2010). In sum, the scientific field has had difficulty establishing efficacy of behavioral interventions specifically for HIV positive gay men, despite several well-conceived research trials.

Even with a handful of interventions that could be disseminated to HIV positive gay men, a common challenge across behavioral interventions is their complexity and length. Multi-session interventions that require a skilled counselor have been challenging, though not impossible, to scale-up, particularly in communities that lack well-established AIDS Service Organizations or where those organizations are struggling financially. Baseline data from the Healthy Living Project showed that only one-third of the HIV positive MSM in the trial reported receiving prevention programming in the 3 months prior to enrolling in the study, and that MSM were significantly less likely to report receiving prevention programming than non-MSM study participants (Steward et al., 2008). The potential for behavioral interventions to impact community-level outcomes must be questioned, given this data on low access to prevention services and the implementation challenges associated with bringing efficacious interventions to scale. The field has made some progress toward scale-up of efficacious interventions, such as the successful implementation of Healthy Relationships, a prevention intervention for people living with HIV (although not specific to MSM) across multiple community based organizations (CBOs) (Heitgerd et al., 2011). While there was great heterogeneity in the participants across the implementing CBOs, Healthy Relationships demonstrated reductions in sexual risk behavior across all groups and this effect was most pronounced among MSM compared to non-MSM groups.

One can look at the data and the fact that gay men have been among the most impacted by HIV in the USA for the past three decades and one could draw several different, but not mutually exclusive, conclusions: (1) there are not enough efficacious interventions for the most impacted members of the gay community (e.g., gay men of color), (2) the public health system has failed gay men and MSM by not adequately scaling up behavioral interventions, (3) there are other societal factors that reduce the impact of behavioral interventions that remain unaddressed among gay men and MSM—i.e., we don't have the right interventions, and (4) the biological reality of HIV transmission via anal sex, along with the background HIV prevalence that reduce the impact of behavioral interventions—makes behavioral interventions necessary but not sufficient. We have made significant progress, but perhaps we need different behavioral approaches to include as part of a combination prevention package, which might include new behavioral theories that postulate novel intervention targets.

Partner-Related Strategies

A comprehensive prevention package should not only target HIV positive gay men, but it should also encompass their sex and relationship partners. Extending a comprehensive prevention package to the partners of HIV positive gay men is consonant with a sexual health framework, which encourages us to conceptualize transmission risk behavior within the broader context of men's sexual scripts and intimate relationships. Partner- and couple-based strategies additionally follow from a combination prevention approach, by extending beyond individual-level approaches to incorporate interventions delivered at the level of social relationships. Furthermore, partner- and couple-based prevention strategies should be fundamental to any comprehensive prevention approach, because it is inside these connections that HIV risk behavior and transmission actually occurs.

Under a comprehensive and combination approach to HIV prevention, HIV negative sexual partners of HIV positive gay men might consider pre-exposure prophylaxis (PrEP) as a complement to condom-protected sex and treatment-as-prevention. PrEP represents a novel HIV prevention strategy in which uninfected individuals take a daily antiretroviral medication regimen as chemoprophylaxis. Clinical trials have proven that oral PrEP is safe, well tolerated, and efficacious for preventing HIV transmission (Baeten et al., 2012; Grant et al., 2010; Thigpen et al., 2012). This included a large-scale international trial which enrolled MSM and transgender women who have sex with men (iPrEx trial; Grant et al., 2010), although that trial had relatively few US participants. In establishing proof-of-concept for PrEP as an HIV prevention tool, these trials have provided a historic expansion of proven HIV prevention strategies. The US FDA approved the first-ever HIV preventive oral medicine (emtricitabine and tenofovir disoproxil fumarate, or "Truvada") in 2012.

Clinical guidelines recommend PrEP for individuals at substantial risk of HIV infection, and this includes individuals in HIV serodiscordant relationships. PrEP use by HIV negative gay men who are in relationships with HIV positive gay men could help to further reduce transmission risks in these couples. There is some question about the value of PrEP in an HIV serodiscordant couple where the HIV positive partner maintains durable viral suppression, since treatment-as-prevention is highly effective (Cohen et al., 2016; Rodger et al., 2016). However, PrEP use may provide some solace to members of gay serodiscordant couples, since research indicates members of these couples frequently worry about transmission issues throughout the course of their relationship (Remien, Carballo-Dieguez, & Wagner, 1995). Oral PrEP may additionally provide an interesting opportunity for an HIV negative man to share and mutually support the demands of daily medication use with his HIV positive relationship partner, if that partner is taking ART for HIV treatment. Just like the importance of adherence for HIV treatment outcomes, strong adherence to

PrEP regimens is necessary to maximize the preventive benefits of PrEP. In the iPrEx trial, participants who adhered more closely to the daily PrEP regimen showed greater reductions in the risk of HIV infection (Grant et al., 2010).

In addition to serodiscordant partners, HIV positive gay men may also have sero-concordant partners—and there are indications that some HIV positive gay men prefer or purposefully seek HIV positive peers as sex and relationship partners (Frost, Stirratt, & Ouellette, 2008). HIV positive gay men may seek seroconcordant partners for a variety of reasons, which include the desire to facilitate feelings of intimacy with their partner, to hold mutually shared experiences and perspectives, and to avoid experiences of HIV prejudice and stigma when seeking partners (Frost et al., 2008). Although we would not encourage it as a specific prevention strategy, another reason that some HIV positive gay men seek seroconcordant partners is a desire to reduce HIV transmission risks and anxiety about any potential for HIV transmission to uninfected partners (Frost et al., 2008). Although many HIV positive MSM with seroconcordant partners may still have condom-protected sex to avoid STI transmission, a study conducted with a large sample of HIV positive MSM found that unprotected sex was substantially more likely to occur with HIV concordant partners than serodiscordant partners (McConnell et al., 2010). This approach—tailoring unprotected sex to partner serostatus—has been described as a seroadaptive strategy (Snowden, Raymond, & McFarland, 2011). Seroadaptive strategies are common among MSM (Wei et al., 2011) but there may be important differences between the intention to use them and their actual practice. In one study (McFarland et al., 2012), 56% of HIV positive MSM agreed with the statement, "I will always use a condom unless I know for a fact that my partner has the same serostatus as me"—but only 5% of HIV positive men and 3% of HIV negative men consistently adhered to this practice over the span of 1 year, in the sense that many still had condom-protected sex with concordant partners, or non-condom-protected sex with discordant partners. Accurate diagnosis and mutual disclosure of HIV serostatus is critical for any HIV positive gay men who may seek condomless sex with seroconcordant partners. Some MSM report seeking information about the HIV status of their partners by checking online profiles and discussing HIV status before or after sex, in addition to making assumptions (Horvath, Nygaard, & Rosser, 2010). MSM who chose to have condomless sex with seroconcordant partners must also recognize that this brings risks for STI transmission, and that STI transmission could subsequently facilitate HIV transmission with any serodiscordant partners.

Community Empowerment Approaches and Addressing Social, Structural, and Legal/Policy Determinants

Gay men and other MSM with men were early leaders in the response to the HIV epidemic. Once the accurate knowledge about the HIV virus and transmission were known, many communities of gay men changed their behavior, resulting in dramatic declines in HIV incidence rates. This kind of broad community response could once again drive down incidence rates and reverse the troubling trends in HIV incidence among gay men in the USA. There is a need to renew the social movement that has been evident since the start of the HIV epidemic, but perhaps with greater awareness and coordination globally (Trapence et al., 2012), especially since one of the recent biomedical advances—PrEP—has shown proof of concept in MSM and transgender women. Early in the epidemic, the community response was not only a reaction to HIV disease, but it also involved a social movement to address the insufficient government and policy response from public health agencies. Thus, a human rights approach was infused at the earliest stages (Wright, 2013). In 1983, the Denver principles were drafted to address the issue of labeling people living with AIDS as victims and to call for greater recognition and involvement of people living with AIDS in the response to the epidemic (The Denver Principles, 1983; Wright, 2013). Due to the lack of an effective early response from governments, civil society banded together to enact behavior change and to provide structural and social support to those community members who were sick, dying, or grieving. The AIDS Coalition to Unleash Power (ACT UP) was among the groups to explicitly identify the issue of homophobia as tied to the lack of a rapid and adequate government response. A significant component of current combination prevention has to be utilizing those coalitions and social advocacy groups that are linked with AIDS Service Organizations and CBOs. These groups were responsible for critical changes to the regulatory approval of products, lowering the prices of licensed HIV medicines and national legislation to provide HIV-related programs and services (FasterCures & HCM Strategies, 2011; France, 2016; Trapence et al., 2012).

History shows that addressing the epidemic among gay men will take more than approaches targeting individuals or communities. Interventions must address those macro-level forces that impact the access to, scale-up, and efficacy of HIV prevention. The Global Commission on HIV and the Law maintains a database of the many governmental laws and policies that impede the HIV prevention efforts globally (www.hivlawcommission.org). For HIV positive gay men, there are two broad sets of laws and policies, those targeting people living with HIV and those targeting same-sex sexual activity, that serve as potential barriers to access to care and uptake of services. Moreover, laws criminalizing same-sex sexual activity and HIV transmission foster stigma and social isolation, both found to impact health behavior, quality of life, and mental health (Hatzenbuehler, O'Cleirigh, Mayer, Mimiaga, & Safren, 2011). HIV-associated stigma negatively impacts individuals, and it may also serve to fracture communities. A review found that HIV-associated stigma may be causing divisions in the gay community between HIV positive and HIV negative men (Smit et al., 2012). Given the historical importance of social mobilization and collective action to HIV prevention within the gay community, the suggestion that HIV-associated stigma may be fracturing the community is particularly concerning.

There are several aspects of social, structural, and policy factors that influence HIV prevention efforts for HIV positive gay men. Stigma associated with HIV/ AIDS or with gay identity has a deleterious impact on HIV prevention efforts and HIV treatment engagement and adherence. Efforts to stem HIV stigma should therefore be regarded as critical. Other structural factors such as housing have been demonstrated to impact the health of all people living with HIV, not specifically HIV positive gay men, and may provide prevention benefit in some circumstances through the positive relationship between stable housing and adherence to medications (Wolitski et al., 2010). There has also been study of the influence of particular laws and policies on HIV-associated outcomes, such as criminalization of HIV transmission and marriage rights for same-sex couples (Hatzenbuehler et al., 2012; Morris & Little, 2011; O'Byrne, 2011; Voelker, 2012). While challenging to study, this work indicates that policy, legal, and structural environments may influence the HIV epidemic, particularly among gay men.

Moving Forward: Building the Prevention Table

We have charted a comprehensive, multicomponent approach to prevention with HIV positive gay men through four overarching domains: improving HIV diagnosis and treatment cascade participation; enhancing risk reduction through counseling and treatment of comorbid conditions; engaging partner-related prevention strategies; and mobilizing communities and structural interventions. Under the combination prevention concept, these four domains could be considered as "four legs" on which HIV positive gay men and MSM can build a "table" to support and sustain comprehensive prevention. Efforts to effectively address prevention with HIV positive gay men and MSM will only be made weaker and more unstable for failing to incorporate one or more of these four posts of support.

Research is urgently needed to strengthen the four legs of the prevention table for HIV positive gay men and MSM. In some domains, there is an overall dearth of research evidence—and in others, the available evidence is derived largely from HIV positive individuals in general, or from groups other than HIV positive gay men or MSM. What are some critical research priorities, to help fill gaps in the evidence base for these approaches, individually or in combination?

Developing Novel Strategies to Advance Prevention Goals

One priority for future research is the further generation of novel HIV prevention tools and approaches. The aim is to continue expansion of available evidence-based prevention approaches for HIV positive gay men, their sexual and romantic partners, and MSM more generally. Research in many areas could be promising here; we will cite only three possible examples.

The development and testing of novel HIV prevention interventions using a positive sexual health approach is one area of focus. There is a relative dearth of proven, evidence-based risk reduction interventions for HIV positive gay men. This may reflect methodological challenges, and perhaps also a heavy disease focus in prior prevention interventions. Efforts to move from disease-focused work toward more holistic and constructive sexual health approaches could be helpful. Such efforts might include the creation of developmentally appropriate interventions that promote healthy sexual and relationship development among young gay men, and particularly HIV positive gay men and gay men of color. Efforts to build social support resources and resiliency among young gay men and HIV positive gay men might assist in improving prevention and care engagement for these groups. The combination prevention and sexual health promotion paradigms also suggest that development of novel biomedical prevention tools that integrate well with the sexual lives of HIV positive gay men could be helpful. The development of an effective rectal microbicide for HIV prevention would be an important advance. Such a microbicide could potentially be used in concert with sexual lubricants and/or anal douching, which are already common components of sexual scripts among many gay men (McGowan, 2011), thereby potentially improving uptake and consistent use. Fresh innovations in existing biomedical prevention approaches could also be helpful. For example, consistent and correct condom use might be improved through the use of condom "fit-kits," which help customize condom size to individual men to provide better fit and sensation.

Further research on HIV treatment engagement, retention, and adherence is particularly important for the prevention agenda among HIV positive gay men and MSM (Sullivan et al., 2012). Sustained involvement in the HIV treatment cascade has proven to be challenging for all populations of individuals living with HIV, and HIV positive gay men are no exception. Evidence of racial/ethnic and age-related disparities in treatment adherence and outcomes among HIV positive gay men are particularly concerning, and must be addressed. Very limited research has been conducted on effective strategies for timely HIV care linkage and sustained HIV care retention in any group, much less among HIV positive gay men or MSM more generally. How can we develop culturally competent health care services and support programs to help ensure consistent and sustained involvement in the full HIV treatment cascade by HIV positive gay men? The treatment-as-prevention concept also opens a fresh opportunity to improve HIV treatment engagement, adherence, and outcomes. Could HIV positive gay men's documented interests in protecting others from HIV transmission help to promote voluntary ART initiation and adherence? Recent advancements in mobile technologies and electronic drug monitoring additionally offer new avenues for adherence promotion, and early technology adopters often include gay men. Could ART adherence among HIV positive gay men be strengthened through technologies that provide real-time adherence monitoring and engage adherence support through online social networks? Lastly, important structural changes in health care provision and coverage have occurred in the USA in recent years. How will the Affordable Care Act and the evolving health care policy landscape influence HIV diagnosis, care engagement, and treatment adherence among MSM in the future?

Last but far from least, another critical priority for prevention research is the development of novel approaches to identify undiagnosed HIV infections among MSM, and particularly among MSM of color. We are deeply concerned by surveillance data which indicates that large numbers of young MSM and MSM of color in the USA remain unaware of their HIV infection (Wejnert et al., 2013). The lack of HIV diagnosis in these groups denies their access to lifesaving HIV treatment, jeopardizes risk reduction and prevention goals, and reinforces disparities in HIV incidence. Rapid home HIV tests may provide one novel way to expand access to HIV testing; this and other new advancements in strategies to improve the timely identification of HIV infection among gay men and MSM are urgently needed.

Implementation Research to Improve Access and Effectiveness of Current Prevention Strategies

Future research with HIV positive gay men and MSM should not only address prevention development, but also prevention delivery. Research is needed to strengthen the real-world implementation of proven HIV prevention interventions, in addition to identifying ways to expand their uptake and reach. Substantial gaps in the availability and effective provision of prevention interventions and services have been documented (Sullivan et al., 2012). Many HIV positive MSM in the USA are not currently being reached by prevention services (Steward et al., 2008), are poorly engaged in HIV treatment (Hall et al., 2012), and do not have access to necessary mental health treatment (Safren, Blashill, et al., 2011). Although efforts to understand individual-level factors may shed light on why some individuals do not better engage with available care and prevention services, we also need implementation science and operations research to identify organizational and structural factors that either facilitate or impede the scale-up and effective provision of preventive services and care. In implementation science and operations research, the unit of analysis is often at the level of HIV outpatient clinics, community organizations, institutions, or even states. What training programs, funding opportunities, and policy approaches could be designed—and what implementation strategies are presently underway—which would target these entities in an effort to optimize outcomes such as the adoption of evidence-based interventions, the delivery of interventions with fidelity or cultural competency, the number of individuals served or reached, or even community viral load or local HIV incidence rates?

A related question is how best to field combination prevention intervention approaches among HIV positive gay men and among MSM overall. In this chapter, we have outlined four core domains for prevention activities among HIV positive MSM and their partners—and each includes a number of important sub-strategies. It has been argued that combination prevention approaches with MSM are most likely to succeed if they simultaneously employ behavioral, biomedical, and structural approaches to address multiple junctures that facilitate HIV transmission (Sullivan et al., 2012). But fundamental questions remain: How much effort and resources should be invested in any one strategy? Are there particular combinations that would be more effective than others? How do local epidemiological and contextual issues inform the selection of combination prevention approaches?

Questions can also emerge when particular strategies are combined. For example, in the current era of antiretroviral-based prevention, how much of a prevention benefit might be provided by PrEP if one's HIV positive relationship partner already maintains durably suppressed viral load through ART treatment? New research is needed to help target, field, and evaluate such combination prevention approaches with HIV positive MSM. The use of modeling could be highly advantageous in this regard, along with efforts to leverage existing national, state, community, and clinic-level data, as well as "natural experiments" that may be underway when prevention services are scaled-up and rolled out in a sequential or stepped fashion.

Research on Social, Structural, and Policy Factors

Finally, further research to evaluate social factors and structural interventions, policy, and laws would be invaluable for advancing HIV prevention among HIV positive gay men and MSM. The vast preponderance of HIV prevention research to date has been conducted at the individual-level. This represents important, foundational research—but its impact may ultimately be constrained by resource limitations for the wide-scale delivery of individual-level interventions, and also by the increasing recognition that HIV transmission is importantly influenced by broader contextual factors, such as community viral load and social networks and mixing patterns. The next generation of HIV prevention research should therefore seek to better address social, structural, and environmental factors that drive HIV incidence and influence prevention. This would likely involve less focus on individual risk behavior and more focus on contexts that may promote transmission risks, including social networks, venues, neighborhoods, and political and legal systems. As one example, how might laws regarding the criminalization of HIV transmission, hate crime prosecution, or same-sex marriage affect HIV prevention with gay men or HIV positive gay men? Prevention interventions would benefit from a greater understanding of political and legal systems and other structural factors that may drive HIV incidence, because structural-level factors could serve as novel targets for intervention.

In terms of social factors, research is needed to not only determine the deleterious effects of forces like homophobia, racism, and HIV stigma on HIV prevention—but also to more clearly document the precise mechanisms and mediators through which these social dynamics compromise prevention and treatment—so that appropriate interventions can be developed. An interesting example is provided by research on food insecurity among HIV positive individuals. Food insecurity—defined as having uncertain or limited availability of nutritionally adequate or safe food—is widely prevalent among HIV positive individuals in both US and global settings, and it has been consistently associated with incomplete viral suppression, reduced CD4 count, and greater mortality (Weiser, Bangsberg, et al., 2009; Weiser, Frongillo, et al., 2009; Weiser et al., 2013). But how exactly does food insecurity foster negative HIV treatment outcomes? This is not yet clear, but it might occur through multiple pathways, including poor nutrition, compromised mental health (such as increased anxiety and depression), or behavioral factors (such as challenges to treatment adherence and retention) (Weiser et al., 2011). Research is underway to understand these pathways, and the results will help inform the optimal interventional response—e.g., to interrupt the negative impacts of food insecurity on HIV treatment outcomes, would it be best to provide HIV positive individuals with food supplementation, nutritional counseling, mental health treatment, income-generation programs, or some combination of the above? Knowledge of the precise mechanisms will be key to developing evidence-based intervention programs and policies; the same applies to research designed to address the impact of social forces such as HIV stigma, homophobia, and racism on prevention with HIV positive gay men.

The field of HIV prevention now stands at a turning point. New approaches such as antiretroviral-based prevention have prompted a sense that we may be in a better position than ever before to truly turn the tide on the HIV epidemic. While there are good reasons for hope, it can be very clearly stated that the HIV/AIDS epidemic will never be brought to a close until we are able to more effectively advance HIV prevention and care with HIV positive gay men, and all gay men. In opening this chapter by noting the leadership of HIV positive gay men in the response to the epidemic, we will close by returning to this point. What are the next prevention innovations that will come from HIV positive gay men? How can we engage the community mobilization efforts among gay men that were evident at the start of the epidemic, to help bring it to end? As we go forward together, let us continue to recognize, research, and support the prevention practices and commitment of HIV positive gay men.

References

Amico, K. R., Harman, J. J., & Johnson, B. T. (2006). Efficacy of antiretroviral therapy adherence interventions: A research synthesis of trials, 1996 to 2004. *Journal of Acquired Immune Deficiency Syndromes, 41*(3), 285–297.

Ayala, G., Bingham, T., Kim, J., Wheeler, D. P., & Millett, G. A. (2012). Modeling the impact of social discrimination and financial hardship on the sexual risk of HIV among Latino and Black men who have sex with men. *American Journal of Public Health, 102*(S2), S242–S249.

Baeten, J. M., Donnell, D., Ndase, P., Mugo, N. R., Campbell, J. D., Wangisi, J., ... Partners PrEP Study Team. (2012). Antiretroviral prophylaxis for HIV prevention in heterosexual men and women. *New England Journal of Medicine, 367*(5), 399–410.

Baggaley, R. F., White, R. G., & Boily, M. C. (2010). HIV transmission risk through anal intercourse: Systematic review, meta-analysis and implications for HIV prevention. *International Journal of Epidemiology, 39*(4), 1048–1063.

Bekker, L. G., Beyrer, C., & Quinn, T. C. (2012). Behavioral and biomedical combination strategies for HIV prevention. *Cold Spring Harbor Perspectives in Medicine, 2*, 1–23.

Beyrer, C., Sullivan, P. S., Sanchez, J., Dowdy, D., Altman, D., Trapence, G., ... Mayer, K. H. (2012). A call to action for comprehensive HIV services for men who have sex with men. *Lancet, 380*(9839), 424–438.

Bogart, L. M., Galvan, F. H., Wagner, G. J., & Klein, D. J. (2011). Longitudinal association of HIV conspiracy beliefs with sexual risk among black males living with HIV. *AIDS and Behavior, 15*(6), 1180–1186.

Bogart, L. M., Wagner, G., Galvan, F. H., & Banks, D. (2010). Conspiracy beliefs about HIV are related to antiretroviral treatment nonadherence among African American men with HIV. *Journal of Acquired Immune Deficiency Syndromes, 53*(5), 648–655.

Bogart, L. M., Wagner, G. J., Galvan, F. H., & Klein, D. J. (2010). Longitudinal relationships between antiretroviral treatment adherence and discrimination due to HIV-serostatus, race, and sexual orientation among African-American men with HIV. *Annals of Behavioral Medicine, 40*(2), 184–190.

Carballo-Dieguez, A., Frasca, T., Dolezal, C., & Balan, I. (2012). Will gay and bisexually active men at high risk of infection use over-the-counter rapid HIV tests to screen sexual partners? *Journal of Sex Research, 49*(4), 379–387.

Carrico, A. W., Chesney, M. A., Johnson, M. O., Morin, S. F., Neilands, T. B., Remien, R. H., … Stover, E. (2009). Randomized controlled trial of a cognitive-behavioral intervention for HIV-positive persons: An investigation of treatment effects on psychosocial adjustment. *AIDS and Behavior, 13*(3), 555–563.

Centers for Disease Control & Prevention. (2011a). Vital signs: HIV prevention through care and treatment—United States. *Morbidity and Mortality Weekly Report, 60*(47), 1618–1623.

Centers for Disease Control & Prevention. (2011b). HIV testing among men who have sex with men—21 cities, United States, 2008. *Morbidity and Mortality Weekly Report, 60*(21), 694–699.

Centers for Disease Control & Prevention. (2014). *Recommendations for HIV prevention with adults and adolescents with HIV in the United States.* Retrieved from http://stacks.cdc.gov/view/cdc/26062.

Centers for Disease Control & Prevention. (2015). Diagnoses of HIV infection in the United States and dependent areas, 2014. *HIV Surveillance Report; 26.*

Centers for Disease Control & Prevention. (2016). HIV infection risk, prevention, and testing behaviors among men who have sex with men—National HIV Behavioral Surveillance, 20 U.S. cities, 2014. *HIV Surveillance Special Report; 15.*

Choi, K. H., Paul, J., Ayala, G., Boylan, R., & Gregorich, S. E. (2013). Experiences of discrimination and their impact on the mental health among African American, Asian and Pacific Islander, and Latino men who have sex with men. *American Journal of Public Health, 103*(5), 868–874.

Christopoulos, K. A., Das, M., & Colfax, G. N. (2011). Linkage and retention in HIV care among men who have sex with men in the United States. *Clinical Infectious Diseases, 52*(Supplement 2), S214–S222.

Coates, T. J., Richter, L., & Caceres, C. (2008). Behavioural strategies to reduce HIV transmission: How to make them work better. *Lancet, 372*, 669–684.

Cohen, M. S., Chen, Y. Q., McCauley, M., Gamble, T., Hosseinipour, M. C., Kumarasamy, N., … HPTN 052 Study Team. (2011). Prevention of HIV-1 infection with early antiretroviral therapy. *New England Journal of Medicine, 365*(6), 493–505.

Cohen, M. S., Chen, Y. Q., McCauley, M., Gamble, T., Hosseinipour, M. C., Kumarasamy, N., … HPTN 052 Study Team. (2016). Antiretroviral therapy for the prevention of HIV-1 transmission. *New England Journal of Medicine, 375*(9), 830–839.

Cohen, M. S., Hoffman, I. F., Royce, R. A., Kazembe, P., Dyer, J. R., Daly, C. C., … Eron, J. J. (1997). Reduction of concentration of HIV-1 in semen after treatment of urethritis: Implications for prevention of sexual transmission of HIV-1. *Lancet, 349*(9069), 1868–1873.

Coleman, E. (2011). What is sexual health? Articulating a sexual health approach to HIV prevention for men who have sex with men. *AIDS and Behavior, 15*(Suppl 1), S18–S24.

Courtenay-Quirk, C., Wolitski, R. J., Hoff, C., Parsons, J. T., & Seropositive Urban Men's Study Team. (2003). Interests in HIV prevention topics of HIV-seropositive men who have sex with men. *AIDS Education and Prevention, 15*(5), 401–412.

Cox, J., Beauchemin, J., & Allard, R. (2004). HIV status of sexual partners is more important than antiretroviral treatment related perceptions for risk taking by HIV positive MSM in Montreal, Canada. *Sexually Transmitted Infections, 80*(6), 518–523.

Craw, J. A., Gardner, L. I., Marks, G., Rapp, R. C., Bosshart, J., Duffus, W. A., … Schmitt, K. (2008). Brief strengths-based case management promotes entry into HIV medical care: Results of the antiretroviral treatment access study-II. *Journal of Acquired Immune Deficiency Syndromes, 47*(5), 597–606.

Crepaz, N., Lyles, C. M., Wolitski, R. J., Passin, W. F., Rama, S. M., Herbst, J. H., … HIV/AIDS Prevention Research Synthesis (PRS) Team. (2006). Do prevention interventions reduce HIV risk behaviours among people living with HIV? A meta-analytic review of controlled trials. *AIDS, 20*(2), 143–157.

Crepaz, N., Tang, T., Marks, G., Mugavero, M. J., Espinoza, L., & Hall, H. I. (2016). Durable viral suppression and transmission risk potential among persons with diagnosed HIV infection: United States, 2012-2013. *Clinical Infectious Diseases*, *63*(7), 976–983.

Das, M., Chu, P. L., Santos, G. M., Scheer, S., Vittinghoff, E., McFarland, W., & Colfax, G. N. (2010). Decreases in community viral load are accompanied by reductions in new HIV infections in San Francisco. *PloS One*, *5*(6), e11068.

Ekstrand, M. L., & Coates, T. J. (1990). Maintenance of safer sexual behaviors and predictors of risky sex: The San Francisco Men's Health Study. *American Journal of Public Health*, *80*(8), 973–977.

FasterCures & HCM Strategies. (2011). *Back to basics: HIV/AIDS advocacy as a model for catalyzing change*. Retrieved from http://www.fastercures.org/assets/Uploads/PDF/Back2BasicsFinal.pdf.

France, D. (2016). *How to survive a plague: The inside story of how citizens and science tamed AIDS*. New York, NY: Knopf.

Frost, D. M., Stirratt, M. J., & Ouellette, S. C. (2008). Understanding why gay men seek HIV-seroconcordant partners: Intimacy and risk reduction motivations. *Culture, Health and Sexuality*, *10*(5), 513–527.

Gardner, L. I., Marks, G., Craw, J. A., Wilson, T. E., Drainoni, M. L., Moore, R. D., ... Retention in Care Study Group. (2012). A low-effort, clinic-wide intervention improves attendance for HIV primary care. *Clinical Infectious Diseases*, *55*(8), 1124–1134.

Gardner, E. M., McLees, M. P., Steiner, J. F., del Rio, C., & Burman, W. J. (2011). The spectrum of engagement in HIV care and its relevance to test-and-treat strategies for prevention of HIV infection. *Clinical Infectious Diseases*, *52*(6), 793–800.

Gardner, L. I., Metsch, L. R., Anderson-Mahoney, P., Loughlin, A. M., del Rio, C., Strathdee, S., ... Antiretroviral Treatment and Access Study Group. (2005). Efficacy of a brief case management intervention to link recently diagnosed HIV-infected persons to care. *AIDS*, *19*(4), 423–431.

Goldhammer, H., & Mayer, K. H. (2011). Focusing on sexual health promotion to enhance preventive behaviors among gay men and other men who have sex with men: Report from a state-of-the-art conference. *AIDS and Behavior*, *15*(Suppl 1), S1–S8.

Grant, R. M., Lama, J. R., Anderson, P. L., McMahan, V., Liu, A. Y., Vargas, L., ... iPrEx Study Team. (2010). Preexposure chemoprophylaxis for HIV prevention in men who have sex with men. *New England Journal of Medicine*, *363*(27), 2587–2599.

Grossman, C. I., Forsyth, A., Purcell, D. W., Allison, S., Toledo, C., & Gordon, C. M. (2011). Advancing novel HIV prevention intervention research with MSM—Meeting report. *Public Health Reports*, *126*(4), 472–479.

Halkitis, P. N., & Wilton, L. (2005). The meanings of sex for HIV-positive gay and bisexual men: Emotions, physicality, and affirmations of self. In P. N. Halkitis, C. A. Gomez, & R. J. Wolitski (Eds.), *HIV+ sex: The psychological and interpersonal dynamics of HIV-seropositive gay and bisexual men's relationships* (pp. 21–38). Washington, DC: American Psychological Association.

Hall, H. I., Frazier, E. L., Rhodes, P., Holtgrave, D. R., Furlow-Parmley, C., Tang, T., ... Skarbinski, J. (2013). Differences in human immunodeficiency virus care and treatment among subpopulations in the United States. *JAMA Internal Medicine*, *173*(14), 1337–1344.

Hall, H. I., Gray, K. M., Tang, T., Li, J., Shouse, L., & Mermin, J. (2012). Retention in care of adults and adolescents living with HIV in 13 U.S. areas. *Journal of Acquired Immune Deficiency Syndromes*, *60*(1), 77–82.

Hatzenbuehler, M. L., O'Cleirigh, C., Grasso, C., Mayer, K., Safren, S., & Bradford, J. (2012). Effect of same-sex marriage laws on health care use and expenditures in sexual minority men: A quasi-natural experiment. *American Journal of Public Health*, *102*(2), 285–291.

Hatzenbuehler, M. L., O'Cleirigh, C., Mayer, K. H., Mimiaga, M. J., & Safren, S. A. (2011). Prospective associations between HIV-related stigma, transmission risk behaviors, and adverse mental health outcomes in men who have sex with men. *Annals of Behavioral Medicine*, *42*(2), 227–234.

Healthy Living Project Team. (2007). Effects of a behavioral intervention to reduce risk of transmission among people living with HIV: The healthy living project randomized controlled study. *Journal of Acquired Immune Deficiency Syndromes*, *44*(2), 213–221.

Heitgerd, J. L., Kalayil, E. J., Patel-Larson, A., Uhl, G., Williams, W. O., Griffin, T., & Smith, D. (2011). Reduced sexual risk behaviors among people living with HIV: Results from the Healthy Relationships Outcome Monitoring Project. *AIDS and Behavior, 15*(8), 1677–1690.

Higa, D. H., Marks, G., Crepaz, N., Liau, A., & Lyles, C. M. (2012). Interventions to improve retention in HIV primary care: A systematic review of U.S. studies. *Current HIV/AIDS Reports, 9*(4), 313–325.

Hightow-Weidman, L. B., Jones, K., Phillips, G., Wohl, A., Giordano, T. P., & YMSM of Color SPNS Initiative Study Group. (2011). Baseline clinical characteristics, antiretroviral therapy use, and viral load suppression among HIV-positive young men of color who have sex with men. *AIDS Patient Care and STDs, 25*(Suppl 1), S9–14.

Hightow-Weidman, L. B., Jones, K., Wohl, A. R., Futterman, D., Outlaw, A., Phillips, G., … YMSM of Color SPNS Initiative Study Group. (2011). Early linkage and retention in care: Findings from the outreach, linkage, and retention in care initiative among young men of color who have sex with men. *AIDS Patient Care and STDs, 25*(Suppl 1), S31–S38.

Holtgrave, D. R., & Curran, J. W. (2006). What works, and what remains to be done, in HIV prevention in the United States. *Annual Review of Public Health, 27*, 261–275.

Horvath, K. J., Nygaard, K., & Rosser, B. R. (2010). Ascertaining partner HIV status and its association with sexual risk behavior among internet-using men who have sex with men. *AIDS and Behavior, 14*(6), 1376–1383.

Horvath, K. J., Oakes, J. M., Rosser, B. R., Danilenko, G., Vezina, H., Amico, K. R., … Simoni, J. (2013). Feasibility, acceptability and preliminary efficacy of an online peer-to-peer social support ART adherence intervention. *AIDS and Behavior, 17*(6), 2031–2044.

Janssen, R. S., Holtgrave, D. R., Valdisseri, R. O., Shepherd, M., Gayle, H. D., & De Cock, K. M. (2001). The serostatus approach to fighting the HIV epidemic: Prevention strategies for infected individuals. *American Journal of Public Health, 91*(7), 1019–1024.

Johnson, W. D., Diaz, R. M., Flanders, W. D., Goodman, M., Hill, A. N., Holtgrave, D., … McClellan, W. M. (2008). Behavioral interventions to reduce risk for sexual transmission of HIV among men who have sex with men. *The Cochrane Database of Systematic Reviews, 3*, CD001230. doi:10.1002/14651858.CD001230.pub2

Koblin, B. A., Mayer, K. H., Eshleman, S. H., Wang, L., Mannheimer, S., del Rio, C., … HPTN 061 Protocol Team. (2013). Correlates of HIV acquisition in a cohort of Black men who have sex with men in the United States: HIV Prevention Trials Network (HPTN) 061. *PloS One, 8*, e70413. doi:10.1371/journal.pone.0070413.

Kurth, A. E., Celum, C., Baeten, J. M., Vermund, S. H., & Wasserheit, J. N. (2011). Combination HIV prevention: Significance, challenges, and opportunities. *Current HIV/AIDS Reports, 8*(1), 62–72.

Labarga, P. (2012). New DHHS guidelines recommend antiretroviral therapy to all HIV-infected persons. *AIDS Reviews, 14*(2), 154.

Lewis, M. A., Uhrig, J. D., Bann, C. M., Harris, J. L., Furberg, R. D., Coomes, C., & Kuhns, L. M. (2012). Tailored text messaging intervention for HIV adherence: A proof-of- concept study. *Health Psychology, 32*(3), 248–253.

Lima, V. D., Harrigan, R., Bangsberg, D. R., Hogg, R. S., Gross, R., Yip, B., & Montaner, J. S. (2009). The combined effect of modern highly active antiretroviral therapy regimens and adherence on mortality over time. *Journal of Acquired Immune Deficiency Syndromes, 50*(5), 529–536.

Lorenc, T., Marrero-Guillamon, I., Aggleton, P., Cooper, C., Llewellyn, A., Lehmann, A., & Lindsay, C. (2011). Promoting the uptake of HIV testing among men who have sex with men: Systematic review of effectiveness and cost-effectiveness. *Sexually Transmitted Infections, 87*(4), 272–278.

Magnus, M., Jones, K., Phillips, G., Binson, D., Hightow-Weidman, L. B., Richards-Clarke, C., … YMSM of Color Special Projects of National Significance Initiative Study Group. (2010). Characteristics associated with retention among African American and Latino adolescent HIV-positive men: Results from the outreach, care, and prevention to engage HIV-seropositive young MSM of Color Special Projects of National Significance Initiative. *Journal of Acquired Immune Deficiency Syndromes, 53*(4), 529–536.

Marks, G., Crepaz, N., & Janssen, R. S. (2006). Estimating sexual transmission of HIV from persons aware and unaware that they are infected with the virus in the USA. *AIDS*, *20*(10), 1447–1450.

Marks, G., Gardner, L. I., Craw, J., & Crepaz, N. (2010). Entry and retention in medical care among HIV-diagnosed persons: A meta-analysis. *AIDS*, *24*(17), 2665–2678.

Mayer, K. H., Bekker, L. G., Stall, R., Grulich, A. E., Colfax, G., & Lama, J. R. (2012). Comprehensive clinical care for men who have sex with men: An integrated approach. *Lancet*, *380*(9839), 378–387.

McConnell, J. J., Bragg, L., Shiboski, S., & Grant, R. M. (2010). Sexual seroadaptation: Lessons for prevention and sex research from a cohort of HIV-positive men who have sex with men. *PloS One*, *5*(1), e8831. doi:10.1371/journal.pone.0008831

McFarland, W., Chen, Y. H., Nguyen, B., Grasso, M., Levine, D., Stall, R., ... Raymond, H. F. (2012). Behavior, intention or chance? A longitudinal study of HIV seroadaptive behaviors, abstinence and condom use. *AIDS and Behavior*, *16*(1), 121–131.

McGowan, I. (2011). Rectal microbicides: Can we make them and will people use them? *AIDS and Behavior*, *15*(Suppl 1), S66–S71.

Millett, G. A., Crowley, J. S., Koh, H., Valdiserri, R. O., Frieden, T., Dieffenbach, C. W., ... Fauci, A. S. (2010). A way forward: The National HIV/AIDS strategy and reducing HIV incidence in the United States. *Journal of Acquired Immune Deficiency Syndromes*, *55*(Suppl 2), S144–S147.

Millett, G. A., Ding, H., Marks, G., Jeffries, W. L., Bingham, T., Lauby, J., ... Stueve, A. (2011). Mistaken assumptions and missed opportunities: Correlates of undiagnosed HIV infection among black and Latino men who have sex with men. *Journal of Acquired Immune Deficiency Syndromes*, *58*(1), 64–71.

Mills, E. J., Nachega, J. B., Buchan, I., Orbinski, J., Attaran, A., Singh, S., ... Bangsberg, D. R. (2006). Adherence to antiretroviral therapy in sub-Saharan Africa and North America: A meta-analysis. *JAMA*, *296*(6), 679–690.

Mimiaga, M. J., O'Cleirigh, C., Biello, K. B., Robertson, A. M., Safren, S. A., Coates, T. J., ... Mayer, K. H. (2015). The effect of psychosocial syndemic production on 4-year HIV incidence and risk behavior in a large cohort of sexually active men who have sex with men. *Journal of Acquired Immune Deficiency Syndromes*, *68*(3), 329–336.

Montaner, J. S., Lima, V. D., Barrios, R., Yip, B., Wood, E., Kerr, T., ... Kendall, P. (2010). Association of highly active antiretroviral therapy coverage, population viral load, and yearly new HIV diagnoses in British Columbia, Canada: A population-based study. *Lancet*, *376*(9740), 532–539.

Morin, S. F., Shade, S. B., Steward, W. T., Carrico, A. W., Remien, R. H., Rotheram-Borus, M. J., ... Healthy Living Project Team. (2008). A behavioral intervention reduces HIV transmission risk by promoting sustained serosorting practices among HIV-infected men who have sex with men. *Journal of Acquired Immune Deficiency Syndromes*, *49*(5), 544–551.

Morris, S. R., & Little, S. J. (2011). MSM: Resurgent epidemics. *Current Opinion in HIV and AIDS*, *6*(4), 326–332.

Mustanski, B. S., Newcomb, M. E., Du Bois, S. N., Garcia, S. C., & Grov, C. (2011). HIV in young men who have sex with men: A review of epidemiology, risk and protective factors, and interventions. *Journal of Sex Research*, *48*(2-3), 218–253.

Nakagawa, F., Lodwick, R. K., Smith, C. J., Smith, R., Cambiano, V., Lundgren, J. D., ... Phillips, A. N. (2012). Projected life expectancy of people with HIV according to timing of diagnosis. *AIDS*, *26*(3), 335–343.

Nakagawa, F., May, M., & Phillips, A. (2012). Life expectancy living with HIV: Recent estimates and future implications. *Current Opinion in Infectious Diseases*, *26*(1), 17–25.

Nelson, K. M., Thiede, H., Hawes, S. E., Golden, M. R., Hutcheson, R., Carey, J. W., ... Jenkins, R. A. (2010). Why the wait? Delayed HIV diagnosis among men who have sex with men. *Journal of Urban Health*, *87*(4), 642–655.

O'Byrne, P. (2011). The potential public health effects of a police announcement about HIV non-disclosure: A case scenario analysis. *Policy, Politics & Nursing Practice*, *12*(1), 55–63.

O'Cleirigh, C., Mimiaga, M., Safren, S., Stall, R., & Mayer, K. H. (2010). *Synergistic effects of psychosocial and substance use problems on increased sexual transmission risk among HIV-infected men who have sex with men*. Paper presented at the XVII International AIDS Conference, Vienna.

O'Cleirigh, C., Skeer, M., Mayer, K. H., & Safren, S. A. (2009). Functional impairment and health care utilization among HIV-infected men who have sex with men: The relationship with depression and post-traumatic stress. *Journal of Behavioral Medicine, 32*, 466–477.

Oh, D. L., Sarafian, F., Silvestre, A., Brown, T., Jacobson, L., Badri, S., & Detels, R. (2009). Evaluation of adherence and factors affecting adherence to combination antiretroviral therapy among White, Hispanic, and Black men in the MACS Cohort. *Journal of Acquired Immune Deficiency Syndromes, 52*(2), 290–293.

Ortego, C., Huedo-Medina, T. B., Llorca, J., Sevilla, L., Santos, P., Rodriguez, E., ... Vejo, J. (2011). Adherence to highly active antiretroviral therapy (HAART): A meta-analysis. *AIDS and Behavior, 15*(7), 1381–1396.

Osborn, C. Y., Paasche-Orlow, M. K., Davis, T. C., & Wolf, M. S. (2007). Health literacy: An overlooked factor in understanding HIV health disparities. *American Journal of Preventive Medicine, 33*(5), 374–378.

Oster, A. M., Wiegand, R. E., Sionean, C., Miles, I. J., Thomas, P. E., Melendez-Morales, L., ... Millett, G. A. (2011). Understanding disparities in HIV infection between black and white MSM in the United States. *AIDS, 25*(8), 1103–1112.

Parsons, J. T., Grov, C., & Golub, S. A. (2012). Sexual compulsivity, co-occurring psychosocial health problems, and HIV risk among gay and bisexual men: Further evidence of a syndemic. *American Journal of Public Health, 102*(1), 156–162.

Purcell, D. W., Johnson, C. H., Lansky, A., Prejean, J., Stein, R., Denning, P., ... Crepaz, N. (2012). Estimating the population size of men who have sex with men in the United States to obtain HIV and syphilis rates. *Open AIDS Journal, 6*, 98–107.

Quinn, T. C., Wawer, M. J., Sewankambo, N., Serwadda, D., Li, C., Wabwire-Mangen, F., ... Gray, R. H. (2000). Viral load and heterosexual transmission of human immunodeficiency virus type 1. Rakai Project Study Group. *New England Journal of Medicine, 342*(13), 921–929.

Rausch, D., Dieffenbach, C., Cheever, L., & Fenton, K. A. (2011). Towards a more coordinated federal response to improving HIV prevention and sexual health among men who have sex with men. *AIDS and Behavior, 15*(Suppl 1), S107–S111.

Remien, R. H., & Borkowski, T. M. (2005). Wishful thinking? HIV treatment optimism and sexual behavior among HIV-positive gay and bisexual men. In P. N. Halkitis, C. A. Gomez, & R. J. Wolitski (Eds.), *HIV+ sex: The psychological and interpersonal dynamics of HIV-seropositive gay and bisexual men's relationships* (pp. 201–215). Washington, DC: American Psychological Association.

Remien, R. H., Carballo-Dieguez, A., & Wagner, G. (1995). Intimacy and sexual risk behaviour in serodiscordant male couples. *AIDS Care, 7*(4), 429–438.

Remien, R. H., Stirratt, M. J., Dognin, J., Day, E., El-Bassel, N., & Warne, P. (2006). Moving from theory to research to practice: Implementing an effective dyadic intervention to improve antiretroviral adherence for clinic patients. *Journal of Acquired Immune Deficiency Syndromes, 43*(Supplement 1), S69–S78.

Remien, R. H., Stirratt, M. J., Dolezal, C., Dognin, J. S., Wagner, G. J., Carballo-Dieguez, A., & Jung, T. M. (2005). Couple-focused support to improve HIV medication adherence: A random-ized controlled trial. *AIDS, 19*(8), 807–814.

Rodger, A. J., Cambiano, V., Bruun, T., Vernazza, P., Collins, S., van Lunzen, J., ... PARTNER Study Group. (2016). Sexual activity without condoms and risk of HIV transmission in serodif-ferent couples when the HIV-positive partner is using suppressive antiretroviral therapy. *JAMA, 316*(2), 171–181.

Rosser, B. R., Hatfield, L. A., Miner, M. H., Ghiselli, M. E., Lee, B. R., & Welles, S. L. (2010). Effects of a behavioral intervention to reduce serodiscordant unsafe sex among HIV positive men who have sex with men: The positive connections randomized controlled trial study. *Journal of Behavioral Medicine, 33*(2), 147–158.

Royce, R. A., Sena, A., Cates, W., Jr., & Cohen, M. S. (1997). Sexual transmission of HIV. *New England Journal of Medicine, 336*(15), 1072–1078.

Safren, S. A., Blashill, A. J., & O'Cleirigh, C. M. (2011). Promoting the sexual health of MSM in the context of comorbid mental health problems. *AIDS and Behavior, 15*(Suppl 1), S30–S34.

Safren, S. A., O'Cleirigh, C., Skeer, M. R., Driskell, J., Goshe, B. M., Covahey, C., & Mayer, K. H. (2011). Demonstration and evaluation of a peer-delivered, individually-tailored, HIV prevention intervention for HIV-infected MSM in their primary care setting. *AIDS and Behavior, 15*(5), 949–958.

Safren, S. A., Otto, M. W., Worth, J. L., Salomon, E., Johnson, W., Mayer, K., & Boswell, S. (2001). Two strategies to increase adherence to HIV antiretroviral medication: Life-steps and medication monitoring. *Behaviour Research and Therapy, 39*(10), 1151–1162.

Sandfort, T. G. M., & Ehrhardt, A. A. (2004). Sexual health: A useful public health paradigm or a moral imperative? *Archives of Sexual Behavior, 33*(3), 181–187.

Simoni, J. M., Huh, D., Frick, P. A., Pearson, C. R., Andrasik, M. P., Dunbar, P. J., & Hooton, T. M. (2009). Peer support and pager messaging to promote antiretroviral modifying therapy in Seattle: A randomized controlled trial. *Journal of Acquired Immune Deficiency Syndromes, 52*(4), 465–473.

Simoni, J. M., Huh, D., Wilson, I. B., Shen, J., Goggin, K., Reynolds, N. R., … Liu, H. (2012). Racial/ethnic disparities in ART adherence in the United States: Findings from the MACH14 study. *Journal of Acquired Immune Deficiency Syndromes, 60*(5), 466–472.

Simoni, J. M., Pearson, C. R., Pantalone, D. W., Marks, G., & Crepaz, N. (2006). Efficacy of interventions in improving highly active antiretroviral therapy adherence and HIV-1 RNA viral load. A meta-analytic review of randomized controlled trials. *Journal of Acquired Immune Deficiency Syndromes, 43*(Supplement 1), S23–S35.

Skarbinski, J., Rosenberg, E., Paz-Bailey, G., Hall, H. I., Viall, A. H., Fagan, J. L., … Mermin, J. H. (2015). Human immunodeficiency virus transmission at each step of the care continuum in the United States. *JAMA Internal Medicine, 175*(4), 588–596.

Smit, P. J., Brady, M., Carter, M., Fernandes, R., Lamore, L., Meulbroek, M., … Thompson, M. (2012). HIV-related stigma within communities of gay men: A literature review. *AIDS Care, 24*(4), 405–412.

Snowden, J. M., Raymond, H. F., & McFarland, W. (2011). Seroadaptive behaviours among men who have sex with men in San Francisco: The situation in 2008. *Sexually Transmitted Infections, 87*(2), 162–164.

Stall, R. D., Coates, T. J., & Hoff, C. (1988). Behavioral risk reduction for HIV infection among gay and bisexual men. A review of results from the United States. *American Psychologist, 43*(11), 878–885.

Stall, R., Mills, T. C., Williamson, J., Hart, T., Greenwood, G., Paul, J., … Catania, J. A. (2003). Association of co-occurring psychosocial health problems and increased vulnerability to HIV/AIDS among urban men who have sex with men. *American Journal of Public Health, 93*(6), 939–942.

Steward, W. T., Charlebois, E. D., Johnson, M. O., Remien, R. H., Goldstein, R. B., Wong, F. L., & Morin, S. F. (2008). Receipt of prevention services among HIV-infected men who have sex with men. *American Journal of Public Health, 98*(6), 1011–1014.

Sullivan, P. S., Carballo-Dieguez, A., Coates, T., Goodreau, S. M., McGowan, I., Sanders, E. J., … Sanchez, J. (2012). Successes and challenges of HIV prevention in men who have sex with men. *Lancet, 380*(9839), 388–399.

The Denver Principles. (1983). Retrieved from http://www.actupny.org/documents/Denver.html.

Thigpen, M. C., Kebaabetswe, P. M., Paxton, L. A., Smith, D. K., Rose, C. E., Segolodi, T. M., … TDF2 Study Group. (2012). Antiretroviral preexposure prophylaxis for heterosexual HIV transmission in Botswana. *New England Journal of Medicine, 367*(5), 423–434.

Thompson, M. A., Mugavero, M. J., Amico, K. R., Cargill, V. A., Chang, L. W., Gross, R., … Nachega, J. B. (2012). Guidelines for improving entry into and retention in care and antiretroviral adherence for persons with HIV: Evidence-based recommendations from an International Association of Physicians in AIDS Care panel. *Annals of Internal Medicine, 156*(11), 817–833.

Trapence, G., Collins, C., Avrett, S., Carr, R., Sanchez, H., Ayala, G., ... Baral, S. D. (2012). From personal survival to public health: Community leadership by men who have sex with men in the response to HIV. *Lancet, 380*(9839), 400–410.

Tripathi, A., Gardner, L. I., Ogbuanu, I., Youmans, E., Stephens, T., Gibson, J. J., & Duffus, W. (2011). Predictors of time to enter medical care after a new HIV diagnosis: A statewide population-based study. *AIDS Care, 23*(11), 1366–1373.

Voelker, R. (2012). Punitive laws undermine HIV prevention, says report. *JAMA, 308*(7), 661.

Wei, C., Raymond, H. F., Guadamuz, T. E., Stall, R., Colfax, G. N., Snowden, J. M., & McFarland, W. (2011). Racial/ethnic differences in seroadaptive and serodisclosure behaviors among men who have sex with men. *AIDS and Behavior, 15*(1), 22–29.

Weiser, S. D., Bangsberg, D. R., Kegeles, S., Ragland, K., Kushel, M. B., & Frongillo, E. A. (2009). Food insecurity among homeless and marginally housed individuals living with HIV/AIDS in San Francisco. *AIDS and Behavior, 13*(5), 841–848.

Weiser, S. D., Frongillo, E. A., Ragland, K., Hogg, R. S., Riley, E. D., & Bangsberg, D. R. (2009). Food insecurity is associated with incomplete HIV RNA suppression among homeless and marginally housed HIV-infected individuals in San Francisco. *Journal of General Internal Medicine, 24*(1), 14–20.

Weiser, S. D., Hatcher, A., Frongillo, E. A., Guzman, D., Riley, E. D., Bangsberg, D. R., & Kushel, M. B. (2013). Food insecurity is associated with greater acute care utilization among HIV-infected homeless and marginally housed individuals in San Francisco. *Journal of General Internal Medicine, 28*(1), 91–98.

Weiser, S. D., Young, S. L., Cohen, C. R., Kushel, M. B., Tsai, A. C., Tien, P. C., ... Bangsberg, D. R. (2011). Conceptual framework for understanding the bidirectional links between food insecurity and HIV/AIDS. *American Journal of Clinical Nutrition, 94*(6), 1729S–1739S.

Weissman, D. (Producer), & Weber, B., & Weissman, D. (Co-Directors). (2011). *We were here* [Motion picture]. (Available from https://wewereherefilm.com)

Wejnert, C., Le, B., Rose, C. E., Oster, A. M., Smith, A. J., Zhu, J., ... for the NHBS Study Group. (2013). HIV infection and awareness among men who have sex with men—20 cities, United States, 2008 and 2011. *PloS One, 8*(10), e76878. doi:10.1371/journal.pone.0076878.

White House Office of National AIDS Policy. (2010). *National HIV/AIDS strategy for the United States*. Washington, DC: The White House National Office of AIDS Policy.

White House Office of National AIDS Policy. (2015). *National HIV/AIDS strategy for the United States: Updated to 2020*. Washington, DC: The White House National Office of AIDS Policy.

Williams, J. K., Wyatt, G. E., Rivkin, I., Ramamurthi, H. C., Li, X., & Liu, H. (2008). Risk reduction for HIV-positive African American and Latino men with histories of childhood sexual abuse. *Archives of Sexual Behavior, 37*(5), 763–772.

Wilton, L. (2009). Men who have sex with men of color in the age of AIDS: The sociocultural contexts of stigma, marginalization, and structural inequalities. In V. Stone, B. Ojikutu, K. Rawlings, & K. Smith (Eds.), *HIV/AIDS in U.S. communities of color* (pp. 179–212). New York: Springer.

Wolitski, R. J., & Fenton, K. A. (2011). Sexual health, HIV, and sexually transmitted infections among gay, bisexual, and other men who have sex with men in the United States. *AIDS and Behavior, 15*(Suppl 1), S9–17.

Wolitski, R. J., Kidder, D. P., Pals, S. L., Royal, S., Aidala, A., Stall, R., ... Housing and Health Study Team. (2010). Randomized trial of the effects of housing assistance on the health and risk behaviors of homeless and unstably housed people living with HIV. *AIDS and Behavior, 14*(3), 493–503.

Wright, J. (2013). Only your calamity: The beginnings of activism by and for people with AIDS. *American Journal of Public Health, 103*(10), 1788–1798.

Yard, S. S., Huh, D., King, K. M., & Simoni, J. M. (2011). Patient-level moderators of the efficacy of peer support and pager reminder interventions to promote antiretroviral adherence. *AIDS and Behavior, 15*(8), 1596–1604.

Chapter 7
HIV-Infected Gay Men and Adherence to HIV Antiretroviral Therapies

Jaclyn M. White Hughto, Janna R. Gordon, and Matthew J. Mimiaga

Epidemiology of ART Adherence Among Gay, Bisexual, and Other MSM in the US

Comprising just 2% of the US population, gay, bisexual, and other men who have sex with men (MSM) accounted for greater than 60% of incident HIV infections in the US and 78% of infections among all newly infected men in 2010 (CDC, 2013). Moreover, MSM represented 489,121, or 56%, of the estimated 873,430 persons living with an HIV diagnosis that same year (CDC, 2013). Advances in medical treatment, specifically antiretroviral medications, have resulted in precipitous declines in HIV-associated morbidity and mortality in the US (CASCADE Collaboration, 2000; CDC, 2013; Crum et al., 2006; Montaner et al., 2006; Palella et al., 2006), allowing for HIV-infected persons to manage their HIV infection as a

J.M. White Hughto (✉)
Department of Chronic Disease Epidemiology, Yale School of Public Health,
New Haven, CT, USA

The Fenway Institute, Fenway Health, Boston, MA, USA
e-mail: jwhite@fenwayhealth.org

J.R. Gordon
Joint Doctoral Program in Clinical Psychology, University of California, San Diego (UCSD)/
San Diego State University (SDSU), San Diego, CA, USA

M.J. Mimiaga
The Fenway Institute, Fenway Health, Boston, MA, USA

Departments of Epidemiology and Behavioral & Social Health Sciences, Brown School of
Public Health, Providence, RI, USA

Department of Psychiatry & Human Behavior, Alpert Medical School, Brown University,
Providence, RI, USA

© Springer Science+Business Media LLC 2017   151
L. Wilton (ed.), *Understanding Prevention for HIV Positive Gay Men*,
DOI 10.1007/978-1-4419-0203-0_7

chronic, rather than imminently life-threatening disease. However, the success of antiretroviral therapies (ART) such as Highly Active Antiretroviral Therapy (HAART) rely on patient adherence to medications.

Studies have shown that high rates of adherence (i.e., taking at least 80% of medication doses as prescribed) are necessary to achieving therapeutic success (an undetectable viral load) (Bangsberg, 2006; Kleeberger et al., 2001; Martin et al., 2008; Paterson et al., 2000; Shuter, Sarlo, Kanmaz, Rode, & Zingman, 2007). While optimal adherence rates differ by drug class (95% adherence is considered optimal for HAART vs. 80% adherence for newer boosted protease inhibitors) (Bangsberg, 2006; Kobin & Sheth, 2011; Martin et al., 2008; Paterson et al., 2000), patients who are highly adherent to ART typically suppress their viral load, increase their CD4 lymphocyte count, reduce their likelihood of developing opportunistic infections, and have lower levels of hospitalization (Halkitis, Palamar, & Mukherjee, 2008; Paterson et al., 2000; Wood et al., 2004). Moreover, individuals who suppress their viral load to an undetectable level are less likely to transmit the virus to their sexual partners, thereby lowering community viral load and incident cases (Ambrosioni, Calmy, & Hirschel, 2011). In contrast, suboptimal ART adherence can compromise the health of an HIV-infected individual by producing a rapid increase in HIV viral load, decrease in CD4 count, and the potential for the development of drug resistant virus (Bangsberg, 2008; Kiertiburanakul & Sungkanuparph, 2009; Nachega et al., 2011; Robbins et al., 2007). Drug resistance, or the ability of HIV to mutate and reproduce itself in the presence of antiretroviral drugs, often occurs during periods of nonadherence when the virus is given the opportunity to replicate. The consequences of drug resistance include treatment failure, increased costs associated with the need for more costly second-line treatments, the spread of resistant strains of HIV, and ultimately the potential for increased HIV incidence at the population level (Kleeberger et al., 2001; Wainberg & Zaharatos, 2012; WHO, 2013). Adherence has therefore proven to be the crux of secondary prevention success with antiretroviral medications.

Medication adherence difficulties are not specific to any one population and are often influenced by a variety of individual, interpersonal, and contextual factors. Indeed, research has shown that adherence rates tend to be highly variable across diverse study samples (Catz, Kelly, Bogart, Benotsch, & McAuliffe, 2000; Chesney, 2000; Halkitis et al., 2008; Ickovics & Meade, 2002; Kalichman et al., 2010; Thrasher, Earp, Golin, & Zimmer, 2008; Weidle et al., 1999) as well as among gay and bisexual men specifically (Halkitis, Parsons, Wolitski, & Remien, 2003; Halkitis et al., 2008; Thrasher et al., 2008; Wagner, 2002). Nonetheless, studies among HIV-infected men and women demonstrated that gay and bisexual men are more likely to be adherent than their heterosexual counterparts (Thrasher et al., 2008; Wagner, Remien, Carballo-Diéguez, & Dolezal, 2002). In a national sample of 1886 HIV-infected men and women (57% MSM) in the US, researchers found that heterosexually-identified participants self-reported poorer medication adherence in the past 7 days than did gay and lesbian individuals ($p < 0.001$) (Thrasher et al., 2008). Moreover, when compared to men who had contracted HIV through sex with other men, all other risk groups were less likely to be adherent (injection drug users: $p = 0.003$; and male to female sexual contact; $p < 0.001$). Similarly, in a small mixed gender and sexual orientation sample (19 gay men, 14 heterosexual men and 7 heterosexual women), Wagner and colleagues found that the mean self-reported adherence rate (past 3 days) for gay men (99%) was significantly higher than the rates for heterosexual men (94%) and heterosexual women (87%) ($p < 0.01$) (Wagner et al., 2002). Additionally, a greater proportion of gay men (79%) reported perfect adherence in the past 3 days than heterosexual men (36%) or heterosexual women (14%).

While some studies have found that gay, bisexual, and other MSM have higher rates of adherence than heterosexual populations, studies with samples comprised exclusively of gay and bisexual men have produced variable rates of adherence (Du Bois & McKirnan, 2012; Halkitis, Kutnick, & Slater, 2005; Halkitis & Palamar, 2008; Halkitis et al., 2008; Kleeberger et al., 2001). In a study assessing adherence among a sample of 276 gay and bisexual men in New York City, average adherence to medications in the past 2 months was 90% as measured by MEMS (Medication Event Management System) Track Cap (Halkitis et al., 2008). Similarily, in a study of 300 HIV-infected gay and bisexual men in New York City, adherence to ART medication in the past 2 weeks ranged from 71.2 to 95.2% based on the method of assessment (self-report yielded higher rates than MEMS Track Cap) (Halkitis & Palamar, 2008). However, given the high levels of adherence required for treatment success, researchers have frequently dichotomized adherence rates in order to examine correlates of optimal vs. suboptimal adherence among samples of gay and bisexual men. For example, researchers examined perfect adherence (i.e., took all doses and numbers of pills as prescribed by a health care provider) in a sample of 539 gay and bisexual men enrolled in the Multicenter AIDS Cohort Study (MACS) across four US cities, and found that the majority (77.7%) of participants reported 100% adherence over a 4-day recall period, with adherence data tending to correlate with biological levels of HIV viral load (Kleeberger et al., 2001). Similarly, in a study of 300 HIV-infected gay and bisexual men in New York City, researchers found that 60% of participants had adherence rates of 95% or greater via both self-report and the MEMS Track Cap System (Halkitis, Kutnick, et al., 2005), while only 51.3% of MSM in a Chicago sample reported 95% adherence or more in the past week (Du Bois & McKirnan, 2012). These results highlight the variability of adherence rates among MSM, which may differ by sample and geographical location as well as the definition and assessment method used.

Adherence Measurement

Given that suboptimal adherence can lead to drug failure (Knobel et al., 2001; Mannheimer et al., 2002), measuring adherence is necessary to evaluating treatment efficacy in both research and clinical settings. Halkitis and Palamar (2008) defined adherence as, "the extent to which a patient's behavior coincides with medical advice, including the dosing and instructions of specific medications." While most researchers and clinicians would agree with this definition, accurate measurement of ART adherence remains an ongoing challenge, and few studies are consistent in their classification (Bosworth, Oddone, & Weinberger, 2005; Reisner et al., 2009). Indeed, rates of adherence have been shown to differ substantially based on measurement period (e.g., missed doses in past month, past week, past day) and measurement format (e.g., interview, anonymous self-report, pill counts, electronic measurement) (Chesney, 2003; Halkitis, Parsons, et al., 2003). Adherence measurement may be classified into three categories described in detail below: (1) subjective measures; (2) pharmacologic measures; and (3) physiological measures.

Subjective Measures

Patient self-reported measurement (e.g., qualitative interviews and quantitative questionnaires) is among the most widely used method of assessing ART adherence in clinical and research settings due to its practicality, low cost, minimal participant burden, ease of administration, and flexibility in administration and timing of assessments (Berg & Arnsten, 2006; Simoni, Kurth, et al., 2006; Wagner & Miller, 2004). Moreover, when measured against nonsubjective measures such as pill count or viral load, studies have shown that the specificity of self-report measures is high (i.e., patients' self-reported adherence to medication is generally reliable) (Bangsberg, Hecht, Clague, et al., 2001; Kleeberger et al., 2001; Nieuwkerk & Oort, 2005; Simoni, Kurth, et al., 2006). A systematic review of 77 studies employing various self-report adherence measures found that self-reported adherence was significantly correlated with HIV viral load in 84% of recall periods (Nieuwkerk & Oort, 2005). Among gay and bisexual men specifically, an observational study of 393 HIV-infected men across four US cities demonstrated that self-report may be a valid tool for assessing patient adherence as 48.2% of the men who were 100% adherent to their HIV medication in the past 4 days (i.e., took all doses and numbers of pills as prescribed by a health care provider) had undetectable viral loads, compared to 33.7% in the lower adherence group ($p = 0.015$) (Kleeberger et al., 2001). Nonetheless, participant biases tend to positively skew self-report measures as patients may be unable to accurately recall their medication use (i.e., recall bias) or may report greater adherence for fear of provider chastisement (i.e., social desirability bias) (Berg & Arnsten, 2006; Simoni, Kurth, et al., 2006; Wilson, Carter, & Berg, 2009). In fact, a study among HIV-infected drug users found that self-reports predictably overestimate adherence by as much as 20% (Arnsten et al., 2001). Overestimated adherence rates can result in imprecise assessments of patient health, delays in addressing adherence issues, and inaccurate assessments of efficacy in adherence intervention trials (Berg & Arnsten, 2006).

Pharmacologic Measures

Due to the limitations of self-report, some researchers have suggested that less sub-jective, pharmacological methods may be preferable to self-report for assessing adherence, especially in intervention trials (Berg & Arnsten, 2006; Miller & Hays, 2000a; Simoni, Kurth, et al., 2006). Pharmacologic measures include electronic drug monitoring (EDM), pill count and pharmacy refill records. EDM utilizes monitoring devices, such as the MEMS—a pill bottle cap with an embedded microprocessor that records the time and date of each bottle opening as an inferred dose and then stores the data until it is downloaded manually with a microprocessor-reading device. Benefits of EDM include the ability to examine patterns of adherence and detailed aspects of medication taking, including the percentage of doses taken for one drug and the accuracy of the timing of doses (Berg & Arnsten, 2006; Mayer et al., 2008). While there is not a "gold standard" adherence measurement, EDM is often treated as such because it correlates strongest with virologic outcomes (Berg & Arnsten, 2006) and has been demonstrated in cross-validation studies (Arnsten et al., 2001; Deschamps et al., 2004; Hugen et al., 2002; Liu et al., 2001) to be the most sensitive measure of adherence (Deschamps et al., 2008). Nonetheless, the expense and devia-tion from some patients' preferred storage systems (e.g., pill boxes) (Kalichman, Cain, Cherry, Kalichman, & Pope, 2005) often make electronic drug monitoring problematic for daily use (Berg & Arnsten, 2006; Bova et al., 2005; Deschamps et al., 2008; Mayer et al., 2008). Moreover, procedural, quality control, and data management issues can impact EDM adherence estimates. For example, the removal of a cap does not necessarily correspond to the ingestion of the medication in the pill bottle and periods of nonuse do not always indicate that a patient was nonadherent (Berg & Arnsten, 2006; Mayer et al., 2008). In addition, such methods only allow the monitoring of one medication per pill bottle cap. If individuals are taking a combina-tion therapy in which different medications are ingested at different times during the day, EDM typically is unable to accurately assess the other pills being taken without the utilization of additional pill bottles. However, the more recent availability of the Wisepill® medication dispenser addresses this limitation and offers researchers a more reliable and feasible means of measuring adherence. Pill-taking (i.e., opening of pill box) is captured via a built-in SIM card that wirelessly transmits data over the Internet in real time (Wisepill®, http://www.wisepill.com/mediscern/). This form of EDM is a more proximate measure of adherence, utilizes a more preferred means of pill storage, and better accommodates combination therapy. Unfortunately, the cost and limited production to-date limit the feasibility of this measure in real-world settings.

Other forms of pharmacological measurement include pill count and pharmacy records. However, in general, pill counts are not ideal as they provide no informa-tion regarding the accuracy of the timing of doses taken and no evidence that the medication doses were actually consumed. Moreover, social desirability in clinical settings could lead to "pill dumping" or the emptying of bottles without ingestion, which could lead to overestimates of adherence (Berg & Arnsten, 2006; Ickovics &

Meisler, 1997; Mayer et al., 2008; Miller & Hays, 2000b). Unannounced pill counts, in which researchers come to the homes of participants to count pills, have been shown to be an accurate measure of adherence, correlating well with HIV viral load levels (Bangsberg, Hecht, Charlebois, Chesney, & Moss, 2001; Bangsberg, Hecht, Clague, et al., 2001; Berg & Arnsten, 2006; Mayer et al., 2008). However, time, cost, and other logistical issues make it hard to implement home-based pill counts in non-research settings. Pharmacy records offer another form of objective measurement in which adherence rates from pharmacy refill records are determined by comparing actual to expected refill dates or by identifying periods of time during which the patient's supply of medication is thought to have been depleted (Berg & Arnsten, 2006). Protections against social desirability and reporting biases as well as limited participant burden make pharmacy refill records a less subjective measurement tool; however, obtaining access to records introduces challenges in clinic settings and this method is unable to account for the sharing of medication, missed doses, medication interuptions, and other gaps in treatment (Acri, TenHave, Chapman, Bogner, & Gross, 2010; Berg & Arnsten, 2006; Reynolds, 2004).

Physiological Measures

Physiological measures of adherence include viral load tests, CD4 count, and direct measurement of drug or drug markers in the blood, urine, or hair. Biological assays, in particular, provide the most objective measures of adherence; however, drug monitoring is expensive, invasive, and therefore impractical in most clinical settings (Berg & Arnsten, 2006; Holzemer et al., 1999). Moreover, assays provide little information about the consistency of medication taking (Gao, Nau, Rosenbluth, Scott, & Woodward, 2000) and typically only measure recent doses; thus, adherence may be overestimated if patients are more conscientious about taking their medication before a clinic visit (Chesney, 2000). Other physiological methods include the measurement of HIV-1 RNA viral load and CD4 lymphocyte count. However, with these measures, there is no clear causal linkage between lab results and actual adherence behaviors; thus, these measures are often combined with other methods such as self-report or EDM in order to provide more robust measures of adherence (Simoni, Kurth, et al., 2006). Techniques that combine information from multiple measures reduce the error associated with any single measure and are thus used frequently in research settings. However, high costs and logistical issues often make combining multiple measures largely impractical in clinic settings. Future research is needed to determine how best to integrate combined measures into clinical care.

Factors Affecting ART Adherence

Despite the abundance of research assessing correlates of adherence, no single factor or combination of factors has been shown to consistently predict optimal medication adherence in any one individual or group of people, including gay men. Specific factors such as body image (Blashill & Vander Wal, 2010) and methamphetamine use (Chartier et al., 2010; Marquez, Mitchell, Hare, John, & Klausner, 2009) may be particularly salient among gay and bisexual men; however, the literature suggests that many of the same issues impacting the general population affect gay and bisexual men as well (e.g., demographic, psychosocial, interpersonal and system-level factors) (Halkitis, Parsons, et al., 2003; Halkitis et al., 2008; Kleeberger et al., 2001). This section explores the numerous factors associated with adherence among diverse samples, particularly the patient-, interpersonal-, and structural-level contexts that enhance or undermine ART adherence among HIV-infected gay, bisexual, and other men who have sex with men.

Patient-Level Characteristics

Demographic Factors

A variety of demographic factors, including race/ethnicity, age, and socioeconomic status (SES), have been found to impact adherence rates among gay, bisexual, and other MSM (Halkitis et al., 2008; Kleeberger et al., 2004; Millett, Flores, Peterson, & Bakeman, 2007; Oh et al., 2009). Although these characteristics have not been shown to consistently predict adherence, there is evidence that certain demographic factors may put some individuals at greater risk for adherence failure. Age, for example, has been found to be associated with medication adherence, with studies indicating that older gay and bisexual men may be more adherent to medication than younger men (Halkitis et al., 2008; Oh et al., 2009). A longitudinal study of gay, bisexual, and other MSM found that being under the age of 40 was significantly associated with decreased ART adherence over time (Kleeberger et al., 2004). Similarly, in a longitudinal study of 300 HIV-infected gay, bisexual, and other MSM, participants over the age of 50 had significantly better rates of baseline medication adherence than those under 50 (Solomon & Halkitis, 2008). In addition to increased access to medical care (Cohen & Bloom, 2010; Cohen, Martinez, & Free, 2008) being older may confer other benefits that facilitate adherence, such as more stable schedules that allow for set dosing schedules and increased knowledge about drug regimens (Wellons et al., 2002).

Race and ethnicity have also been linked to adherence outcomes, with gay and bisexual men of color often reporting suboptimal medication adherence (Halkitis, Parsons, et al., 2003; Halkitis, Kutnick, et al., 2005; Oh et al., 2009). In a sample of 214 African American men with HIV, many of whom reported sex with other men, adherence rates were generally low, with less than 25% of participants adhering to their medication at the level necessary to prevent virologic failure and drug resistance (Bogart, Wagner, Galvan, & Banks, 2010). In comparing adherence rates across groups, a longitudinal study of 1102 gay and bisexual men enrolled in the MAC study found that race was a significant predictor of medication adherence, with Black and Latino participants each at greater odds of reporting suboptimal adherence over the previous 4 days than White participants (Oh et al., 2009). Similarly, Halkitis, Kutnick, et al. (2005) found that three times as many African American men and twice as many Latino men had <80% adherence compared to White men. The association between race and nonadherence has not been consistently found across studies, however, as a study of 456 gay and bisexual men in San Francisco and New York found that African American men were no less adherent than other men, although African American men were less likely to be on ART than men of other ethnicities (Halkitis, Parsons, et al., 2003). Findings suggest that the relationship between racial/ethnic minority status and ART adherence is complex and often impacted by individual- and structural-level factors. For example, beliefs about treatment, health care discrimination, and corresponding mistrust of health care providers may contribute to nonadherence individually (Stall et al., 1996; Thrasher et al., 2008), while structurally, there is evidence that access to health care access may mediate the relationship between race and adherence (Halkitis, Parsons, et al., 2003; Halkitis, Kutnick, et al., 2005). Such factors will be explored later in this chapter (see "Access to HIV/Medical Care" section).

At the patient level, SES may play a role in the relationship between race/ethnicity and medication adherence among gay, bisexual, and other MSM, as individuals who lack private health insurance, or those who struggle to afford medications, may experience challenges in remaining adherent. This was supported by Oh and colleagues, who found that Black and Latino gay and bisexual men reported significantly more financial difficulty and lower income than their White counterparts; moreover, higher ART cost and financial difficulties were associated with nonadherence (Oh et al., 2009). These findings are consistent with the work of Kleeberger and colleagues, who demonstrated differences in adherence rates between gay and bisexual men making over $50,000 and those earning less than $50,000 annually (Kleeberger et al., 2001). Factors associated with low SES such as unstable housing may also contribute to suboptimal ART adherence as individuals living in short-term shelters, hostels, or motels routinely report poorer adherence to ART compared to those living in more stable environments, including long-term housing (for a meta-analysis, see Leaver, Bargh, Dunn, & Hwang, 2007). For low-income individuals infected with HIV, living in unstable housing may influence set schedules and other forms of support (e.g., social support, financial resources) that are beneficial for optimal adherence.

Level of educational attainment might also serve as a moderator between race, age, SES, and medication adherence, as having a lower level of education has been found to be a determinant of suboptimal adherence among gay and bisexual men (e.g., Kleeberger et al., 2004). Indeed, individuals with more education may have greater knowledge about the disease and therefore better understand the importance of initiating and remaining adherent to treatment, than those with limited education. Additionally, those with more education may be better equipped to manage complex treatment regimens and dosing instructions, than those lacking education. This is evidenced by Gonzalez et al. (2007), who found that level of education was positively associated with level of adherence in a diverse cohort of men and women living with HIV. Similarly, Kleeberger et al. (2001) found that the rates of adherence among gay, bisexual, and other MSM in the sample (77.7% of men reported 100% adherence) exceeded the rates reported in other studies, with researchers attributing superior adherence rates to educational attainment (56% of the sample had completed at least a college degree or higher). Health literacy may further moderate the relationship between medication adherence and specific demographic characteristics such as age, race, and SES (e.g., Gonzalez et al., 2007; Kalichman, Catz, & Ramachandran, 1999; Thrasher et al., 2008) as health literacy was also found to be an important factor in HIV medication adherence among 184 men and women with HIV (70% men, % MSM not reported) in one study (Kalichman et al., 1999). Among participants in the sample, Kalichman et al. (1999) found that those with limited health literacy reported suboptimal rates of adherence, often citing confusion and misguided beliefs about HIV medications (e.g., wanting to "cleanse" their body) as reasons for missing doses. Providing accessible information and counseling regarding HIV, health, and medication regimens to those with lower educational attainment may support individuals in making the best choices for their health, including adhering to prescribed treatments.

While studies demonstrating associations between demographic characteristics and medication adherence may be of use in determining which groups are in need of adherence interventions, there is much variability when it comes to the predictive nature of demographic factors on adherence. Bartlett (2002) warns against the use of such assumptions as a means of "nonadherence profiling," as these assumptions may lead to overestimates of adherence among men of higher socioeconomic status, for example, and underestimates of adherence among men of color. Although demographic characteristics may highlight specific factors that have an impact in individuals' lives, the traits themselves are not necessarily indicators of adherence. For instance, in a sample of HIV positive homeless and transiently housed individuals, Bangsberg et al. (2000) noted that rates of adherence were better than anticipated, with nearly 40% of the population demonstrating over 90% pill count adherence. It is therefore important to understand the relationship between demographic factors and adherence in the context of other interpersonal (e.g., caregiver relationship, patient-provider relationship) and structural factors (e.g., access to care) that may facilitate or impede adherence to ART (Halkitis, Kutnick, et al., 2005). Such factors will be discussed in depth throughout this chapter.

Treatment and Disease Factors

Patients on ART are required to adhere to treatment regimens that may include numerous medications, varying dosing schedules, dietary restrictions, and specific storage requirements (Stone et al., 2001; U.S. Department of Health and Human Services, 2012). Not surprisingly, the complex and confusing nature of these regimens has been shown to contribute to nonadherence in some samples (Bartlett, DeMasi, Quinn, Moxham, & Rousseau, 2001; Halkitis & Palamar, 2008; Kleeberger et al., 2001; Trotta et al., 2002). For example, researchers found that a greater number of pills taken was associated with lower adherence in a sample of gay and bisexual men enrolled in the MACS cohort, while certain drug combinations (3TC, SQV, RTV and d4T) with complex storage requirements were also found to be associated with lower adherence (Kleeberger et al., 2001). Similarly, Halkitis et al. (2008) found that the number of pills prescribed per day was a predictor of adherence among a sample of 300 gay and bisexual men in New York City (e.g., as the daily number of pills increased, adherence to one's medication decreased). Treatment complexity has not consistently been shown to be associated with nonadherence, however, as a study of 456 ethnically diverse gay and bisexual men found that adherence was unrelated to the number of different HIV medications taken, with no differences in adherence rates between those on mono-therapy and those on dual and triple class therapies (Halkitis, Parsons, et al., 2003). While these results appear inconsistent, findings suggest that adherence issues may not be the result of treatment complexity alone, but rather the degree to which patients are able to integrate complex regimens into their lifestyles (Brion & Menke, 2008). This was supported by participants in the MACS cohort who cited changes to daily routines as a common explanation for missed doses (Kleeberger et al., 2001). Likewise, in a national sample of 1186 men and women (57% MSM), Thrasher et al. (2008) found that the difficulty participants reported integrating their medications into their lives had the strongest direct effect on self-reported nonadherence in the past 7 days.

Medication side effects have also been found to be associated with nonadherence among diverse populations (Cooper, Gellaitry, Hankins, Fisher, & Horne, 2009; Corless, Nicholas, Davis, Dolan, & McGibbon, 2005; Duran et al., 2001; Gagnon, Welles, & Japour, 2007; Gay et al., 2011; Kleeberger et al., 2001; Remien et al., 2003). Among HIV-infected gay and bisexual men, for example, Kleeberger et al. (2001) found that side effects were associated with lower adherence to medication. For many patients, nonadherence may be intentional, as individuals may purposely skip medication doses in order to avoid negative side effects. For example, participants in a mixed sample of 110 men and women (35% were men who reported having sex with other men) reported that antiretroviral medications produced a wide range of negative symptoms (e.g., nausea, diarrhea, irritability, headaches, fatigue, joint pain, and insomnia), which resulted in the deliberate skipping of doses and even the discontinuation of treatment altogether (Remien et al., 2003). Side effects may not always lead to nonadherence, however, as disease-related symptomatology and/or the stage of disease may also play a role in one's decision to remain adherent to treatment.

Studies have shown that the stage and severity of infection, including the physical symptoms of the disease, are associated with treatment adherence, although these factors may have differential effects on adherence. For example, individuals in the later stages of HIV disease may tolerate medication side effects as the effects of treatment may not be as severe as the symptoms of the disease itself. Conversely, those in the earlier stages of HIV disease, who are otherwise asymptomatic, may find the side effects of treatment acute and consequently suspend or terminate use (Bartlett, 2002; Cooper et al., 2009; Gao et al., 2000). Research has also shown that physical symptoms may motivate individuals to adhere to their medication as poor physical health serves as a cue to treatment for some individuals (Remien et al., 2003). Conversely, physical symptoms may discourage other individuals and even lead to depression, which may have an impact on adherence behaviors (see Gonzalez, Batchelder, Psaros, & Safren, 2011 for a review). Still, some studies have failed to show an association between adherence and medication side effects, especially when studied longitudinally, as it is possible that some individuals may adapt to the negative effects of medications or side effects may subside over time (see Fogarty et al., 2002 for a review). The literature on disease-related factors is thus variable and dependent on the stage of HIV infection, type of symptoms experienced, and individual beliefs regarding the significance of these disease factors.

HIV Treatment Beliefs

Long-standing research suggests that the beliefs one holds about their HIV treatment regimen are among the most reliable and proximate determinants of adherence (Chesney, 2003; Ickovics & Meade, 2002; Richter, Sowell, & Pluto, 2002; Viswanathan, Anderson, & Thomas, 2005). Indeed, those that believe that treatment is beneficial to survival and that failure to take medications will lead to illness are likely to take their HIV medications as prescribed (e.g., Gonzalez et al., 2007; Remien et al., 2003; Thrasher et al., 2008). This was evidenced by participants in a qualitative study of 110 HIV-infected women, MSM, and male injection drug users, many of whom credited their medication adherence to the fact that the medicines facilitated their recovery from serious illness (Remien et al., 2003). Similarly, in a national longitudinal study of 1886 HIV-infected men and women (57% MSM), treatment beliefs predicted participants' level of adherence, such that those who endorsed beliefs that HIV medications would lengthen their lifespan and improve their quality of life were at significantly greater odds of being adherent to their medications than those who did not endorse such beliefs (Thrasher et al., 2008). Stall et al. (1996) found similar results in a study of gay and bisexual men, with those adhering to their HIV medications at significantly greater odds of perceiving the effectiveness of these treatments than nonadherers. Moreover, treatment toxicity beliefs were inversely associated with adherence, such that participants who were not adherent were more likely to harbor antiretroviral toxicity beliefs than those who were adherent (Stall et al., 1996). In fact, treatment toxicity beliefs have been shown to impact adherence in several studies of MSM (e.g., Gonzalez et al., 2007; Kalichman et al., 2009), with participants endorsing toxicity beliefs in one study displaying worse adherence over time than those without such concerns (Gonzalez et al., 2007).

In addition to beliefs about medication toxicity, conspiracy beliefs regarding the origin of HIV and the government's role in its creation and transmission have also been associated with ART nonadherence, particularly among African Americans (see Bogart et al., 2010). In a sample of 214 African American men (78% identified as gay or bisexual), Bogart et al. (2010) found that HIV-related conspiracy beliefs were associated with nonadherence. In fact, research has consistently shown that Black men are more likely to have negative opinions about HIV treatment (e.g., believe that the medications are toxic), which may in part explain the low rates of adherence across samples of gay and bisexual men of color (e.g., Halkitis, Kutnick, et al., 2005; Halkitis, Shrem, & Martin, 2005; Oh et al., 2009; Thrasher et al., 2008). Intervention research that addresses inaccurate beliefs about HIV treatment should take into account the cultural factors and historical contexts that guide myths and misconceptions among specific populations (e.g., history of slavery, segregation, racism, and involvement in the Tuskegee syphilis experiments among African Americans) and identify how beliefs about HIV treatment may be respectfully challenged to ensure uptake and adherence to lifesaving medications (for more on intervention work targeting cultural beliefs among African Americans see Bogart et al., 2010; Raja, McKirnan, & Glick, 2007; Jones et al., 2008; Wilton et al., 2009).

Beliefs about oneself may also have important implications for adherence to ART in those living with HIV. Self-efficacy, or the belief in one's ability to successfully perform a task as necessary, has been linked to the management of HIV and adherence to ART across diverse samples (Arnsten et al., 2007; Halkitis, Kutnick, et al., 2005; Johnson et al., 2007). For example, Halkitis, Kutnick, et al. (2005), in a sample of 300 gay, bisexual, and other MSM, found that endorsing greater adherence self-efficacy was associated with better adherence to one's ART treatment plan. Conversely, those that believed they lacked the ability to take medications correctly and on time reported suboptimal adherence to HIV medications. Given these findings, interventions that help individuals develop the skills necessary to take medications as prescribed, as well as identify and challenge certain cognitions that inhibit self-efficacy, may empower individuals to become more adherent to their HIV medications (see "Mental Health" section for more on self-efficacy).

Researchers have sought to examine the pathways for the relationship between ART use and sexual behavior, with many studies demonstrating that the beliefs individuals hold about ART efficacy are stronger predictors of sexual risk behavior than ART use itself. Indeed, there is evidence that those who believe they are less infectious due to ART treatment may behaviorally compensate by engaging in greater HIV risk behavior (Halkitis, Wilton, Parsons, & Hoff, 2004; Kalichman et al., 2010; Ostrow et al., 2002; Stolte, Dukers, Geskus, Coutinho, & Wit, 2004; Vanable, Ostrow, & McKirnan, 2003). For example, Halkitis and colleagues (2004) found that beliefs about decreased risk as a result of taking antiretrovirals were significantly associated with unprotected anal sex among gay men. Similarly, Ostrow et al. (2002) found that HIV-infected MSM who were less concerned about transmitting HIV to sexual partners, due to the availability of ART, were up to six times more likely to engage in unprotected insertive anal intercourse. Kalichman et al. (2010) also supported these findings; in a mixed sample of HIV-infected men (55% MSM), holding the belief that an undetectable viral load leads to lower infectiousness was associated with greater number of partners, having an HIV-uninfected partner and lower condom use. Moreover, men who had an undetectable viral load and believed that having an undetectable viral load reduces their infectiousness were at significantly greater odds of having contracted a recent STI. Results suggest that beliefs about HIV transmissibility while on ART are critically important to sexual decision-making and may serve to explain differences in sexual risk behaviors among HIV-infected gay and bisexual men taking antiretroviral medications.

When examining associations between sexual behavior and adherence specifically, the literature appears to be more consistent. For example, among mixed gender samples, Diamond et al. (2005) found that consistent antiretroviral adherence was associated with a lower likelihood of unprotected sex, while Kalichman et al. (2010) found that nonadherence to ART was associated with greater number of sex partners, engaging in unprotected and protected anal intercourse, and illicit substance use. While it is possible that other individual or contextual factors may influence nonadherence and sexual risk behaviors, Kalichman and colleagues (2010) postulate that nonadherence and sexual risk behavior may be members of the same group of health harming behaviors. Similarly, Diamond et al. (2005) theorized that individuals who are adherent to ART may actually be more health-conscious, aware of the risks of unprotected sex (e.g., HIV and STI transmission risk), and ultimately more risk-averse than those not adherent to ART. Thus, while a subset of men may believe that adherence to ART mitigates the risks involved in sexual encounters, men who are adherent are in fact less likely to engage in such behavior. Such findings indicate the complex interplay between personal beliefs, behavioral norms, and actual behaviors, underscoring the need for research that explores the multiple factors influencing sexual behavior and medication adherence among gay, bisexual, and other MSM.

Mental Health

Mental health problems are prevalent among HIV-infected individuals, with estimates indicating that 50% of HIV-infected persons experience one or more comorbid psychiatric disorders (Bing et al., 2001). Depression, in particular, is one of the most common mental health problems experienced by HIV-infected adults (Rabkin, 2008; Zanjani, Saboe, & Oslin, 2007), with large-scale, nationally representative studies estimating that up to 36% of individuals living with HIV also experience depression (Asch et al., 2003; Bing et al., 2001)—a prevalence approximately five times greater than that found in the general population (Bing et al., 2001; SAMHSA, 1996). Among gay, bisexual, and other MSM, there is evidence that those with HIV have higher risk of depression than those without (for a review, see Ciesla & Roberts, 2001), with the frequency of depression in gay and bisexual men living with HIV nearly double that of those without the disease.

Depression has been shown to lead to worse health outcomes among gay and bisexual men, with a longitudinal study of 400 HIV-infected gay men in San Francisco finding that those who were depressed at baseline progressed to AIDS on average 1.4 years sooner than those who were not depressed (Page-Shafer, Delorenze, Satariano, & Winkelstein, 1996). Comorbid depression also poses significant implications for ART adherence among gay and bisexual men, as numerous studies have demonstrated the association between depressive symptoms and suboptimal ART adherence among this population (Blashill, Perry, & Safren, 2011; Du Bois & McKirnan, 2012; Halkitis, Parsons, et al., 2003; Kleeberger et al., 2001; Mugavero et al., 2006). For example, lowered adherence and depressive symptoms were linked in the MACS cohort both cross-sectionally (Kleeberger et al., 2001) and longitudinally (Kleeberger et al., 2004), while in another longitudinal study of more than 800 MSM, Du Bois and McKirnan (2012) found that reductions in depression predicted better medication adherence over a 1 year period. Given these findings, identifying and treating depression in gay and bisexual men living with HIV constitutes a substantial concern for those seeking to maximize ART adherence in this population.

While the complexities permeating the relationship between ART adherence and depression are not yet well established, researchers have posited a few possibilities. Depressive symptoms are associated with feelings of worthlessness, hopelessness, loss of interest, concentration problems, and pessimistic thoughts, which likely act as barriers to the self-care behaviors required for optimal health outcomes and disease management, including medication adherence (Kleeberger et al., 2001; Rabkin, 2008). Adhering to ART regimens also requires self-efficacy, or the belief in one's ability to take medications as prescribed by a health care provider. The negative affect experienced by depressed persons may impact self-efficacy and lead to suboptimal medication adherence as depressed individuals may experience diminished confidence in their ability to successfully complete difficult tasks (e.g., Kavanagh & Bower, 1985). The use of avoidant coping to deal with HIV-related stressors (e.g., isolation from others, sleep, indulging in food, having sex, working excessively) has been cited as another possible mediator between depression and medication nonadherence among gay and bisexual men (Halkitis & Palamar, 2008; Halkitis, Parsons, et al., 2003; Halkitis, Kutnick, et al., 2005). Men who use avoidant coping techniques to escape stress may also try to escape the reminders of their HIV status and consequently evade activities related to managing their illness (Halkitis & Kirton, 1999). Thus, interventions to assist HIV-infected individuals in utilizing active, rather than avoidant, coping strategies in managing stress and negative affect may also help to promote adherence to HIV medications.

In addition to depression, individuals living with HIV experience high levels of lifetime stress and trauma (e.g., sexual or physical abuse, unexpected deaths) (Ironson et al., 2005; Leserman, 2008; Leserman, Ironson, O'Cleirigh, Fordiani, & Balbin, 2008; Leserman et al., 2005; Leserman et al., 2007). For example, more than 70% of participants in a sample of HIV-infected adults had experienced more than two lifetime traumatic events and more than 50% reported a history of abuse (Leserman et al., 2005). Among gay and bisexual men, traumatic experiences are common, particularly when it comes to experiences of childhood sexual abuse, with prevalence estimates as high as 47% (Mimiaga et al., 2009; Paul, Catania, Pollack, & Stall, 2001; Welles, Corbin, Rich, Reed, & Raj, 2011; Welles et al., 2009). The high prevalence of trauma poses considerable challenges for HIV-related health outcomes and disease management, as trauma has been shown not only to be associated with HIV disease progression, but also with nonadherence to ART medications (Leserman, 2000; Mugavero et al., 2009). Interestingly, trauma may have an immediate effect on adherence; in one study of gay and bisexual men in New York City, Halkitis and colleagues found a significant increase in the number of missed doses immediately after the traumatic events of September 11th 2001 (Halkitis, Kutnick, Rosof, Slater, & Parsons, 2003). Trauma may also have a cumulative effect on adherence, with a cross-sectional study of HIV-infected men and women finding that medication nonadherence became incrementally more likely with each traumatic event reported (Mugavero et al., 2006).

Although the pathway between trauma and ART adherence is one that demands further exploration, the presence of high levels of stress resulting from trauma may constitute increased vulnerability to specific psychological disorders such as depression and post-traumatic stress disorder (PTSD) (O'Cleirigh, Skeer, Mayer, & Safren, 2009; Vranceanu et al., 2008). In fact, the diagnostic prevalence of PTSD among HIV-infected patients has been estimated to be as high as 27–54% (Bing et al., 2001; O'Cleirigh, Ironson, & Smits, 2007; O'Cleirigh et al., 2009) and MSM may be up to four times more likely to meet criteria for PTSD than heterosexual men in the general population (Kelly, Hoffman, Rompa, & Gray, 1998). Like depression, PTSD symptoms may impact one's ability to manage important self-care behaviors such as the ability to adhere to one's medication regimen (Vranceanu et al., 2008). These findings underscore the importance of psychological screening and treatment to address depression and the cognitive effects of past trauma as a critical component of HIV care.

Body image concerns constitute another means by which mental health stressors can be detrimental to HIV medication adherence among gay, bisexual, and other MSM living with HIV. Body image is defined as an individual's attitudes and perceptions regarding his or her physical appearance and includes both beliefs and behaviors (Cash, 2004). Body image concerns among men living with HIV/AIDS are common, with 31% of HIV-infected men in one study reporting dissatisfaction with their bodies (Sharma et al., 2007). Changes in body fat composition associated with HAART-induced lipodystrophy (Giralt et al., 2006; Guaraldi et al., 2006; Marín et al., 2006) is thought to contribute to the high rates of body dissatisfaction as the fat atrophy associated with lipodystrophy has been found to significantly and negatively impact men's views of their own bodies (Giralt et al., 2006; Guaraldi et al., 2006; Guaraldi et al., 2008; Huang et al., 2006; Martinez, Kemper, Diamond, & Wagner, 2005; Santos et al., 2005; Sharma et al., 2007). Although with newer ART regimens, lipodystrophy is less common, gay and bisexual men may be particularly vulnerable to body image concerns. Indeed, gay communities tend to report greater body dissatisfaction than heterosexual populations (see Morrison, Morrison, & Sager, 2004 for a review) and societal and cultural norms and expectations calling for muscular physiques appear to be highly prevalent among gay men more generally (Blashill & Vander Wal, 2009; Halkitis, 2001; Halkitis, Green, & Wilton, 2004; McCreary, Saucier, & Courtenay, 2005; Schwartz & Tylka, 2008).

Body dissatisfaction among gay and bisexual men may have important implications for the uptake of HIV treatment, as body dissatisfaction has been linked to

ART nonadherence among diverse samples both cross-sectionally (e.g., Corless et al., 2005) and longitudinally (Glass et al., 2010; Plankey et al., 2009). In a sample of MSM, for instance, Blashill and Vander Wal (2010) found that appearance concerns were positively associated with suboptimal ART adherence, with those endorsing greater appearance-related concerns reporting significantly worse HIV medication adherence than those with less severe body dissatisfaction. While few studies have examined the link between appearance concerns and nonadherence, studies by Blashill and Vander Wal (2010) and Blashill, Gordon, and Safren (2012b) have identified depression as one potential factor mediating the relationship between body dissatisfaction and medication adherence. Specifically, body dissatisfaction was found to contribute to depression severity, in turn influencing individuals' ability to adhere to their medications. Although research in this area is preliminary, a substantial amount of literature supports this model, as depression has been widely associated with negative body image and appearance concerns (Blashill, Gordon, & Safren, 2012a; Marín et al., 2006; Sharma, Howard, Schoenbaum, Buono, & Webber, 2006; Sharma et al., 2007; Wagner & Rabkin, 1999) as well as HIV medication nonadherence among diverse populations (see Gonzalez et al., 2011 for a review). Interventions that simultaneously address ART adherence and the underlying mental health conditions that impede adherence (e.g., depression, trauma, body dissatisfaction) could help to improve the mental and physical health of HIV-infected gay and bisexual men and may also confer benefits for secondary HIV prevention.

Substance use

Substance use is common among individuals living with HIV (Bing et al., 2001; McGowan et al., 2011; Mellins et al., 2009; Pence, Miller, Whetten, Eron, & Gaynes, 2006) and has been found to impact the ability of HIV-infected people in maintaining adherence to medication regimens (e.g., Halkitis, Shrem, et al., 2005). For example, Tegger et al. (2008) found that patients with substance use disorders were significantly less likely to initiate ART than those without, while HIV-infected drug users in another study were at four times greater odds of demonstrating suboptimal ART adherence (measured via electronic pill monitoring) than those who did not use drugs (Hinkin et al., 2007). Substance use and abuse may impact adherence both directly and indirectly. For example, substance use may promote lapses in adherence as recreational drugs and alcohol can lead to impaired judgment, short-term memory loss, decline in cognitive function, and disruption in one's daily schedule, thus decreasing the ability of individuals to take their medications correctly (Halkitis, Kutnick, et al., 2005). In addition, substance use has been found to be related to psychological distress and maladaptive behaviors such as avoidant coping, which, as previously discussed in this chapter, may place individuals at risk for ART nonadherence (e.g., Halkitis, Palamar, & Mukherjee, 2007; Mimiaga et al., 2013).

The impact of drug use and abuse on adherence may be a particularly salient concern for gay and bisexual men on ART, as substance use is common among this population (Halkitis et al., 2007; Morin et al., 2005; Ostrow & Stall, 2008; Skeer et al., 2012). In a multicenter cohort study of HIV-infected patients ($N = 3413$; 84% male, 46% racial/ethnic minority) engaged in HIV care in four US cities, 24% of patients reported current use of marijuana, 9% amphetamines, 9% crack/cocaine, 2% opiates; 3.8% IDU; and 10.3% concurrent drug use and nonadherence to antiretroviral therapy was associated with use of any substance (p-values < 0.05), except marijuana (Mimiaga et al., 2013). In another study of 503 MSM in primary care, 52% of those interviewed reported using at least one drug in the past 3 months, 20% reported using multiple drugs, and nearly one-third reported drug abuse as defined by the Patient Health Questionnaire (Kroenke, Spitzer, & Williams, 2003). Indeed, substance use and HIV medication adherence have been shown to be associated with decreased adherence to HIV medications among MSM in numerous studies, regardless of measurement technique (e.g., self-report, electronic medication monitoring) (Halkitis, Parsons, et al., 2003; Halkitis, Kutnick, et al., 2005; Halkitis et al., 2008; Kleeberger et al., 2004; Skeer et al., 2012). Two substances in particular have been cited as being particularly prevalent and with important implications for ART adherence among gay, bisexual, and other MSM: alcohol and crystal methamphetamine.

The prevalence of alcohol use among HIV-infected individuals have been found to be nearly double that of the general population (Galvan et al., 2002) and research has suggested that gay and bisexual men are at greater risk for developing substance use problems than heterosexual individuals (Green & Feinstein, 2012). Indeed, alcohol use is prevalent among HIV-infected MSM, with approximately half of HIV-infected MSM reporting drinking alcohol in the past 3 months and nearly 20% also reporting excessive alcohol use (Skeer et al., 2012). Moreover, alcohol use has consistently been found to be detrimental to medication adherence among those living with HIV (Azar, Springer, Meyer, & Altice, 2010; Hendershot, Stoner, Pantalone, & Simoni, 2009), including gay and bisexual men (e.g., Skeer et al., 2012). For example, one study found that heavy alcohol use was significantly associated with decreased ART adherence among MSM in the sample (Halkitis, Parsons, et al., 2003).

One possible pathway for medication nonadherence among HIV-infected alcohol users is depression, as elevated depressive symptoms have been directly associated with increased levels of alcohol use among those living with HIV (Ghebremichael et al., 2009; Sullivan et al., 2008; Velasquez et al., 2009). A recent longitudinal study of HIV-infected alcohol users found that level of drinking influenced depressive symptoms, such that individuals who increased or decreased their alcohol use experienced higher and lower levels of depressive symptoms, respectively (Sullivan, Goulet, Justice, & Fiellin, 2011). A substantial body of literature in the general population suggests that HIV-infected individuals may use alcohol as a means of coping with negative affect (see Conner, Pinquart, & Gamble, 2009 and Thornton et al., 2012 for meta-analyses) and as a means of escaping distress. The high comorbidity of depression and alcohol use, coupled with the high prevalence of adherence failure in these contexts, underscore the necessity of adherence interventions that contain the requisite flexibility to address multiple, overlapping mental health issues.

Like alcohol, crystal methamphetamine use among gay, bisexual, and other MSM is prevalent (Shoptaw, 2006; Solomon, Halkitis, Moeller, & Pappas, 2012), with some studies showing the prevalence of methamphetamine use among MSM to be 20 times greater than that of the general population (Colfax & Shoptaw, 2005; Fernández et al., 2005; Mimiaga et al., 2008; SAMHSA, 2001; Stall & Purcell, 2000). Methamphetamine use places uninfected men at risk for HIV as its use facilitates sexual encounters and risk taking (Mimiaga et al., 2008; Mimiaga et al., 2010; Mimiaga, Closson, et al., 2012; Rajasingham et al., 2012; Reback, Larkins, & Shoptaw, 2004). In fact, MSM who use crystal methamphetamine are at greater odds of engaging in a number of sexual risk activities, including unprotected anal sex (Bousman et al., 2009; Forrest et al., 2010; Mansergh et al., 2006; Mayer et al., 2010), group sex (Halkitis, Shrem, et al., 2005), multiple sex partners (Bousman et al., 2009; Forrest et al., 2010; Marquez et al., 2009; Wohl, Frye, & Johnson, 2008), sex with an injection drug user (Bousman, et al., 2009), and substance use during sex (Bousman, et al., 2009; Forrest et al., 2010), compared to MSM who do not use crystal methamphetamine, regardless of HIV status (Mimiaga et al., 2008; Mimiaga et al., 2010; Mimiaga, Closson, et al., 2012; Rajasingham et al., 2012). Sexual risk behavior in the context of methamphetamine use often leads to HIV infection, which in part accounts for disparities in HIV incidence between MSM who use methamphetamine and those who do not (prevalence of HIV among MSM methamphetamine users are nearly double that of non-methamphetamine users) (Buchacz et al., 2005). However, there is also evidence that HIV-infected MSM are at greater odds of using methamphetamine than are uninfected MSM (Forrest et al., 2010), although this estimate may be conflated by the predictive relationship between methamphetamine use and HIV acquisition. For some MSM who use methamphetamine, the experience of being diagnosed with HIV may lead to continued or increased use, while others may begin using methamphetamine as a means of mitigating HIV-related depression and negative affect (Gorman & Carroll, 2000; Robinson & Rempel, 2006; Semple, Patterson, & Grant, 2002).

Methamphetamine use among MSM has been shown to be significantly associated with poor ART adherence (Carrico, Johnson, Colfax, & Moskowitz, 2010; Colfax et al., 2007; Gorbach et al., 2008; Hinkin et al., 2007; Marquez et al., 2009; Reback, Larkins, & Shoptaw, 2003). A cross-sectional study of HIV-infected patients (39% MSM) showed that methamphetamine use in the prior 4 weeks was associated with poor ART adherence (Marquez et al., 2009). Similarly, in a diverse sample of HIV-infected individuals (65% MSM), Hinkin et al. (2007) found that HAART adherence was poorest among active stimulant users compared to users of other drugs, with active stimulant users at seven times greater odds of having poor adherence compared to drug-free participants. While the study did not analyze adherence among crystal methamphetamine users specifically, researchers found that those who used methamphetamine and cocaine together had a trend toward poorer adherence compared to those who used cocaine alone (54.5% vs. 68.1%, $p = 0.06$).

While few studies have examined factors associated with poor adherence among HIV-infected gay and bisexual men who use methamphetamine, Reback et al. (2003) found that lapses in ART adherence among MSM methamphetamine users may be intentional, and motivated by the desire to regain control over one's life, or unintentional, and related to the effects of methamphetamine use. For example, methamphetamine users may avoid taking medications in an effort to prevent the mixing of drugs or to feel liberated, while at other times, nonadherence may be unplanned and the result of methamphetamine-related sleep or appetite disturbances. A qualitative study of 20 HIV-infected MSM who believed they had sero-converted in the context of methamphetamine use supported the relationship between methamphetamine use and unplanned nonadherence, as participants reported that methamphetamine use often compromised their ability to care for themselves by eating correctly, sleeping regularly and taking medications as prescribed by a health care provider (Mimiaga et al., 2008). Moreover, some participants had lost jobs as a result of methamphetamine abuse, become estranged from family and friends, and were homeless and/or experienced chronic depression—outcomes that may have significant implications for ART adherence. Indeed, methamphetamine use has been linked with depression following the cessation of use (Meredith, Jaffe, Ang-Lee, & Saxon, 2005; Mimiaga et al., 2008; Peck, Shoptaw, Rotheram-Fuller, Reback, & Bierman, 2005), with individuals reporting symptoms of apathy and depression within the first several days of methamphetamine use cessation (Newton, Kalechstein, Duran, Vansluis, & Ling, 2004). There is also evidence that depressive symptoms may persist for many months following the discontinuation of methamphetamine use (Zweben et al., 2004). Additionally, despite having stopped their use of methamphetamine, former methamphetamine users have reported the persistence of other forms of cognitive impairment, which barred their ability to take medications as prescribed (Mimiaga et al., 2008). Psychological impairment may therefore serve as a pathway for nonadherence among HIV-infected men who use methamphetamine.

To improve ART adherence among gay men, effective interventions are needed which simultaneously address the motivations for use and psychological effects of cessation, which may impede one's ability to be fully adherent to HIV medications. Early research in this area has been promising; one intervention combined contingency management, a widely used intervention for stimulant use, with behavioral activation, commonly used to treat depression (Mimiaga, Closson, et al., 2012; Mitty, Closson, Pantalone, et al., 2012). Pilot testing revealed that the combined contingency management intervention yielded reductions in stimulant use, cravings and depressive symptoms among HIV positive stimulant users; further research using this approach in a randomized controlled efficacy trial is currently underway.

Interpersonal Characteristics

Patient-Provider Relationship

The patient-provider relationship has important implications for retention in care, beliefs in treatment efficacy, and adherence to HIV treatment. Qualitative research with sexual minority men has identified the commonality of feeling judged by providers due to their sexuality and encountering homophobic providers, as well as the desire to find providers who are more understanding of and sensitive to social and sexual contexts and identities (Schilder et al., 2001). Interestingly, however, men who reported having a positive, caring relationship with their provider also tended to report that they had better access to medication and the support needed to stay on ART medications. In a study of young MSM, Magnus et al. (2010) found that patients who felt a connection with their provider and felt respected at the clinic were likely to be retained in care. Similarly, Stall et al. (1996), in a sample of more than 400 HIV-infected gay and bisexual men, found that adherent men were at significantly greater odds of reporting a good relationship with their provider and believing in the efficacy of early ART intervention, compared to those who were not adherent. Additionally, men who trusted their physicians were more likely to follow the standard of care guidelines for HIV. The valence of patient-provider interaction may therefore play an important role in the success of HIV treatment.

As positive relationships may engender proper facilitation of ART medication, while poor experiences with HIV medical providers may have an impact on patient mistrust in health care and affect ART medication adherence (see Christopoulos, Das, & Colfax, 2011 for a review). Consistent with these findings, Thrasher et al. (2008) found that those who experienced more discrimination in the health care environment had greater distrust in their medical provider and in the efficacy of treatment than those who did not experience discrimination. In turn, these factors were related to poorer ART treatment adherence, with decreased beliefs in ART benefits partially accounting for worse adherence. Such findings underscore the need for cultural competence among medical providers, as well as professional training tailored to increase awareness and understanding of the unique needs of MSM. For gay, bisexual, and other MSM living with HIV, having a HIV care provider who promotes a sense of respect, trust, and support within the patient-provider dynamic may facilitate medication adherence among this population.

Caregiver Relationship

In addition to the patient-provider relationship, relationships with friends, partners, and other caregivers may impact medication adherence. Indeed, adequate social support is an important factor affecting medication adherence and has been shown to promote ART adherence among MSM (Halkitis, Parsons, et al., 2003; Stall et al., 1996; Wrubel, Stumbo, & Johnson, 2010). Halkitis, Parsons, et al. (2003) found that individuals with more HIV-infected friends missed fewer days of their medications, while those who were uncomfortable talking to their partners about HIV had worse adherence. Likewise, Stall et al. (1996) found that adherent men were more likely to report having the necessary social support to take their ART medications compared to those who were nonadherent. However, there is evidence that the type of social support one receives matters, with practical support for adherence serving a prominent role in enhancing medication adherence (see Vervoort, Borleffs, Hoepelman, & Grypdonck, 2007 for a review). Wrubel, Stumbo, and Johnson (2008) analyzed the type of practical support being given in the relationships of gay men and found that it was largely comprised of three components: (1) reminders to take medications (e.g., at a certain time each day or during different circumstances, such as when their partner is tired); (2) coaching (e.g., problem-solving to manage side effects or make adherence a routine); and (3) instrumental helping (e.g., bringing medication, setting out medications, or ordering refills). These support strategies used among gay male couples have been found to remain consistent regardless of serostatus concordance (i.e., whether one or both partners have HIV) (Wrubel et al., 2008; Wrubel et al., 2010). Given the benefit of practical social support in medication adherence, understanding which strategies are most helpful may provide important possibilities for intervention development.

Whereas Wrubel et al. (2008) have identified positive implications of close interpersonal relationships for ART adherence, there are other aspects of partner relationships that may negatively impact treatment adherence, such as intimate partner violence (IPV). Ramachandran, Yonas, Silvestre, and Burke (2010) found that rates of IPV among MSM attending an HIV clinic were among the highest in the sample, with nearly a third of the men reporting sexual or physical abuse. In another study, the majority (73%) of HIV-infected MSM reported experiencing psychological abuse from their partner in the past year (Craft & Serovich, 2005). While IPV among gay men is an emergent phenomenon in the literature, IPV has been shown to have important implications for ART adherence among diverse samples (Illangasekare et al., 2012; Lopez, Jones, Villar-Loubet, Arheart, & Weiss, 2010). For example, Pantalone, Hessler, and Simoni (2010) found that partner violence was connected to suboptimal medication adherence, with those who had experienced IPV demonstrating worse adherence than those who did not experience partner violence. Negative mental health outcomes from experiencing abuse likely mediate adherence; however, there is evidence that even when controlling for psychiatric status, the link between traumatic experiences and suboptimal adherence remains (Mugavero et al., 2006), indicating that the relationship between IPV and adherence may persist despite existing mental health problems. Given the prevalence of IPV in male, same-sex intimate relationships and its implications for adherence as well as general mental health, researchers (e.g., Pantalone et al., 2010) recommend that health care providers regularly screen HIV-infected gay patients for abuse. Such precautions would assist in providing support to gay men experiencing IPV and likely mitigate outcomes that are further detrimental to long-term health (e.g., nonadherence to HIV medications).

Environmental/Structural-Level Characteristics

Access to HIV Medical Care

Engagement in medical care is essential for the proper management of HIV treatment regimens (Christopoulos et al., 2011). Access to health care providers and quality care is necessary for obtaining prescriptions for ART as well as proper dosing instructions. Moreover, health care access allows for the identification and treatment of other medical and mental health issues that can affect medication adherence and long-term health outcomes (e.g., problematic side effects or symptoms, depression, trauma), as well as access to social services that may facilitate uptake of ART by easing certain societal issues that have the potential to impede optimal adherence (e.g., unstable housing). Indeed, ART medication adherence has been found to significantly correspond with type of care, frequency of care, access to health insurance, as well as perceived access to medications in MSM (Halkitis, Parsons, et al., 2003; Halkitis, Kutnick, et al., 2005). For example, Halkitis, Parsons, et al. (2003) found that those with health insurance, who were receiving HIV care at private facilities and who perceived uncomplicated access to HIV medications, were at significantly greater odds of being on ART treatment regimens than those who indicated that they did not have insurance, received HIV care at public facilities, or did not perceive readily available HIV medications. In 2005, Halkitis and colleagues found that adherence was also related to the type of health care coverage one has, with individuals with private health insurance demonstrating greater adherence than those in public care. In addition, Kleeberger et al. found in both cross-sectional (Kleeberger et al., 2001) and longitudinal (Kleeberger et al., 2004) studies that outpatient visits were associated with adherence among gay and bisexual men, such that individuals who saw their HIV care provider in the preceding year were more likely to be adherent to their ART medications than those with a lower level of engagement in medical care. It is possible that individuals receiving private HIV care may have longer-term and more secure relationships with their providers, which has been shown to increase trust in both ART efficacy as well as one's ability to adhere to ART regimens (see the "Patient-Provider Relationship" section). In addition, those with private health care and insurance may be in a better position to utilize health care due to fewer concerns regarding cost or insurance coverage, whereas those without insurance, or those receiving public assistance, may be more uncertain about seeking health care due to concerns about affording treatment. Lastly, health care access may serve as a proxy in these studies for other factors discussed in this chapter, including low SES and mental health issues. Nonetheless, the association between public care and nonadherence is critical given the vast number of HIV-infected persons receiving public HIV care in the US (Bhattacharya, Goldman, & Sood, 2003).

As discussed earlier, race, social class, and education disparities are associated with ART nonadherence among MSM and these factors may be moderated by access to care. For example, Halkitis, Kutnick, et al. (2005) examined the role of racial disparities in HIV care and treatment among gay men and found that 65% of White respondents had access to private HIV care, while only 15% of Latino and 12% of African American men had similar access. Such findings are suggestive of disparities and inequities in HIV medical care access and quality, which translate into disparities in ART medication adherence rates as well as differences in the overall health of MSM of color in comparison to their White counterparts. Racial differences among HIV-infected MSM may further manifest at the socioeconomic level as ability to afford care and medications and may limit health care access (e.g., McKirnan, Du Bois, Alvy, & Jones, 2012). For example, McKirnan and colleagues (2012) found that limited health care access among MSM was associated with being African American and/or Latino and having lower income. Similarly Oh et al. (2009) found marked SES differences between racial groups, with Black and Latino men reporting significantly more financial difficulty than White men. Level of educational attainment might also serve as a moderator between race, SES, and ART medication adherence since, as noted above, having a lower level of education has been associated with decreased adherence among MSM (e.g., Kleeberger et al., 2004). Indeed, individuals with more education may be better able to access care, better equipped to identify and navigate (e.g., logistically, financially) potential sources of health care, and better able to understand complex medication regimens. Given the implications of race, SES, and education, future adherence interventions should address structural factors, while taking into account specific populations at risk for suboptimal adherence, in order to improve access to care and ART adherence among diverse populations of MSM (for more about the need for structural interventions, see Millett et al., 2007 and Christopoulos et al., 2011).

Overall, findings suggest that ART medication adherence is a complex and fluid phenomenon that is impacted by numerous individual, interpersonal, and structural factors situated in the lives of HIV-infected gay men and other MSM. While no intervention is sure to be a "one size fits all" approach, research would benefit from the development of holistic interventions that address the multilevel barriers to ART adherence among this group of men.

Interventions to Improve ART Adherence

Patient-, interpersonal-, and structural-level factors interact to impact medication adherence among gay men living with HIV. By identifying such factors, researchers have been able to develop strategies to improve ART adherence in nonadherent individuals or those at risk for poor adherence. To date, the majority of interventions implemented among gay men and other MSM have targeted patient-level factors of nonadherence. For example, interventions have incorporated strategies to guard against forgetting to take one's medication (e.g., Lewis et al., 2012; Safren, Hendriksen, Desousa, Boswell, & Mayer, 2003); patient education to provide information about HIV, ART, and the importance of adherence (e.g., Rathbun, Farmer, Stephens, & Lockhart, 2005; Rawlings et al., 2003); motivational interviewing (MI) (see Hill & Kavookjian, 2012 for a preliminary review of the efficacy of MI); and counseling to support individuals in identifying personal barriers to adherence and problem-solving skills to assist individuals in overcoming these obstacles (e.g., Henderson, Hindman, Johnson, Valuck, & Kisser, 2011; Safren et al., 2001). In fact, Safren, Otto, and Worth (1999), combined many of these strategies into a single-session intervention (Life-Steps), which included patient education, cognitive behavioral and problem-solving techniques for adherence (e.g., obtaining medications, coping with side effects, creating cues for adherence), and motivational interviewing. Individuals who received the Life-Steps intervention and maintained a medication diary displayed faster gains in adherence than those who only completed medication diaries; moreover, this improvement was maintained after 3 months (Safren et al., 2001; 67% MSM). More recently, interventions utilizing technology have also shown promise. For example, Lewis et al. (2012) sent MSM text message reminders to take their medications as well as messages reinforcing continued adherence among those with consistent or improved adherence. Lewis and colleagues found a statistically significant decrease in the number of days participants missed, as well as a decrease in the number of participants reporting they forgot, were busy, or slept through dose times.

Given the high comorbidity of psychological concerns among gay men and other MSM living with HIV, as well as the detrimental effects these conditions have on ART medication adherence, interventions have also targeted mental health and substance use issues among HIV-infected individuals with some preliminary success (e.g., Safren et al., 2009; Safren et al., 2012; Parsons, Rosof, & Mustanski, 2007; Mimiaga, Closson, et al., 2012; Mimiaga, Reisner, et al., 2012). For depression, Safren et al. (2009) combined the cognitive behavioral therapy (CBT)/problem-solving intervention described earlier (Life-Steps) with CBT for adherence and depression (CBT-AD) and compared it against a control condition (enhanced treatment as usual; ETAU—receiving the single session of Life-Steps alone) in a randomized controlled trial with HIV-infected individuals with comorbid depression (82% MSM). While both the CBT-AD and ETAU groups received the Life-Steps intervention aimed at increasing ART treatment adherence, the experimental intervention received the full CBT intervention, which integrated adherence counseling into a modular treatment for depression. After 3 months, participants in the CBT-AD condition were less depressed and more adherent to ART than participants in the ETAU condition; moreover, these results were generally maintained at 6- and 12-month follow-up visits.

Researchers have also addressed interpersonal factors in ART adherence; for example, Remien et al. (2005) and Simoni, Pantalone, Plummer, and Huang (2007) have incorporated social support in their adherence interventions. Remien et al. (2005; 18% MSM) provided couples counseling to cultivate active social support for adherence from HIV-uninfected partners in addition to problem-solving strategies and partner-communication exercises to combat barriers to adherence. Compared to the usual standard of care condition (i.e., education and follow-up with one's primary care provider), HIV-infected participants receiving the couples-based intervention obtained higher mean medication adherence post-intervention, as measured by electronic pill cap, and were more likely to achieve levels of adherence over 80%, 90%, and 95% than those receiving the standards of care condition.

To date, few studies have evaluated interventions targeting structural-level issues affecting medication adherence among HIV-infected gay, bisexual, and other MSM (see Christopoulos et al., 2011 for a review). However, recent programs have worked to increase linkage and retention in care for gay and bisexual men. For example, the Positive Health Access to Services and Treatment intervention at the San Francisco General Hospital (Christopoulos, Geng, & Jones, 2010) successfully linked newly diagnosed gay, bisexual, and other MSM to care and facilitated timely appointments with an HIV care provider. The National Institutes of Health has also embraced the concept of "test, link to care and treat" (TLC+) and is currently implementing a large-scale, nationally representative 3-year feasibility study in cities across the US that provides financial incentives to individuals who remain in care and achieve viral suppression (Branson, 2010).

Overall, adherence interventions have been shown to be effective in increasing medication adherence among individuals living with HIV (Simoni, Pearson, Pantalone, Marks, & Crepaz, 2006); however, challenges in intervention development and implementation remain. Leeman et al. (2010) noted that in order for an intervention to change individuals' behavior, individuals must "enroll in the intervention, attend sessions, and continue to participate over time" and that "these steps may be influenced by characteristics of the participant, intervener, intervention and setting" (p. 3). Randomized controlled trials testing the efficacy of interventions are thus inherently limited by their success in enrolling and retaining participants in the intervention over the follow-up period. Further, individuals affected by structural-level barriers to adherence may be less likely to participate in interventions. As such, the efficacy of any given intervention may vary as a function of external factors, and different populations may require various supportive features not inherent to the intervention content itself (e.g., flexible scheduling; Leeman et al., 2010).

In addition to challenges in the implementation of intervention content, the broad nature of strategies used within interventions poses a challenge for developing future interventions better tailored to the diverse needs of gay men. Many interventions address multiple correlates of adherence at once, or have no specific target at all (see Sandelowski, Voils, Chang, & Lee, 2009; Simoni, Pearson, et al., 2006), thus making it difficult to discern which components of interventions are likely to impact adherence. Moreover, interventions measure adherence to ART in various manners, creating further difficulties in comparing results across studies. As the literature expands rapidly with interventions targeting ART adherence among HIV-infected individuals, research should seek to include some degree of standardization of assessment, inquiry into the efficacy of core components, as well as sensitivity to study population and context. With this knowledge, researchers may then begin to identify and incorporate best practices in order to promote ART adherence among diverse subsets of gay men.

ART as Prevention

Improved adherence to ART is critical for improving the health of HIV-infected gay men as well as reducing the likelihood of HIV transmission among serodiscordant partners. Achieving an undetectable viral load has taken on increased importance with regard to HIV prevention given recent findings illustrating that individuals on ART with a suppressed viral load are less likely to sexually transmit HIV to their uninfected partners, relative to those without a suppressed viral load (Cohen et al., 2011). Newer uses of ART for primary prevention provide an opportunity to more effectively combat the HIV epidemic, namely, post-exposure prophylaxis (PEP) and pre-exposure prophylaxis (PrEP). These antiretroviral drugs, when used as prevention, can reduce the likelihood of acquiring HIV infection among people exposed to the virus. Recommended for use by the US Public Health Service in 1996, PEP is a 28-day regimen provided to individuals within 72 h after HIV exposure and is used for both occupational (e.g., work place exposures) and non-occupational exposures (e.g., sexual and injection drug use exposures) (Panlilio, Cardo, Grohskopf, Heneine, & Ross, 2005). In November 2010, the iPrEx study established that a once-daily tablet containing a fixed-dose combination of tenofovir disoproxil fumarate and emtricitabine (TDF-FTC) could successfully reduce the risk of HIV acquisition among at-risk MSM compared to a placebo control (Grant et al., 2010), thereby confirming the efficacy of oral PrEP in this population. PrEP is taken prior to exposure and is currently FDA-approved for daily use (CDC, 2012). While these drugs provide an important stop gap in the HIV epidemic, particularly among gay and bisexual men, similar to ART as treatment, these medicines must be taken according to the proper dosing indications, with adherence failure resulting in diminished protection against HIV acquisition, as well as the potential development of drug resistance (van de Vijver & Boucher, 2010). Moreover, suboptimal adherence can impact HIV incidence outcomes in PrEP efficacy trials, as lack of adherence may compromise trial results (e.g., underestimation of the true effect) and undermine the effectiveness of biomedical prevention methods for real-world use (Stirratt & Gordon, 2008).

Nonadherence is particularly relevant in the context of PrEP use; as, similiary to ART, individuals may take PrEP daily for an indefinite period of time. While contextual research examining nonadherence among PrEP users is fairly preliminary, much of the current research indicates that many of the same factors impacting ART treatment adherence among HIV-infected persons may also influence adherence to antiretrovirals as prevention (Grant et al., 2010; Mimiaga, Closson, Kothary, & Mitty, 2014; Taylor, Safren, Elsesser, Mimiaga, & Mayer, 2012). For example, as with ART, side effects have been shown to impact adherence, as nonadherence was linked to differential symptomatology (i.e., men who were assigned to take PrEP reported more initial nausea than those assigned to the placebo) among participants in the iPrEx study (Grant et al., 2010). Other possible explanations for nonadherence among iPrEx participants include lifestyle barriers, substance use, and individual beliefs regarding the amount of medication necessary for effective HIV transmission prevention. Qualitative studies among MSM have demonstrated similar findings, with men reporting limited knowledge regarding PrEP efficacy and use, substance use, mood, HIV stigma, and provider and caregiver concerns as potential barriers to PrEP adherence (Mimiaga et al., 2014; Mitty, Closson, Rowley, Mayer, & Mimiaga, 2012; Taylor et al., 2012). As PrEP becomes more widely disseminated as an HIV prevention tool, effective interventions are needed to address the barriers to PrEP use and adherence among at-risk gay, bisexual, and other MSM.

Future Considerations

Despite more than two decades of research on ART adherence, there is still a need for improved measurement technologies to accurately assess adherence in both clinical and research settings. Pill count and pharmacy fill monitoring offer more objective measures of adherence, but these methods tend to be labor intensive and thus largely unfeasible outside of research contexts. Electronic dose monitoring as well as physiological measures, such as blood assay levels, are highly accurate, but these technologies tend to be expensive and therefore infrequently used to measure adherence among patients in HIV care. Due to its low cost and feasibility, patient self-report remains the most widely used measure of adherence across settings. While there are concerns about inaccurate measurement due to reporting bias, reviews of the literature indicate that clinicians and researchers can confidently proceed with the use of self-report measures as patient report has been found to be strongly associated with more reliable, indirect markers of adherence (e.g., viral load) (Simoni, Kurth, et al., 2006; Wilson et al., 2009). Rather than reject self-report for more advanced technological measures of adherence, experts have provided recommendations on how to improve the validity of self-report. To reduce social desirability, researchers suggest that researchers and clinicians explore patient explanations for missed doses; limit their measurement to recent behavior and/or a specific time frame; use their authority to substantiate and normalize suboptimal adherence behaviors; and perform post-hoc reliability tests to ensure the accuracy of self-report data (see Simoni, Kurth, et al., 2006and Miller & Hays, 2000a, 2000b for a full list of recommendations). The use of computer-assisted technology has also been suggested as a strategy to improve the accuracy of self-reported adherence as such technology has been shown to improve the quality and validity of responses for other sensitive behaviors (e.g., sex and drug use) (Schroder, Carey, & Vanable, 2003). The measurement of biological markers of adherence may also be used to supplement self-reported adherence as these methods are often readily available in both research and real-world settings. Some experts recommend the use of multiple measures of adherence, especially in intervention research, as the inclusion of less subjective measures of adherence (e.g., electronic drug monitoring) may be necessary to adequately assess intervention effects (Berg & Arnsten, 2006; Ickovics & Meisler, 1997; Liu et al., 2001; Simoni, Kurth, et al., 2006; Simoni, Person, et al., 2006; Wilson et al., 2009). Thus, in order to help HIV medical providers and researchers more accurately assess patient adherence, future research is needed to determine the most definitive and accurate measures of medication adherence across settings.

While medication adherence interventions generally appear to be efficacious among HIV-infected adults (Amico, Harman, & Johnson, 2006; Simoni, Pearson, et al., 2006), suboptimal adherence still persists. The literature highlights the enormity of factors associated with adherence among gay and bisexual men, with rates varying according to demographic factors such as age, education, SES, and race. Much of the research highlights the impact of highly prevalent psychosocial issues such as depression, trauma, body image concerns, and drug and alcohol use on medication adherence among MSM. These conditions, in particular, have the ability to undermine even the most effective intervention, as impaired judgment, memory loss, disrupted sleep-wake cycles, reduced self-efficacy, and other consequences can lessen one's ability to take medications as prescribed (Du Bois & McKirnan, 2012; Halkitis, Kutnick, et al., 2005). Structural-level factors may also lead to nonadherence among specific sub-groups of MSM, as lack of insurance, limited access to quality HIV medical care, or discrimination in health care can create difficulties for HIV-infected gay and bisexual men, leading to suboptimal adherence and poor health outcomes (Hatzenbuehler, O'Cleirigh, Mayer, Mimiaga, & Safren, 2011). This research highlights the importance of understanding adherence to ART from a contextual perspective. Continued efforts must be made to develop tailored and culturally appropriate interventions for gay and bisexual men; moreover, the adherence strategies used in rigorous clinical intervention trials must be translated into practice in order to improve adherence and secondary prevention outcomes among HIV-infected gay, bisexual, and other MSM and their sexual partners.

References

Acri, T., TenHave, T., Chapman, J., Bogner, H., & Gross, R. (2010). Lack of association between retrospectively collected pharmacy refill data and electronic drug monitoring of antiretroviral adherence. *AIDS and Behavior, 14*(4), 748–754.

Ambrosioni, J., Calmy, A., & Hirschel, B. (2011). HIV treatment for prevention. *Journal of the International AIDS Society, 14*, 28.

Amico, K., Harman, J. J., & Johnson, B. T. (2006). Efficacy of antiretroviral therapy adherence interventions: A research synthesis of trials, 1996 to 2004. *JAIDS Journal of Acquired Immune Deficiency Syndromes, 41*(3), 285–297.

Arnsten, J. H., Demas, P. A., Farzadegan, H., Grant, R. W., Gourevitch, M. N., Chang, C. J., … Schoenbaum, E. E. (2001). Antiretroviral therapy adherence and viral suppression in HIV-infected drug users: Comparison of self-report and electronic monitoring. *Clinical Infectious Diseases, 33*(8), 1417–1423.

Arnsten, J. H., Li, X., Mizuno, Y., Knowlton, A. R., Gourevitch, M. N., Handley, K., … INSPIRE Study Team (2007). Factors associated with antiretroviral therapy adherence and medication errors among HIV-infected injection drug users. *JAIDS Journal of Acquired Immune Deficiency Syndromes, 46*(Suppl 2), S64–S71.

Asch, S. M., Kilbourne, A. M., Gifford, A. L., Burnam, M. A., Turner, B., Shapiro, M. F., …
HCSUS Consortium. (2003). Underdiagnosis of depression in HIV: Who are we missing?
Journal of General Internal Medicine, 18(6), 450–460.

Azar, M. M., Springer, S. A., Meyer, J. P., & Altice, F. L. (2010). A systematic review of the impact
of alcohol use disorders on HIV treatment outcomes, adherence to antiretroviral therapy and
health care utilization. *Drug and Alcohol Dependence, 112*(3), 178–193.

Bangsberg, D. R. (2006). Less than 95% adherence to nonnucleoside reverse-transcriptase inhibitor therapy can lead to viral suppression. *Clinical Infectious Diseases, 43*(7), 939–941.

Bangsberg, D. R. (2008). Prevention HIV antiretroviral resistance through better monitoring of
treatment adherence. *Journal of Infectious Diseases, 15*, s272–s278.

Bangsberg, D. R., Hecht, F., Charlebois, E., Chesney, M., & Moss, A. (2001). Comparing objective measures of adherence to HIV antiretroviral therapy: Electronic medication monitors and
unannounced pill counts. *AIDS and Behavior, 5*(3), 275–281.

Bangsberg, D. R., Hecht, F., Charlebois, E., Zolopa, A., Holodniy, M., Sheiner, L., … Moss, A.
(2000). Adherence to protease inhibitors, HIV-1 viral load, and development of drug resistance
in an indigent population. *AIDS, 14*, 357–366.

Bangsberg, D. R., Hecht, F. M., Clague, H., Charlebois, E. D., Ciccarone, D., Chesney, M., &
Moss, A. (2001). Provider assessment of adherence to HIV antiretroviral therapy. *Journal of
Acquired Immune Deficiency Syndromes, 26*(5), 435–442.

Bartlett, J. A. (2002). Addressing the challenges of adherence. *Journal of Acquired Immune
Deficiency Syndromes, 29*, s2–10.

Bartlett, J. A., DeMasi, R., Quinn, J., Moxham, C., & Rousseau, F. (2001). Overview of the effectiveness of triple combination therapy in antiretroviral-naive HIV-1 infected adults. *AIDS,
15*(11), 1369–1377.

Berg, K. M., & Arnsten, J. H. (2006). Practical and conceptual challenges in measuring antiretroviral adherence. *Journal of Acquired Immune Deficiency Syndromes, 43*, S79–S87.

Bhattacharya, J., Goldman, D., & Sood, N. (2003). The link between public and private insurance
and HIV-related mortality. *Journal of Health Economics, 22*(6), 1105–1122.

Bing, E. G., Burnam, M. A., Longshore, D., Fleishman, J. A., Sherbourne, C. D., London, A. S.,
… Shapiro, M. (2001). Psychiatric disorders and drug use among human immunodeficiency
virus-infected adults in the United States. *Archives of General Psychiatry, 58*(8), 721–728.

Blashill, A., Gordon, J., & Safren, S. (2012a). Appearance concerns and psychological distress
among HIV-infected individuals with injection drug use histories: Prospective analyses. *AIDS
Patient Care and STDs, 26*(9), 557–561.

Blashill, A., Gordon, J., & Safren, S. (2012b). Depression longitudinally mediates the association
of appearance concerns to ART non-adherence in HIV-infected individuals with a history of
injection drug use. *Journal of Behavioral Medicine, 37*(1), 166–172.

Blashill, A., Perry, N., & Safren, S. (2011). Mental health: A focus on stress, coping, and mental
ilness as it relates to treatment retention, adherence, and other health outcomes. *Current HIV/
AIDS Reports, 8*(4), 215–222.

Blashill, A., & Vander Wal, J. (2009). Mediation of gender role conflict and eating pathology in gay
men. *Psychology of Men & Masculinity, 10*, 204–217.

Blashill, A., & Vander Wal, J. (2010). The role of body image dissatisfaction and depression on
HAART adherence in HIV positive men: Tests of mediation models. *AIDS and Behavior,
14*(2), 280–288.

Bogart, L. M., Wagner, G., Galvan, F. H., & Banks, D. (2010). Conspiracy beliefs about HIV
are related to antiretroviral treatment nonadherence among African American men with HIV.
Journal of Acquired Immune Deficiency Syndromes, 53(5), 648–655.

Bosworth, H. B., Oddone, E. Z., & Weinberger, M. (2005). *Patient treatment adherence: Concepts,
interventions, and measurement.* Mahwah, NJ: Lawrence Erlbaum Association.

Bousman, C. A., Cherner, M., Ake, C., Letendre, S., Atkinson, J. H., Patterson, T. L., … HNRC
Group (2009). Negative mood and sexual behavior among non-monogamous men who have
sex with men in the context of methamphetamine and HIV. *Journal of Affective Disorders,
119*(1–3), 84–91.

Bova, C., Fennie, K., Knafl, G., Dieckhaus, K., Watrous, E., & Williams, A. (2005). Use of electronic monitoring devices to measure antiretroviral adherence: Practical considerations. *AIDS and Behavior, 9*(1), 103–110.

Branson, B. (2010). HPTN 065 TLC-Plus: A study to evaluate the feasibility of an enhanced test, link to care, plus treat approach for HIV prevention in the United States. *A Study of the HIV Prevention Trials Network.* Retrieved from http://www.hptn.org/web%20documents/HPTN065/HPTN065ProtocolFINALVer1_01Mar10.pdf.

Brion, J. M., & Menke, E. M. (2008). Perspectives regarding adherence to prescribed treatment in highly adherent HIV-infected gay men. *Journal of the Association of Nurses in AIDS Care, 19*(3), 181–191.

Buchacz, K., McFarland, W., Kellogg, T., Loeb, L., Holmberg, S., Dilley, J., & Klausner, J. D. (2005). Amphetamine use is associated with increased HIV incidence among men who have sex with men in San Francisco. *AIDS, 19,* 1423–1424.

Carrico, A., Johnson, M., Colfax, G., & Moskowitz, J. (2010). Affective correlates of stimulant use and adherence to anti-retroviral therapy among HIV-positive methamphetamine users. *AIDS and Behavior, 14*(4), 769–777.

CASCADE Collaboration. (2000). Survival after introduction of HAART in people with known duration of HIV-1 infection. *Lancet, 355,* 1158–1159.

Cash, T. (2004). Body image: Past, present, and future. *Body Image, 1,* 1–15.

Catz, S. L., Kelly, J. A., Bogart, L. M., Benotsch, E. G., & McAuliffe, T. L. (2000). Patterns, correlates, and barriers to medication adherence among persons prescribed new treatments for HIV disease. *Health Psychology, 19*(2), 124–133.

CDC. (2012, July 16). *CDC statement on FDA approval of drug for HIV prevention.* Retrieved from http://www.cdc.gov/hiv/prep/pdf/CDC_FDA_Approval_Truvada.pdf.

CDC. (2013). HIV Mortality (through 2009). *Mortality Slide Series.* Retrieved from http://www.cdc.gov/hiv/topics/surveillance/resources/slides/mortality/.

Chartier, M., Vinatieri, T., DeLonga, K., McGlynn, L. M., Gore-Felton, C., & Koopman, C. (2010). A pilot study investigating the effects of trauma, experiential avoidance, and disease management in HIV-positive MSM using methamphetamine. *Journal of the International Association of Providers of AIDS Care, 9*(2), 78–81.

Chesney, M. A. (2000). Factors affecting adherence to antiretroviral therapy. *Clinical Infectious Diseases, 30*(Supplement 2), S171–S176.

Chesney, M. (2003). Adherence to HAART regimens. *AIDS Patient Care and STDs, 17,* 169–177.

Christopoulos, K. A., Das, M., & Colfax, G. N. (2011). Linkage and retention in HIV care among men who have sex with men in the United States. *Clinical Infectious Diseases, 52*(suppl 2), S214–S222.

Christopoulos, K. A., Geng, E., & Jones, D. (2010). *A model linkage to care program for rapid HIV testing in the emergency department.* Paper presented at the XVIII International AIDS Conference, Vienna, Austria.

Ciesla, J. A., & Roberts, J. E. (2001). Meta-analysis of the relationship between HIV infection and risk for depressive disorders. *American Journal of Psychiatry, 158*(5), 725–730.

Cohen, R. A., & Bloom, B. (2010). Access to and utilization of medical care for young adults ages 20–29 years: United States, 2008. *NCHS Data Brief, 29,* 1–8.

Cohen, M. S., Chen, Y. Q., McCauley, M., Gamble, T., Hosseinipour, M. C., Kumarasamy, N., … HPTN 052 Study Team (2011). Prevention of HIV-1 infection with early antiretroviral therapy. *New England Journal of Medicine, 365*(6), 493–505.

Cohen, R. A., Martinez, M. E., & Free, H. L. (2008). *Health insurance coverage: Early release of estimates from the National Health Interview Survey, 2007.* Retrieved from http://www.cdc.gov/nchs/nhis.htm.

Colfax, G., & Shoptaw, S. (2005). The methamphetamine epidemic: Implications for HIV prevention and treatment. *Current HIV/AIDS Reports, 2*(4), 194–199.

Colfax, G. N., Vittinghoff, E., Grant, R., Lum, P., Spotts, G., & Hecht, F. M. (2007). Frequent methamphetamine use is associated with primary non-nucleoside reverse transcriptase inhibitor resistance. *AIDS, 21*(2), 239–241.

Conner, K. R., Pinquart, M., & Gamble, S. A. (2009). Meta-analysis of depression and substance use among individuals with alcohol use disorders. *Journal of Substance Abuse Treatment, 37*(2), 127–137.

Cooper, V., Gellaitry, G., Hankins, M., Fisher, M., & Horne, R. (2009). The influence of symptom experiences and attributions on adherence to highly active anti-retroviral therapy (HAART): A six-month prospective, follow-up study. *AIDS Care, 21*(4), 520–528.

Corless, I. B., Nicholas, P. K., Davis, S. M., Dolan, S. A., & McGibbon, C. A. (2005). Symptom status, medication adherence, and quality of life in HIV disease. *Journal of Hospice & Palliative Nursing, 7*(3), 129–138.

Craft, S. M., & Serovich, J. M. (2005). Family-of-origin factors and partner violence in the intimate relationships of gay men who are HIV positive. *Journal of Interpersonal Violence, 20*(7), 777–791.

Crum, N. F., Riffenburgh, R. H., Wegner, S., Agan, B. K., Tasker, S. A., Spooner, K. M., … Triservice AIDS Clinical Consortium. (2006). Comparisons of causes of death and mortality rates among HIV-infected persons: Analysis of the pre-, early, and late HAART (highly active antiretroviral therapy) eras. *Journal of Acquired Immune Deficiency Syndromes, 41*(2), 194–200.

Deschamps, A. E., De Geest, S., Vandamme, A. M., Bobbaers, H., Peetermans, W. E., & Van Wijngaerden, E. (2008). Diagnostic value of different adherence measures using electronic monitoring and virologic failure as reference standards. *AIDS Patient Care and STDs, 22*(9), 735–743.

Deschamps, A. E., Graeve, V. D., van Wijngaerden, E., De Saar, V., Vandamme, A. M., van Vaerenbergh, K., … de Geest, S. (2004). Prevalence and correlates of nonadherence to antiretroviral therapy in a population of HIV patients using Medication Event Monitoring System. *AIDS Patient Care and STDs, 18*(11), 644–657.

Diamond, C., Richardson, J. L., Milam, J., Stoyanoff, S., McCutchan, J. A., Kemper, C., … California Collaborative Trials Group. (2005). Use of and adherence to antiretroviral therapy is associated with decreased sexual risk behavior in HIV clinic patients. *Journal of Acquired Immune Deficiency Syndromes, 39*(2), 211–218.

Du Bois, S. N., & McKirnan, D. J. (2012). A longitudinal analysis of HIV treatment adherence among men who have sex with men: A cognitive escape perspective. *AIDS Care, 24*, 1–7.

Duran, S., Spire, B., Raffi, F., Walter, V., Bouhour, D., Journot, V., … APROCO Cohort Study Group. (2001). Self-reported symptoms after initiation of a protease inhibitor in HIV-infected patients and their impact on adherence to HAART. *HIV Clinical Trials, 2*(1), 38–45.

Fernández, M. I., Bowen, G. S., Varga, L. M., Collazo, J. B., Hernandez, N., Perrino, T., & Rehbein, A. (2005). High rates of club drug use and risky sexual practices among Hispanic men who have sex with men in Miami, Florida. *Substance Use & Misuse, 40*(9–10), 1347–1362.

Fogarty, L., Roter, D., Larson, S., Burke, J., Gillespie, J., & Levy, R. (2002). Patient adherence to HIV medication regimens: A review of published and abstract reports. *Patient Education and Counseling, 46*(2), 93–108.

Forrest, D., Metsch, L., LaLota, M., Cardenas, G., Beck, D., & Jeanty, Y. (2010). Crystal methamphetamine use and sexual risk behaviors among HIV-positive and HIV-negative men who have sex with men in South Florida. *Journal of Urban Health, 87*(3), 480–485.

Gagnon, J., Welles, S., & Japour, A. (2007). *Predictors of low adherence to HAART among indigent HIV-infected men who have sex with men in Miami/Dade County's HIV Drug Assistance Program*. Paper presented at the American Public Health Association 132nd Annual Meeting and Exposition, Washington, DC.

Galvan, F. H., Bing, E. G., Fleishman, J. A., London, A. S., Caetano, R., Burnam, M. A., … Shapiro, M. (2002). The prevalence of alcohol consumption and heavy drinking among people with HIV in the United States: Results from the HIV Cost and Services Utilization Study. *Journal of Studies on Alcohol and Drugs, 63*(2), 179–186.

Gao, X., Nau, D. P., Rosenbluth, S. A., Scott, V., & Woodward, C. (2000). The relationship of disease severity, health beliefs and medication adherence among HIV patients. *AIDS Care, 12*(4), 387–398.

Gay, C., Portillo, C. J., Kelly, R., Coggins, T., Davis, H., Aouizerat, B. E., … Lee, K. A. (2011). Self-reported medication adherence and symptom experience in adults with HIV. *Journal of the Association of Nurses in AIDS Care, 22*(4), 257–268.

Ghebremichael, M., Paintsil, E., Ickovics, J. R., Vlahov, D., Schuman, P., Boland, R., … Zhang, H. (2009). Longitudinal association of alcohol use with HIV disease progression and psychological health of women with HIV. *AIDS Care, 21*(7), 834–841.

Giralt, M., Domingo, P., Guallar, J. P., Rodriguez de la Concepción, M. L., Alegre, M., & Villarroya, F. (2006). HIV-1 infection alters gene expression in adipose tissue, which contributes to HIV-1/HAART-associated lipodystrophy. *Antiviral Therapy, 11*(6), 729.

Glass, T. R., Battegay, M., Cavassini, M., De Geest, S., Furrer, H., Vernazza, P. L., … Swiss HIV Cohort Study. (2010). Longitudinal analysis of patterns and predictors of changes in self-reported adherence to antiretroviral therapy: Swiss HIV Cohort Study. *Journal of Acquired Immune Deficiency Syndromes, 54*(2), 197–203.

Gonzalez, J. S., Batchelder, A. W., Psaros, C., & Safren, S. A. (2011). Depression and HIV/AIDS treatment nonadherence: A review and meta-analysis. *Journal of Acquired Immune Deficiency Syndromes, 58*, 181–187.

Gonzalez, J., Penedo, F., Llabre, M., Durán, R., Antoni, M., Schneiderman, N., & Horne, R. (2007). Physical symptoms, beliefs about medications, negative mood, and long-term HIV medication adherence. *Annals of Behavioral Medicine, 34*(1), 46–55.

Gorbach, P. M., Drumright, L. N., Javanbakht, M., Pond, S. L., Woelk, C. H., Daar, E. S., & Little, S. J. (2008). Antiretroviral drug resistance and risk behavior among recently HIV-infected men who have sex with men. *Journal of Acquired Immune Deficiency Syndromes, 47*(5), 639–643.

Gorman, E. M., & Carroll, R. T. (2000). Substance abuse and HIV: Considerations with regard to methamphetamines and other recreational drugs for nursing practice and research. *Journal of the Association of Nurses in AIDS Care, 11*(2), 51–62.

Grant, R. M., Lama, J. R., Anderson, P. L., McMahan, V., Liu, A. Y., Vargas, L., … iPrEx Study Team. (2010). Preexposure chemoprophylaxis for HIV prevention in men who have sex with men. *New England Journal of Medicine, 363*(27), 2587–2599.

Green, K. E., & Feinstein, B. A. (2012). *Substance use in lesbian, gay, and bisexual populations: An update on empirical research and implications for treatment* (Vol. 26). Washington, DC: American Psychological Association.

Guaraldi, G., Murri, R., Orlando, G., Giovanardi, C., Squillace, N., Vandelli, M., … Wu, A. W. (2008). Severity of lipodystrophy is associated with decreased health-related quality of life. *AIDS Patient Care and STDs, 22*(7), 577–585.

Guaraldi, G., Orlando, G., Murri, R., Vandelli, M., De Paola, M., Beghetto, B., … Wu, A. W. (2006). Quality of life and body image in the assessment of psychological impact of lipodystrophy: Validation of the Italian version of assessment of body change and distress questionnaire. *Quality of Life Research, 15*(1), 173–178.

Halkitis, P. N. (2001). An exploration of perceptions of masculinity among gay men living with HIV. *Journal of Men's Health, 9*, 413–429.

Halkitis, P. N., Green, K. A., & Wilton, L. (2004). Masculinity, body image, and sexual behavior in HIV-seropositive gay men: A two-phase formative behavioral investigation using the internet. *International Journal of Men's Health, 3*, 27–42.

Halkitis, P. N., & Kirton, C. (1999). Self-strategies as means of enhancing adherence to HIV antiretroviral therapies. *Journal of the New York State Nurses Association, 14*, 1–5.

Halkitis, P. N., Kutnick, A. H., Rosof, E., Slater, S., & Parsons, J. P. (2003). Adherence to HIV medications in a cohort of men who have sex with men: Impact of September 11th. *Journal of Urban Health, 80*(1), 161.

Halkitis, P. N., Kutnick, A. H., & Slater, S. (2005). The social realities of adherence to prote-
ase inhibitor regimens: Substance use, health care and psychological states. *Journal of Health Psychology, 10*(4), 545–558.

Halkitis, P. N., & Palamar, J. (2008). A mediation model to explain HIV antiretroviral adherence among gay and bisexual men. *Journal of Gay and Lesbian Social Services, 19*(1), 35–55.

Halkitis, P. N., Palamar, J. J., & Mukherjee, P. P. (2007). Poly-club-drug use among gay and bisex-ual men: A longitudinal analysis. *Drug and Alcohol Dependence, 89*(2–3), 153–160.

Halkitis, P. N., Palamar, J., & Mukherjee, P. (2008). Analysis of HIV medication adherence in rela-tion to person and treatment characteristics using hierarchical linear modeling. *AIDS Patient Care and STDs, 22*(4), 323–335.

Halkitis, P. N., Parsons, J. T., Wolitski, R. J., & Remien, R. H. (2003). Characteristics of HIV anti-retroviral treatments, access and adherence in an ethnically diverse sample of men who have sex with men. *AIDS Care, 15*(1), 89–102.

Halkitis, P. N., Shrem, M., & Martin, F. (2005). Sexual behavior patterns of methamphetamine-using gay and bisexual men. *Substance Use & Misuse, 40*(5), 703–719.

Halkitis, P. N., Wilton, L., Parsons, J. T., & Hoff, C. (2004). Correlates of sexual risk-taking behav-iour among HIV seropositive gay men in concordant primary partner relationships. *Psychology, Health & Medicine, 9*(1), 99–113.

Hatzenbuehler, M., O'Cleirigh, C., Mayer, K., Mimiaga, M., & Safren, S. (2011). Prospective asso-ciations between HIV-related stigma, transmission risk behaviors, and adverse mental health outcomes in men who have sex with men. *Annals of Behavioral Medicine, 42*(2), 227–234.

Hendershot, C. S., Stoner, S. A., Pantalone, D. W., & Simoni, J. M. (2009). Alcohol use and antiretroviral adherence: Review and meta-analysis. *Journal of Acquired Immune Deficiency Syndromes, 52*(2), 180–202.

Henderson, K. C., Hindman, J., Johnson, S. C., Valuck, R. J., & Kisser, J. J. (2011). Assessing the effectiveness of pharmacy-based adherence interventions on antiretroviral adherence in persons with HIV. *AIDS Patient Care and STDs, 25*(4), 221–228.

Hill, S., & Kavookjian, J. (2012). Motivational interviewing as a behavioral intervention to increase HAART adherence in patients who are HIV-positive: A systematic review of the lit-erature. *AIDS Care, 24*(5), 583–592.

Hinkin, C., Barclay, T., Castellon, S., Levine, A., Durvasula, R., Marion, S., … Longshore, D. (2007). Drug use and medication adherence among HIV-1 infected individuals. *AIDS and Behavior, 11*(2), 185–194.

Holzemer, W. L., Corless, I. B., Nokes, K. M., Turner, J. G., Brown, M. A., Powell-Cope, G. M., … Portillo, C. J. (1999). Predictors of self-reported adherence in persons living with HIV disease. *AIDS Patient Care and STDs, 13*(3), 185–197.

Huang, J. S., Lee, D., Becerra, K., Santos, R., Barber, E., & Mathews, W. C. (2006). Body image in men with HIV. *AIDS Patient Care and STDs, 20*(10), 668–677.

Hugen, P., Langebeek, N., Burger, D. M., Zomer, B., van Leusen, R., Schuurman, R., … Hekster, Y. A. (2002). Assessment of adherence to HIV protease inhibitors: Comparison and combina-tion of various methods, including MEMS (electronic monitoring), patient and nurse report, and therapeutic drug monitoring. *Journal of Acquired Immune Deficiency Syndromes, 30*(3), 324.

Ickovics, J. R., & Meade, C. S. (2002). Adherence to antiretroviral therapy among patients with HIV: A critical link between behavioral and biomedical sciences. *JAIDS Journal of Acquired Immune Deficiency Syndromes, 31*(Suppl 3), S98–S102.

Ickovics, J. R., & Meisler, A. W. (1997). Adherence in AIDS clinical trials: A framework for clini-cal research and clinical care. *Journal of Clinical Epidemiology, 50*(4), 385–391.

Illangasekare, S., Tello, M., Hutton, H., Moore, R., Anderson, J., Baron, J., & Chander, G. (2012). Clinical and mental health correlates and risk factors for intimate partner violence among HIV-positive women in an inner-city HIV clinic. *Women's Health Issues, 22*(6), e563–e569.

Ironson, G., O'Cleirigh, C., Fletcher, M. A., Laurenceau, J. P., Balbin, E., Klimas, N., … Solomon, G. (2005). Psychosocial factors predict CD4 and viral load change in men and women with human immunodeficiency virus in the era of highly active antiretroviral treatment. *Psychosomatic Medicine*, *67*(6), 1013–1021.

Johnson, M. O., Neilands, T. B., Dilworth, S. E., Morin, S. F., Remien, R. H., & Chesney, M. A. (2007). The role of self-efficacy in HIV treatment adherence: Validation of the HIV Treatment Adherence Self-Efficacy Scale (HIV-ASES). *Journal of Behavioral Medicine*, *30*(5), 359–370.

Jones, K. T., Gray, P., Whiteside, Y. O., Wang, T., Bost, D., Dunbar, E., … Johnson, W. D. (2008). Evaluation of an HIV prevention intervention adapted for black men who have sex with men. *American Journal of Public Health*, *98*(6), 1043–1050.

Kalichman, S. C., Amaral, C. M., White, D., Swetsze, C., Pope, H., Kalichman, M. O., … Eaton, L. (2009). Prevalence and clinical implications of interactive toxicity beliefs regarding mixing alcohol and antiretroviral therapies among people living with HIV/AIDS. *AIDS Patient Care and STDs*, *23*(6), 449–454.

Kalichman, S. C., Cain, D., Cherry, C., Kalichman, M., & Pope, H. (2005). Pillboxes and antiretroviral adherence: Prevalence of use, perceived benefits, and implications for electronic medication monitoring devices. *AIDS Patient Care and STDs*, *19*(12), 833–839.

Kalichman, S. C., Catz, S., & Ramachandran, B. (1999). Barriers to HIV/AIDS treatment and treatment adherence among African-American adults with disadvantaged education. *Journal of the National Medical Association*, *91*(8), 439–446.

Kalichman, S. C., Cherry, C., Amaral, C. M., Swetzes, C., Eaton, L., Macy, R., … Kalichman, M. O. (2010). Adherence to antiretroviral therapy and HIV transmission risks: Implications for test-and-treat approaches to HIV prevention. *AIDS Patient Care and STDs*, *24*(5), 271–272.

Kavanagh, D. J., & Bower, G. H. (1985). Mood and self-efficacy: Impact of joy and sadness on perceived capabilities. *Cognitive and Behavioral Practice*, *9*(5), 507–525.

Kelly, J. A., Hoffman, R. G., Rompa, D., & Gray, M. (1998). Protease inhibitor combination therapies and perceptions of gay men regarding AIDS severity and the need to maintain safer sex. *AIDS*, *12*(10), F91–F95.

Kiertiburanakul, S., & Sungkanuparph, S. (2009). Emerging of HIV drug resistance: Epidemiology, diagnosis, treatment and prevention. *Current HIV Research*, *7*(3), 273–278.

Kleeberger, C. A., Buechner, J., Palella, F., Detels, R., Riddler, S., Godfrey, R., & Jacobson, L. P. (2004). Changes in adherence to highly active antiretroviral therapy medications in the multicenter AIDS cohort study. *AIDS*, *18*(4), 683–688.

Kleeberger, C. A., Phair, J. P., Strathdee, S. A., Detels, R., Kingsley, L., & Jacobson, L. P. (2001). Determinants of heterogeneous adherence to HIV-antiretroviral therapies in the Multicenter AIDS Cohort Study. *Journal of Acquired Immune Deficiency Syndromes*, *26*(1), 82–92.

Knobel, H., Guelar, A., Carmona, A., Espona, M., González, A., López-Colomés, J. L., … Díez, A. (2001). Virologic outcome and predictors of virologic failure of highly active antiretroviral therapy containing protease inhibitors. *AIDS Patient Care and STDs*, *15*(4), 193–199.

Kobin, A. B., & Sheth, N. U. (2011). Levels of adherence required for virologic suppression among newer antiretroviral medications. *Annals of Pharmacotherapy*, *45*(3), 372–379.

Kroenke, K., Spitzer, R. L., & Williams, J. B. W. (2003). The Patient Health Questionnaire-2: Validity of a two-item depression screener. *Medical Care*, *41*(11), 1284–1292.

Leaver, C., Bargh, G., Dunn, J., & Hwang, S. (2007). The effects of housing status on health-related outcomes in people living with HIV: A systematic review of the literature. *AIDS and Behavior*, *11*(6 Suppl), 85–100.

Leeman, J., Chang, Y., Lee, E., Voils, C., Crandell, J., & Sandelowski, M. (2010). Implementation of antiretroviral therapy adherence interventions: A realist synthesis of evidence. *Journal of Advanced Nursing*, *66*(9), 1915–1930.

Leserman, J. (2000). The effects of depression, stressful life events, social support, and coping on the progression of HIV infection. *Current Psychiatry Reports*, *2*(6), 495–502.

Leserman, J. (2008). Role of depression, stress, and trauma in HIV disease progression. *Psychosomatic Medicine*, *70*(5), 539–545.

Leserman, J., Ironson, G., O'Cleirigh, C., Fordiani, J. M., & Balbin, E. (2008). Stressful life events and adherence in HIV. *AIDS Patient Care and STDs, 22*(5), 403–411.

Leserman, J., Pence, B. W., Whetten, K., Mugavero, M. J., Thielman, N. M., Swartz, M. S., & Stangl, D. (2007). Relation of lifetime trauma and depressive symptoms to mortality in HIV. *American Journal of Psychiatry, 164*(11), 1707–1713.

Leserman, J., Whetten, K., Lowe, K., Stangl, D., Swartz, M. S., & Thielman, N. M. (2005). How trauma, recent stressful events, and PTSD affect functional health status and health utilization in HIV-infected patients in the south. *Psychosomatic Medicine, 67*(3), 500–507.

Lewis, M. A., Uhrig, J. D., Bann, C. M., Harris, J. L., Furberg, R. D., Coomes, C., & Kuhns, L. M. (2012). Tailored text messaging intervention for HIV adherence: A proof-of-concept study. *Health Psychology, 32*(3), 248–253.

Liu, H., Golin, C. E., Miller, L. G., Hays, R. D., Beck, C. K., Sanandaji, S., … Wenger, N. S. (2001). A comparison study of multiple measures of adherence to HIV protease inhibitors. *Annals of Internal Medicine, 134*(10), 968–977.

Lopez, E. J., Jones, D. L., Villar-Loubet, O. M., Arheart, K. L., & Weiss, S. M. (2010). *Violence, coping, and consistent medication adherence in HIV-positive couples* (Vol. 22). New York, NY: Guilford.

Magnus, M., Jones, K., Phillips, G., Binson, D., Hightow-Weidman, L. B., Richards-Clarke, C., … YMSM of color Special Projects of National Significance Initiative Study Group. (2010). Characteristics associated with retention among African American and Latino adolescent HIV-positive men: Results from the outreach, care, and prevention to engage HIV-seropositive young MSM of color special project of national significance initiative. *Journal of Acquired Immune Deficiency Syndromes, 53*(4), 529–536.

Mannheimer, S., Friedland, G., Matts, J., Child, C., Chesney, M., & Terry Beirn Community Programs for Clinical Research on AIDS. (2002). The consistency of adherence to antiretroviral therapy predicts biologic outcomes for human immunodeficiency virus—Infected persons in clinical trials. *Clinical Infectious Diseases, 34*(8), 1115–1121.

Mansergh, G., Shouse, R. L., Marks, G., Guzman, R., Rader, M., Buchbinder, S., … Colfax, G. N. (2006). Methamphetamine and sildenafil (Viagra) use are linked to unprotected receptive and insertive anal sex, respectively, in a sample of men who have sex with men. *Sexually Transmitted Infections, 82*(2), 131–134.

Marín, A., Casado, J., Aranzabal, L., Moya, J., Antela, A., Dronda, F., … Moreno, S. (2006). Validation of a specific questionnaire on psychological and social repercussions of the lipodystrophy syndrome in HIV-infected patients. *Quality of Life Research, 15*(5), 767–775.

Marquez, C., Mitchell, S. J., Hare, C. B., John, M., & Klausner, J. D. (2009). Methamphetamine use, sexual activity, patient–provider communication, and medication adherence among HIV-infected patients in care, San Francisco 2004–2006. *AIDS Care, 21*(5), 575–582.

Martin, M., Del Cacho, E., Codina, C., Tuset, M., De Lazzari, E., Mallolas, J., … Ribas, J. (2008). *Relationship between adherence level, type of the antiretroviral regimen, and plasma HIV type 1 RNA viral load: A prospective cohort study* (Vol. 24). New Rochelle, NY: Liebert.

Martinez, S. M., Kemper, C. A., Diamond, C., & Wagner, G. (2005). Body image in patients with HIV/AIDS: Assessment of a new psychometric measure and its medical correlates. *AIDS Patient Care and STDs, 19*(3), 150–156.

Mayer, K. H., Mimiaga, M. J., Cohen, D., Grasso, C., Bill, R., Van Derwarker, R., & Fisher, A. (2008). Tenofovir DF plus lamivudine or emtricitabine for nonoccupational postexposure prophylaxis (NPEP) in a Boston Community Health Center. *Journal of Acquired Immune Deficiency Syndromes, 47*(4), 494–499.

Mayer, K. H., O'Cleirigh, C., Skeer, M., Covahey, C., Leidolf, E., Vanderwarker, R., & Safren, S. A. (2010). Which HIV-infected men who have sex with men in care are engaging in risky sex and acquiring sexually transmitted infections: Findings from a Boston community health centre. *Sexually Transmitted Infections, 86*(1), 66–70.

McCreary, D. R., Saucier, D. M., & Courtenay, W. H. (2005). The drive for muscularity and masculinity: Testing the associations among genderrole traits, behaviors, attitudes, and conflict. *Psychology of Men & Masculinity, 6*, 83–94.

McGowan, C. C., Weinstein, D. D., Samenow, C. P., Stinnette, S. E., Barkanic, G., Rebeiro, P. F., … Hulgan, T. (2011). Drug use and receipt of highly active antiretroviral therapy among HIV-infected persons in two U.S. clinic cohorts. *PloS One, 6*(4), e18462.

McKirnan, D. J., Du Bois, S. N., Alvy, L. M., & Jones, K. (2012). Health care access and health behaviors among men who have sex with men: The cost of health disparities. *Health Education & Behavior, 40*(1), 32–41.

Mellins, C. A., Havens, J., McDonnell, C., Lichtenstein, C., Uldall, K., Chesney, M., … Bell, J. (2009). Adherence to antiretroviral medications and medical care in HIV-infected adults diagnosed with mental and substance abuse disorders. *AIDS Care, 21*(2), 168–177.

Meredith, C. W., Jaffe, C., Ang-Lee, K., & Saxon, A. J. (2005). Implications of chronic methamphetamine use: A literature review. *Harvard Review of Psychiatry, 13*(3), 141–154.

Miller, L. G., & Hays, R. D. (2000a). Adherence to combination antiretroviral therapy: Synthesis of the literature and clinical implications. *The AIDS Reader, 10*(3), 177–185.

Miller, L. G., & Hays, R. D. (2000b). Measuring adherence to antiretroviral medications in clinical trials. *HIV Clinical Trials, 1*(1), 36–46.

Millett, G. A., Flores, S. A., Peterson, J. L., & Bakeman, R. (2007). Explaining disparities in HIV infection among black and white men who have sex with men: A meta-analysis of HIV risk behaviors. *AIDS, 21*(15), 2083–2091.

Mimiaga, M. J., Closson, E. F., Kothary, V., & Mitty, J. A. (2014). Sexual partnerships and considerations for HIV antiretroviral pre-exposure prophylaxis utilization among high-risk substance using MSM. *Archives of Sexual Behavior, 43*(1), 99–10.

Mimiaga, M. J., Closson, E. F., Pantalone, D. W., Taylor, S. W., Garber, M., Safren, S. A., Mitty, J. A. (2012) *An open phase pilot of behavioral activation to sustain and enhance the effect of contingency management for reducing stimulant use among HIV-infected patients*. Poster presented at the Society of Behavioral Medicine 33rd Annual Meeting and Scientific Sessions, New Orleans, LA.

Mimiaga, M. J., Fair, A. D., Mayer, K. H., Karestan, K., Gortmaker, S., Tetu, A. M., … Safren, S. A. (2008). Experiences and sexual behaviors of HIV-infected MSM who acquired HIV in the context of crystal methamphetamine use. *AIDS Education and Prevention, 20*(1), 30–41.

Mimiaga, M. J., Noonan, E., Donnell, D., Safren, S., Koenen, K., Gortmaker, S., … Mayer, K. H. (2009). Childhood sexual abuse is highly associated with HIV risk-taking behavior and infection among MSM in the EXPLORE Study. *JAIDS Journal of Acquired Immune Deficiency Syndromes, 51*(3), 340–348.

Mimiaga, M. J., Reisner, S. L., Grasso, C., Crane, H. M., Safren, S. A., Kitahata, M. M., … Mayer, K. H. (2013). Substance use among HIV-infected patients engaged in primary care in the United States: Findings from the Centers for AIDS Research Network of Integrated Clinical Systems cohort. *American Journal of Public Health, 103*(8), 1457–1467.

Mimiaga, M. J., Reisner, S. L., Pantalone, D. W., O'Cleirigh, C., Mayer, K. H., & Safren, S. A. (2010). *An open phase pilot of behavioral activation therapy and risk reduction counseling for MSM with crystal methamphetamine abuse at risk for HIV infection*. Paper presented at the Society of Behavioral Medicine 31st Annual Meeting and Scientific Sessions, Seattle, WA.

Mimiaga, M., Reisner, S., Pantalone, D., O'Cleirigh, C., Mayer, K., & Safren, S. (2012). A pilot trial of integrated behavioral activation and sexual risk reduction counseling for HIV-uninfected men who have sex with men abusing crystal methamphetamine. *AIDS Patient Care and STDs, 26*(11), 683–693.

Mitty, J. A., Closson, E. F., Pantalone, D. W., Garber, M., Taylor, S. W., Safren, S. A., & Mimiaga, M. J. (2012). *Improvements in medication adherence and health care utilization as evidenced from a pilot intervention combining contingency management and behavioral activation to reduce stimulant use among HIV-infected individuals*. Paper presented at the International Association of Physicians in AIDS Conference, Miami, FL.

Mitty, J. A., Closson, E. F., Rowley, B., Mayer, K., & Mimiaga, M. J. (2012). *Preference for daily versus intermittent PrEP dosing among substance-dependent high-risk MSM*. Paper presented at the International Association of Physicians in AIDS Conference, Miami, FL.

Montaner, J. S., Hogg, R., Wood, E., Kerr, T., Tyndall, M., Levy, A. R., & Harrigan, P. R. (2006). The case for expanding access to highly active antiretroviral therapy to curb the growth of the HIV epidemic. *Lancet, 368*(9534), 531–536.

Morin, S. F., Steward, W. T., Charlebois, E. D., Remien, R. H., Pinkerton, S. D., Johnson, M. O., … Chesney, M. A. (2005). Predicting HIV transmission risk among HIV-infected men who have sex with men: Findings from the healthy living project. *Journal of Acquired Immune Deficiency Syndromes, 40*(2), 226–235.

Morrison, M. A., Morrison, T. G., & Sager, C.-L. (2004). Does body satisfaction differ between gay men and lesbian women and heterosexual men and women?: A meta-analytic review. *Body Image, 1*(2), 127–138.

Mugavero, M., Ostermann, J., Whetten, K., Leserman, J., Swartz, M., Stangl, D., & Thielman, N. (2006). Barriers to antiretroviral adherence: The importance of depression, abuse, and other traumatic events. *AIDS Patient Care and STDs, 20*(6), 418–428.

Mugavero, M. J., Raper, J. L., Reif, S., Whetten, K., Leserman, J., Thielman, N. M., & Pence, B. W. (2009). Overload: Impact of incident stressful events on antiretroviral medication adherence and virologic failure in a longitudinal, multisite human immunodeficiency virus cohort study. *Psychosomatic Medicine, 71*(9), 920–926.

Nachega, J. B., Marconi, V. C., van Zyl, G. U., Gardner, E. M., Preiser, W., Hong, S. Y., … Gross, R. (2011). HIV treatment adherence, drug resistance, virologic failure: Evolving concepts. *Infectious Disorders-Drug Targets, 11*(2), 167–174.

Newton, T. F., Kalechstein, A. D., Duran, S., Vansluis, N., & Ling, W. (2004). Methamphetamine abstinence syndrome: Preliminary findings. *American Journal on Addictions, 13*(3), 248–255.

Nieuwkerk, P. T., & Oort, F. J. (2005). Self-reported adherence to antiretroviral therapy for HIV-1 infection and virologic treatment response: A meta-analysis. *Journal of Acquired Immune Deficiency Syndromes, 38*(4), 445–448.

O'Cleirigh, C., Ironson, G., & Smits, J. A. J. (2007). Does distress tolerance moderate the impact of major life events on psychosocial variables and behaviors important in the management of HIV? *Behavior Therapy, 38*(3), 314–323.

O'Cleirigh, C., Skeer, M., Mayer, K., & Safren, S. (2009). Functional impairment and health care utilization among HIV-infected men who have sex with men: The relationship with depression and post-traumatic stress. *Journal of Behavioral Medicine, 32*(5), 466–477.

Oh, D. L., Sarafian, F., Silvestre, A., Brown, T., Jacobson, L., Badri, S., & Detels, R. (2009). Evaluation of adherence and factors affecting adherence to combination antiretroviral therapy among White, Hispanic, and Black men in the MACS Cohort. *Journal of Acquired Immune Deficiency Syndromes, 52*(2), 290–293.

Ostrow, D. E., Fox, K. J., Chmiel, J. S., Silvestre, A., Visscher, B. R., Vanable, P. A., … Strathdee, S. A. (2002). Attitudes towards highly active antiretroviral therapy are associated with sexual risk taking among HIV-infected and uninfected homosexual men. *AIDS, 16*(5), 775–780.

Ostrow, D. G., & Stall, R. (2008). Alcohol, tobacco, and drug use among gay and bisexual men. In R. J. Wolitski, R. Stall, & R. O. Valdiserri (Eds.), *Unequal opportunity: Health disparities affecting gay and bisexual men in the United States*. New York, NY: Oxford University Press.

Page-Shafer, K., Delorenze, G. N., Satariano, W. A., & Winkelstein, W. (1996). Comorbidity and survival in HIV-infected men in the San Francisco Men's Health Survey. *Annals of Epidemiology, 6*(5), 420–430.

Palella Jr, F. J., Baker, R. K., Moorman, A. C., Chmiel, J. S., Wood, K. C., Brooks, J. T., … HIV Outpatient Study Investigators. (2006). Mortality in the highly active antiretroviral therapy era: Changing causes of death and disease in the HIV outpatient study. *Journal of Acquired Immune Deficiency Syndromes, 43*(1), 27–34.

Panlilio, A. L., Cardo, D. M., Grohskopf, L. A., Heneine, W., & Ross, C. S. (2005). Updated U.S. Public Health Service guidelines for the management of occupational exposures to HIV and recommendations for postexposure prophylaxis. *Morbidity and Mortality Weekly Report, 54*(RR-9), 1–17.

Pantalone, D. W., Hessler, D. M., & Simoni, J. M. (2010). Mental health pathways from interpersonal violence to health-related outcomes in HIV-positive sexual minority men. *Journal of Consulting and Clinical Psychology, 78*(3), 387–397.

Parsons, J. T., Rosof, E., & Mustanski, B. (2007). Patient-related factors predicting HIV medication adherence among men and women with alcohol problems. *Journal of Health Psychology, 12*(2), 357–370.

Paterson, D., Swindells, S., Mohr, J., Vergis, E., Squire, C., Wagener, M., … Singh, N. (2000). Adherence to protease inhibitor therapy and outcomes in patients with HIV infection. *Annals of Behavioral Medicine, 133*, 21–30.

Paul, J. P., Catania, J., Pollack, L., & Stall, R. (2001). Understanding childhood sexual abuse as a predictor of sexual risk-taking among men who have sex with men: The Urban Men's Health Study. *Child Abuse & Neglect, 25*(4), 557–584.

Peck, J. A., Shoptaw, S., Rotheram-Fuller, E., Reback, C. J., & Bierman, B. (2005). HIV-associated medical, behavioral, and psychiatric characteristics of treatment-seeking, methamphetamine-dependent men who have sex with men. *Journal of Addictive Diseases, 24*(3), 115–132.

Pence, B. W., Miller, W. C., Whetten, K., Eron, J. J., & Gaynes, B. N. (2006). Prevalence of DSM-IV-defined mood, anxiety, and substance use disorders in an HIV clinic in the southeastern United States. *Journal of Acquired Immune Deficiency Syndromes, 42*(3), 298–306.

Plankey, M., Bacchetti, P., Chengshi, J., Grimes, B., Hyman, C., Cohen, M., … Tien, P. C. (2009). Self-perception of body fat changes and HAART adherence in the Women's interagency HIV study. *AIDS and Behavior, 13*(1), 53–59.

Rabkin, J. (2008). HIV and depression: 2008 review and update. *Current HIV/AIDS Reports, 5*(4), 163–171.

Raja, S., McKirnan, D., & Glick, N. (2007). The treatment advocacy program-sinai: A peer-based HIV prevention intervention for working with African American HIV-infected persons. *AIDS and Behavior, 11*(1), 127–137.

Rajasingham, R., Mimiaga, M., White, J., Pinkston, M., Baden, R., & Mitty, J. (2012). A systematic review of behavioral and treatment outcome studies among HIV-infected men who have sex with men who abuse crystal methamphetamine. *AIDS Patient Care and STDs, 26*(1), 36–52.

Ramachandran, S., Yonas, M. A., Silvestre, A. J., & Burke, J. G. (2010). Intimate partner violence among HIV-positive persons in an urban clinic. *AIDS Care, 22*(12), 1536–1543.

Rathbun, R., Farmer, K. C., Stephens, J. R., & Lockhart, S. M. (2005). Impact of an adherence clinic on behavioral outcomes and virologic response in treatment of HIV infection: A prospective, randomized, controlled pilot study. *Clinical Therapeutics, 27*(2), 199–209.

Rawlings, K. M., Thompson, M. A., Farthing, C. F., Brown, L. S., Racine, J., Scott, R. C., … NZTA4006 Helping to Enhance Adherence to Antiretroviral Therapy (HEART) Study Team (2003). Impact of an educational program on efficacy and adherence with a twice-daily Lamivudine/Zidovudine/Abacavir regimen in underrepresented HIV-infected patients. *Journal of Acquired Immune Deficiency Syndromes, 34*(2), 174–183.

Reback, C. J., Larkins, S., & Shoptaw, S. (2003). Methamphetamine abuse as a barrier to HIV medication adherence among gay and bisexual men. *AIDS Care, 15*(6), 775–785.

Reback, C. J., Larkins, S., & Shoptaw, S. (2004). Changes in the meaning of sexual risk behaviors among gay and bisexual male methamphetamine abusers before and after drug treatment. *AIDS and Behavior, 8*(1), 87–98.

Reisner, S. L., Mimiaga, M. J., Skeer, M., Perkovich, B., Johnson, C. V., & Safren, S. A. (2009). A review of HIV antiretroviral adherence and intervention studies among HIV-infected youth. *Topics in HIV Medicine, 17*(1), 14–25.

Remien, R. H., Hirky, A. E., Johnson, M. O., Weinhardt, L. S., Whittier, D., & Le, G. M. (2003). Adherence to medication treatment: A qualitative study of facilitators and barriers among a diverse sample of HIV+ men and women in four US cities. *AIDS and Behavior, 7*(1), 61–72.

Remien, R. H., Stirratt, M. J., Dolezal, C., Dognin, J. S., Wagner, G. J., Carballo-Dieguez, A., … Jung, T. M. (2005). Couple-focused support to improve HIV medication adherence: A randomized controlled trial. *AIDS, 19*(8), 807–814.

Reynolds, N. R. (2004). Adherence to antiretroviral therapies: State of the science. *Current HIV Research, 2*(3), 207–214.

Richter, D. L., Sowell, R. L., & Pluto, D. M. (2002). Attitudes towards antiretroviral therapy among African American women. *American Journal of Health Behavior, 26*, 25–33.

Robbins, G. K., Daniels, B., Zheng, H., Chueh, H., Meigs, J. B., & Freedberg, K. A. (2007). Predictors of antiretroviral treatment failure in an urban HIV clinic. *Journal of Acquired Immune Deficiency Syndromes, 44*(1), 30.

Robinson, L., & Rempel, H. (2006). Methamphetamine use and HIV symptom self-management. *Journal of the Association of Nurses in AIDS Care, 17*(5), 7–14.

Safren, S. A., Hendriksen, E. S., Desousa, N., Boswell, S. L., & Mayer, K. H. (2003). Use of an on-line pager system to increase adherence to antiretroviral medications. *AIDS Care, 15*(6), 787–793.

Safren, S. A., O'Cleirigh, C., Tan, J. Y., Raminani, S. R., Reilly, L. C., Otto, M. W., … Mayer, K. H. (2009). A randomized controlled trial of cognitive behavioral therapy for adherence and depression (CBT-AD) in HIV-infected individuals. *Health Psychology, 28*(1), 1–10.

Safren, S. A., O'Cleirigh, C. M., Bullis, J. R., Otto, M. W., Stein, M. D., & Pollack, M. H. (2012). Cognitive behavioral therapy for adherence and depression (CBT-AD) in HIV-infected injection drug users: A randomized controlled trial. *Journal of Consulting and Clinical Psychology, 80*(3), 404–415.

Safren, S. A., Otto, M. W., & Worth, J. L. (1999). Life-steps: Applying cognitive behavioral therapy to HIV medication adherence. *Cognitive and Behavioral Practice, 6*(4), 332–341.

Safren, S. A., Otto, M. W., Worth, J., Salomon, E., Johnson, W., Mayer, K., & Boswell, S. (2001). Two strategies to increase adherence to HIV antiretroviral medication: Life-steps and medication monitoring. *Behaviour Research and Therapy, 39*, 1151–1162.

SAMHSA. (1996). *National household survey on drug abuse: Population estimates.* Rockville, MD: Substance Abuse and Mental Health Services Administration.

SAMHSA. (2001). *Summary of findings from the 2000 National Household Survey on Drug Abuse.* Rockville, MD, Substance Abuse and Mental Health Services Administration. Office of Applied Studies, NHSDA Series H-13.

Sandelowski, M., Voils, C. I., Chang, Y., & Lee, E. J. (2009). A systematic review comparing antiretroviral adherence descriptive and intervention studies conducted in the USA. *AIDS Care, 21*(8), 953–966.

Santos, C. P., Felipe, Y. X., Braga, P. E., Ramos, D., Lima, R. O., & Segurado, A. C. (2005). Self-perception of body changes in persons living with HIV/AIDS: Prevalence and associated factors. *AIDS, 19*(Suppl 4), S14–S21.

Schilder, A. J., Kennedy, C., Goldstone, I. L., Ogden, R. D., Hogg, R. S., & O'Shaughnessy, M. V. (2001). "Being dealt with as a whole person." Care seeking and adherence: The benefits of culturally competent care. *Social Science & Medicine, 52*(11), 1643–1659.

Schroder, K., Carey, M., & Vanable, P. (2003). Methodological challenges in research on sexual risk behavior: II. Accuracy of self-reports. *Annals of Behavioral Medicine, 26*(2), 104–123.

Schwartz, J. P., & Tylka, T. L. (2008). Exploring entitlement as a moderator and mediator of the relationship between masculine gender role conflict and men's body esteem. *Psychology of Men & Masculinity, 9*, 67–81.

Semple, S. J., Patterson, T. L., & Grant, I. (2002). Motivations associated with methamphetamine use among HIV men who have sex with men. *Journal of Substance Abuse Treatment, 22*(3), 149–156.

Sharma, A., Howard, A. A., Klein, R. S., Schoenbaum, E. E., Buono, D., & Webber, M. P. (2007). Body image in older men with or at-risk for HIV infection. *AIDS Care, 19*(2), 235–241.

Sharma, A., Howard, A. A., Schoenbaum, E. E., Buono, D., & Webber, M. P. (2006). Body image in middle-aged HIV-infected and uninfected women. *AIDS Care, 18*(8), 998–1003.

Shoptaw, S. (2006). Methamphetamine use in urban gay and bisexual populations. *Topics in HIV Medicine, 14*(2), 84–87.

Shuter, J., Sarlo, J. A., Kanmaz, T. J., Rode, R. A., & Zingman, B. S. (2007). HIV-infected patients receiving lopinavir/ritonavir-based antiretroviral therapy achieve high rates of virologic suppression despite adherence rates less than 95%. *JAIDS Journal of Acquired Immune Deficiency Syndromes, 45*(1), 4–8.

Simoni, J. M., Kurth, A. E., Pearson, C. R., Pantalone, D. W., Merrill, J. O., & Frick, P. A. (2006). Self-report measures of antiretroviral therapy adherence: A review with recommendations for HIV research and clinical management. *AIDS and Behavior, 10*(3), 227–245.

Simoni, J. M., Pantalone, D. W., Plummer, M. D., & Huang, B. (2007). A randomized controlled trial of a peer support intervention targeting antiretroviral medication adherence and depressive symptomatology in HIV-positive men and women. *Health Psychology, 26*(4), 488–495.

Simoni, J. M., Pearson, C. R., Pantalone, D. W., Marks, G., & Crepaz, N. (2006). Efficacy of interventions in improving highly active antiretroviral therapy adherence and HIV-1 RNA viral load: A meta-analytic review of randomized controlled trials. *Journal of Acquired Immune Deficiency Syndromes, 43*, S23–S35.

Skeer, M. R., Mimiaga, M. J., Mayer, K. H., O'Cleirigh, C., Covahey, C., & Safren, S. A. (2012). Patterns of substance use among a large urban cohort of HIV-infected men who have sex with men in primary care. *AIDS and Behavior, 16*(3), 676–689.

Solomon, T., & Halkitis, P. (2008). Cognitive executive functioning in relation to HIV medication adherence among gay, bisexual, and other men who have sex with men. *AIDS and Behavior, 12*(1), 68–77.

Solomon, T. M., Halkitis, P. N., Moeller, R. W., & Pappas, M. K. (2012). Levels of methamphetamine use and addiction among gay, bisexual, and other men who have sex with men. *Addiction Research & Theory, 20*(1), 21–29.

Stall, R., Hoff, C., Coates, T. J., Paul, J., Phillips, K. A., Ekstrand, M., … Diaz, R. (1996). Decisions to get HIV tested and to accept antiretroviral therapies among gay/bisexual men: Implications for secondary prevention efforts. *JAIDS Journal of Acquired Immune Deficiency Syndromes, 11*(2), 151–160.

Stall, R., & Purcell, D. (2000). Intertwining epidemics: A review of research on substance use among men who have sex with men and its connection to the AIDS epidemic. *AIDS and Behavior, 4*, 181–192.

Stirratt, M., & Gordon, C. (2008). Adherence to biomedical HIV prevention methods: Considerations drawn from HIV treatment adherence research. *Current HIV/AIDS Reports, 5*(4), 186–192.

Stolte, I. G., Dukers, N. H., Geskus, R. B., Coutinho, R. A., & Wit, J. B. (2004). Homosexual men change to risky sex when perceiving less threat of HIV/AIDS since availability of highly active antiretroviral therapy: A longitudinal study. *AIDS, 18*(2), 303–309.

Stone, V. E., Hogan, J. W., Schuman, P., Rompalo, A. M., Howard, A. A., Korkontzelou, C., … HERS Study (2001). Antiretroviral regimen complexity, self-reported adherence, and HIV patients' understanding of their regimens: Survey of women in the HER study. *Journal of Acquired Immune Deficiency Syndromes, 28*(2), 124–131.

Sullivan, L. E., Goulet, J. L., Justice, A. C., & Fiellin, D. A. (2011). Alcohol consumption and depressive symptoms over time: A longitudinal study of patients with and without HIV infection. *Drug and Alcohol Dependence, 117*(2–3), 158–163.

Sullivan, L. E., Saitz, R., Cheng, D. M., Libman, H., Nunes, D., & Samet, J. H. (2008). The impact of alcohol use on depressive symptoms in human immunodeficiency virus-infected patients. *Addiction, 103*(9), 1461–1467.

Taylor, S. W., Safren, S. A., Elsesser, S. M., Mimiaga, M. J., & Mayer, K. H. (2012). *Enhancing pre-exposure prophylaxis adherence in men who have sex with men: Determining optimal content for a PrEP adherence package*. Paper presented at the International Association of Physicians in AIDS Conference, Miami, FL.

Tegger, M. K., Crane, H. M., Tapia, K. A., Uldall, K. K., Holte, S. E., & Kitahata, M. M. (2008). The effect of mental illness, substance use, and treatment for depression on the initiation of highly active antiretroviral therapy among HIV-infected individuals. *AIDS Patient Care and STDs*, *22*(3), 233–243.

Thornton, L. K., Baker, A. L., Lewin, T. J., Kay-Lambkin, F. J., Kavanagh, D., Richmond, R., … Johnson, M. P. (2012). Reasons for substance use among people with mental disorders. *Addictive Behaviors*, *37*(4), 427–434.

Thrasher, A. D., Earp, J. A. L., Golin, C. E., & Zimmer, C. R. (2008). Discrimination, distrust, and racial/ethnic disparities in antiretroviral therapy adherence among a national sample of HIV-infected patients. *Journal of Acquired Immune Deficiency Syndromes*, *49*(1), 84–93.

Trotta, M. P., Ammassari, A., Melzi, S., Zaccarelli, M., Ladisa, N., Sighinolfi, L., … AdICoNA Study Group. (2002). Treatment-related factors and highly active antiretroviral therapy adherence. *Journal of Acquired Immune Deficiency Syndromes*, *31*, S128–S131..

U.S. Department of Health and Human Services. (2012). Limitations to treatment safety and efficacy: Adherence to antiretroviral therapy. *Guidelines for the use of antiretroviral agents in HIV-1-infected adults and adolescents*. Retrieved from http://www.aidsinfo.nih.gov/guidelines/html/1/adult-and-adolescent-arv-guidelines/30/adherence-to-art.

van de Vijver, D. A., & Boucher, C. A. (2010). The risk of HIV drug resistance following implementation of pre-exposure prophylaxis. *Current Opinion in Infectious Diseases*, *23*(6), 621–627.

Vanable, P. A., Ostrow, D. G., & McKirnan, D. J. (2003). Viral load and HIV treatment attitudes as correlates of sexual risk behavior among HIV-positive gay men. *Journal of Psychosomatic Research*, *54*(3), 263–269.

Velasquez, M. M., von Sternberg, K., Johnson, D. H., Green, C., Carbonari, J. P., & Parsons, J. (2009). *Reducing sexual risk behaviors and alcohol use among HIV-positive men who have sex with men: A randomized clinical trial* (Vol. 77). Washington, DC: American Psychological Association.

Vervoort, S. C., Borleffs, J. C., Hoepelman, A. I., & Grypdonck, M. H. (2007). Adherence in antiretroviral therapy: A review of qualitative studies. *AIDS*, *21*(3), 271–281.

Viswanathan, H., Anderson, R., & Thomas, J. (2005). Evaluation of an antiretroviral medication attitude scale and relationships between medication attitudes and medication nonadherence. *AIDS Patient Care and STDs*, *19*, 306–316.

Vranceanu, A. M., Safren, S. A., Lu, M., Coady, W. M., Skolnik, P. R., Rogers, W. H., & Wilson, I. B. (2008). The relationship of post-traumatic stress disorder and depression to antiretroviral medication adherence in persons with HIV. *AIDS Patient Care and STDs*, *22*(4), 313–321.

Wagner, G. J. (2002). Predictors of antiretroviral adherence as measured by self-report, electronic monitoring, and medication diaries. *AIDS Patient Care and STDs*, *16*(12), 599–608.

Wagner, G., & Miller, L. G. (2004). Is the influence of social desirability on patients' self-reported adherence overrated? *Journal of Acquired Immune Deficiency Syndromes*, *35*(2), 203–204.

Wagner, G. J., & Rabkin, J. G. (1999). Development of the Impact of Weight Loss Scale (IWLS): A psychometric study in a sample of men with HIV/AIDS. *AIDS Care*, *11*(4), 453–457.

Wagner, G. J., Remien, R. H., Carballo-Diéguez, A., & Dolezal, C. (2002). Correlates of adherence to combination antiretroviral therapy among members of HIV-positive mixed status couples. *AIDS Care*, *14*(1), 105–109.

Wainberg, M. A., & Zaharatos, G. J. (2012). Development and transmission of HIV drug resistance. *Sande's HIV/AIDS Medicine: Medical Management of AIDS 2012*, 155.

Weidle, P. J., Ganea, C. E., Irwin, K. L., McGowan, J. P., Ernst, J. A., Olivo, N., & Holmberg, S. D. (1999). Adherence to antiretroviral medications in an inner-city population. *JAIDS Journal of Acquired Immune Deficiency Syndromes*, *22*(5), 498–502.

Welles, S. L., Baker, A. C., Miner, M. H., Brennan, D. J., Jacoby, S., & Rosser, B. S. (2009). History of childhood sexual abuse and unsafe anal intercourse in a 6-city study of HIV-positive men who have sex with men. *American Journal of Public Health*, *99*(6), 1079–1086.

Welles, S. L., Corbin, T. J., Rich, J. A., Reed, E., & Raj, A. (2011). Intimate partner violence among men having sex with men, women, or both: Early-life sexual and physical abuse as antecedents. *Journal of Community Health, 36*(3), 477–485.

Wellons, M. F., Sanders, L., Edwards, L. J., Bartlett, J. A., Heald, A. E., & Schmader, K. E. (2002). HIV infection: Treatment outcomes in older and younger adults. *Journal of the American Geriatrics Society, 50*(4), 603–607.

WHO. (2013). *HIV drug resistance.* Retrieved from http://www.who.int/hiv/topics/drugresistance/en/index.html.

Wilson, I. B., Carter, A. E., & Berg, K. M. (2009). Improving the self-report of HIV antiretroviral medication adherence: Is the glass half full or half empty? *Current HIV/AIDS Reports, 6*(4), 177–186.

Wilton, L., Herbst, J. H., Coury-Doniger, P., Painter, T. M., English, G., Alvarez, M. E., … Carey, J. W. (2009). Efficacy of an HIV/STI prevention intervention for black men who have sex with men: Findings from the Many Men, Many Voices (3MV) project. *AIDS and Behavior, 13*(3), 532–544.

Wohl, A. R., Frye, D. M., & Johnson, D. F. (2008). Demographic characteristics and sexual behaviors associated with methamphetamine use among MSM and non-MSM diagnosed with AIDS in Los Angeles County. *AIDS and Behavior, 12*(5), 705–712.

Wood, E., Hogg, R. S., Yip, B., Harrigan, P. R., O'Shaughnessy, M. V., & Montaner, J. S. G. (2004). The impact of adherence on CD4 cell count responses among HIV-infected patients. *JAIDS Journal of Acquired Immune Deficiency Syndromes, 35*(3), 261–268.

Wrubel, J., Stumbo, S., & Johnson, M. O. (2008). Antiretroviral medication support practices among partners of men who have sex with men: A qualitative study. *AIDS Patient Care and STDs, 22*(11), 851–858.

Wrubel, J., Stumbo, S., & Johnson, M. O. (2010). Male same-sex couple dynamics and received social support for HIV medication adherence. *Journal of Social and Personal Relationships, 27*(4), 553–572.

Zanjani, F., Saboe, K., & Oslin, D. (2007). Age difference in rates of mental health/substance abuse and behavioral care in HIV-positive adults. *AIDS Patient Care and STDs, 21*(5), 347–355.

Zweben, J. E., Cohen, J. B., Christian, D., Galloway, G. P., Salinardi, M., Parent, D., … Methamphetamine Treatment Project. (2004). Psychiatric symptoms in methamphetamine users. *American Journal on Addictions, 13*(2), 181–190.

Chapter 8
Emerging and Innovative Prevention Strategies for HIV Positive Gay Men

John A. Schneider and Alida M. Bouris

This chapter will focus primarily on secondary HIV prevention—incorporating novel and emerging structural, behavioral, and biomedical strategies—for the reduction of onwards HIV transmission among HIV positive gay men and men who have sex with men (MSM). Because the current HIV epidemic in the USA consists of marked racial/ethnic disparities in HIV prevalence and transmission rates, our inquiry parallels such realities by focusing disproportionately on prevention strategies for these "dual minority" status populations—that is underrepresented and sexual minority populations. We first begin with a brief review of existing prevention interventions and discuss what features are common among successful interventions, as well as those that have failed. Also, we identify notable prevention intervention lacunae, both with respect to limited interventions that target MSM of color, younger MSM, and other MSM who are HIV infected—prevention for positives. We then examine several contemporary social forces that will affect the trajectory of the HIV epidemic and how these forces are or could be leveraged for intervention: minority stress and syndemic morbidities; marriage equality; healthcare reform; increasing digital communication technology; and an aging infected population. We then describe several promising novel or emerging prevention strategies that leverage networks as we move over the next three decades to near elimination of new HIV transmission among MSM in the USA.

J.A. Schneider (✉)
Departments of Medicine and Public Health Sciences, Chicago Center for HIV Elimination, University of Chicago, Chicago, IL, USA
e-mail: jschnei1@medicine.bsd.uchicago.edu

A.M. Bouris
School of Social Service Administration, Chicago Center for HIV Elimination, University of Chicago, Chicago, IL, USA

© Springer Science+Business Media LLC 2017
L. Wilton (ed.), *Understanding Prevention for HIV Positive Gay Men*,
DOI 10.1007/978-1-4419-0203-0_8

Background

MSM continue to be a group representing the largest number of individuals living with HIV in the USA (Centers for Disease Control and Prevention, 2012). Within MSM, people of color comprise the majority of new HIV transmission cases and currently represent the largest HIV infected subgroups (Prejean et al., 2011). While there is increasing excitement about biomedical approaches such as treatment as prevention (Cohen et al., 2011) for HIV positive MSM to limit onward transmission within MSM networks, there is a critical need for additional study of biomedical approaches within these networks, as well as efforts to increase the potency of targeted behavioral, public health, and structural approaches to limiting onwards transmission of HIV, sexually transmitted infection (STI) acquisition and prolongation of life among HIV positive MSM. This becomes critically important given the context of individuals that are HIV infected and aware of their status being associated with almost half of new HIV infections in the USA (Marks, Crepaz, Senterfitt, & Janssen, 2005).

Prevention Strategies: The Extant Literature

Behavioral

There are numerous behavioral interventions tested to prevent the transmission of HIV among MSM. According to the Centers for Disease Control and Prevention (CDC) "Effective Behavioral Interventions" (EBI) that were specifically designed for MSM include Mpowerment (Kegeles, Hays, & Coates, 1996) and for Black MSM d-UP (Jones et al., 2008) and 3MV (Many Men, Many Voices) (Wilton et al., 2009). Among EBIs, there were no Latino MSM specific interventions and none specifically targeting HIV infected MSM. There are several other effective behavioral interventions designed for other HIV infected populations, which have also been applied to MSM, such as CLEAR (Rotheram-Borus et al., 2004).

Other interventions for HIV infected MSM have generally been intensive interventions that involve multiple individual and/or group sessions (Kelly et al., 1993; Mausbach, Semple, Strathdee, Zians, & Patterson, 2007; Morin et al., 2008; Rosser et al., 2010; Safren, O'Cleirigh, Skeer, Elsesser, & Mayer, 2012; Wolitski, Gomez, & Parsons, 2005). Although one of these was found to be efficacious, it consisted of fifteen 90-min sessions with a counselor (Morin et al., 2008), which is not practical in most HIV primary care or community-based settings. Another brief intervention demonstrated some potential benefit to nondepressed HIV infected MSM (Safren et al., 2012). Behavioral interventions that combine skills training and cultural or interactive engagement of participants have been found to be more effective when compared to those depending upon didactic messaging. While such behavioral interventions are of great interest, biologic endpoints are of importance when determining initial efficacy (Pequegnat & Szapocznik, 2000). For example, d-UP (Jones et al., 2008), a prevention intervention targeting Black MSM is based upon the Community Popular Opinion Leader (C-POL) model, which has improved behavior in many settings; however, evidence of change in HIV seroprevalence using C-POL has been elusive when evaluated (Rosser et al., 2010; Schneider & Laumann, 2011). Further rigor is also needed when evaluating such interventions as d-UP did not utilize randomization procedures to measure behavioral outcomes and did not use biologic endpoints (Kelly et al., 1991). Additionally, few interventions are related to clinic settings where integration of biomedical and behavioral prevention can occur (Safren et al., 2012). Notably, there also are no interventions targeting bisexual men.

Biomedical

The greatest biomedical intervention for primary prevention, and potentially secondary prevention, targeting HIV infected MSM has been antiretroviral (ARV) therapy. ARVs have been found to prevent AIDS among HIV infected MSM, including MSM of color, through the reduction of HIV virus and concomitant increase in CD-4 T-cell percentage (Office of AIDS Research Advisory Council, 2015). This primary AIDS prevention is one of the greatest advancements in the history of HIV, and is certainly dependent upon excellent adherence to ARVs (Paterson et al., 2000). Adherence to ARVs among MSM is one of several factors in the treatment cascade following successful linkage and retention in HIV primary care (Gardner, McLees, Steiner, Del Rio, & Burman, 2011). While data exist for MSM on individual- and provider-level correlates of adherence to HIV care (CDPH, 2008; Oh et al., 2009; Schneider, Kaplan, Greenfield, Li, & Wilson, 2004), there is a lack of research on younger MSM of color (Belzer, Fuchs, Luftman, & Tucker, 1999; Harper, Fernandez, Bruce, Hosek, & Jacobs, 2011; Macdonell, Naar-King, Murphy, Parsons, & Harper, 2010). Studies show that Black and Latino YMSM have poorer rates of retention than Whites (Christopoulos, Das, & Colfax, 2011) and that poor retention is associated with reduced ARV adherence and increased risk for virologic failure (Giordano et al., 2007). Although it is recommended that HIV-infected youth see a healthcare provider every 3–4 months, one study found that the cumulative probability for males to be retained in care after an initial visit declined to 45% after 2 months, 24% after 1 year, and 10% after 2 years (Harris et al., 2003). Whereas some research has found that Latino MSM have better retention in care than other HIV positive Latinos (Gebo et al., 2005), one project found that Latino YMSM had poorer retention than Black YMSM (Magnus et al., 2010), suggesting that additional retention research is needed for both groups.

Maximizing retention and adherence to ARVs may have additional value to sexual risk reduction by attenuating onward transmission given the high-degree of within-group mixing (sex partnering based upon race) (Cohen et al., 2011), especially within racially segregated environments (Doherty, Schoenbach, & Adimora, 2009). Racially segregated environments, such as the South Side of

Chicago, can consolidate risk within the community and provide greater opportunities for individuals at higher and lower HIV risk to mix (Laumann, Ellingson, Mahay, Paik, & Youm, 2004). Thus, maximizing retention and adherence to ARVs in these contexts could have a major impact. This treatment as prevention approach has not been adequately studied among MSM (Cohen et al., 2011), with some models optimistic about this strategy's potential for secondary prevention among MSM in general (Sorensen et al., 2012).

Structural and Public Health

Structural and public health interventions have received little attention in HIV prevention research, despite their potential for population level impact. Most of these interventions target populations broadly; however, they can still have significant impact upon HIV infected MSM and, in particular, MSM who have few financial resources. For example, healthcare coverage (Schneider, McFadden, Laumann, et al., 2012; Schneider, Michaels, Gandham, et al., 2012; Schneider, Walsh, et al., 2012) and stable housing (Robertson et al., 2004) may be effective and least costly interventions for preventing onward HIV transmission (Adimora & Auerbach, 2010). For example, in a study with 2149 adolescents and adults living with HIV/AIDS, of which 34.2% were MSM, homeless and unstably housed persons were two times more likely to report sexual exchange, recent drug use, and needle use at baseline than were their stably housed peers. Follow-up data collected 6–9 months later showed that improvements in housing status were associated with significant decreases in needle use, needle sharing, and unprotected sexual intercourse. Moreover, individuals whose housing status worsened over time were five times more likely to report exchanging sex than were those whose housing remained stable (Wolitski et al., 2010). However, a subsequent randomized controlled trial of rental assistance for homeless persons living with HIV/AIDS had positive benefits on self-reported depression, physical health, and perceived stress but no impact on sexual risk behaviors, healthcare access, and adherence (Aidala, Cross, Stall, Harre, & Sumartojo, 2005). Thus, while the extant research points to the importance of stable housing for persons at risk for and living with HIV/AIDS, additional research is needed to better understand which types of housing interventions are most efficacious and the precise mechanism of change. Condom distribution programs have been found to be efficacious in meta-analyses of populations that include MSM (Charania et al., 2011). Partner services are also important interventions applied to HIV infected MSM and include various levels of contact tracing (Centers for Disease Control and Prevention, 2008). These programs, many of which are led by local Departments of Public Health, utilize organically derived sex networks to locate, educate, test, and refer sex partners of newly infected persons. Partner notification has been around for nearly 80 years (Parran, 1961), longer than most HIV prevention programs, however, very little evaluation has been conducted to determine best practices (Brown et al., 2011; Samoff, Koumans, Katkowsky, Shouse, & Markowitz, 2007). These programs are often limited in their scope and do not discriminate between individuals who are chronically versus recently infected. More sophisticated network-based tracing and interventions that are emerging and under development will be discussed in the final section of this chapter.

In sum, there are considerable needs with respect to MSM-based interventions that target those who are HIV infected and, in particular, HIV infected MSM of color. A recent review of behavioral, biomedical, structural, and public health interventions in the USA aimed at reducing HIV transmission racial disparities (Hemmige, McFadden, Cook, Tang, & Schneider, 2012) found only 2 out of 76 targeting MSM of color (Operario, Smith, Arnold, & Kegeles, 2010; Somerville, Diaz, Davis, Coleman, & Taveras, 2006). Neither of these were targeting HIV infected MSM of color. Remarkably, 31 years after the first cases of HIV were identified among MSM (Auerbach, Darrow, Jaffe, & Curran, 1984; MMWR, 1981), there are limited interventions for secondary prevention among HIV infected MSM and none for MSM of color. Urgent attention to this lacunae is required if we hope to fulfill the promise of eliminating new cases among MSM in the next 30 years.

Contextual and Core Issues Related to Emerging and Innovative Prevention Strategies

Minority Stress and Syndemic Comorbidities

One contextual factor that must be addressed in prevention with HIV positive MSM is the role of social discrimination. Despite increases in public acceptance of homosexuality and support of same-sex marriage (Baunach, 2011; Becker, 2012; Smith, 2011), homophobia and heterosexism remain serious social problems. In addition, HIV/AIDS continues to be a highly stigmatized illness, which further complicates the delivery of effective prevention services. As research on the role of social discrimination in the development and maintenance of health disparities has grown, minority stress (Meyer, 1995; Meyer, 2003, 2007) and syndemic theories (Stall, Friedman, & Catania, 2008; Stall et al., 2003) of health have emerged as critical conceptual frameworks for understanding the disproportionate impact of HIV/AIDS on MSM. Originally developed by Brooks (Brooks, 1981) for lesbians and expanded by Meyer (Meyer, 1995; Meyer, 2003) to the larger lesbian, gay, bisexual, and transgender (LGBT) population, minority stress theory posits that sexual minorities experience heightened levels of stress resulting from experiences with homophobia, stigmatization, and violence. These experiences, in turn, are thought to increase vulnerability to a range of poor health outcomes. Indeed, a large body of research has found that MSM are at greater risk than their heterosexual peers for a range of negative health problems, including substance use, depression, and suicidality (Institute of Medicine, 2011). While additional research is needed to understand the precise mechanism through which experiences with discrimination increase vulnerability to HIV/AIDS, research points to the potential relationships between social stressors and psychological distress (Choi, Paul, Ayala, Boylan, & Gregorich, 2013; Hatzenbuehler, Nolen-Hoeksema, & Erickson, 2008), coping styles (Wilson & Yoshikawa, 2004), and sexual risk behaviors (Ayala, Bingham, Kim, Wheeler, & Millett, 2012; Meyer & Dean, 1998).

The presence of multiple psychosocial health problems that interact to increase vulnerability to poor health is known as a syndemic. Although first applied to the overlapping problems of substance abuse, violence, and AIDS in inner-city communities (Singer, 1996), syndemics refer to "the concentration and deleterious interaction of two or more diseases, or other health conditions, in a population, especially as a consequence of social inequity and the unjust exercise of power"(Singer, 2009). Stall's Theory of the Syndemic Production emphasizes the impact of early experiences with social marginalization on the psychosocial and behavioral health of MSM over the life course (Stall et al., 2003). Experiences with social marginalization are synergistic, such that adverse experiences have an additive impact on poor health over time. In addition, these psychosocial health problems have been associated with increased likelihood of unprotected anal intercourse among HIV positive MSM (VanDevanter et al., 2011).

Among HIV infected MSM, experiences with minority stress and the presence of multiple epidemics (i.e., syndemic comorbidities) have implications for the prevention of onward transmission. At a minimum, interventions need to be sensitive to the potential presence and synergistic interactions between social conditions and psychosocial health problems among HIV infected MSM (Christopoulos et al., 2011) and should seek to deliver comprehensive services (i.e., services that not only focus on managing HIV and preventing onward transmission), but also on addressing other health conditions and the root causes behind them (Mayer et al., 2012). This includes attending to issues related to substance use, mental health, and violence, as well as factors such as homelessness, under- and unemployment, lack of access to care, and incarceration. In addition, there is increasing attention on resilience among MSM as an untapped resource in HIV/AIDS prevention (Herrick et al., 2011). A recent study found that resilience among HIV infected MSM was associated with a reduced odds of unprotected anal intercourse (Kurtz, Buttram, Surratt, & Stall, 2012). Although this research is growing, intervention strategies that focus on the strengths of HIV infected MSM, many of whom have experienced significant adversity over the life course, would be a welcome addition to current prevention packages.

Marriage Equality

Another contextual factor that may affect future interventions with HIV infected MSM is marriage equality. In 2015, the United States Supreme Court ruled in *Obergefell v. Hodges* that same-sex couples have a fundamental right to marry under both the Equal Protection Clause and the Due Process Clause of the 14th Amendment to the United States Constitution. Although research on how marriage equality will affect HIV infected MSM is limited, emerging studies point to a number of benefits. First, legal recognition of same-sex partnerships as marriages confers social, legal, and health benefits from which LGBT people have long been excluded (Buffie, 2011; Ponce, Cochran, Pizer, & Mays, 2010). With the advent of marriage equality, same-sex couples now have access to employer-sponsored healthcare through their spouse. Prior to the *Obergefell v Hodges* (2015) decision, in contrast, employers could deny employees the ability to purchase healthcare for same-sex partners or impose residential or financial requirements on same-sex couples that are not required of heterosexual married couples (Ponce et al., 2010).

There also is research to suggest that marriage may have a health promoting effect beyond access to social and legal protections. For example, Klausner and colleagues conducted a population-based telephone survey with 2881 gay men residing in Chicago, New York, Los Angeles, and San Francisco (Klausner, Pollack, Wong, & Katz, 2006). Study results indicated that men in domestic partnerships reported significantly lower rates of sexual risk behaviors (e.g., multiple sexual partners, unprotected anal intercourse with a non-primary partner, and "one night stands") than did men without a primary partner or men with non-domestic steady partners (Klausner et al., 2006). Still other scholars have discussed marriage equality as an important structural determinant of gay men's health (Halkitis, 2012), especially for the potential to reduce stigma and increase social tolerance, which may have downstream effects on LGBT people's health and well-being. For example, Hatzenbuehler and colleagues found the state bans on same-sex marriage were associated with increased rates of mental health problems among LGB adults (Hatzenbuehler, McLaughlin, Keyes, & Hasin, 2010). Similarly, Francis and Mialon (2010) examined how tolerance was related to HIV and found that society-wide tolerance of gay people was inversely related to the rate of HIV infections. Additional research is needed to better understand how marriage equality may specifically affect prevention and treatment efforts for men living with HIV.

Healthcare Reform

On September 23, 2010, President Obama signed into law the Patient Protection and Affordable Care Act (ACA), which was subsequently upheld by the U.S. Supreme Court on June 28, 2012. Because a full discussion of ACA and its impact on HIV care is outside the purview of this chapter, we briefly highlight key provisions likely to affect HIV positive MSM (Martin & Schackman, 2012; Owens, 2012; Sherer, 2012). For additional details, please visit HIV Healthcare Reform at http://www.hivhealthreform.org/. Of particular note is that access to healthcare for all Americans will increase via (1) the expansion of Medicaid coverage to individuals with incomes that are ≤133% of the federal poverty level, (2) the creation of state-based health insurance exchanges, and (3) tax credits. Medicaid expansion is expected to be the greatest source of increased care for persons living with HIV.

A number of provisions of the ACA affect HIV positive MSM. First, individuals with a preexisting condition such as HIV can no longer be denied insurance coverage. In order to help uninsured individuals obtain coverage prior to 2014, ACA included a provision that enables individuals living with HIV to join a "Pre-Existing Condition Insurance Plan," further expanding access to care (for more information, see: http://www.pcip.gov). Second, dependent young adults can now remain on their parent's private health insurance up to age 26. Although it is unknown how many YMSM living with HIV have utilized this option, the expanded years of coverage overlap with a developmental period during which YMSM, especially youth of color, are at highest risk for HIV (Martin & Schackman, 2012). However, despite increased opportunities for access, the most recent data on health insurance coverage show that 46.4% of Latino and 32.3% Black young adults aged 19–25 are uninsured compared to 16.7% of their White peers (Cohen & Martinez, 2012). Finally, ACA will gradually eliminate the "donut hole" in prescription drug coverage in Medicare Part D, which is expected to greatly reduce costs for antiretroviral medications (Martin & Schackman, 2012).

Despite these benefits, there is uncertainty about how the ACA will affect MSM at risk for or living with HIV/AIDS. This uncertainty is especially heightened in early 2017, as the incoming Republican administration has made the repeal of the ACA a cornerstone of their political platform. Furthermore, both Medicaid and Medicare are subject to intense political debate and both programs may change under a new administration. It also is unclear how the pending repeal of the ACA and current efforts to cut taxes and increase spending on other programs may affect services covered under the Ryan White CARE Act, such as the AIDS Drug Assistance Program (ADAP). Thus, the benefits afforded to many American citizens may be rolled back and it is unclear how pending changes in healthcare policy will affect healthcare and future intervention efforts for MSM living with HIV.

Epidemic Shift

While HIV has always disproportionately affected MSM, there have been shifts within this subpopulation with respect to the epidemiology of new cases and access to care. According to the CDC, from 2006 to 2009, the largest percentage increase in HIV incidence was among young Black MSM, aged 13–29, at 48%, with HIV incidence unchanged among young White and Latino MSM (Prejean et al., 2011). In several urban centers like Chicago, this disparity is even higher—young Black men have 7 times the rate of HIV infection as young men with similar sexual behavior and substance use patterns (CDPH, 2008). These alarming disparities represent a public health emergency and require bold interventions that work in partnership with Black communities and their leadership. Partnership between academic and community units that are researching new strategies for HIV prevention locally are just one component. For example, the Chicago Black Gay Men's Caucus and several units within the University of Chicago including the Urban Health Initiative, the Sexually

Transmitted Infection and HIV Network, and the Center for HIV Elimination have Black leaders and their allies engaged with the community affected by one of the major domestic HIV epidemics ("Chicago Black Gay Men's Caucus. http://chiblackgaycaucus.org/ (Last accessed April 18, 2013)"; "Chicago Center for HIV Elimination. http://hivelimination.uchicago.edu/ (Last Accessed, April 18 2013); "STI and HIV Intervention Network. http://ssascholars.uchicago.edu/shine. Last accessed April 18, 2013.").

Several drivers of these epidemiologic findings which suggest widening disparities have been explored in great detail (Millett, Peterson, Wolitski, & Stall, 2006; Millett et al., 2012). One of the key factors relate to social and sexual networks of communities of color, such as African Americans. Some research has explained disparities in HIV rates by examining sexual network mixing patterns within and between racial subgroups (Rothenberg, Hoang, Muth, & Crosby, 2007; Stoner, Whittington, Hughes, Aral, & Holmes, 2000). Previously, Edward Laumann demonstrated that higher rates of sexually transmitted infections within the African American community were related to sexual network mixing patterns (Laumann & Youm, 1999). Higher levels of disassortative mixing—core high-risk groups mixing with peripheral low-risk groups—within the African American community, combined with limited inter-racial mixing, was a major contributor for the disproportionately higher rates of sexually transmitted infections among Blacks when compared to Whites. Similar sexual network mixing explanations have been demonstrated among Blacks in the North Carolina (Doherty et al., 2009) and Black MSM in Chicago (Schneider et al., 2013). Drug use behavior was found to be highly assortative (like behavior with like), while sex behavior in the form of concurrent (or simultaneous) partnerships was minimally assortative.

Younger MSM are embedded in nonsexual networks that may influence their risk/risk reduction behaviors. Influential confidants include kin, friends, boyfriends, girlfriends, teachers, counselors, and clergy; such people can promote or discourage an individual's risk/risk reduction behaviors and alter the intensity and impact of "social drivers" of the HIV/AIDS epidemic among young Black MSM. These network members/influences may also move between nonsexual and sexual network membership over time, further altering the social context within which sex and drug use behavior occur (Montgomery et al., 2002). The effects of such network dynamics on sex partner selection, sexual/drug related practices, and risk reduction behaviors are poorly understood. Moreover, given the high rates of poverty in several urban centers, macro-level structural problems (e.g., arrest for drug use, commercial sex work, theft, and gang activities and other petty crimes) are common (Voisin & Neilands, 2010). Disproportionate rates of incarceration and release of Black men and young Black MSM into these neighborhoods, from detention and prison where rates of HIV is high, contribute to the emergence of HIV epicenters (Mauer, 1999). Thus, structural barriers, sex partner characteristics (network phenomenon), and HIV care outcomes are associated with HIV infection and disparities among Black MSM. Elimination of disparities among Black MSM cannot be accomplished without addressing structural barriers or differences in HIV clinical care access and outcomes (Millett et al., 2012).

Aging

Shifting demographics in the HIV epidemic as infected populations live longer will likely affect secondary prevention efforts, as well as primary prevention of non-AIDS related comorbidities (Halkitis, 2010). Higher mortality is evident among HIV infected populations older than 50 years of age when compared to younger than 50 years of age, as it is in non-HIV infected populations. There are increased rates of non-AIDS defining illnesses including cardiovascular disease, liver disease, renal impairment, and malignancy among elderly HIV infected patients (Sackoff, Hanna, Pfeiffer, & Torian, 2006). Older patient responses to antiretroviral therapy, however, are comparable to younger individuals (Perez & Moore, 2003; Tumbarello et al., 2003; Wellons et al., 2002). The relative contribution of HIV medication toxicities and immune senescence to the natural aging process is unknown and an area of continued interest (Effros et al., 2008).

While there are important issues that older HIV infected MSM face compared to the general HIV infected population, the biology of aging is likely similar. For primary prevention, we recommend that providers of HIV infected MSM follow the evidence-based guidelines of the United States Preventive Services Task Force (see Moyer & on behalf of the United States Preventive Services Task Force, 2013). Specific MSM preventive care include assessments of sexual function and sexual health, screening of cancers such as anal cancer, lung, and colon cancer (given increased rates of smoking among MSM), liver cancer, eating disorders, and body image dissatisfaction (Applebaum, 2008). Stereotypes of older MSM being lonely or more isolated are generally not true; however, for those MSM who are HIV infected, they may have lived through partners or close friends dying from AIDS. Screening for anxiety and depression should be considered in multiple settings, i.e., medical doctors, social service settings, and senior centers. Additionally, special consideration of the multiple layers of stigma experienced by "quadruple minority" men (MSM, Black, HIV infected and over 50 years of age) (Haile, Padilla, & Parker, 2011) needs to be given during the development of any prevention intervention that includes older MSM.

Technology

Digital communication technologies (DCT) such as cell phones and the Internet are rapidly becoming ubiquitous even in technology-limited communities. In 2009, nearly 80% of US homes reported having at least one cell phone and 74% of Americans reported use of the Internet (Blumberg & Luke, 2010; Rainie, 2010). That such technologies have begun to replace traditional communication technologies is evident by the rapidly increasing number of homes with only a cell phone (no landline), which grew from 7.3% in 2005 (January to June) to 20.2% in 2008 (July to December) (Blumberg & Luke, 2010).

DCT presents both opportunities and challenges for HIV treatment, research in disease management, survey-based health data collection, and HIV prevention interventions. DCT can overcome barriers in traditional healthcare and research methodologies, including facilitator issues (i.e., discomfort with topics, incomplete implementation) and participation obstacles (i.e., transportation, insurance, physical limitations). In addition, HIV education interventions can be individually tailored, increasing relevance, and content can be quickly and easily updated (Ybarra & Bull, 2007). By using DCT to overcome these barriers, providers and researchers are able to reach a larger and more geographically dispersed audience. For example, personalized, interactive, daily SMS reminders for younger HIV infected MSM have been recently found to be feasible, acceptable, and can significantly improve self-reported antiretroviral adherence (Dowshen, Kuhns, Johnson, Holoyda, & Garofalo, 2012).

Spirituality

Spirituality has been associated with improved health among individuals living with a range of chronic illnesses, including HIV/AIDS (McClain, Rosenfeld, & Breitbart, 2003; Pardini, Plante, Sherman, & Stump, 2000; Woods, Antoni, Ironson, & Kling, 1999). Spiritual beliefs, practices, and communities are thought to improve an individual's ability to cope with adverse life events, such as managing a chronic illness like HIV/AIDS. Among HIV infected MSM, religious coping has been associated with reduced rates of depression and religious behaviors have been associated with higher T-cell and CD4 cell counts (Woods et al., 1999). In addition, connections to a faith community may increase access to social support, a formidable force in the health of HIV infected persons (D'Augelli, Pilkington, & Hershberger, 2002; Green, 1993; Pescosolido, Wright, Alegría, & Vera, 1998; Tobin, German, Spikes, Patterson, & Latkin, 2011). In one study, social support was the only psychosocial predictor of nonattendance in HIV care and was a greater predictor of retention when compared to factors such as physician consistency (Catz, McClure, Jones, & Brantley, 1999). Finally, although more research is needed, emerging evidence suggests that interventions that incorporate Eastern spiritual practices, such as meditation and mindfulness, may have potential health benefits for HIV infected individuals (Creswell, Myers, Cole, & Irwin, 2009; Gayner et al., 2011; Robinson, Mathews, & Witek-Janusek, 2003).

Taken together, the extant evidence suggests that spirituality in the lives of HIV positive gay men warrants additional attention. However, despite calls for greater attention to faith-based initiatives for MSM (Hill & McNeely, 2013; Malebranche, 2003), few interventions have utilized spirituality or faith-based communities as a context through which to limit onward transmission of HIV (Francis & Liverpool, 2009; Williams, Palar, & Derose, 2011). The lack of research in this domain may reflect concerns that religious institutions often serve as a source of stress, abuse, and stigmatization for MSM (Miller, 2007; Williams, Wyatt, Resell, Peterson, & Asuan-O'Brien, 2004;

Wilson, Wittlin, Muñoz-Laboy, & Parker, 2011). Despite this, many MSM living with HIV view spirituality as an important dimension in their lives, and a particularly strong value has been observed among Black MSM (Miller, 2007). Studies show that many Black MSM are involved in a faith-based community and value spirituality, even in the context of institutional endorsement of homophobia or difficulty integrating their religious identity with their sexual behavior or sexual identity (Foster, Arnold, Rebchook, & Kegeles, 2011; Miller, 2007; Seegers, 2007).

Black churches remain vital social and political institutions in Black/African American communities throughout the USA, and research with religious leaders has highlighted the need to build on the strengths of faith-based communities. Black church leaders have articulated a strong interest in implementing HIV services (Nunn et al., 2012; Smith, Simmons, & Mayer, 2005) but have limited capacity and financial resources to do so (Smith et al., 2005). Although the effects of integrating HIV services in faith-based communities on HIV prevention interventions is understudied, such approaches would likely be embraced among diverse groups of HIV infected gay men and could have additional benefits, such as increasing religious leaders' comfort with discussing issues of homosexuality (Pichon et al., 2012), reducing homophobia and HIV/AIDS-related stigma, and mobilizing faith-based communities in the fight against HIV/AIDS.

Emerging and Innovative Prevention Strategies

Network-Based

The centrality of a network approach to prevention among HIV infected MSM is becoming increasingly clear (Latkin et al., 2011; Schneider, McFadden, Laumann, et al., 2012; Schneider, Michaels, & Bouris, 2012; Schneider, Michaels, Gandham, et al., 2012; Schneider, Walsh, et al., 2012). Social network *oriented* interventions have been effective in preventing high-risk behavior that leads to HIV infection (Kelly, 2004; Latkin, Sherman, & Knowlton, 2003). Some have demonstrated that organic support networks are effective in preventing high risk sexual behavior in adolescents (Bouris, Guilamo-Ramos, Jaccard, et al., 2010; Guilamo-Ramos et al., 2009; Guilamo-Ramos et al., 2011), and are likely to be effective in HIV prevention targeting younger Black MSM, for example (Bouris, Guilamo-Ramos, Pickard, et al. 2010; Garofalo, Mustanski, & Donenberg, 2008b; Schneider et al., 2011). However, these innovative interventions have yet to be tested *after* a new HIV diagnosis has been made—an effort that could strengthen components within the HIV treatment cascade such as retention in care. Moreover, utilization of rigorous social and sexual network assessments that map directly onto interventions—a *social network intervention*—has promise for eliminating new cases of HIV transmission.

Project Engage is just one example of emerging efforts to utilize endogenous social networks to improve outcomes along the HIV treatment spectrum. Project

Engage is an ongoing NIMH-funded randomized controlled trial examining the effect of a key social network member intervention on the antiretroviral adherence and retention in care of an HIV infected MSM. This approach is a personalized network intervention that aims to activate a network member to motivate an index client. The approach has its roots in similar efforts to recruit social network members to have an impact on identified high-risk men in India (Bouris et al., 2013; Schneider, McFadden , Laumann, et al., 2012; Schneider, Michaels, Gandham, et al., 2012; Schneider, Walsh, et al., 2012).

A recent National Institutes of Drug Abuse Avant-Garde award to Samuel Friedman in 2012 funded an innovative approach to preventing HIV transmission by the recently infected. One of the three intervention populations is HIV infected MSM in South Chicago. Intervention approaches against HIV transmission during the recent infection period will use a combination of sexual- and social-network-based contact tracing methods; community alerts in the networks and venues of recent infectees; and the logic of going "up" and "down" infection chains. Newly infected "seeds," defined as younger Black MSM who have recently been infected will initially be identified through repeated HIV testing using techniques to identify recently and acutely infected study participants. Following this, the intervention will target members of seeds' networks and people who attend their venues. These individuals will also be tested for acute and recent infection, and be alerted to the probability that their networks contain highly-infectious members so they should reduce their risk and transmission behaviors for the next several months to minimize their chances of getting infected. This may also reduce transmission by untested people with recent infection (Nikolopoulos et al., 2016).

Family-Based Interventions

There has been a critical void in family-based interventions for HIV infected MSM in the USA. To date, most research with MSM has focused on negative family dynamics, such as rejection (Bouris, Guilamo-Ramos, Pickard, et al. 2010; Garofalo, Mustanski, & Donenberg, 2008a; Garofalo et al., 2008b; Ryan, Huebner, Diaz, & Sanchez, 2009), resulting in research and practice paradigms that have overlooked the potentially protective role of families. Although many MSM experience rejection from their family of origin, studies suggest that MSM are coming out to their families at younger ages and report high levels of family acceptance and/or tolerance (Garofalo et al., 2008a, 2008b). However, family rejection remains a concern and research has examined support from members outside of one's family of origin, i.e., family of choice (Cohen & Wills, 1985; Collins & Laursen, 2004; Hays, Chauncey, & Tobey, 1990). More recent studies have documented the evolution and importance of non-kin family structures in the Ball community, where MSM come together in Houses led by "mothers" and "fathers" who serve a parent-like role and provide social support, guidance, and material aid to MSM (Arnold & Bailey, 2009; Bailey, 2011; Bailey, 2013).

A central question in all family-based research is how to define a family? Research with MSM has tended to define family in two primary ways: (1) "family of origin" which refers to parents, siblings, and other members related by blood or marriage or (2) "family of choice" which refers to individuals not related by blood but who serve a family-like role via the provision of closeness, support, and mutual aid. Although it has been suggested that families of choice are more important for MSM than are families of origin (Diamond & Butterworth, 2008), we believe a more nuanced approach is necessary. In our research with HIV infected MSM, we define family as a *"network of mutual commitment,"* using the definition first offered by the NIMH in 1990 and utilized by the NIMH Consortium on Families and HIV/AIDS since 1997 (Anhalt & Morris, 1998; Pequegnat, 2012; Pequegnat & Bray, 1997). A focus on mutual commitment moves beyond the dichotomy of family of origin versus family of choice by allowing MSM to define what family means to them and thus captures a greater diversity of family networks available to MSM.

As scholars call for greater attention to the role of families in HIV research with MSM (Mustanski, Hunter, Pequegnat, & Bell, 2011), a growing body of research is finding that closeness to family is negatively associated with HIV-risk (Bouris, Guilamo-Ramos, Jaccard, et al., 2010; Bouris, Guilamo-Ramos, Pickard, et al. 2010; Garofalo et al., 2008a). In our work with HIV negative and positive Black MSM, we found that having a greater proportion of family members in one's close personal network (i.e., having 2 or more *family of origin* members in the close network) was negatively associated with sex-drug use and group sex, positively associated with having a regular primary care physician, and positively associated with discouraging group sex and sex-drug use among one's MSM friend network (Schneider, Michaels, et al., 2012). Further, increased male but not female family network proportion was associated with less HIV-risk and greater discouragement of HIV-risk among MSM friends. The role of male family members differs from research with heterosexual youth, where mothers have been viewed as the primary agents of change (Pequegnat, Bell, Dancy, & DiIorio, 2012); it also highlights the need to better understand the types of family supports available to HIV positive MSM and how family-based interventions could best prevent onward transmission of HIV.

The lack of family-based interventions for HIV infected MSM represents a critical gap in existing prevention services and programs (Bouris, Guilamo-Ramos, Jaccard, et al., 2010; Bouris, Guilamo-Ramos, Pickard, et al. 2010; Garofalo et al., 2008a). Future research and interventions with families could pursue several approaches. First, there is a clear opportunity to build on supportive family relationships, be they family of origin or choice, in the delivery of services to HIV infected gay men. Although additional research is needed to develop such interventions, these prevention strategies would be an innovative addition to the existing prevention with positives landscape. Second, there are opportunities to work with MSM and their families who are struggling; such interventions could help MSM to disclose their sexual orientation and/or their HIV status to their families, offer services to families who struggle with learning about their love one's sexual orientation and/or HIV status, and, when appropriate, help to repair strained family relationships. Although untested, such approaches warrant future consideration. The families of HIV infected MSM represent *organic social systems* for which we have remarkably little understanding given the past 30 years of HIV treatment and prevention research. This research becomes especially important given the rapid changes in acceptance of homosexuality and same-sex marriage in the US population (Keleher & Smith, 2012).

Disclosure Interventions

Knowledge and disclosure of HIV status is critical to the prevention of onward transmission. A number of studies have found that sexual risk behaviors tend to decline when individuals know their HIV status (CDC, 2006; MacKellar et al., 2005). In addition, serosorting (i.e., selecting sexual partners with the same HIV status) and seropositioning (i.e., selecting sexual positions that minimize the likelihood of transmission between serodiscordant partners), both require that MSM know their HIV status and disclose it to their sexual partners (Butler & Smith, 2007; Parsons et al., 2005; Steward et al., 2009; Wilson et al., 2010). In the absence of such disclosure, serosorting and seropositioning have been associated with increased HIV transmission (Butler & Smith, 2007; Eaton et al., 2007; Golden, Stekler, Hughes, & Wood, 2008). In addition, disclosure may lead to increased social support, which has been positively correlated with retention and adherence to ARVs (Wohl et al., 2010). At the same time, disclosure could have deleterious effects if the environment where disclosure occurs is dominated by stigma or is otherwise hostile. HIV/AIDS remains a highly stigmatized illness and disclosure of HIV status has been identified as one of the greatest challenges experienced by HIV positive MSM (Kalichman, DiMarco, Austin, Luke, & DiFonzo, 2003).

Despite the important role of disclosure in reducing the risk on onward transmission, relatively few disclosure interventions have been developed for HIV infected MSM. Novel approaches that warrant additional consideration include the use of technology to support disclosure and interventions to foster disclosure to casual sexual partners. Although few disclosure interventions have been delivered via DCT, there is some evidence to suggest that such approaches are feasible and efficacious. Chiasson and colleagues implemented a brief video-based intervention delivered online. Men were recruited via banner ads posted on the largest subscription-based sexual meeting websites for gay men (Chiasson, Shaw, Humberstone, Hirshfield, & Hartel, 2009). The ad asked "Is HIV Still a Big Deal?" and was followed by large "No" and "Yes" buttons. Clicking a button led MSM to a website, http://www.hivbigdeal.org, where they completed study forms and watched "The Morning After," a 9-min video designed to foster critical thinking about disclosure and other health factors (Chiasson et al., 2009). Large numbers of MSM were reached through this approach: 522 MSM viewed the video and completed the 3 month follow-up. Furthermore, significant increases in disclosure of HIV status and significant decreases in both unprotected anal intercourse and reports of casual sexual partners were observed (Chiasson et al., 2009). Although not an RCT, the intervention is a novel way to reach large numbers of MSM who might not otherwise be reached through individual or group-based interventions. At the same time, Black and other MSM of color were underrepresented in the sample, suggesting that additional work is needed to reach these men online. Future approaches could consider more tailored approaches, implementing risk assessments online, and directing MSM to videos that have been specifically tailored to meet the disclosure needs of diverse MSM.

In another pilot study, Serovich and colleagues evaluated the efficacy of a brief intervention designed to support disclosure to casual sex partners (Serovich, Reed, Grafsky, & Andrist, 2009). The intervention was delivered across four sessions with content on (1) goal setting and disclosure triggers and strategies, (2) the pros and cons of disclosure and exercises to help MSM maximize disclosure benefits and minimize disclosure costs, (3) behavioral skills rehearsal and the evaluation of disclosure strategies and ways to handle reactions to disclosure, and (4) additional behavioral skills rehearsal (i.e., reinforcement and practice from session three) (Serovich et al., 2009). A total of 77 HIV infected MSM were randomly assigned to one of three study conditions: a waitlist control group, a facilitator only group where all activities were completed face-to-face with a trained facilitator, or a facilitator + computer group where baseline assessment and paper-and-pencil exercises were completed electronically and all other activities with a facilitator. Results indicated that both disclosure and sexual risk behavior outcomes tended to be significantly better in the facilitator only group relative to both the waitlist and facilitator + computer groups at the 3-month follow-up (Serovich et al., 2009). In addition, there were notable reductions in sexual risk behavior among MSM with multiple sexual partners, suggesting that the intervention was especially effective for higher risk MSM (Serovich et al., 2009). Although promising, additional research is needed, especially to reach MSM of color, who were underrepresented in the sample.

Community Mobilization

Community mobilization has played a critical role in the fight against HIV/AIDS since the earliest days of the epidemic (Campbell & Cornish, 2010). Domestically and globally, community mobilization efforts such as ACT-UP, Gay Men's Health Crisis (GMHC), Gay Men of African Descent (GMAD), NAESM Inc., and the Treatment Action Campaign have resulted in dramatic positive impacts on the health of HIV infected persons (Landers, Pickett, Rennie, & Wakefield, 2011; Trapence et al., 2012). The Chicago Black Gay Men's Caucus aims to mobilize Black gay men, including those HIV infected to better their well-being. The Lifestyles Guide and the HIS intervention (Health Is Sexy) are two examples of this local approach ("Chicago Black Gay Men's Caucus. http://chiblackgaycaucus.org/ (Last accessed April 18, 2013),"). In other HIV positive gay populations such as in San Francisco, mobilization of has been credited as a major force in controlling the epidemic (Katz, 1997). One of the largest community mobilization interventions currently underway is "Connect To Protect (C2P)," a community mobilization and structural intervention designed to reduce the incidence and prevalence of HIV among urban youth that is being conducted via the Adolescent Trials Network (ATN) (Ziff et al., 2006). Although a full discussion of *C2P* is outside the scope of this chapter, we briefly review the purpose below. For more information, see http://www.connect2protect.org/.

The purpose of *C2P* is to mobilize urban communities to examine the root causes of HIV and to develop and implement structural changes that will prevent HIV among youth aged 12–24 (Ziff et al., 2006). *C2P* began in 2002 and is being implemented in 15 urban areas in the USA and Puerto Rico (Harper et al., 2012). At each site, ATN researchers partner with a diverse group of community organizations to form a coalition and to develop a local strategic plan to reduce HIV risk among youth. Each site then implements structural interventions designed to change practices, environments, programs, laws, and policies at the community, city, and state levels (Ziff et al., 2006). A number of recent publications have highlighted the power and challenges of this approach to address HIV/AIDS among YMSM of color (Robles-Schrader et al., 2012) and in the House Ball community (Castillo et al., 2012). Evaluation of *C2P* on individual HIV risk behaviors and on epidemiological surveillance indicators (i.e., the incidence of HIV and other STIs) is currently underway, with data collection to be completed by 2016.

Biomedical

Two existing biomedical interventions are being tested specifically in MSM: circumcision and microbicides. Circumcision and vaginal microbicides have been found to be efficacious in preventing HIV acquisition among heterosexual populations for men and women respectively; however, the utility of such modalities in MSM is not yet understood. Circumcision is being studied as an HIV prevention intervention among insertive MSM in China (Wiysonge et al., 2011), however, such an intervention targeting only insertive MSM may be stigmatizing, especially in societies where marriage to women is common among MSM (Schneider, McFadden, Laumann, et al. 2012; Schneider, Michaels, Gandham, et al. 2012; Schneider, Walsh, et al. 2012). Circumcision at birth for all men may be an alternative (Task Force on Circumcision, 2012). Moreover, as in heterosexual populations, it is unclear whether the receptive male partner will receive any benefit. Importantly for HIV infected MSM, the utility of circumcision is even less clear. Will benefits in reducing acquisition of other STIs, such as Human Papilloma Virus, occur as in heterosexual populations, and if so, will such a benefit be worth undergoing a minor surgical procedure?

Rectal microbicides, products usually in gel form that are applied intra-rectally, are currently being studied as an HIV prevention intervention for HIV uninfected men and women. A full review is beyond the scope of this chapter; however, a comprehensive resource for scientists and community members is IRMA (international rectal microbicide advocates; http://www.rectalmicrobicides.org/). The use of rectal microbicides, especially in HIV positive MSM, is not clear. It is possible that use of such products by the receptive partner may prevent transmission to insertive MSM, but this has not been studied even in the case of vaginal microbicides. Moreover, current formulations of antiretroviral-based rectal microbicides are unlikely to have an effect on other sexually transmitted disease acquisition among HIV positive MSM. In fact, some have suggested that use of some lubricant products may increase vulnerability to STIs (Gorbach et al., 2012). The majority of Phase II rectal microbicide research has been conducted in Pittsburgh, San Francisco, and Boston, and careful attention must be made towards including MSM of color in such research. This is especially important given that MSM of color will likely be a target of this biomedical intervention and potentially have much to benefit; but MSM of color have largely not been included as study participants in the development of this potentially important prevention intervention (*Lunchtime HIV prevention research session*, 2012).

Primary biomedical prevention recommendations for HIV positive men are similar to the general population. For example, HIV positive MSM with compromised immune systems are susceptible to opportunistic infections and should follow Department of Health and Human Services recommendations for prevention and treatment of these infections (Kaplan et al., 2009). As discussed previously, aging HIV positive MSM should be screened for comorbidities according to the U.S. Preventive Services Task Force. Additional attention to lipid profiles as well as kidney function should be considered for HIV positive MSM on ARVs, and in particular those men taking protease inhibitors and/or Tenofovir. Other behaviors and conditions that are more common among MSM should be screened for and treated (i.e., tobacco use, depression). While there are many interventions for such conditions, research suggests that targeting subpopulations is more likely to be effective (Hemmige et al., 2012). Project Exhale, for example, is an evaluation of a tailored smoking cessation program for HIV positive Black MSM which produced follow-up quit rates ranging from 6 to 24%, with treatment completers having better outcomes (Matthews, Kuhns, Conrad, & Vargas, 2011). This first of its kind intervention for HIV positive African American MSM was feasible, acceptable, and showed benefit for reducing smoking behaviors and depression scores. This targeted intervention as well as other promising interventions for the general population will become increasingly important with the concomitant aging among HIV positive MSM, as well as societal forces in the USA that are moving towards greater acceptance and assimilation of MSM.

References

Adimora, A. A., & Auerbach, J. D. (2010). Structural interventions for HIV prevention in the United States. *Journal of Acquired Immune Deficiency Syndromes, 55*, S132–S135.

Aidala, A., Cross, J. E., Stall, R., Harre, D., & Sumartojo, E. (2005). Housing status and HIV risk behaviors: Implications for prevention and policy. *AIDS and Behavior, 9*(3), 251–265. doi:10.1007/s10461-005-9000-7

Anhalt, K., & Morris, T. L. (1998). Developmental and adjustment issues of gay, lesbian, and bisexual adolescents: A review of the empirical literature. *Clinical Child and Family Psychology Review, 1*, 215.

Applebaum, J. S. (2008). Late adulthood and aging: Clinical approaches. In H. J. Makadon, K. H. Mayer, J. Potter, & H. Goldhammer (Eds.), *Fenway guide to lesbian, gay, bisexual and transgender health*. Philadelphia: American College of Physicians.

Arnold, E. A., & Bailey, M. M. (2009). Constructing home and family: How the ballroom community supports African American GLBTQ youth in the face of HIV/AIDS. *Journal of Gay & Lesbian Social Services, 21*, 171–188.

Auerbach, D. M., Darrow, W. W., Jaffe, H. W., & Curran, J. W. (1984). Cluster of cases of the acquired immune deficiency syndrome. Patients linked by sexual contact. *The American Journal of Medicine, 76*(3), 487–492.

Ayala, G., Bingham, T., Kim, J., Wheeler, D. P., & Millett, G. A. (2012). Modeling the impact of social discrimination and financial hardship on the sexual risk of HIV among Latino and Black men who have sex with men. *American Journal of Public Health, S2*, S242–S249.

Bailey, M. M. (2011). Gender/Racial realness: Theorizing the gender system in ballroom culture. *Feminist Studies, 37*, 365–384.

Bailey, M. M. (2013). *Butch queens up in pumps: Gender, performance, and ballroom culture in Detroit*. Ann Arbor: University of Michigan Press.

Baunach, D. M. (2011). Decomposing trends in attitudes toward gay marriage, 1988–2006*. *Social Science Quarterly, 92*(2), 346–363. doi:10.1111/j.1540-6237.2011.00772.x

Becker, A. B. (2012). What's marriage (and family) got to do with it? Support for same-sex marriage, legal unions, and gay and lesbian couples raising children. *Social Science Quarterly, 93*(4), 1007–1029. doi:10.1111/j.1540-6237.2012.00844.x

Belzer, M. E., Fuchs, D. N., Luftman, G. S., & Tucker, D. J. (1999). Antiretroviral adherence issues among HIV-positive adolescents and young adults. *The Journal of Adolescent Health, 25*(5), 316–319.

Blumberg, S., & Luke, J. (2010). *Wireless substitution: Early release of estimates from the National Health Interview Survey, July–December 2009*. Retrieved from http://www.cdc.gov/nchs/data/nhis/earlyrelease/wireless201005.pdf.

Bouris, A., Guilamo-Ramos, V., Jaccard, J., McCoy, W., Aranda, D., Pickard, A., & Boyer, C. B. (2010). The feasibility of a clinic-based parent intervention to prevent HIV, sexually transmitted infections, and unintended pregnancies among Latino and African American adolescents. *AIDS Patient Care and STDs, 24*(6), 381–387. doi:10.1089/apc.2009.0308

Bouris, A., Guilamo-Ramos, V., Pickard, A., Shiu, C., Loosier, P., Dittus, P., … Michael Waldmiller, J. (2010). A systematic review of parental influences on the health and well-being of lesbian, gay, and bisexual youth: Time for a new public health research and practice agenda. *The Journal of Primary Prevention, 31*(5–6), 273–309. doi:10.1007/s10935-010-0229-1

Bouris, A., Voisin, D., Pilloton, M., Flatt, N., Eavou, R., Hampton, K., … Schneider, J. A. (2013). Project nGage: Network supported HIV care engagement for younger Black men who have sex with men and transgender persons. *Journal of AIDS & Clinical Research, 4*. doi:10.4172/2155-6113.1000236

Brooks, V. R. (1981). *Minority stress and lesbian women*. Lexington, MA: D.C. Health.

Brown, L. B., Miller, W. C., Kamanga, G., Nyirenda, N., Mmodzi, P., Pettifor, A., … Hoffman, I. F. (2011). HIV partner notification is effective and feasible in Sub-Saharan Africa: Opportunities for HIV treatment and prevention. *Journal of Acquired Immune Deficiency Syndromes, 56*(5), 437–442. doi:10.1097/Qai.0b013e318202bf7d

Buffie, W. C. (2011). Public health implications of same-sex marriage. *Journal Information, 101*(6), 986–990.

Butler, D. M., & Smith, D. M. (2007). Serosorting can potentially increase HIV transmissions. *AIDS, 21*(9), 1218–1220. doi:10.1097/QAD.0b013e32814db7bf

Campbell, C., & Cornish, F. (2010). Towards a "fourth generation" of approaches to HIV/AIDS management: Creating contexts for effective community mobilisation. *AIDS Care, 22*(S2), 1569–1579.

Castillo, M., Palmer, B. J., Rudy, B. J., Fernandez, M. I., & Adolescent Medicine Trials Network for HIV/AIDS Interventions. (2012). Creating partnerships for HIV prevention among YMSM: The connect to protect project and house and ball community in Philadelphia. *Journal of Prevention & Intervention in the Community*, *40*(2), 165–175.

Catz, S. L., McClure, J. B., Jones, G. N., & Brantley, P. J. (1999). Predictors of outpatient medical appointment attendance among persons with HIV. *AIDS Care*, *11*(3), 361–373. doi:10.1080/09540129947983

CDC. 2006. *Revised recommendations for HIV testing of adults, adolescents, and pregnant women in health-care settings*. *55*(RR14), 1–17.

CDPH. (2008). *HIV prevalence and unrecognized infection among men who have sex with men— Chicago*. Chicago: Chicago Department of Public Health.

Centers for Disease Control and Prevention. (2008). Recommendations for partner services programs for HIV infection, syphilis, gonorrhea, and chlamydial infection. MMWR Recommendations and Reports, 57(RR-9), 1–83; quiz CE81–84.

Centers for Disease Control and Prevention. (2012). Estimated HIV incidence among adults and adolescents in the United States, 2007–2010. *HIV Surveillance Supplemental Report, 17*(No. 4), 1–26. Retrieved January 4, 2015.

Charania, M. R., Crepaz, N., Guenther-Gray, C., Henny, K., Liau, A., Willis, L. A., & Lyles, C. M. (2011). Efficacy of structural-level condom distribution interventions: A meta-analysis of US and international studies, 1998–2007. *AIDS and Behavior*, *15*(7), 1283–1297. doi:10.1007/s10461-010-9812-y

Chiasson, M. A., Shaw, F. S., Humberstone, M., Hirshfield, S., & Hartel, D. (2009). Increased HIV disclosure three months after an online video intervention for men who have sex with men (MSM). *AIDS Care, 21*(9), 1081–1089. doi:10.1080/09540120902730013

Chicago Black Gay Men's Caucus. (n.d.). Retrieved from http://chiblackgaycaucus.org/.

Chicago Center for HIV Elimination. (n.d.). Retrieved from http://hivelimination.uchicago.edu/.

Choi, K. H., Paul, J., Ayala, G., Boylan, R., & Gregorich, S. E. (2013). Experiences of discrimination and their impact on the mental health among African American, Asian and Pacific Islander, and Latino men who have sex with men. *American Journal of Public Health, 103*(5), 868–874.

Christopoulos, K. A., Das, M., & Colfax, G. N. (2011). Linkage and retention in HIV care among men who have sex with men in the United States. *Clinical Infectious Diseases, 52*(suppl 2), S214–S222. doi:10.1093/cid/ciq045

Cohen, M.S., Chen, Y.Q., McCauley, M., Gamble, T., Hosseinipour, M.C., Kumarasamy, N., … HPTN 052 Study Team. (2011). Prevention of HIV-1 infection with early antiretroviral therapy. *The New England Journal of Medicine, 365*(6), 493–505. doi:10.1056/NEJMoa1105243.

Cohen, R.A., & Martinez, M.E. (2012). *Health insurance coverage: Early release of estimates from the National Health Interview Survey, 2011* (Vol. June 2012). National Center for Health Statistics.

Cohen, S., & Wills, T. A. (1985). Stress, social support, and the buffering hypothesis. *Psychological Bulletin, 98*, 310.

Collins, W. A., & Laursen, B. (2004). Changing relationships, changing youth: Interpersonal contexts of adolescent development. *Journal of Early Adolescence, 24*, 55.

Creswell, J. D., Myers, H. F., Cole, S. W., & Irwin, M. R. (2009). Mindfulness meditation training effects on CD4+ T lymphocytes in HIV-1 infected adults: A small randomized controlled trial. *Brain, Behavior, and Immunity, 23*(2), 184–188.

D'Augelli, A. R., Pilkington, N. W., & Hershberger, S. L. (2002). Incidence and mental health impact of sexual orientation victimization of lesbian, gay, and bisexual youths in high school. *School Psychology Quarterly, 17*, 148.

Diamond, L. M., & Butterworth, M. (2008). The close relationships of sexual minorities: Partners, friends, and family. In J. M. C. Smith & T. G. Reio (Eds.), *Handbook of research on adult development and learning* (pp. 348–375). Mahwah, NJ: Lawrence Erlbaum.

Doherty, I. A., Schoenbach, V. J., & Adimora, A. A. (2009). Sexual mixing patterns and hetero-sexual hiv transmission among African Americans in the Southeastern United States. *Journal of Acquired Immune Deficiency Syndromes, 52*(1), 114–120.

Dowshen, N., Kuhns, L. M., Johnson, A., Holoyda, B. J., & Garofalo, R. (2012). Improving adherence to antiretroviral therapy for youth living with HIV/AIDS: A pilot study using personalized, interactive, daily text message reminders. *Journal of Medical Internet Research, 14*(2), e51. doi:10.2196/jmir.2015

Eaton, L. A., Kalichman, S. C., Cain, D. N., Cherry, C., Stearns, H. L., Amaral, C. M., … Pope, H. L. (2007). Serosorting sexual partners and risk for HIV among men who have sex with men. *American Journal of Preventive Medicine, 33*(6), 479–485.

Effros, R.B., Fletcher, C.V., Gebo, K., Halter, J.B., Hazzard, W.R., Horne, F.M., … High, K. P. (2008). Aging and infectious diseases: Workshop on HIV infection and aging: What is known and future research directions. *Clinical Infectious Diseases, 47*(4), 542–553.

Foster, M. L., Arnold, E., Rebchook, G., & Kegeles, S. M. (2011). 'It's my inner strength': Spirituality, religion and HIV in the lives of young African American men who have sex with men. *Culture, Health & Sexuality, 13*(9), 1103–1117.

Francis, S. A., & Liverpool, J. (2009). A review of faith-based HIV prevention programs. *Journal of Religion and Health, 48*(1), 6–15.

Francis, A. M., & Mialon, H. M. (2010). Tolerance and HIV. *Journal of Health Economics, 29*(2), 250–267.

Gardner, E. M., McLees, M. P., Steiner, J. F., Del Rio, C., & Burman, W. J. (2011). The spectrum of engagement in HIV care and its relevance to test-and-treat strategies for prevention of HIV infection. *Clinical Infectious Diseases, 52*(6), 793–800. doi:10.1093/cid/ciq243

Garofalo, R., Mustanski, B., & Donenberg, G. (2008a). Parents know and parents matter; is it time to develop family-based Hiv prevention programs for young men who have sex with men? *The Journal of Adolescent Health, 43*(2), 201–204.

Garofalo, R., Mustanski, B., & Donenberg, G. (2008b). HIV prevention with young men who have sex with men: Parents know and parents matter; is it time to develop family-based programs for this vulnerable population? *The Journal of Adolescent Health, 43*(2), 201.

Gayner, B., Esplen, M. J., DeRoche, P., Wong, J., Bishop, S., Kavanagh, L., & Butler, K. (2011). A randomized controlled trial of mindfulness-based stress reduction to manage affective symptoms and improve quality of life in gay men living with HIV. *Journal of Behavioral Medicine, 35*(3), 272–285.

Gebo, K. A., Fleishman, J. A., Conviser, R., Reilly, E. D., Korthuis, P. T., Moore, R. D., … Mathews, W. C. (2005). Racial and gender disparities in receipt of highly active antiretroviral therapy persist in a multistate sample of HIV patients in 2001. *Journal of Acquired Immune Deficiency Syndromes, 38*(1), 96–103.

Giordano, T. P., Gifford, A. L., White, A. C., Jr., Suarez-Almazor, M. E., Rabeneck, L., Hartman, C., … Morgan, R. O. (2007). Retention in care: A challenge to survival with HIV infection. *Clinical Infectious Diseases, 44*(11), 1493–1499.

Golden, M. R., Stekler, J., Hughes, J. P., & Wood, R. W. (2008). HIV serosorting in men who have sex with men: Is it safe? *Journal of Acquired Immune Deficiency Syndromes, 49*(2), 212–218. doi:10.1097/QAI.0b013e31818455e8

Gorbach, P.M., Weiss, R.E., Fuchs, E., Jeffries, R.A., Hezerah, M., Brown, S., … Cranston, R.D. (2012). The slippery slope: Lubricant use and rectal sexually transmitted infections: A newly identified risk. *Sexually Transmitted Diseases, 39*(1), 59–64.

Green, G. (1993). Social support and HIV. *AIDS Care, 5*(1), 87–104.

Guilamo-Ramos, V., Bouris, A., Jaccard, J., Gonzalez, B., McCoy, W., & Aranda, D. (2011). A parent-based intervention to reduce sexual risk behavior in early adolescence: Building alliances between physicians, social workers, and parents. *The Journal of Adolescent Health, 48*(2), 159–163.

Guilamo-Ramos, V., Bouris, A., Jaccard, J., Lesesne, C. A., Gonzalez, B., & Kalogerogiannis, K. (2009). Family mediators of acculturation and adolescent sexual behavior among Latino youth. *The Journal of Primary Prevention, 30*(3–4), 395–419.

Haile, R., Padilla, M. B., & Parker, E. A. (2011). 'Stuck in the quagmire of an HIV ghetto': The meaning of stigma in the lives of older black gay and bisexual men living with HIV in New York City. *Culture, Health & Sexuality, 13*(4), 429–442.

Halkitis, P. N. (2010). Reframing HIV prevention for gay men in the United States. *American Psychologist, 65*, 752–763.

Halkitis, P. N. (2012). Obama, marriage equality, and the health of gay men. *American Journal of Public Health, 102*(9), 1628–1629.

Harper, G., Fernandez, I., Bruce, D., Hosek, S. G., & Jacobs, R. (2011). The role of multiple identities in adherence to medical appointments among gay/bisexual male adolescents living with HIV. *AIDS and Behavior, 17*(1), 213–223. doi:10.1007/s10461-011-0071-3

Harper, G. W., Willard, N., Ellen, J. M., & Adolescent Medicine Trials Network for HIV/AIDS Interventions. (2012). Connect to protect®: Utilizing community mobilization and structural change to prevent HIV infection among youth. *Journal of Prevention & Intervention in the Community, 40*(2), 81–86.

Harris, S. K., Samples, C. L., Keenan, P. M., Fox, D. J., Melchiono, M. W., & Woods, E. R. (2003). Outreach, mental health, and case management services: Can they help to retain HIV-positive and at-risk youth and young adults in care? *Maternal and Child Health Journal, 7*(4), 205–218.

Hatzenbuehler, M. L., McLaughlin, K. A., Keyes, K. M., & Hasin, D. S. (2010). The impact of institutional discrimination on psychiatric disorders in lesbian, gay, and bisexual populations: A prospective study. *American Journal of Public Health, 100*(3), 452.

Hatzenbuehler, M. L., Nolen-Hoeksema, S., & Erickson, S. J. (2008). Minority stress predictors of HIV risk behavior, substance use, and depressive symptoms: Results from a prospective study of bereaved gay men. *Health Psychology, 27*(4), 455–462.

Hays, R. B., Chauncey, S., & Tobey, L. A. (1990). The social support networks of gay men with AIDS. *Journal of Community Psychology, 18*(4), 374–385.

Hemmige, V., McFadden, R., Cook, S., Tang, H., & Schneider, J. A. (2012). HIV prevention interventions to reduce racial disparities in the United States: A systematic review. *Journal of General Internal Medicine, 27*(8), 1047–1067.

Herrick, A. L., Lim, S. H., Wei, C., Smith, H., Guadamuz, T., Friedman, M. S., & Stall, R. (2011). Resilience as an untapped resource in behavioral intervention design for gay men. *AIDS and Behavior, 15*, 25–29.

Hill, W., & McNeely, C. (2013). HIV/AIDS disparity between African-American and Caucasian men who have sex with men: Intervention strategies for the Black church. *Journal of Religion and Health, 52*, 475–487.

Institute of Medicine. (2011). *The health of lesbian, gay, bisexual, and transgender people: Building a foundation for better understanding*. Washington, DC: National Academies Press.

Jones, K. T., Gray, P., Whiteside, Y. O., Wang, T., Bost, D., Dunbar, E., … Johnson, W. D. (2008). Evaluation of an HIV prevention intervention adapted for Black men who have sex with men. *American Journal of Public Health, 98*(6), 1043–1050.

Kalichman, S. C., DiMarco, M., Austin, J., Luke, W., & DiFonzo, K. (2003). Stress, social support, and HIV-status disclosure to family and friends among HIV-positive men and women. *Journal of Behavioral Medicine, 26*(4), 315–332.

Kaplan, J.E., Benson, C., Holmes, K.H., Brooks, J.T., Pau, A., Masur, H., … HIV Medicine Association of the Infectious Diseases Society of America. (2009). Guidelines for prevention and treatment of opportunistic infections in HIV-infected adults and adolescents: Recommendations from CDC, the National Institutes of Health, and the HIV Medicine Association of the Infectious Diseases Society of America. MMWR Recommendations and Reports, 58(RR-4), 1–207; quiz CE201–204.

Katz, M. H. (1997). AIDS epidemic in San Francisco among men who report sex with men: Successes and challenges of HIV prevention. *Journal of Acquired Immune Deficiency Syndromes, 14*, S38.

Kegeles, S. M., Hays, R. B., & Coates, T. J. (1996). The Mpowerment Project: A community-level HIV prevention intervention for young gay men. *American Journal of Public Health, 86*(8), 1129–1136.

Keleher, A., & Smith, E. R. A. N. (2012). Growing support for gay and lesbian equality since 1990. *Journal of Homosexuality, 59*(9), 1307–1326.

Kelly, J. A. (2004). Popular opinion leaders and HIV prevention peer education: Resolving discrepant findings, and implications for the development of effective community programmes. *AIDS Care, 16*(2), 139–150.

Kelly, J. A., Lawrence, J. S. S., Diaz, Y. E., Stevenson, L. Y., Hauth, A. C., Brasfield, T. L., ... Andrew, M. E. (1991). Hiv risk behavior reduction following intervention with key opinion leaders of population—An experimental-analysis. *American Journal of Public Health, 81*(2), 168–171.

Kelly, J. A., Murphy, D. A., Bahr, G. R., Kalichman, S. C., Morgan, M. G., Stevenson, L. Y., ... Bernstein, B. M. (1993). Outcome of cognitive-behavioral and support group brief therapies for depressed, HIV-infected persons. *The American Journal of Psychiatry, 150*(11), 1679–1686.

Klausner, J. D., Pollack, L. M., Wong, W., & Katz, M. H. (2006). Same-sex domestic partnerships and lower-risk behaviors for STDs, including HIV infection. *Journal of Homosexuality, 51*(4), 137–144.

Kurtz, S. P., Buttram, M. E., Surratt, H. L., & Stall, R. D. (2012). Resilience, syndemic factors, and serosorting behaviors among HIV-positive and HIV-negative substance-using MSM. *AIDS Education and Prevention, 24*(3), 193–205.

Landers, S., Pickett, J., Rennie, L., & Wakefield, S. (2011). Community perspectives on developing a sexual health agenda for gay and bisexual men. *AIDS and Behavior, 15,* 101–106.

Latkin, C. A., Sherman, S., & Knowlton, A. (2003). HIV prevention among drug users: Outcome of a network-oriented peer outreach intervention. *Health Psychology, 22*(4), 332–339.

Latkin, C., Yang, C., Tobin, K., Penniman, T., Patterson, J., & Spikes, P. (2011). Differences in the social networks of African American men who have sex with men only and those who have sex with men and women. *American Journal of Public Health, 101*(10), e18–e23. doi:10.2105/AJPH.2011.300281

Laumann, E. O., Ellingson, S., Mahay, J., Paik, A., & Youm, Y. (2004). *The sexual organization of the city.* Chicago: University of Chicago.

Laumann, E. O., & Youm, Y. (1999). Racial/ethnic group differences in the prevalence of sexually transmitted diseases in the United States: A network explanation. *Sexually Transmitted Diseases, 26*(5), 250–261.

Lunchtime HIV prevention research session. (2012). Paper presented at the 2012 National African American MSM Leadership Conference on HIV/AIDS and other Health Disparities, Atlanta.

Macdonell, K. E., Naar-King, S., Murphy, D. A., Parsons, J. T., & Harper, G. W. (2010). Predictors of medication adherence in high risk youth of color living with HIV. *Journal of Pediatric Psychology, 35*(6), 593–601.

MacKellar, D.A., Valleroy, L.A., Secura, G.M., Behel, S., Bingham, T., Celentano, D. D., ... Young Men's Survey Study Group. (2005). Unrecognized HIV infection, risk behaviors, and perceptions of risk among young men who have sex with men: Opportunities for advancing HIV prevention in the third decade of HIV/AIDS. *Journal of Acquired Immune Deficiency Syndromes, 38*(5), 603–614.

Magnus, M., Jones, K., Phillips, G., 2nd, Binson, D., Hightow-Weidman, L. B., Richards-Clarke, C., ... Hidalgo, J. (2010). Characteristics associated with retention among African American and Latino adolescent HIV-positive men: Results from the outreach, care, and prevention to engage HIV-seropositive young MSM of color special project of national significance initiative. *Journal of Acquired Immune Deficiency Syndromes, 53*(4), 529–536.

Malebranche, D. J. (2003). Black men who have sex with men and the HIV epidemic: Next steps for public health. *American Journal of Public Health, 93*(6), 862.

Marks, G., Crepaz, N., Senterfitt, J. W., & Janssen, R. S. (2005). Meta-analysis of high-risk sexual behavior in persons aware and unaware they are infected with HIV in the United States:

Implications for HIV prevention programs. *Journal of Acquired Immune Deficiency Syndromes*, *39*(4), 446–453.

Martin, E. G., & Schackman, B. R. (2012). What does US health reform mean for HIV clinical care? *Journal of Acquired Immune Deficiency Syndromes*, *60*(1), 72.

Matthews, A.K., Kuhns, L., Conrad, M., & Vargas, M. (2011). *Project exhale: Preliminary evaluation of a tailored smoking cessation treatment for HIV+African American Smokers*. Paper presented at the Annual Meeting of the Gay and Lesbian Medical Association (GLMA), Atlanta, GA.

Mauer, M. (1999). *Race to incarcerate*. New York, NY: The New Press.

Mausbach, B. T., Semple, S. J., Strathdee, S. A., Zians, J., & Patterson, T. L. (2007). Efficacy of a behavioral intervention for increasing safer sex behaviors in HIV-positive MSM methamphetamine users: Results from the EDGE study. *Drug and Alcohol Dependence*, *87*(2–3), 249–257. doi:10.1016/j.drugalcdep.2006.08.026

Mayer, K. H., Bekker, L. G., Stall, R., Grulich, A. E., Colfax, G., & Lama, J. R. (2012). Comprehensive clinical care for men who have sex with men: An integrated approach. *The Lancet*, *380*(9839), 378–387.

McClain, C. S., Rosenfeld, B., & Breitbart, W. (2003). Effect of spiritual well-being on end-of-life despair in terminally-ill cancer patients. *The Lancet*, *361*(9369), 1603–1607.

Meyer, I. H. (1995). Minority stress and mental health in gay men. *Journal of Health and Social Behavior*, *36*, 38–56.

Meyer, I. H. (2003). Prejudice, social stress, and mental health in lesbian, gay, and bisexual populations: Conceptual issues and research evidence. *Psychological Bulletin*, *129*(5), 674–697.

Meyer, I. H. (2007). Prejudice and discrimination as social stressors. In I. H. Meyer & M. E. Northridge (Eds.), *The health of sexual minorities* (pp. 242–267). New York: Springer.

Meyer, I. H., & Dean, L. (1998). Internalized homophobia, intimacy, and sexual behavior among gay and bisexual men. In G. M. Herek (Ed.), *Stigma and sexual orientation: Understanding prejudice against lesbians, gay men, and bisexuals* (pp. 160–186). Thousasand Oaks, CA: Sage.

Miller, R. L., Jr. (2007). Legacy denied: African American gay men, AIDS, and the black church. *Social Work*, *52*(1), 51–61.

Millett, G.A., Peterson, J.L., Flores, S.A., Hart, T.A., Jeffries, W. L. 4th, Wilson, P.A., ... Remis, R.S. (2012). Comparisons of disparities and risks of HIV infection in black and other men who have sex with men in Canada, UK, and USA: A meta-analysis. Lancet, 380(9839), 341–348.

Millett, G. A., Peterson, J. L., Wolitski, R. J., & Stall, R. (2006). Greater risk for HIV infection of black men who have sex with men: A critical literature review. *American Journal of Public Health*, *96*(6), 1007–1019. doi:10.2105/Ajph.2005.066720

MMWR. (1981). Pneumocystis pneumonia—Los Angeles. *MMWR. Morbidity and Mortality Weekly Report*, *30*(21), 250–252.

Montgomery, S. B., Hyde, J., DeRosa, C., Rohrbach, L., Ennett, S., Harvey, S. M., ... Kipke, M. (2002). Gender differences in HIV risk behaviors among youth injectors and their social network menbers. *American Journal of Drug and Alcohol Abuse*, *28*(3), 453–475.

Morin, S.F., Shade, S.B., Steward, W.T., Carrico, A.W., Remien, R.H., Rotheram-Borus, M.J., ... Healthy Living Project Team. (2008). A behavioral intervention reduces HIV transmission risk by promoting sustained serosorting practices among HIV-infected men who have sex with men. *Journal of Acquired Immune Deficiency Syndromes*, *49*(5), 544–551.

Moyer, V. A., & on behalf of the United States Preventive Services Task Force. (2013). Screning for HIV: U.S. preventive servies task force recommendation statement. *Annals of Internal Medicine*, *159*(1), 51–60.

Mustanski, B., Hunter, J., Pequegnat, W., & Bell, C. (2011). Parents as agents of HIV prevention for gay, lesbian, and bisexual youth. In W. Pequegnat & C. C. Bell (Eds.), *Family and HIV/AIDS: Cultural and contextual issues in prevention and treatment* (p. 249). New York: Springer.

Nikolopoulos, G. K., Pavlitina, E., Muth, S. Q., Schneider, J., Psichogiou, M., Williams, L. D., ... Korobchuk, A. (2016). A network intervention that locates and intervenes with recently HIV-infected persons: The Transmission Reduction Intervention Project (TRIP). *Scientific Reports, 6*, 38100.

Nunn, A., Cornwall, A., Chute, N., Sanders, J., Thomas, G., James, G., … Flanigan, T. (2012). Keeping the faith: African American faith leaders' perspectives and recommendations for reducing racial disparities in HIV/AIDS infection. *PloS One, 7*(5), e36172.

Office of AIDS Research. (2015). *Guidelines for the use of antiretroviral agents in HIV-1-infected adults and adolescents.* Department of Health and Human Services. Retrieved February 1, 2015, from http://www.aidsinfo.nih.gov/contentfiles/lvguidelines/adultandadolescentgl.pdf.

Oh, D. L., Sarafian, F., Silvestre, A., Brown, T., Jacobson, L., Badri, S., & Detels, R. (2009). Evaluation of adherence and factors affecting adherence to combination antiretroviral therapy among White, Hispanic, and Black men in the MACS Cohort. *Journal of Acquired Immune Deficiency Syndromes, 52*(2), 290–293.

Operario, D., Smith, C. D., Arnold, E., & Kegeles, S. (2010). The Bruthas Project: Evaluation of a community-based HIV prevention intervention for African American men who have sex with men and women. *AIDS Education and Prevention, 22*(1), 37–48.

Owens, A. P. (2012). The affordable care act: Implications for African Americans living with HIV. *Journal of Human Behavior in the Social Environment, 22*(3), 319–333.

Pardini, D. A., Plante, T. G., Sherman, A., & Stump, J. E. (2000). Religious faith and spirituality in substance abuse recovery: Determining the mental health benefits. *Journal of Substance Abuse Treatment, 19*(4), 347–354.

Parran, T. (1961). *The eradication of syphilis; Task force report to Surgeon General. United States.* Washington, DC: U. S. Department of Health, Education, and Welfare, Public Health Service.

Parsons, J. T., Schrimshaw, E. W., Wolitski, R. J., Halkitis, P. N., Purcell, D. W., Hoff, C. C., & Gomez, C. A. (2005). Sexual harm reduction practices of HIV-seropositive gay and bisexual men: Serosorting, strategic positioning, and withdrawal before ejaculation. *AIDS, 19*, S13.

Paterson, D. L., Swindells, S., Mohr, J., Brester, M., Vergis, E. N., Squier, C., … Singh, N. (2000). Adherence to protease inhibitor therapy and outcomes in patients with HIV infection. *Annals of Internal Medicine, 133*(1), 21–30.

Pequegnat, W. (2012). Family and HIV/AIDS: First line of health promotion and disease prevention. In W. Pequegnat & C. C. Bell (Eds.), *Family and HIV/AIDS* (pp. 3–45). New York: Springer.

Pequegnat, W., Bell, C. C., Dancy, B., & DiIorio, C. (2012). Mothers: The major force in preventing HIV/STD risk behaviors. In *Family and HIV/AIDS* (pp. 121–134). New York: Springer.

Pequegnat, W., & Bray, J. H. (1997). Families and HIV/AIDS: Introduction to the special section. *Journal of Family Psychology, 11*(1), 3–10.

Pequegnat, W., & Szapocznik, J. (2000). *Working with families in the era of HIV/AIDS.* Thousand Oaks: Sage.

Perez, J. L., & Moore, R. D. (2003). Greater effect of highly active antiretroviral therapy on survival in people aged >= 50 years compared with younger people in an urban observational cohort. *Clinical Infectious Diseases, 36*(2), 212–218.

Pescosolido, B. A., Wright, E. R., Alegría, M., & Vera, M. (1998). Social networks and patterns of use among the poor with mental health problems in Puerto Rico. *Medical Care, 36*(7), 1057–1072.

Pichon, L. C., Griffith, D. M., Campbell, B., Allen, J. O., Williams, T. T., & Addo, A. Y. (2012). Faith leaders' comfort implementing an HIV prevention curriculum in a faith setting. *Journal of Health Care for the Poor and Underserved, 23*(3), 1253–1265.

Ponce, N. A., Cochran, S. D., Pizer, J. C., & Mays, V. M. (2010). The effects of unequal access to health insurance for same-sex couples in California. *Health Affairs, 29*(8), 1539–1548.

Prejean, J., Ruiguang, S., Hernandez, A., Ziebell, R., Green, T. A., Walker, F., … Irene Hall, H. (2011). Estimated HIV incidence in the United States, 2006–2009. *PloS One, 6*(8), e17502. doi:10.1371/journal.pone.0017502

Rainie, L. (2010). *Internet, broadband, and cell phone statistics.* Pew Research Center. Retrieved from http://pewinternet.org/~/media/Files/Reports/2010/PIP_December09_update.pdf.

Robertson, M. J., Clark, R. A., Charlebois, E. D., Tulsky, J., Long, H. L., Bangsberg, D. R., & Moss, A. R. (2004). HIV seroprevalence among homeless and marginally housed adults in San Francisco. *American Journal of Public Health, 94*(7), 1207–1217.

Robinson, F. P., Mathews, H. L., & Witek-Janusek, L. (2003). Psycho-endocrine-immune response to mindfulness-based stress reduction in individuals infected with the human immunodeficiency virus: A quasiexperimental study. *The Journal of Alternative & Complementary Medicine, 9*(5), 683–694.

Robles-Schrader, G. M., Harper, G. W., Purnell, M., Monarrez, V., Ellen, J. M., & Adolescent Medicine Trials Network for HIV/AIDS Interventions. (2012). Differential challenges in coalition building among HIV prevention coalitions targeting specific youth populations. *Journal of Prevention & Intervention in the Community, 40*(2), 131–148.

Rosser, B. R., Hatfield, L. A., Miner, M. H., Ghiselli, M. E., Lee, B. R., Welles, S. L., & Positive Connections Team. (2010). Effects of a behavioral intervention to reduce serodiscordant unsafe sex among HIV positive men who have sex with men: The positive connections randomized controlled trial study. *Journal of Behavioral Medicine, 33*(2), 147–158.

Rothenberg, R., Hoang, T. D. M., Muth, S. Q., & Crosby, R. (2007). The Atlanta urban adolescent network study: A network view of STD prevalence. *Sexually Transmitted Diseases, 34*(8), 525–531.

Rotheram-Borus, M. J., Swendeman, D., Comulada, W. S., Weiss, R. E., Lee, M., & Lightfoot, M. (2004). Prevention for substance-using HIV-positive young people: Telephone and in-person delivery. *Journal of Acquired Immune Deficiency Syndromes, 37*(Suppl 2), S68–S77.

Ryan, C., Huebner, D., Diaz, R. M., & Sanchez, J. (2009). Family rejection as a predictor of negative health outcomes in white and Latino lesbian, gay, and bisexual young adults. *Pediatrics, 123*(1), 346–352. doi:10.1542/peds.2007-3524

Sackoff, J. E., Hanna, D. B., Pfeiffer, M. R., & Torian, L. V. (2006). Causes of death among persons with AIDS in the era of highly active antiretroviral therapy: New York City. *Annals of Internal Medicine, 145*(6), 397–406.

Safren, S. A., O'Cleirigh, C. M., Skeer, M., Elsesser, S. A., & Mayer, K. H. (2012). Project enhance: A randomized controlled trial of an individualized HIV prevention intervention for HIV-infected men who have sex with men conducted in a primary care setting. *Health Psychology, 32*(2), 171–179. doi:10.1037/a0028581

Samoff, E., Koumans, E. H., Katkowsky, S., Shouse, R. L., & Markowitz, L. E. (2007). Contact-tracing outcomes among male syphilis patients in Fulton County, Georgia, 2003. *Sexually Transmitted Diseases, 34*(7), 456–460.

Schneider, J. A., Cornwell, B., Ostrow, D., Michaels, S., Friedman, S. R., & Laumann, E. O. (2011). *Formal network analyses illuminate opportunities for personal network intervention on sex and sex drug use behavior of African American men who have sex with men (AA-MSM).* Paper presented at the 6th IAS Conference on HIV Pathogenesis, Treatment and Prevention, Rome, Italy.

Schneider, J. A., Cornwell, B., Ostrow, D., Michaels, S., Schumm, P., Laumann, E. O., & Friedman, S. (2013). Network mixing and network influences most linked to HIV infection and risk behavior in the HIV epidemic among black men who have sex with men. *American Journal of Public Health, 103*(1), e28–e36. doi:10.2105/AJPH.2012.301003

Schneider, J., Kaplan, S. H., Greenfield, S., Li, W., & Wilson, I. B. (2004). Better physician-patient relationships are associated with higher reported adherence to antiretroviral therapy in patients with HIV infection. *Journal of General Internal Medicine, 19*(11), 1096–1103.

Schneider, J. A., & Laumann, E. O. (2011). Alternative explanations for negative findings in the community popular opinion leader multisite trial and recommendations for improvements of health interventions through social network analysis. *Journal of Acquired Immune Deficiency Syndromes, 56*(4), e119–e120. doi:10.1097/QAI.0b013e318207a34c

Schneider, J. A., McFadden, R. B., Laumann, E. O., Prem Kumar, S. G., Gandham, S. R., & Oruganti, G. (2012). Candidate change agent identification among men at risk for HIV infection. *Social Science & Medicine, 75*(7), 1192–1201.

Schneider, J. A., Michaels, S., & Bouris, A. (2012). Family network proportion and HIV risk among black men who have sex with men. *Journal of Acquired Immune Deficiency Syndromes, 61*, 627–635.

Schneider, J. A., Michaels, S., Gandham, S. R., McFadden, R., Liao, C. H., Yeldandi, V. V., & Oruganti, G. (2012). A protective effect of circumcision among receptive male sex partners of indian men who have sex with men. *AIDS and Behavior, 16*(2), 350–359.

Schneider, J. A., Walsh, T., Cornwell, B., Ostrow, D., Michaels, S., & Laumann, E. O. (2012). HIV health center affiliation networks of black men who have sex with men: Disentangling fragmented patterns of HIV prevention service utilization. *Sexually Transmitted Diseases, 39*(8), 598–604.

Seegers, D. L. (2007). Spiritual and religious experiences of gay men with HIV illness. *Journal of the Association of Nurses in AIDS Care, 18*(3), 5–12.

Serovich, J. M., Reed, S., Grafsky, E. L., & Andrist, D. (2009). An intervention to assist men who have sex with men disclose their serostatus to casual sex partners: Results from a pilot study. *AIDS Education and Prevention, 21*(3), 207.

Sherer, R. (2012). The future of HIV care in the USA. *Sexually Transmitted Infections, 88*(2), 106–111.

Singer, M. (1996). A dose of drugs, a touch of violence, a case of AIDS: Conceptualizing the SAVA syndemic. *Free Inquiry in Creative Sociology, 24*, 99–110.

Singer, M. (2009). *Introduction to syndemics: A critical systems approach to public and community health*. San Francisco: Jossey-Bass Inc.

Smith, T. (2011). *Public attitudes toward homosexuality*. Chicago, IL: National Opinion Research Council.

Smith, J., Simmons, E., & Mayer, K. H. (2005). HIV/AIDS and the black church: What are the barriers to prevention services? *Journal of the National Medical Association, 97*(12), 1682.

Somerville, G. G., Diaz, S., Davis, S., Coleman, K. D., & Taveras, S. (2006). Adapting the popular opinion leader intervention for Latino young migrant men who have sex with men. *AIDS Education and Prevention, 18*(4 Suppl A), 137–148. doi:10.1521/aeap.2006.18.supp.137

Sorensen, S. W., Sansom, S. L., Brooks, J. T., Marks, G., Begier, E. M., Buchacz, K., … Kilmarx, P. H. (2012). A mathematical model of comprehensive test-and-treat services and HIV incidence among men who have sex with men in the United States. *PloS One, 7*(2), e29098. doi:10.1371/journal.pone.0029098

Stall, R., Friedman, M., & Catania, J. A. (2008). Interacting epidemics and gay men's health: A theory of syndemic production among urban gay men. In R. J. Wolitski, R. Stall, & R. O. Valdiserri (Eds.), *Unequal opportunity: Health disparities affecting gay and bisexual men in the United States* (pp. 251–274). Oxford: Oxford University Press.

Stall, R., Mills, T. C., Williamson, J., Hart, T., Greenwood, G., Paul, J., … Catania, J. A. (2003). Association of co-occurring psychosocial health problems and increased vulnerability to HIV/AIDS among urban men who have sex with men. *American Journal of Public Health, 93*(6), 939–942.

Steward, W., Remien, R., Higgins, J., Dubrow, R., Pinkerton, S., Sikkema, K., … Morin, S. (2009). Behavior change following diagnosis with acute/early HIV infection—A move to serosorting with other HIV-infected individuals. The NIMH Multisite Acute HIV Infection Study: III. *AIDS and Behavior, 13*(6), 1054–1060.

STI and HIV Intervention Network. (n.d.). Retrieved from http://ssascholars.uchicago.edu/shine.

Stoner, B. P., Whittington, W. L., Hughes, J. P., Aral, S. O., & Holmes, K. K. (2000). Comparative epidemiology of heterosexual gonococcal and chlamydial networks—Implications for transmission patterns. *Sexually Transmitted Diseases, 27*(4), 215–223.

Task Force on Circumcision. (2012). Circumcision policy statement. *Pediatrics, 130*(3), 585. doi:10.1542/peds.2012-1989

Tobin, K. E., German, D., Spikes, P., Patterson, J., & Latkin, C. (2011). A comparison of the social and sexual networks of crack-using and non-crack using african american men who have sex with men. *Journal of Urban Health, 88*(6), 1052–1062. doi:10.1007/s11524-011-9611-4

Trapence, G., Collins, C., Avrett, S., Carr, R., Sanchez, H., Ayala, G., ... Baral, S. D. (2012). From personal survival to public health: Community leadership by men who have sex with men in the response to HIV. *The Lancet, 380*(9839), 400–410. doi:10.1016/S0140-6736(12)60834-4

Tumbarello, M., Rabagliati, R., Donati, K. D., Bertagnolio, S., Tamburrini, E., Tacconelli, E., & Cauda, R. (2003). Older HIV-positive patients in the era of highly active antiretroviral therapy: Changing of a scenario. *AIDS, 17*(1), 128–131.

VanDevanter, N., Duncan, A., Burrell-Piggott, T., Bleakley, A., Birnbaum, J., Siegel, K., ... Ramjohn, D. (2011). The influence of substance use, social sexual environment, psychosocial factors, and partner characteristics on high-risk sexual behavior among young Black and Latino men who have sex with men living with HIV: A qualitative study. *AIDS Patient Care and STDs, 25*(2), 113–121.

Voisin, D. R., & Neilands, T. B. (2010). Community violence and health risk factors among adolescents on Chicago's southside: Does gender matter? *Journal of Adolescent Health, 46*(6), 600–602.

Wellons, M. F., Sanders, L., Edwards, L. J., Bartlett, J. A., Heald, A. E., & Schmader, K. E. (2002). HIV infection: Treatment outcomes in older and younger adults. *Journal of the American Geriatrics Society, 50*(4), 603–607.

Williams, M. V., Palar, K., & Derose, K. P. (2011). Congregation-based programs to address HIV/AIDS: Elements of successful implementation. *Journal of Urban Health, 88*(3), 517–532.

Williams, J. K., Wyatt, G. E., Resell, J., Peterson, J., & Asuan-O'Brien, A. (2004). Psychosocial issues among gay-and non-gay-identifying HIV-seropositive African American and Latino MSM. *Cultural Diversity and Ethnic Minority Psychology, 10*(3), 268.

Wilson, D. P., Regan, D. G., Heymer, K.-J., Jin, F., Prestage, G. P., & Grulich, A. E. (2010). Serosorting may increase the risk of HIV acquisition among men who have sex with men. *Sexually Transmitted Diseases, 37*(1), 13–17. doi:10.1097/OLQ.1090b1013e3181b35549

Wilson, P. A., Wittlin, N. M., Muñoz-Laboy, M., & Parker, R. (2011). Ideologies of Black churches in New York City and the public health crisis of HIV among Black men who have sex with men. *Global Public Health, 6*(Suppl 2), S227–S242.

Wilson, P. A., & Yoshikawa, H. (2004). Experiences of and responses to social discrimination among Asian and Pacific Islander gay men: Their relationship to HIV risk. *AIDS Education and Prevention, 16*(1), 68–83.

Wilton, L., Herbst, J. H., Coury-Doniger, P., Painter, T. M., English, G., Alvarez, M. E., ... Carey, J. W. (2009). Efficacy of an HIV/STI prevention intervention for black men who have sex with men: Findings from the Many Men, Many Voices (3MV) Project. *AIDS and Behavior, 13*(3), 532–544.

Wiysonge, C. S., Kongnyuy, E. J., Shey, M., Muula, A. S., Navti, O. B., Akl, E. A., & Lo, Y. R. (2011). Male circumcision for prevention of homosexual acquisition of HIV in men. *Cochrane Database of Systematic Reviews, 6*, CD007496. doi:10.1002/14651858.Cd007496.Pub2

Wohl, A. R., Galvan, F. H., Myers, H. F., Garland, W., George, S., Witt, M., ... Carpio, F. (2010). Social support, stress and social network characteristics among HIV-positive Latino and African American women and men who have sex with men. *AIDS and Behavior, 14*(5), 1149–1158.

Wolitski, R. J., Gomez, C. A., & Parsons, J. T. (2005). Effects of a peer-led behavioral intervention to reduce HIV transmission and promote serostatus disclosure among HIV-seropositive gay and bisexual men. *AIDS, 19*(Suppl 1), S99–109.

Wolitski, R.J., Kidder, D.P., Pals, S.L., Royal, S., Aidala, A., Stall, R., ... Housing and Health Study Team. (2010). Randomized trial of the effects of housing assistance on the health and risk behaviors of homeless and unstably housed people living with HIV. *AIDS and Behavior, 14*(3), 493–503.

Woods, T. E., Antoni, M. H., Ironson, G. H., & Kling, D. W. (1999). Religiosity is associated with affective and immune status in symptomatic HIV-infected gay men. *Journal of Psychosomatic Research, 46*(2), 165–176.

Ybarra, M. L., & Bull, S. S. (2007). Current trends in internet- and cell phone-based HIV prevention and intervention programs. *Current HIV/AIDS Reports, 4*(4), 201–207.

Ziff, M. A., Harper, G. W., Chutuape, K. S., Deeds, B. G., Futterman, D., Francisco, V. T., ... Ellen, J. M. (2006). Laying the foundation for connect to protect®: A multi-site community mobilization intervention to reduce HIV/AIDS incidence and prevalence among urban youth. *Journal of Urban Health, 83*(3), 506–522.

Part III
Communities

Chapter 9
Working with Asian American/Pacific Islander Gay Men Living with HIV/AIDS: Promoting Effective and Culturally Appropriate Approaches

Kevin L. Nadal and Ben Cabangun

Introduction

Many scholars have contended that research focusing on lesbian, gay, bisexual, transgender, and queer (LGBTQ) issues tends to exclude the experiences of LGBTQ persons of color, particularly LGBTQ Asian Americans and Pacific Islanders (AAPIs) (Chan, 1989, 1992, 1995; Chung & Szymanski, 2006; Nadal, 2010; Nadal & Corpus, 2012). Specifically, while there has been an increase in literature focusing on White gay men, African American gay men, and Latino gay men, there has been a dearth of research concentrating on the experiences of Asian American gay men (Nadal, 2010; Nadal & Corpus, 2012). Furthermore, some scholars have described how studies pertaining to LGBTQ AAPIs and other people of color tend to emphasize the "deficit model" (i.e., focusing primarily on the negative aspects of LGBTQ AAPIs' and other people of color's experiences), instead of focusing on macro-level and sociopolitical experiences that influence LGBTQ mental health, physical health, and behaviors (Akerlund & Chung, 2000). Accordingly, the experiences of AAPI gay men tend to be marginalized in the academic literature in general, resulting in practitioners' and educators' inability to work with this population in effective or culturally competent ways. Second, an overemphasis is placed on the shortcomings or faults of AAPI gay men, often resulting in the pathologizing of their experiences, instead of highlighting the group's strengths and potential for optimal physical and mental health.

The purpose of this chapter is to describe the experiences of AAPI gay men living with HIV/AIDS. First, we will introduce fundamental information about the AAPI

K.L. Nadal (✉)
Department of Psychology, John Jay College of Criminal Justice—City
University of New York, New York, NY, USA
e-mail: knadal@jjay.cuny.edu

B. Cabangun
Asian & Pacific Islander American Health Forum, Oakland, CA, USA

© Springer Science+Business Media LLC 2017
L. Wilton (ed.), *Understanding Prevention for HIV Positive Gay Men*,
DOI 10.1007/978-1-4419-0203-0_9

population, which will be followed by a discussion about the various factors that may impact AAPI gay men's identity development and mental health. Then, we will provide current epidemiological findings involving gay men living with HIV and AIDS, as well as the types of experiences that this community may face in their everyday lives. Finally, we will conclude with recommendations for providing effective and culturally appropriate approaches in working with Asian American/ Pacific Islander gay men living with HIV and AIDS.

Who Are Asian Americans and Pacific Islanders?

Before we describe the experiences of AAPI gay men, it is necessary to first understand who is included in the AAPI population. The term "Asian American" refers to persons who have common ancestral roots in Asia and the Pacific Islands, with a similar physical appearance and cultural values. The Asian American racial category comprises of over 40 distinct ethnicities, which may include Chinese, Asian Indian, Filipino, Vietnamese, Korean, Japanese, Hmong, and Cambodian. While Pacific Islanders are separated from Asian Americans in the US Census, they are often lumped into this category when discussing multicultural issues, forming broader racial categorizations such as "Asian/Pacific Islander" (or API), "Asian Americans/Pacific Islanders" (or AAPI), or "Asian Pacific Americans" (or APA).

According to the 2010 US Census, Asian Americans are the fastest growing racial/ethnic minority group in the USA (Hoeffel, Rastogi, Kim, & Shahid, 2012). As a group, Asian Americans have multiplied eightfold from 1.4 million in 1970 to 11.9 million in 2000, and are projected to increase to 20 million by 2020 (Nadal & Sue, 2009). In fact, the Asian population grew faster than any other racial group in the USA between 2000 and 2010, increasing by 43% from 10.2 million to 14.7 million (Hoeffel et al., 2012). Meanwhile, the 2010 Census revealed that the Native Hawaiian and other Pacific Islander populations increased three times faster than the general US population, resulting in a population of 540,000 people (Hixson, Hepler, & Kim, 2012). According to the 2010 US Census, the largest ethnic group within the Asian American population is Chinese American, with 3.7 million individuals in the USA, which is followed by Filipino Americans (3.4 million), Asian Indian (3.1 million), Vietnamese Americans (1.7 million), and Korean Americans (1.7 million). Nearly half of the population lived on the West Coast, while 22% lived in the South, 20% in the Northwest, and 12% in the Midwest (Hoeffel et al., 2012). Asian Americans also contribute greatly to immigration to the USA, accounting for one-third of all arrivals since the 1970s (Nadal & Sue, 2009).

Based on this population data, it is critical to note the heterogeneity of the AAPI community. First, there are hundreds of languages within the AAPI population, including Tagalog, Farsi, Cantonese, Mandarin, Vietnamese, and Japanese. Second, there are over 20 major religions within the Asian American racial group, including Buddhism, Sikhism, Hinduism, Taoism, Confucianism, and Christianity. Third, there are many physical differences between the major Asian subgroups.

For example, while East Asians (e.g., Chinese, Japanese, and Korean) may have a lighter peach skin tone and smaller eyes, Filipino Americans and Southeast Asians (e.g., Vietnamese, Cambodian, Laotian) may have a light to dark brown skin tone, and South Asians (e.g., Asian Indians, Pakistanis) may have a very dark brown skin tone and larger eyes. Because of this heterogeneity and lack of cohesion between Asian countries, it is common for Asian Americans to identify in terms of their ethnicity (e.g., "Indian," "Filipino," "Korean"), instead of the broader racial category of Asian or Asian American (Nadal & Sue, 2009). As a result, some individuals may not be included in AAPI statistics, may purposefully separate themselves from the pan-ethnic AAPI community and associate only with others in their ethnic group. Importantly, research which makes broad generalizations about AAPIs may not reflect the identities and experiences of all people who would fit under the racial umbrella.

Furthermore, it is important to note that because of different historical, religious, and colonial experiences in their home countries, Asian Americans may prescribe to various cultural worldviews and values. Asian and Asian American ethnic groups may have a range of common cultural values (e.g., collectivism, saving face, emphasis on family), while the unique sociohistorical experiences of each Asian ethnic group will influence these values. For instance, because of English colonization on India and Spanish/American colonization on the Philippines, these two ethnic groups may have both similar and unique cultural values than groups like Chinese or Japanese Americans who may be more heavily influenced by Buddhist or Confucian teachings (Nadal, 2011; Nadal & Sue, 2009).

Asian Americans and Gender Roles

In order to understand AAPI gay men, it is first important to understand how gender is generally conceptualized and understood in AAPI cultures. While gender is defined as "a socially constructed identity that is usually determined by one's biological sex (or whether one has male or female reproductive organs" (Nadal, 2013, p. 35), gender roles are "expectations defined within specific societies and cultures about culturally appropriate behaviors, norms, and values for men and women, based on gender" (Nadal, 2013, p. 35). Gender roles are derived from a spectrum of factors, including (a) traditional gender stereotypes; (b) messages about dress and clothing; (c) messages about career choices or family roles; and (d) expectations of personality, traits, interests, or behaviors. Across AAPI ethnic groups, there are some similarities in the ways that gender roles and sexuality are constructed. First, in terms of gender, Asian American families tend to assign men a higher status as compared with women, give older generations an elevated status, and designate the father as the dominant member of the household with unquestioned authority (Tewari & Alvarez, 2009). For example, in some Asian countries, there has been a history of "son preference," in which male babies are considered a prize because they can continue on the family name and legacy, while female babies are considered a burden because they cannot (Chung, 2007; Mahalingam & Balan, 2008). As a result, boys and men may learn that there is an expectation to continue on the family name and legacy; bring honor to the family; and to be dominant and strong members in their families. When boys and men who do not assume traditional gender roles that are prescribed in their families and communities (e.g., individuals who identify as gay), they may experience gender role conflict, often resulting in varying amounts of psychological distress (Nadal, 2010).

There are also many ways that gender role expectations manifest differently for the various Asian American ethnic groups. For example, some scholars have asserted that Chinese and Chinese American gender roles emphasize the dominance of males and the submissiveness or obedience of women (Chia, Moore, Lam, & Chuang, 1994). Conversely, Filipinos and Filipino Americans tend to have a more complex experience with gender role expectations (Nadal & Corpus, 2012). First, the Philippines advocates for a gender-neutral society, in which women are encouraged to succeed in careers as much as men, and in which women are often the leaders, disciplinarians, and financial decision-makers in the family. In fact, the Philippines was one of the few Asian countries to elect a woman as president. However, as a result of Spanish colonization, Filipino men are still taught to be ultramasculine and Filipina women are taught to be ultrafeminine (Nadal & Corpus, 2012). Accordingly, Filipino and Filipino Americans may learn messages about gender that are both similar and unique to other Asian Americans.

Furthermore, in Asian and Asian American cultures, it is quite common for gender, gender identity, and sexuality to be used interchangeably (Jackson, 1999; Nadal & Corpus, 2012). For instance, in Thailand, there is a strong presence of "ladyboys" or *kathoey* (drag queens, cross-dressers, transgender male-to-female) who are often viewed as sexual objects who work as entertainers or commercial sex workers (Jackson, 1999). As a result, many Thai people (and people of other Asian countries) may assume that all gay men are feminine and identify as transgender women, or both. Perhaps one reason why AAPI men who have sex with men (MSM) may not identify with the terms "gay" or "bisexual" is because they view themselves as masculine and as "real" men, assuming that gay men must behave otherwise.

Asian Americans and Sexual Orientation Identity

Some scholars have described the psychological stressors that AAPI gay men may experience as a result of their intersectional identities (i.e., the intersection of their sexual orientation, racial, ethnic identities). First, many studies support that Asian Americans and other LGBTQ persons of color are often forced and/or expected to choose between their racial/ethnic identity (e.g., Asian American, Cambodian American) and sexual orientation identity (e.g., gay or lesbian). Previous authors have revealed that individuals may desire to identify with both their racial/ethnic and sexual orientation identities, but may struggle because they feel negative repercussions from both of their groups (Chan, 1989, 1992, 1995; Nadal & Corpus, 2012;

Operario, Han, & Choi, 2008). Moreover, many studies have found that it was common for LGBTQ Asian Americans to be the subject of racial stereotyping in general LGBTQ social circles, while enduring homophobia in their ethnic families and communities (Han, 2008; Nadal & Corpus, 2012).

Regarding sexual orientation identity development, there are myriad ways that identity development processes may be different for AAPI gay men. First, while numerous Western/American models of sexual orientation identity development label the "coming out" process as an imperative, developmental stage for gay/bisexual individuals (Nadal, 2010), many LGBTQ people of color (particularly those from immigrant communities) may view coming out (or announcing one's sexual orientation to one's family and friends) as superfluous and unnecessary (Chan, 1989, 1992, 1995; Nadal, 2010; Nadal & Corpus, 2012). Many LGBTQ individuals may not feel the need to officially proclaim their sexual orientation for numerous reasons, including the desire to avoid family conflict or the resentment that heterosexuals do not have to proclaim their sexualities (Nadal, 2010).

For AAPI gay men, there is an array of real or perceived repercussions that may occur if one chooses to "come out" in traditional Western/American ways. Previous research has indicated that many Asian Americans may hide their sexual identities from their families and communities because of the shame that accompanies it (Chan, 1989, 1992, 1995; Nadal & Corpus, 2012; Operario et al., 2008). Shame may impact LGBTQ children who do not want to disgrace or dishonor their family, while also affecting parents of LGBTQ people who fear that they may be blamed for not raising their child heterosexual (Chan, 1992; Operario et al., 2008). Similarly, open disclosure about one's sexual orientation for AAPI gay men may also be viewed as disrespectful because in doing so, one is openly announcing that he is rejecting one's traditional gender roles (Chan, 1992). As a result, many AAPI gay men may maintain a "public self" and a "private self" (Chan, 1995); the public self is one that is revealed to one's family and ethnic community, while the private self is reserved for the individual's personal life and intimate social circles.

Religion may also be a major factor that may prevent many AAPI gay men from accepting their sexual orientation identities. Most Asian countries have had a strong presence of organized religion in their histories and cultures. For example, Hinduism is widespread in India, Buddhism is prevalent in Thailand, Islam is customary in Indonesia, and Christianity is present in Korea (Chung & Singh, 2008). Each of these religions promotes varying levels of negative teachings of homosexuality and bisexuality, which may further result in AAPI gay men resisting their true sexual orientation identities.

Current Findings of AAPI Gay Men Living with HIV/AIDS

Now that we have provided a contextualized scope of some of the core experiences of AAPI gay men's communities, we will now describe how HIV/AIDS has affected AAPI gay men as well as AAPI MSM. At mere surface glance, the epidemiological profile of HIV/AIDS in the USA indicates a low prevalence in AAPI communities. In 2015, AAPIs had the lowest rates of HIV/AIDS out of all racial minority groups, comprising only 5.5% for every 100,000 cases (Centers for Disease Control and Prevention [CDC], 2017). For Black/African Americans, the rates were 44.3%, rates for people of multiple races were 12.2%, rates for Latino/as were 16.4%, rates for Native Hawaiians/other Pacific Islanders were 14.1%, rates for American Indians/Alaska Natives were 8.8%, and rates for Whites were 5.3% (CDC, 2017). There have been several studies that have found that HIV prevalence estimates among the AAPI MSM population to be quite low. For instance, a CDC (2008a) report on new infections found that only 2% of AAPIs were infected with HIV/AIDS. Studies that included AAPI MSM participants listed HIV prevalence rates for this group as between 6 and 10% (Catania et al., 2001; Nemoto, Iwamoto, Kamitani, Morris, & Sakata, 2011; Raymond & McFarland, 2009). For young AAPI MSM (i.e., individuals between 18 and 29 years old), HIV/AIDS prevalence estimates have been recorded as low as 2.6% (Choi et al., 2004; Do et al., 2005).

Despite this low prevalence, there are many studies that have suggested that HIV/AIDS is still a considerable problem in the AAPI community. First, an analysis from 2001 to 2008 showed that Asian Americans and Pacific Islanders had the highest HIV incidence rates in the nation (at 4.4%), representing the only statistically significant growth among any racial or ethnic group in the same time period; in fact, the HIV incidence rate actually declined for several of the other racial groups (Adih, Campsmith, Williams, Hardnett, & Hughes, 2011). The CDC (2006) found that from 2001 to 2004, AAPIs had the highest estimated annual percentage increase in HIV/AIDS diagnosis rates of all race/ethnicities, particularly for AAPI women (34.5% for males and 68% for females). Two years later, the CDC (2008b) reported that from 2001 to 2006, the largest proportionate increase in HIV/AIDS diagnosis rates (255.6%) was with AAPI MSM aged 13–24 years. More recently, the CDC (2017) reported that while the total number of reported AIDS cases has generally declined over the past 5 years for the White population, it has increased for Asian Americans.

Despite these numbers, AAPIs are still stereotyped as being unaffected by the HIV/AIDS epidemic in comparison to how other communities of color are perceived as being affected by the disease (Sabato & Silverio, 2010). As a result, the funding of HIV/AIDS prevention campaigns, education programs, and research studies for AAPIs has been inadequate. One reason for this lack of advocacy for AAPIs is based on the Model Minority Myth (Sabato & Silverio, 2010). The Model Minority Myth, which contends that Asian Americans are well-educated, successful, and law-abiding citizens in the USA (Nadal & Sue, 2009; Wu, 2003), is problematic for several reasons. First, the myth presumes that every person under the AAPI umbrella is the same; so while there are some parts of the AAPI community that fit the stereotype of the "Model Minority," there are many Asian American subgroups (e.g., Southeast Asians, Filipino Americans, LGBTQ AAPIs) who experience a multitude of health, sociocultural, and educational inequalities that are quite contrary to the myth. Furthermore, the myth perpetuates tensions between AAPIs and other people of color groups. For instance, African Americans are often compared to AAPIs, being told that they need to "work hard" like the Asian Americans; as a result, racial tensions may arise between the two groups. At the same time, AAPIs may be commended for being the "model" which in turn may create a perceived racial hierarchy and discrimination between Asian Americans and other people of color. Finally, regarding HIV/AIDS and other health-related disparities, the myth often creates the view that because many AAPIs are financially successful and educated that they do not experience health problems (including becoming infected with HIV/AIDS).

One of the main reasons for the low HIV/AIDS prevalence and high incidence relates to the cultural stigma among AAPIs. Because of the shame and silence among AAPI communities, many AAPI individuals may experience a lack of access to HIV testing, education, and prevention services (Sabato & Silverio, 2010). In fact, nearly two-thirds of Asian Americans and over 70% of Pacific Islanders have never tested for HIV, and AAPIs have the lowest HIV testing rates of all races and ethnicities (Schiller, Lucas, Ward, and Peregoy, 2012). Some researchers even esti- mate that one in three AAPIs who are living with HIV/AIDS is undiagnosed (Campsmith, Rhodes, Hall, & Green, 2010). Cultural factors may influence the lack of HIV testing for both heterosexual and LGBTQ AAPIs; some studies have found that AAPIs may delay testing and treatment for fear of bringing shame to one's self and one's family, as well as being disowned from one's family because of the stigma of HIV/AIDS (Sabato & Silverio, 2010). Based on these sociocultural factors, low HIV testing rates and increasing HIV incidence among AAPIs suggests that the rates of HIV/AIDS in this community are likely to be higher than currently documented.

Some research has also found that when AAPIs have HIV testing, it is usually at a late stage in the disease's progression, often resulting in an AIDS diagnosis (Wong, Nehl, Han et al., 2012). Another study found that many Asian American MSM participants were diagnosed with HIV/AIDS at later stages, because they never were tested for HIV, citing that some of the reasons for avoiding being tested included perceived low risk, fear of results, and fear of needles (Do et al., 2005). Taken together, while AAPIs have low HIV testing rates, when they do get tested, this often results in a more accelerated progression to AIDS, which, in turn, affects their opportunities for treatment and care.

There are many barriers facing AAPI communities that provide reasons for the prevalence of HIV/AIDS. Because of the lack of culturally sensitive and language appropriate media campaigns, outreach material, and trained clinical staff, there is a lack of access to HIV/AIDS prevention, testing, and education services among AAPI communities (Sabato & Silverio, 2010). In addition, many states with consid- erable AAPI populations have not included Asians or Pacific Islanders in their HIV surveillance reports. For example, according to the CDC (2008b), California only began including AAPIs in their HIV surveillance reports within the past few years. Furthermore, medical professionals who misclassify the race and ethnicity of AAPI patients in medical record intakes contribute to the underreporting of HIV/AIDS of AAPI people (Zaidi et al., 2005). Finally, because HIV researchers tend not to disaggregate AAPI data, there is very little known about AAPI ethnic groups.

Given that there is a vast range of health, educational, and sociocultural disparities that affect different AAPI ethnic groups (Nadal, 2011), there is a potential for ethnic differences with HIV/AIDS experiences that are being neglected or overlooked.

Furthermore, despite the lack of data and underreporting, HIV/AIDS prevention researchers have contended that there is no evidence to suggest that AAPIs are engaging in less risk behaviors (Nemoto et al., 2011; Peterson, Bakeman, & Stokes, 2001). One study revealed that 38% of AAPI MSM participants who self-identified as being HIV positive reported having sex with casual partners under the influence of alcohol, while 62% of the group reported having sex with casual partners under the influence of drugs; findings also showed that approximately two-thirds of them (68%) reported that they did not know their casual partners' HIV status (Nemoto et al., 2011). Another study found 64% of AAPI MSM had multiple sex partners and 47% reported unprotected anal sex in the past 6 months (Choi, et al., 2004). Operario and Hall (2003) also found that 49% of AAPI MSM reported having sex under the influence of substances. Choi et al. (2005) found that within the past 6 months, 32% of API MSM participants reported having sex under the influence of alcohol and 34% had sex while under the influence of drugs. Nemoto, Operario, and Soma (2002) found that Filipino American MSM who used amphetamines were likely to have unprotected sex, were more likely to have sex under the influence of drugs and alcohol and engage in injection drug use, while being less likely to be tested for HIV/AIDS. Operario et al. (2006) found a significant and positive relationship between risky sexual behaviors and substance use. All of these findings are supported by other studies which revealed that AAPI MSM often engage in risky behaviors such as drug use and unprotected sex, which simultaneously often leads to higher exposure to HIV/AIDS (Choi, Han, Hudes, & Kegeles, 2002; McFarland, Chen, Weide, Kohn, & Klausner, 2004; Peterson et al., 2001; Schwarcz et al., 2007).

In addition to risky sexual behaviors, lack of HIV education can also contribute to the spread of the disease. One study found that 85% of AAPI MSM who reported unprotected anal intercourse reported that they were unlikely to contract HIV (Santa Clara County, 2008). Perhaps AAPI gay men believe that they are not susceptible to the disease because they are not educated about HIV risk factors, because HIV/AIDS is not highly visible in their communities, or both.

Finally, a multitude of sociocultural factors may influence the risky sexual behaviors of AAPI MSM. First, because sex is rarely discussed in AAPI families, many AAPI individuals may not learn about the risk factors associated with unprotected sex, as social norms discouraging the discussion of sex are prevalent in many AAPI cultures (Nemoto et al., 2003). For LGBTQ AAPI people, there may not be any opportunities to discuss sex, sexuality, or sexual behaviors, because they do not have any LGBTQ role models, are in the closet, or a number of other reasons. Similarly, sociocultural factors may influence mental health and HIV risk behaviors. Because AAPI MSM may fear being disowned by family or become depressed because they are unable to navigate their LGBTQ identities, they may engage in high HIV risk behavior, deny their potential for risk, and even avoid HIV prevention services at all costs.

Stigma, Discrimination, and Cultural Factors for AAPI Gay Men Living with HIV/AIDS

There are numerous factors that may affect the everyday lives of AAPI gay men living with HIV/AIDS. First, they must live with the stigma and discrimination that all people infected with HIV/AIDS may encounter. Stigma has been found to be a major stressor for individuals living with HIV/AIDS (Swendeman, Rotheram-Borus, Comulada, Weiss, & Ramos, 2006), and stigma has even been found to be a major barrier for HIV prevention (Chesney & Smith, 1999; Wolitski, Pals, Kidder, Courtenay-Quirk, & Holtgrave, 2009). Some researchers have described how gay men living with HIV/AIDS are likely to experience both a "double stigma"—stigma due to their HIV status and stigma due to their gay identity (Chenard, 2007). Because HIV/AIDS is typically stereotyped as being the "gay disease," people tend to blame gay men with HIV/AIDS for their actions, often citing that they deserved to contract the disease (Nadal & Rivera, 2012). Some studies have even supported that members of the general public are more likely to place blame and anger on gay men living with HIV/AIDS than they are with other populations with HIV (Herek & Capitanio, 1999).

For AAPI gay men (and other gay men of color), they may experience a "triple stigma" as a result of their race, sexual identities, HIV status, or some combinations of them all. First, they may experience overt racism, in that they may be the victims of race-based hate crimes, subjected to racial slurs like "chinks," "gooks," or "japs," and denied service because of their race. This group may also be victimized by racial microaggressions, which are defined as subtle or covert behaviors or statements that convey negative slights and insults towards people of color (Sue, Bucceri, Lin, Nadal, & Torino, 2007). For example, people may assume that AAPIs have limited English proficiency, may categorize them as model minorities, or treat them as perpetual foreigners (i.e., assume that they are immigrants, despite their actual citizenship or long family histories in the USA) (Wu, 2003). AAPI gay men may also experience stigma and discrimination based on their sexual orientation. Gay and bisexual men have been reported to be victims to hate crimes (Herek, 2009) and heterosexist prejudice (Meyer, 2003), and may even experience microaggressions (or subtle forms of discrimination) based on their sexual orientation or gender identity and expression (Nadal, Rivera, & Corpus, 2010). Understanding the spectrum of discrimination based on sexual orientation may be especially important for AAPI gay men, given that one study reported that Asian American gay men perceived more discrimination due to sexual orientation and not due to race/ethnicity (Chan, 1989).

Furthermore, AAPI gay men may be susceptible to experiencing stigma and discrimination that is based on the intersections of their race, ethnicity, gender, and sexual identities (Choi, Han, Paul & Ayala, 2011). As previously discussed, it is quite common for LGBTQ people of color to encounter discrimination from their racial/ethnic communities, from the general LGBTQ community, and both. For AAPI gay men specifically, they may be taunted and teased by their family members because of their sexual orientation, invalidated, excluded, or devalued in the general LGBTQ community based on their race. They may also be treated as second-class citizens as a result of both their race and sexual identities. One commonly reported experience for Asian gay men is that they are often exoticized, in that they are treated like sexual objects by other gay men, particularly White gay men (Han, 2006; Nadal & Corpus, 2012). For instance, in a qualitative study of lesbian and gay Filipino Americans, participants shared that they felt exoticized as Asians or Filipinos, in that they were stereotyped as being "oversexual" or "subordinate" (Nadal & Corpus, 2012). AAPI gay men also report feeling invisible in the general LGBTQ community, particularly because they do not fit the White standards of beauty or cultural norms; they are often told (directly and indirectly) that they are not attractive enough (especially in comparison to White men) and/or that they are not "man enough" (Han, 2006; Nadal, 2013). In fact, one study found that 80% of AAPI MSM participants reported instances of racism within the gay community (Dang & Hu, 2005), suggesting that racial discrimination is a common experience for this community.

Furthermore, the stigma and discrimination experienced by AAPI gay males may also negatively impact one's health behaviors, which in turn can affect one's HIV status and health (Ayala, Bingham, Kim, Wheeler, & Millett, 2012). For instance, one qualitative study examined how the intersection of race and sexuality influenced the sexual behaviors of AAPI MSM (Han, 2008). Based on 15 qualitative interviews with AAPI MSM, three major themes that were identified:

1. Racism was seen as a primary factor in the way that API gay men came to view their experiences within the larger gay community.
2. Racism in the gay community led to the creation of a social context of sexual behavior that placed gay API men at a disadvantage in partner selection.
3. The disadvantage resulted in API gay men competing for White male partners that involved taking on the submissive role during sexual intercourse, thus having less ability to negotiate safer sexual behavior with their White partners (Han, 2008, p. 830).

The findings from this study demonstrated how racism contributed to the types of experiences that AAPI MSM men had in their romantic and sexual relationships, as well as their participation in the broader gay community. Furthermore, racism often resulted in AAPI MSM feeling isolated or unwanted, which also had an impact on their selection of sexual partners. Finally, racism resulted in AAPI MSM stereotypically assuming a sexually submissive role (i.e., to be the anal recipient or "bottom"), which increased their risk for HIV and other sexually transmitted infections.

Psychological stressors based on the intersection of race and sexuality may influence AAPI gay men's mental health (Choi, Paul, Ayala, Boylan, & Gregorich, 2013). For instance, one study found that Asian American gay men were more likely than heterosexual Asian American men to have reported a recent suicide attempt (Cochran, Mays, Alegria, Ortega, & Takeuchi, 2007). This finding poses significant considerations for the mental health needs of AAPI gay men. For example, research has shown that multiple gender role expectations that AAPI men experience to be heterosexual, masculine, strong, and individuals who bring honor to the family can be psychologically challenging for those who may be struggling with their sexual identity (Nadal, 2010). AAPI gay men may also develop depressive symptoms as a result of not being able to accept one's sexual identity, which may potentially lead to suicidal ideation (Cochran et al., 2007).

Furthermore, the experiences of discrimination and stigma for AAPI gay men may influence one's susceptibility to mental health issues. For instance, in a study with MSM of color (e.g., African American MSM, Latino MSM, and AAPI MSM), experiences of racism in the general community and homophobia among one's heterosexual friends were related to both depression and anxiety, while homophobia in the general community was related to anxiety (Choi et al., 2013). The results from this study also indicated that AAPI MSM were the only group in which racism in the gay community had a negative influence on their mental health (Choi et al., 2013), suggesting that racism in the gay community is significantly distressful for AAPI gay men. Based on these cultural considerations, AAPI gay men may develop mental health issues because of the racism encountered in LGBTQ communities, racism in the general community, homophobia experienced among friendship circles, and homophobia among the general community. This supports previous literature that has cited that AAPI gay men may be more susceptible to psychological issues than his heterosexual AAPI or gay White counterparts who only have to deal with one type of discrimination (Chan, 1989, 1992, 1995; Chung & Singh, 2008; Chung & Szymanski, 2006; Nadal, 2010; Nadal & Corpus, 2012).

Another problem that may negatively influence AAPI gay men's health behaviors and their increased vulnerability for HIV transmission is substance use and abuse (Nemoto et al., 2011). While one study revealed that AAPI men in general (i.e., heterosexual, gay, and bisexual AAPI men) were least likely as compared to other racial/ethnic groups (i.e., Whites, African Americans, and Latino men) to report use of cocaine, ecstasy, marijuana, and poppers (Grov, Bimbi, Nanin, & Parsons, 2006), there are several studies that support that drug and alcohol use is quite high among AAPI MSM (Toleran, et al., 2012). For example, one study found that AAPI MSMs in San Francisco engaged in more substance use than other racial groups (Greenwood et al., 2001). Operario et al. (2006) reported that alcohol use was very pervasive among AAPI MSMs (94% of participants drank alcohol in their lifetime and 89% drank in the past 6 months); other drugs that were used by majority of the sample included marijuana (61% lifetime, 44% past 6 months) and ecstasy (58% lifetime, 47% past 6 months). Meanwhile, Nemoto et al. (2011) revealed that AAPI MSMs were more likely than heterosexual AAPI substance abusers and AAPI incarcerated offenders to use "club drugs" (i.e., hallucinogens such as MDMA, LSD, and GHB), which are drugs that often used when engaging in unprotected anal sexual intercourse.

Perhaps one main reason why AAPI gay men may turn to substances is to cope with the discrimination that may experience. Because many AAPI men in general may have difficulty connecting to their feelings, have difficulty asking for help, have trouble talking about their insecurities or vulnerable topics, substance use may be a more viable option (Iwamoto, 2010; Nadal, 2000, 2011). In fact, through an analysis of studies focusing on AAPI men in general, Iwamoto (2010) discussed how alcohol use has increased significantly among AAPI men over the past 10 years, citing that stress and cultural factors may be reasons for use. In another study, researchers found that conformity to masculine norms and Asian values influenced substance abuse and discussed how AAPI men may turn to drugs and alcohol in an attempt to escape their problems and alleviate psychological anguish (Liu & Iwamoto, 2007). Further, there has also been some literature that has revealed that substance use is perceived as culturally acceptable in various Asian American ethnic groups, particularly for youth and for AAPI men, and that factors like peer pressure, difficulties with acculturation, and familial pressures to achieve may influence substance use (Fang, Barnes-Ceeney, Lee, & Tao, 2011; Nadal, 2000). Finally, specific to substance use and AAPI MSM, one study reported that drug and alcohol use often increased feelings of sociability and comfort among AAPI MSM (Nemoto et al., 2003), suggesting that AAPI MSM may use substances in order to feel less isolated and to fit in with their peers.

Racism and heterosexism may also influence substance use behaviors among AAPI gay men. First, one study found that when AAPIs (both women and men) were not treated as "Americans," they were likely to be at risk for tobacco use, alcohol use, and substance use (Yoo, Gee, Lowthrop, & Robertson, 2010). Second, a study examining experiences of lesbian, gay, and bisexual (LGB) adults found that individuals who encountered more discrimination would be more likely to develop a substance use disorder (McCabe, Bostwick, Hughes, West, & Boyd, 2010). Finally, in one study that examined Asian adolescents in Canada, it was found that the heterosexual Asians were less likely to engage in illicit drug, marijuana, and alcohol use than their Asian Canadian LGB counterparts (Homma, Chen, Poon, & Saewyc, 2012). While there are many reasons that may influence this disparity, it can be hypothesized that differential experiences due to sexual orientation may be one major influence.

Because AAPI gay men experience a great deal of stigma due to their race and sexual orientation, it may be difficult for them to cope if they become infected with HIV/AIDS. Some authors have cited that disclosure of HIV status may be particularly difficult for AAPIs because of the cultural shame that accompanies it. Because HIV is also often associated with drugs and homosexuality, which are all topics deemed to be "taboo" in Asian cultures, it may be difficult for AAPIs in general to disclose their HIV statuses (Chin & Kroesen, 1999). So when an AAPI gay man actually is infected with HIV, he may experience difficulties in disclosing his status to loved ones seek help, or both. Furthermore, for AAPI gay men who have not disclosed their sexual identity, becoming infected with HIV or developing AIDS further complicates their ability to come to terms with their sexual identity. They may repress their sexual orientations even further, which may influence their risky behaviors, their mental health, or both.

The stigma and shame of HIV/AIDS may be so salient for AAPI gay men who are diagnosed with the disease, that many may even avoid seeking medical care. In fact, one study found that AAPI people who are living with HIV/AIDS avoid

Western medical care due to cultural stigma and shame, but also due to the lack of knowledge of Western medicine (Wilkinson, 1997). Because the mental health field has been traditionally viewed as a Western practice, in that talking about one's problems (particularly with an outsider) is viewed as unnecessary and selfish, many AAPI people may turn to religion, spirituality, or alternative forms of healing as a culturally appropriate way of coping with one's problems (Sue & Sue, 2008). Additionally, AAPIs living with HIV/AIDS may underutilize health care due to the cultural mistrust of American hospitals and medical institutions, the lack of culturally competent services, and language inaccessibility (Chin, Kang, Kim, Martinez, & Eckholdt, 2006; Operario & Hall, 2003). Cultural mistrust refers to the tendency for people of color to mistrust Whites, across a variety of sectors (e.g., mental health practice, hospitals, educational settings), due to the historic mistreatment and discrimination against their racial groups (Bell & Tracey, 2006). Some research has found that cultural mistrust can explain the high rates of premature termination in psychotherapy (Sue & Sue, 2008). Other research supports that LGBT people of color may have a dual cultural mistrust due to their dual identity statuses and the historical mistreatment and discrimination of both LGBT people and people of color (Green, 1997). Finally, some literature describes how LGBT clients are likely to feel less connected to their therapists when they commit microaggressions, or behaviors that convey subtle forms of discrimination or discrimination (Shelton & Deglado-Romero, 2011).

For AAPI MSM immigrants living with HIV/AIDS, there are even more complex factors that influence their views of the health care system and their reasons for seeking or not seeking treatment. First, given that 73% of AAPIs speak a language other than English in their homes (Barnes & Bennett, 2002), language becomes a barrier that can negatively impact HIV knowledge, health education, HIV testing and counseling, and medical treatment. For AAPI MSM immigrants specifically, language deficiencies may negatively influence sexual practices. For instance, one study found that young AAPI MSM are at higher risk for HIV when meeting partners on the Internet because they lack skills to negotiate safer sex in person (Santa Clara County, 2008). For AAPI MSM undocumented immigrants, the fear of deportation may negatively influence one's ability to get tested, seek medical treatment, or utilize other HIV-related services (Chin et al., 2006).

A Critical Response: HIV/AIDS Intervention Strategies and AAPIs

Behavioral interventions have shown to be one of the most powerful tools to reduce the HIV epidemic, particularly through reducing HIV risk behaviors (Lyles et al., 2007). In order to successfully achieve this goal, HIV/AIDS scholars have developed curricular interventions aimed at educating communities at risk for HIV. The Centers for Disease Control and Prevention, along with other federal and private agencies, provides funding for these researchers to develop HIV prevention interventions. Once developed and implemented, these agencies then evaluate the findings and deem these interventions as "effective" in reducing risk behaviors. The CDC then accumulates these proven effective interventions in a compendium, which is known as the Diffusion of Effective Behavioral Interventions (DEBIs). Each of these interventions specifically targets specific populations, among them for example, youth, women, and people of color communities. The CDC provides training and education for community organizations to implement these interventions. The Evidence Based Intervention (EBI) is the adaptation of DEBIs to be effective for implementing in "emerging populations."

Despite the many interventions proven effective by the CDC, there is a lack of prevention interventions designed for, or even adapted for, AAPIs (Han, 2009). Furthermore, while there have been some prevention interventions that have been created for MSMs (e.g., Choi, 1995), there has not been an EBI that has specifically looked at AAPI MSM. As previously discussed, the percentage of diagnoses of HIV infection and AIDS for AAPIs remains relatively small compared to other racial/ethnic groups. However, because of the aforementioned research that supports that AAPI MSMs engage in high-risk behaviors (e.g., McFarland et al., 2004; Nemoto et al., 2011; Schwarcz et al., 2007), evidenced-based interventions are still necessary for this group.

In 2005, the Substance Abuse and Mental Health Services Administration/Center for Substance Abuse Prevention (SAMHSA/CSAP) awarded Minority AIDS Initiative (MAI) grants to only three AAPI organizations of approximately 80 nationwide grantees, but only one of them focused on high-risk groups of adult men who have sex with men. Other organizations such as the CDC provided a similar or smaller percentage of awards to AAPIs in comparison to other racial groups. To the authors' knowledge, there are seven known AAPI-adapted HIV EBIs—four of which have been implemented in San Francisco, California, by the Asian & Pacific Islander Wellness Center. None of these three EBIs have been conducted in geographical regions where large populations of AAPI reside and none included other high-risk populations (i.e., substance users and re-entry individuals).

The limited number or lack of interventions for AAPIs may be due to the aforementioned heterogeneity of the AAPI community. Because the AAPI umbrella comprises diverse ethnicities, nationalities, languages, dialects, cultural histories, and disparate socioeconomic statuses, a universal AAPI intervention may not be appropriate for the entire group. For instance, because a large number of AAPIs live at below the federal poverty level, while many AAPIs belong to a much higher socioeconomic status, some subgroups may respond differently to HIV prevention interventions. Similarly, some qualitative studies have found that there is a community concern for lack of culturally and linguistically appropriate HIV prevention programs for AAPIs (Jemmott, Maula, & Bush, 1999). Thus, tailoring prevention interventions to meet the needs of this culturally and socioeconomically diverse population is a challenge for various institutions.

Furthermore, as previously discussed AAPI health problems are compounded by the low utilization of HIV health services (Ye, Mack, Fry-Johnson, & Parker, 2012). AAPIs access health services less than other racial and ethnic groups due to culture, including values and norms related to family reputation, shames, stigma, denial, taboo surrounding sexuality and drug use, and fear of immigration status (Chin et al., 2006; Operario & Hall, 2003). In order to overcome these issues, adaptation of interventions must address these cultural barriers for people to attend and feel comfortable enough to participate in HIV prevention programs. The prevalence of these diseases and behaviors, deficient number of culturally appropriate HIV, hepatitis, or substance use service providers, social/cultural barriers and decreasing government and private budgets and resources have deterred high-risk AAPI populations from accessing and participating in these integrated prevention services.

There are many additional variables that influence why some interventions have not been effective for AAPI MSMs. Han (2009) conducted focus groups with AAPI MSMs who described the most important issues that needed to be addressed in providing HIV prevention for AAPI gay men. Five themes emerged including: (1) the need to address racism in the gay community, (2) the need to address homophobia in the AAPI community, (3) the need to increase self-esteem, (4) the need to promote a gay AAPI community, and (5) the need to provide positive role models. Based on these participants' experiences, it would be necessary for any intervention program to address racism and homophobia directly, as it appears to be a major factor that may influence AAPI individuals' behaviors and mental health, which in turn can increase risk for HIV infection. Furthermore, based on participants in Han's (2009) study, it would be crucial to promote a healthy gay AAPI identity and expose gay AAPI men to role models and a greater community, in order to endorse healthy psychological well-being.

Finally, some scholars have cited that one of the main reasons why HIV disparities are still prevalent among AAPI communities is because of the lack of funding that provides program development, data collection, and research of AAPI HIV-related issues (Sabato & Silverio, 2010). Because many funding institutions focus on the low prevalence of HIV/AIDS among AAPIs, many may not provide adequate amounts of funding for organizations that focus specific on AAPI populations. Thus, it is necessary for HIV/AIDS researchers, educators, and practitioners to inform others that HIV/AIDS is still an issue affecting AAPIs, particularly MSM who are not getting tested or who are still engaging in risky behaviors. In doing so, it is hoped that others will realize that the epidemic is still affecting the community and that funding can still be made available for them.

Psychological Approaches for Working with AAPI Gay Men Living with HIV/AIDS

In addition to systemic recommendations that are necessary to improve the lives of AAPI gay men living with HIV/AIDS, we conclude this chapter by providing suggestions for individuals who work directly with this population. While we speak specifically about clinicians (e.g., HIV counselors, psychologists, social workers), this section can also be applied to other practitioners including medical doctors, nurses, teachers, health educators, and others. Because there is a dearth of clinical and counseling services for people living with HIV/AIDS (Lam, Naar-King, & Wright, 2007), it is crucial for clinicians and other practitioners to develop strong therapeutic relationships with their clients, in order to prevent treatment dropout rates (Leeman et al., 2010). Furthermore, because LGBT people have reported to drop out of psychotherapy due to cultural insensitivity and stigma (Green, 1997) and because Asian Americans have been known to underutilize mental health services and drop out of psychotherapy as well (Tewari & Alvarez, 2009), it is necessary for clinicians and other practitioners to become culturally competent in working with AAPI gay men who are living with HIV/AIDS. Finally, because gay-related stigma consciousness, or one's ability to perceive heterosexist stigma, has been found to be a significant predictor of depressive symptoms (Lewis, Derlega, Griffin, & Krowinski, 2003), it is crucial for clinicians to manage or minimize their stigma in their therapeutic relationships, in order to provide the most effective treatment for their clients.

Utilizing the multicultural competence model can be beneficial in working with all clients of diverse backgrounds, but particularly gay male clients who are living with HIV/AIDS (Nadal & Rivera, 2012). The model involves three parts: (a) knowledge, (b) awareness, and (c) skills. The knowledge component involves the notion that clinicians have gained appropriate education about cultural topics and identities that are different from their own experiences. Specific to AAPI gay men living with HIV/AIDS, there are many facets of a person's experience that a culturally competent counselor will be knowledgeable. First, the clinician will be educated in HIV research and treatment, in order to understand how a client's HIV status may influence his mental health and everyday experiences. A clinician will have a working knowledge of AAPI cultural values and experiences, as well as familiarity with various issues affecting the LGBT community. For instance, perhaps an understanding of the racial dynamics in gay male interracial relationships will allow a clinician to validate a client's experiences. Having a basic understanding of certain cultural issues (and working to improve this knowledge) is necessary for clinicians and other practitioners because it is important that clients are not spending great amounts of time educating counselors during psychotherapy, when time could be spent on exploring emotions and engaging in therapeutic interventions.

The awareness component of multicultural competence involves a clinician being cognizant of their cultural attitudes, biases, and worldviews, particularly the ways that such perspectives could negatively impact therapeutic relationships. For instance, if a therapist maintains any prejudice against people living with HIV/AIDS (conscious or unconscious), this bias can impede her or his working relationship with the client. If the client perceives a therapist's discomfort, anxiety, or prejudice, it is possible for the client to disengage or even drop out of therapy. Moreover, in working with AAPI gay men, it is possible for clinicians to have multiple biases about the clients' multiple identities. For example, the therapist may have negative stereotypes about gay men or gay male relationships, while also having prejudicial views of Asian American cultural values. If the clinician is unable to admit to, or manage, these biases, it may be difficult for her or him to convey empathy, which in turn may make it difficult for the client to feel trusting or open the clinician.

While it is very difficult for individuals to admit to any prejudicial attitudes, acknowledging these thoughts may be helpful in order to prevent them from affecting one's working relationships.

Finally, the skills component of multicultural competence refers to the notion that therapists learn and practice the most effective approaches or techniques in working with various clients. For clinicians working with AAPI gay men living with HIV/AIDS, this may involve utilizing or adapting the evidence-based treatments that have been empirically supported to be effective. A culturally competent clinician may also adapt techniques that they have found to be useful in their own practice, particularly with certain cultural groups. However, the most competent therapist is one who is able to utilize interventions that are based on a client's multiple identities. Given a client's unique experiences with race, gender, sexual orientation, age, socioeconomic status, HIV status, and other identities, it may be necessary to adapt one's methods from various treatment models in order to most effectively serve their clients.

There are some specific skills that have been recommended for working with AAPI patients or clients. First, one scholar describes the importance of teaching a bicultural approach for care, particularly in working with AAPI clients living with HIV/AIDS. Because AAPI patients and clients, particularly those from immigrant backgrounds, may be less acculturated to American ways of being, it is necessary to respect and validate AAPI patients' cultural ways of doing things (Yu, 1999). Similarly, it is necessary for practitioners to respect traditional forms of healing, particularly with clients who may have a distrust or fear of Western medical models (Yu, 1999). Sometimes, it is necessary for practitioners to be direct with AAPI, particularly because of the shame and stigma that may prevent them from seeking help. For example, some scholars describe how AAPI people must be encouraged to seek medical assistance, even when symptoms are obvious and persistent (Jemmott et al., 1999). Finally, because of the cultural shame and stigma regarding HIV within the AAPI community, it is crucial that practitioners engage the client in an empowerment approach to care (Yu, 1999). Because AAPI culture sometimes tends to encourage deference to authority, it can be common for AAPI patients to not fully comprehend their health issues, to not voice their concerns to a medical practitioner, or to not self-advocate for themselves. Having an open and honest conversation and ensuring that a client understands every aspect of her or his medical or psychotherapeutic treatment can truly empower the client to take control of her or his life.

Conclusions

In this chapter, we aimed to highlight the overall experiences of Asian American and Pacific Islander gay men who are living with HIV/AIDS. Because there is limited research that focuses on this community, we advocate for future research and scholarship to emerge with this group. Based on the review of the literature, one of these core research priorities would be to create culturally appropriate evidence-based interventions for AAPI gay men and MSM. Another key priority would be to examine how racism and homophobia may be related to risky behaviors, particularly unprotected sexual intercourse and substance use. In terms of advocacy, it is necessary for systemic and institutional changes to occur (e.g., national institutes must provide funding, or create treatment models, for this population), while also promoting change on individual levels (e.g., practitioners must attempt to be culturally competent in working with this group). Finally, in order to improve the lives of AAPI gay men, it is important for our society as a whole to recognize the unique needs of this group. Because AAPI gay men experience adversity on many levels (e.g., racism in the LGBTQ community, homophobia in their families, lack of role models and acceptance), it is the role of society as a whole to provide an environment where they are validated and accepted.

References

Adih, W. K., Campsmith, M., Williams, C. L., Hardnett, F. P., & Hughes, D. (2011). Epidemiology of HIV among Asians and Pacific Islanders in the United States, 2001–2008. *Journal of the International Association of Physicians in AIDS Care, 10*(3), 150–159.

Akerlund, M., & Chung, M. (2000). Teaching beyond the deficit model: Gay and lesbian issues among African Americans, Latinos, and Asian Americans. *Journal of Social Work Education, 36*(2), 279–292.

Ayala, G., Bingham, T., Kim, J., Wheeler, D. P., & Millett, G. A. (2012). Modeling the impact of social discrimination and financial hardship on the sexual risk of HIV among Latino and Black men who have sex with men. *American Journal of Public Health, S2,* S242–S249.

Barnes, J. S., & Bennett, C. E. (2002). *The Asian population, 2000.* U.S. Census Brief. Retrieved May 7, 2013 from http://www.census.gov.

Bell, T. J., & Tracey, T. J. G. (2006). The relation of cultural mistrust and psychological health. *Journal of Multicultural Counseling and Development, 34*(1), 2–14.

Campsmith, L., Rhodes, P. H., Hall, H. I., & Green, T. A. (2010). Undiagnosed HIV prevalence among adults and adolescents in the United States at the end of 2006. *Journal of Acquired Immune Deficiency Syndromes, 53*(5), 619–624.

Catania, J. A., Osmond, D., Stall, R. D., Pollack, L., Paul, J. P., Blower, S., … Coates, T. J. (2001). The continuing HIV epidemic among men who have sex with men. *American Journal of Public Health, 91*(6), 907–914.

Centers for Disease Control. (2006). Racial/ethnic disparities in diagnoses of HIV/AIDS—33 states, 2001–2004. *Morbidity and Mortality Weekly Report, 55,* 121–125.

Centers for Disease Control. (2008a). *Estimates of new HIV infections in the United States.* Retrieved from http://www.cdc.gov/nchhstp/newsroom/docs/Fact-Sheet-on-HIV-Estimates.pdf.

Centers for Disease Control. (2008b). Trends in HIV/AIDS diagnoses among men who have sex with men, 33 states, 2001–2006. *Morbidity and Mortality Weekly Report, 57*(25), 681–686. Retrieved April, 2009 from http://www.cdc.gov/mmwr/preview/mmwrhtml/mm5725a2. htm?s_cid=mm5725a2_e.

Centers for Disease Control. (2017). *HIV surveillance report: Diagnoses of HIV infection in the United States and Dependent Areas, 2015* (Vol. 27). Retrieved from https://www.cdc.gov/hiv/pdf/library/reports/surveillance/cdc-hiv-surveillance-report-2015-vol-27.pdf.

Chan, C. (1989). Issues of identity development among Asian-American lesbians and gay men. *Journal of Counseling & Development, 68*(1), 16–20.

Chan, C. (1992). Cultural considerations in counseling Asian American lesbians and gay men. In S. Dworkin & F. Gutierrez (Eds.), *Counseling gay men and lesbians* (pp. 115–124). Alexandria, VA: American Association for Counseling and Development.

Chan, C. (1995). Issues of sexual identity in an ethnic minority: The case of Chinese American lesbians, gay men, and bisexual people. In A. R. D'Augelli & C. J. Patterson (Eds.), *Lesbian, gay, and bisexual identities over the lifespan: Psychological perspectives* (pp. 87–101). Oxford: Oxford University Press.

Chenard, C. (2007). The impact of stigma on the self-care behaviors of HIV-positive gay men striving for normalcy. *Journal of the Association of Nurses in AIDS Care, 18*, 23–32.

Chesney, M. A., & Smith, A. W. (1999). Critical delays in HIV testing and care: The potential role of stigma. *The American Behavioral Scientist, 42*, 1162–1174.

Chia, R. C., Moore, J. L., Lam, K. N., & Chuang, C. J. (1994). Cultural differences in gender role attitudes between Chinese and American students. *Sex Roles, 31*(1-2), 23–30.

Chin, J. J., Kang, E., Kim, J. H., Martinez, J., & Eckholdt, H. (2006). Serving Asians and Pacific Islanders with HIV/AIDS: Challenges and lessons learned. *Journal of Health Care for the Poor and Underserved, 17*, 910–927.

Chin, D., & Kroesen, K. W. (1999). Disclosure of HIV infection among Asian/Pacific Islander American women: Cultural stigma and support. *Cultural Diversity and Ethnic Minority Psychology, 5*(3), 222–235.

Choi, K. H., Coates, T. J., Catania, J. A., Lew, S., & Chow, P. (1995). High HIV risk among gay Asian and Pacific Islander men in San Francisco. *AIDS, 9*(3), 306–308.

Choi, K. H., Han, C. S., Hudes, E. S., & Kegeles, S. (2002). Unprotected sex and associated risk factors among young Asian and Pacific Islander men who have sex with men. *AIDS Education and Prevention, 14*, 472–481.

Choi, K. H., Han, C. S., Paul, J., & Ayala, G. (2011). Strategies for managing racism and homophobia among US ethnic and racial minority men who have sex with men. *AIDS Education and Prevention, 23*, 145–158.

Choi, K. H., McFarland, W., Neilands, T. B., Nguyne, S., Louie, B., Secura, G., ... Valleroy, L. (2004). An opportunity for prevention: Prevalence, incidence, and sexual risk for HIV among young Asian and Pacific Islander men who have sex with men, San Francisco. *Sexually Transmitted Diseases, 31*, 475–480.

Choi, K. H., Operario, D., Gregorich, S. E., McFarland, W., MacKellar, D., & Valleroy, L. (2005). Substance use, substance choice, and unprotected anal intercourse among young Asian American and Pacific Islander men who have sex with men. *AIDS Education and Prevention, 17*, 418–429.

Choi, K. H., Paul, J., Ayala, G., Boylan, R., & Gregorich, S. E. (2013). Experiences of discrimination and their impact on the mental health among African American, Asian and Pacific Islander, and Latino men who have sex with men. *American Journal of Public Health, 103*(5), 868–874.

Chung, W. (2007). The relation of son preference and religion to induced abortion: The case of South Korea. *Journal of Biosocial Science, 39*(05), 707–719.

Chung, Y. B., & Singh, A. A. (2008). Lesbian, gay, bisexual, and transgender Asian Americans. In N. Tewari & A. N. Alvarez (Eds.), *Asian American psychology: Current perspectives* (pp. 233–246). New York: Psychology Press.

Chung, Y. B., & Szymanski, D. M. (2006). Racial and sexual identities of Asian American gay men. *Journal of LGBT Issues in Counseling, 1*(2), 67–93. doi:10.1300/J462v01n02_05

Cochran, S. D., Mays, V. M., Alegria, M., Ortega, A. N., & Takeuchi, D. (2007). Mental health and substance use disorders among Latino and Asian American lesbian, gay, and bisexual adults. *Journal of Consulting and Clinical Psychology, 75*(5), 785–794.

Dang, A., & Hu, M. (2005). *Asian Pacific American lesbian, gay, bisexual and transgender people: A community portrait*. A report from New York's Queer Asian Pacific Legacy Conference, 2004.

Do, T. D., Chen, S., McFarland, W., Secura, G. M., Behel, S. K., MacKellar, D. A., ... Choi, K. (2005). HIV testing patterns and unrecognized HIV infection among young Asian and Pacific Islander men who have sex with men in San Francisco. *AIDS Education and Prevention, 17*(6), 540–554.

Fang, L., Barnes-Ceeney, K., Lee, R., & Tao, J. (2011). Substance use among Asian-American adolescents: Perceptions of use and preferences for prevention programming. *Social Work in Health Care, 50*(8), 606–624.

Green, B. (1997). Ethnic minority lesbians and gay men: Mental health and treatment issues. In B. Greene (Ed.), *Ethnic and cultural diversity among lesbians and gay men* (pp. 216–239). Thousand Oaks, CA: Sage.

Greenwood, G. L., White, E. W., Page-Shafer, K., Bein, E., Osmond, D. H., Paul, J., & Stall, R. D. (2001). Correlates of heavy substance use among young gay and bisexual men: The San Francisco Young Men's Health Study. *Drug and Alcohol Dependence, 61*(2), 105–112.

Grov, C., Bimbi, D. S., Nanin, J. E., & Parsons, J. T. (2006). Exploring racial and ethnic differences in recreational drug use among gay and bisexual men in New York City and Los Angeles. *Journal of Drug Education, 36*(2), 105–123.

Han, C. (2006). Geisha of a different kind: Gay Asian men and the gendering of sexual identity. *Sexuality & Culture: An Interdisciplinary Quarterly, 10*(3), 3–28.

Han, C. (2008). A qualitative exploration of the relationship between racism and unsafe sex among Asian Pacific Islander gay men. *Archives of Sexual Behavior, 37*, 827–837. doi:10.1007/s10508-007-9308-7

Han, C. (2009). Chopsticks don't make it culturally competent: Addressing larger issues for HIV prevention among gay, bisexual, and Queer Asian Pacific Islander Men. *Health and Social Work, 34*(4), 273–281.

Herek, G. M. (2009). Hate crimes and stigma-related experiences among sexual minority adults in the United States: Prevalence estimates from a national probability sample. *Journal of Interpersonal Violence, 24*(1), 54–74.

Herek, G. M., & Capitanio, J. P. (1999). AIDS stigma and sexual prejudice. *American Behavioral Scientist, 42*, 1126–1143.

Hixson, L., Hepler, B. B., & Kim, M. O. (2012). *The native Hawaiian and other Pacific Islander population*. Washington, DC: U.S. Census Bureau. Retrieved March 1, 2013 from http://www.census.gov/prod/cen2010/briefs/c2010br-12.pdf.

Hoeffel, E. M., Rastogi, S., Kim, M. O., & Shahid, H. (2012). *The Asian population: 2010*. Washington, DC: U.S. Census Bureau. Retrieved March 1, 2013 from http://www.census.gov/prod/cen2010/briefs/c2010br-11.pdf.

Homma, Y., Chen, W., Poon, C. S., & Saewyc, E. M. (2012). Substance use and sexual orientation among East and Southeast Asian adolescents in Canada. *Journal of Child & Adolescent Substance Abuse, 21*(1), 32–50.

Iwamoto, D. K. (2010). Alcohol abuse and alcohol-related problems among Asian American men. In W. M. Liu, D. K. Iwamoto, & M. H. Chae (Eds.), *Culturally responsive counseling with Asian American men* (pp. 145–169). New York, NY: Routledge.

Jackson, P. A. (1999). An American death in Bangkok: The murder of Darrell Berrigan and the hybrid origins of gay identity in 1960s Thailand. *GLQ: A Journal of Lesbian and Gay Studies, 5*, 361–411.

Jemmott, L. S., Maula, E. C., & Bush, E. (1999). Hearing our voices: Assessing HIV prevention needs among Asian and Pacific Islander women. *Journal of Transcultural Nursing, 10*, 102–111.

Lam, P. K., Naar-King, S., & Wright, K. (2007). Social support and disclosure as predictors of mental health in HIVpositive youth. *AIDS Patient Care and STDs, 21*, 20–29.

Leeman, J., Chang, Y. K., Lee, E. J., Voils, C. I., Crandell, J., & Sandelowski, M. (2010). Implementation of antiretroviral therapy adherence interventions: A realist synthesis of evidence. *Journal of Advanced Nursing, 66*(9), 1915–1930.

Lewis, R. J., Derlega, V. J., Griffin, J. L., & Krowinski, A. C. (2003). Stressors for gay men and lesbians: Life stress, gay-related stress, stigma consciousness, and depressive symptoms. *Journal of Social and Clinical Psychology, 22*(6), 716–729.

Liu, W. M., & Iwamoto, D. K. (2007). Conformity to masculine norms, Asian values, coping strategies, peer group influences and substance use among Asian American men. *Psychology of Men & Masculinity, 8*(1), 25–39.

Lyles, C. M., Kay, L. S., Crepaz, N., Herbst, J. H., Passin, W. F., Kim, A. S., ... Mullins, M. M. (2007). Best-evidence interventions: Findings from a systematic review of HIV behavioral interventions for US populations at high risk, 2000–2004. *American Journal of Public Health, 97*(1), 133–143. doi:10.2105/AJPH.2005.076182

Mahalingam, R., & Balan, S. (2008). Culture, son preference, and beliefs about masculinity. *Journal of Research on Adolescence, 18*(3), 541–553.

McCabe, S. E., Bostwick, W. B., Hughes, T. L., West, B. T., & Boyd, C. J. (2010). The relationship between discrimination and substance use disorders among lesbian, gay, and bisexual adults in the United States. *American Journal of Public Health, 100*(10), 1946–1952.

McFarland, W., Chen, S., Weide, D., Kohn, R., & Klausner, J. (2004). Gay Asian men in San Francisco follow the International trend: Increases in rates of unprotected anal intercourse and sexually transmitted diseases, 1999–2002. *AIDS Education and Prevention, 16*(1), 13–18.

Meyer, I. H. (2003). Prejudice, social stress, and mental health in lesbian, gay, and bisexual populations: Conceptual issues and research evidence. *Psychological Bulletin, 129*(5), 674–697.

Nadal, K. L. (2000). F/Pilipino American substance abuse: Sociocultural factors and methods of treatment. *Journal of Alcohol and Drug Education, 46*(2), 26–36.

Nadal, K. L. (2010). Sexual orientation and identity development for gay and bisexual Asian American men: Implications for culturally competent counseling. In W. Liu, D. Iwamoto, & M. Chae (Eds.), *Culturally responsive counseling with Asian American men* (pp. 113–134). New York: Routledge Press.

Nadal, K. L. (2011). *Filipino American psychology: A handbook of theory, research, and clinical practice*. New York: Wiley.

Nadal, K. L. (2013). *That's so gay! Microaggressions and the lesbian, gay, bisexual, and transgender community*. Washington, DC: American Psychological Association.

Nadal, K. L., & Corpus, M. J. (2013). "Tomboys" and "baklas": Experiences of lesbian and gay Filipino Americans. *Asian American Journal of Psychology, 4*, 166–175.

Nadal, K. L., & Rivera, D. P. (2012). Stigma and its role in HIV prevention and care of gay and bisexual men: Recommendations for clinical and counseling practices. *Psychology and AIDS Exchange, 37*, 20–22.

Nadal, K. L., Rivera, D. P., & Corpus, M. J. H. (2010). Sexual orientation and transgender microaggressions in everyday life: Experiences of lesbians, gays, bisexuals, and transgender individuals. In D. W. Sue (Ed.), *Microaggressions and marginality: Manifestation, dynamics, and impact* (pp. 217–240). New York: John Wiley & Sons.

Nadal, K. L., & Sue, D. W. (2009). Asian American youth. In C. S. Clauss-Ehlers (Ed.), *Encyclopedia of cross-cultural school psychology* (pp. 116–122). New York: Springer.

Nemoto, T., Iwamoto, M., Kamitani, E., Morris, A., & Sakata, M. (2011). Targeted expansion project for outreach and treatment for substance abuse and HIV risk behaviors in Asian and Pacific Islander communities. *AIDS Education and Prevention, 23*(2), 175–191.

Nemoto, T., Operario, D., & Soma, T. (2002). Risk behaviors of Filipino methamphetamine users in San Francisco: Implications for prevention and treatment of drug use and HIV. *Public Health Reports, 117*, 15–29.

Nemoto, T., Operario, D., Soma, T., Bao, D., Cristosomo, V., & Vajrabukka, A. (2003). HIV risk and prevention among API men who have sex with men: Listen to our voices. *AIDS Education and Prevention, 15*, 7–20.

Operario, D., Choi, K. H., Chu, P. L., McFarland, W., Secura, G. M., Behel, S., ... Valleroy, L. (2006). Prevalence and correlates of substance use among young Asian Pacific Islander men who have sex with men. *Prevention Science, 7*(1), 19–29.

Operario, D., & Hall, V. (2003). *Exploring the cultural and social context of HIV risk among Filipinos in San Francisco*. San Francisco: University of California at San Francisco Center for AIDS Prevention Studies.

Operario, D., Han, C., & Choi, K. (2008). Dual identity among gay Asian Pacific Islander men; Culture. *Health & Sexuality, 10*(5), 447–461.

Peterson, J. L., Bakeman, R., & Stokes, J. (2001). Racial/ethnic patterns of HIV sexual risk behaviors among young men who have sex with men. *Journal of the Gay and Lesbian Medical Association, 5*(4), 155–162.

Raymond, H. F., & McFarland, W. (2009). Racial mixing and HIV risk among men who have sex with men. *AIDS and Behavior, 13*(4), 630–637.

Sabato, T. M., & Silverio, A. Q. (2010). A forgotten population: Addressing comprehensive HIV prevention needs among American Asians and Pacific Islanders. *Journal of the Association of Nurses in AIDS Care, 21*(4), 364–370.

Santa Clara County Comprehensive HIV Planning Council for Prevention and Care. (2008). *Santa Clara County comprehensive HIV prevention and care plan 2009–2011*. Retrieved March 4, 2013 from http://www.sccgov.org/sites/sccphd/en-us/Documents/Comprehensive%20 Plan%202009-11.pdf.

Schiller, J. S., Lucas, J. W., Ward, B. W., & Peregoy, J. A. (2012). Summary health statistics for US adults: National Health Interview Survey, 2010. *Vital and Health Statistics*. 2012;(252): 1–207. Epub 2012/07/28.

Schwarcz, S., Scheer, S., McFarland, W., Katz, M., Valleroy, L., Chen, S., & Catania, J. (2007). Prevalence of HIV infection and predictors of high-transmission sexual risk behaviors among men who have sex with men. *American Journal of Public Health, 97*, 1067–1075.

Shelton, K., & Deglado-Romero, E. A. (2011). Sexual orientation microaggressions: The experiences of lesbian, gay, bisexual, and queer clients in psychotherapy. *Journal of Counseling Psychology, 58*(2), 210–221. doi:10.1037/a0022251

Sue, D. W., Bucceri, J. M., Lin, A. I., Nadal, K. L., & Torino, G. C. (2007). Racial microaggressions and the Asian American experience. *Cultural Diversity and Ethnic Minority Psychology, 13*(1), 72–81.

Sue, D. W., & Sue, D. (2008). *Counseling the culturally diverse*. New York: Wiley.

Swendeman, D., Rotheram-Borus, M. J., Comulada, S., Weiss, R., & Ramos, M. E. (2006). Predictors of HIV-related stigma among young people living with HIV. *Health Psychology, 25*(4), 501–509.

Tewari, N., & Alvarez, A. N. (2009). *Asian American psychology: Current perspectives*. Mahwah, NJ: Lawrence Erlbaum Associates.

Toleran, D. E., Tran, P. D., Cabangun, B., Lam, J., Battle, R. S., & Gardiner, P. (2012). Substance use among Chinese, Filipino, and Vietnamese adult men living in San Jose, Daly City, and San Francisco, and its implications on ATOD prevention services. *Journal of ethnicity in substance abuse, 11*, 86–99.

Wilkinson, W. (1997). HIV/AIDS in Asian and Pacific Islander women. In N. Goldstein & J. Manlowe (Eds.), *The gender politics of HIV/AIDS in women: Perspectives on the pandemic in the United States* (pp. 168–187). New York: New York University Press.

Wolitski, R. J., Pals, S. L., Kidder, D. P., Courtenay-Quirk, C., & Holtgrave, D. R. (2009). The effects of HIV stigma on health, disclosure of HIV status, and risk behavior of homeless and unstably housed persons living with HIV. *AIDS and Behavior, 13*(6), 1222–1232.

Wong, F.Y., Nehl, E.J., Han, J.J., Huang, Z.J., Wu, Y., Young, D., …, MATH Study Consortium. (2012). HIV testing and management: Findings from a national sample of Asian/Pacific Islander men who have sex with men. Public Health Reports, 127, 186–194.

Wu, F. (2003). *Yellow: Race in America beyond Black and White*. New York: Basic Books.

Ye, J., Mack, D., Fry-Johnson, Y., & Parker, K. (2012). Health care access and utilization among US-born and foreign-born Asian Americans. *Journal of Immigrant and Minority Health, 14*, 731–737.

Yoo, H. C., Gee, G. C., Lowthrop, C. K., & Robertson, J. (2010). Self-reported racial discrimination and substance use among Asian Americans in Arizona. *Journal of Immigrant and Minority Health, 12*(5), 683–690.

Yu, D. D. (1999). *Clinician's guide to working with Asians and Pacific Islanders living with HIV*. Retrieved from http://www. aids-ed.org/pdf/curricula/clinicianguide-api.pdf.

Zaidi, I. F., Crepaz, N., Song, R., Wan, C. K., Lin, L. S., Hu, D. J., & Sy, F. S. (2005). Epidemiology of HIV/AIDS among Asians and Pacific Islanders in the United States. *AIDS Education and Prevention, 17*, 405–417.

Chapter 10
An Evolving Epidemic for African American and Latino HIV Positive Gay Men: Understanding the Sociocultural Contexts of Stigma, Marginalization, and Structural Inequalities

Leo Wilton

Introduction

Christopher is a 20-year-old Black gay man who grew up in Harlem in a close-knit family with his mother, younger brother, older sister, and maternal grandmother in the household. In terms of his cultural heritage, Christopher identifies as Caribbean and Afro-Latino in that his mother is from Jamaica and his father is from Puerto Rico. His mother met his father while he lived for some time in Jamaica. Christopher visits his father in Puerto Rico on occasion. His mother immigrated to the United States from Jamaica with their family when he was eight years old. During his formative years, Christopher attended public school in New York City and was enrolled in the "free lunch" program. He was a hard-working and well-liked student in school; however, there were several occasions where he was made fun of, picked on, pushed, and threatened by some of the older male students because of not adhering to perceived ideals of masculine gender norms (i.e., being referred to as a "sissy"). His mother often worked two part-time jobs over the years as a single mom raising three children. However, the majority of the household income came from public assistance. His mother found it challenging to obtain employment due to anti-immigrant sentiments in the United States.

Christopher is a sophomore majoring in history at City College in New York City. He really likes school and is considering a career in law. He is a popular and outgoing student at City College and participates in a number of student organizations, such

L. Wilton (✉)
Department of Human Development, College of Community and Public Affairs (CCPA),
State University of New York at Binghamton, Binghamton, NY, USA

Faculty of Humanities, University of Johannesburg, Johannesburg, South Africa
e-mail: lwilton@binghamton.edu

© Springer Science+Business Media LLC 2017   247
L. Wilton (ed.), *Understanding Prevention for HIV Positive Gay Men*,
DOI 10.1007/978-1-4419-0203-0_10

as the Caribbean Students Association, cricket team, and Thurgood Marshall Pre-Law Society. He spends a lot of time with friends both at school and in his neighborhood. During one of his courses, Christopher was intrigued to learn that he lives in a building directly across the street from where James Baldwin used to reside in Harlem. He receives financial aid and educational loans for tuition and participates in a work-study program that helps to provide some funds. He has had some part-time jobs while in college but is often in-between jobs.

Christopher attended a Baptist church with his family on Sundays while growing up. For the holidays, church members would bring his family food since they often struggled financially. One of Christopher's most memorable experiences in the Church involved some people approaching him and his mother after a service and commented, "We've been wondering about you Christopher. How come a good looking, handsome man like you does not have a girlfriend? Why haven't you settled down yet with a nice young woman? We have just the person for you." He was left feeling despondent. However, Christopher also recalled how his grandmother, after overhearing the conversation, immediately recognized what was happening and changed the nature of the discussion.

Although Christopher does not go to church on a regular basis at the current time, he very much values his relationship with God. He struggles with some of the teachings of the Church related to sexuality (e.g., same-gender practicing people being referred to as an "abomination"). One of the major tensions in Christopher's relationship with his mother involves him not routinely attending Church. However, Christopher always knew that he was attracted to men. He feels very close to his grandmother who has been supportive of his sexuality. He has not shared this information with his mother or siblings for fear of judgment and misunderstanding. At the same time, Christopher experiences challenges related to being the oldest or first-born son in his family based on cultural expectations from his father about establishing a family.

During his sophomore year at City College, Christopher met a young man named David during a Caribbean Students Association program. They enjoyed each other and spent a lot of time together. They were attracted to each other and shortly thereafter became romantically involved. After talking with friends, Christopher decided to be tested for HIV at the student health center on campus; this was his first HIV testing experience. He tested HIV negative. At this visit, Christopher inquired about PrEP (Pre-exposure prophylaxis) since his friends were talking about it. He was not sure about the health benefits of PrEP or how it worked. The health care staff indicated that PrEP was unnecessary for him; they also suggested that his student health insurance did not cover PrEP. David had shared with Christopher that he recently tested HIV negative and had not had sex without condoms during this period. After dating for a number of months, Christopher and David decided to be in an exclusive relationship. They decided not to use condoms during sex. After some months, they separated because the relationship was not working out.

The next year Christopher met another young man, Colin, on an online social media platform. They went on several dates before the relationship became more serious. Christopher and Colin decided that they were going to be in an exclusive relationship. They decided to get tested for HIV. Although Christopher initially received his first HIV test at the student health center, he opted to use a free clinic because of privacy and confidentiality concerns related to being on campus. He thought that it would be more anonymous at a free clinic. Colin went to his primary care provider to get tested for HIV. On the way to the clinic, Christopher was stopped by the police on the street based on the stop-question-and-frisk practice (commonly referred to as stop-and-frisk), which disproportionately racially profiles Black men in New York City (Newberry, 2017). During this procedure, police officers detain, question, and often conduct searches of people. Christopher experienced pervasive disrespect, humiliation, and contempt from the White police officers who ridiculed and used aggressive physical force with him. To say the least, his day was already encumbered with this hostile experience.

When he reached the clinic, Christopher explained to the front-line staff person that he was there to get tested for HIV. He experienced the front-line staff person interfacing with him with a "look of scorn" as if he was invisible. With a disrespectful tone, the front-line staff person directed Christopher to fill out some paperwork and wait until he is called by the nurse. He felt dismissed and that his concerns were not heard. Christopher observed that the front-line staff person was wearing a large gold cross necklace around her neck; he also noted a collection of religious parapher-nalia around her desk. Christopher was reminded of some of the negative experi-ences that he had in Church. He then looked around the crowded waiting room with lots of people. He felt very uncomfortable about the possibility of someone from his community seeing him at the clinic. After about one hour, he was seen by the nurse who also offered him sexually transmitted infection (STI) testing in addition to HIV testing.

When he finally received his test results, Christopher was in disbelief that he was diagnosed with HIV and syphilis—particularly since he had previously tested HIV negative. He remembered that David, his former boyfriend, had told him that he himself tested HIV negative. Christopher was upset and questioned how this could have occurred. He also pondered how he was going to share this information with his partner as well as his family. He was feeling alone, desolate, and downhearted. When he was waiting to be connected to care, Christopher picked up the phone and called David to share the results with him and to ask how this was possible because David was the only person he had anal sex without a condom. During the call, David disclosed to him that he tested positive for HIV within the last four months and was on medication. David told Christopher that he was too ashamed to call him to talk about it. David later explained that he had not realized he was in the window period during the time he was initially tested. David thought that he did not need to retest because he was "always careful" and that he had loved Christopher.

Later that evening, Christopher was scheduled to meet up with Colin at his home for their usual Friday night of "Netflix and chill." On the train ride over to Colin's apartment, a multitude of scenarios continuously played out in his mind about how he was going to disclose this information to Colin. Christopher arrived at Colin's place who was delighted to see him. He had ordered some food for him. Christopher opened up a conversation with Colin and shared the test results with him. Immediately the mood in the room changed. At that moment, Colin said to Christopher "I do not know if I can do this. I'm clean and I want to keep it that way." He ended by saying that "I think that you should leave." Christopher felt that his "world had turned upside down" with his diagnosis. He left Colin's apartment feeling distraught.

David called Christopher the following morning to check on him. He provided Christopher with lots of love and support. He started to talk with Christopher about his experiences of living with HIV and taking medicine. Christopher was concerned about getting into care. Christopher discussed his ongoing challenges about getting into care and taking his medicine at home. Over the next few months, they reconnected and developed a strong friendship. They supported each other based on being diagnosed with HIV. They reconnected because of similar experiences and the prior bond with each other. Christopher had been newly diagnosed and had limited social support to share this information. By reconnecting with David, Christopher would go with him to see his HIV care provider. They supported each other. They got really close. They decided to live together.

The narratives of Christopher, David, and Colin are part of a larger, ongoing, and systemic problem of stigma, marginalization, and structural inequalities experienced by African American and Latino HIV positive gay men and their partners. This overarching theme is interconnected to the critical role of understanding multilayered processes embedded in power relationships based on macro-level or structural disenfranchisement, while simultaneously, the importance of addressing micro-level processes that occur in the everyday based on cultural values and worldviews; cultural constructions of masculinity; gender role socialization; and social, religious, peer, family, and community norms. These narratives illuminate how structural barriers based on socioeconomic indicators (e.g., poverty, education, employment status, income), access to health care and treatment (e.g., un-/underinsured), housing and food instability, incarceration, racialized stigma and discrimination, sexuality-based stigma and discrimination, HIV stigma and discrimination, and immigration status affect the HIV care continuum for African American and Latino gay men. The narratives also point to the salience of strength-based frameworks in communities of color in the form of resiliency or what Bailey (2013) as illustrated as "intraventions" or prevention work that occurs organically within the context of communities for groups that have often experienced multiple forms of exclusion and marginalization.

Based on this context, there has been a critical void in research related to prevention and care for African American and Latino HIV positive gay men (Arreola et al., 2015; Ayala, Bingham, Kim, Wheeler, & Millett, 2012; Bogart, Landrine, Galvan, Wagner, & Klein, 2013; Bonacci & Holtgrave, 2016; Brewer et al., 2014; Galvan, Bogart, Klein, Wagner, & Chen, 2017; García, Lechuga, & Zea, 2012; Hussen, Andes, Gilliard, Del Rio, & Malebranche, 2015; Millett et al., 2012; Nieves-Lugo et al., 2017; Spikes et al., 2009; Zea, Reisen, Poppen, Bianchi, & Echeverry, 2005). Therefore, the primary objective of this chapter is to examine core socio-cultural contexts that influence prevention and care for African American and Latino HIV positive gay men. More specifically, this chapter will explore: (1) prevention and care-related outcomes for African American and Latino HIV positive gay men;

(2) health care delivery for African American and Latino HIV gay men; (3) role of health insurance; (4) theoretical approaches in prevention and care for African American and Latino HIV positive gay men; and (5) psychosocial support needs of African American and Latino HIV positive gay men. This chapter will be situated within culturally relevant frameworks for African American and Latino HIV positive gay men in articulating the need for a paradigm shift in the field of public health with an integration of core theoretical premises of interdisciplinarity, intersectionality, and structural inequalities.

African American and Latino HIV Positive Gay Men and Prevention and Care

Nearly four decades since the onset of the AIDS epidemic in the United States, African American and Latino men who have sex with men (MSM) have represented a significant disproportionate number of cases of HIV and AIDS (CDC, 2015a). It is estimated that 1 of 2 African American MSM and 1 of 4 Latino MSM will be diagnosed with HIV during the course of their lifetime if current epidemiologic trends persist without systematic interventions (CDC, 2016). Epidemiologic research has indicated that African American and Latino HIV positive gay men experience deleterious health outcomes related to the HIV continuum of care (e.g., early diagnosis, linkage to care, retention in care, and viral suppression) (Hall, Holtgrave, Tang, & Rhodes, 2013; Poteat, White, & van Griensven, 2014; Rosenberg, Millett, Sullivan, Del Rio, & Curran, 2014; Seth, Wang, Collins, et al., 2015; Vermund, 2017). Research has also shown that African American and Latino HIV positive gay men have inadequate access to culturally informed HIV care and treatment (Bouris et al., 2013; Cahill et al., 2017; Levy et al., 2014; Martinez et al., 2017; Millett et al., 2012; Peek et al., 2016). Both Healthy People 2020 and the National HIV/AIDS Strategy have recognized African American and Latino MSM as a priority population for addressing HIV-related health inequities (e.g., reducing new HIV infections, increasing HIV care access, and reducing undiagnosed HIV infections) (Millett et al., 2010; Office of National AIDS Policy, 2015; U.S. Department of Health and Human Services, 2015).

Further, prior research has shown that several core factors have influenced HIV-related health inequities for African American and Latino MSM, such as insufficient health care (inadequate HIV prevention and treatment access) (Cahill et al., 2017; Freese, Padwa, Oeser, Rutkowski, & Schulte, 2017; Millett et al., 2012; Poteat et al., 2014; Rosenberg et al., 2014), high undiagnosed HIV/STI (sexually transmitted infection) rates within their sexual networks (Hickson et al., 2017; Latkin et al., 2017; Scott et al., 2015; Tieu, Nandi, Hoover, et al., 2016), not testing for HIV/STIs on a regular basis (e.g., at least once a year or every 3–6 months for those who indicate greater HIV risk behavior as per CDC HIV testing guidelines) (García et al., 2012; Hall et al., 2013; Joseph et al., 2014; Mannheimer et al., 2014), being unaware of their HIV status (Mayer, Wang, Koblin, et al., 2014), acute HIV infection (Hall et al., 2013), and receiving an advanced HIV disease diagnosis (i.e., AIDS) when initially being tested for HIV (Hall et al., 2013). Acute HIV infection and advanced HIV disease have been shown to result in increased viral load (i.e., the amount of the HIV virus in the body) and decreased CD4 levels, reflecting greater HIV disease burden for African American and Latino gay men (Hall et al., 2013). Moreover, research has indicated that other structural barriers, including HIV-related stigma/discrimination in addition to poverty, influence HIV-related health inequities among African American and Latino gay men (Mena, Crosby, & Geter, 2017; Nelson, Wilton, Moineddin, et al., 2016; Quinn et al., 2017; Rodríguez-Díaz, Jovet-Toledo, Ortiz-Sánchez, Rodríguez-Santiago, & Vargas-Molina, 2015; Zea et al., 2005).

African American and Latino Gay Men and HIV-Related Health Care Delivery

One domain that can provide a more comprehensive understanding of HIV-related health inequities for African American and Latino gay men involves HIV-related health care delivery (DeGroote, Korhonen, & Shouse, 2016; Freese et al., 2017; Garcia et al., 2016; Levy et al., 2014; Malebranche, Peterson, Fullilove, & Stackhouse, 2004; Quinn, Voisin, Bouris, & Schneider, 2016). This contemporary significant public health challenge has posed critical implications for the development and implementation of HIV-related health care delivery to address the substantial HIV-related health inequities among African American and Latino HIV positive gay men (Cahill et al., 2017; Levy et al., 2014). In particular, HIV prevention research suggests that high impact prevention services are cost effective in addressing the HIV epidemic among vulnerable populations including communities of color (Gwadz et al., 2017).

In terms of HIV testing and service delivery program data from 61 US health department jurisdictions, a recent CDC (2015b) report found that more than half (54.9%) of all newly identified HIV positive persons (i.e., new positives) were African Americans. In addition, among African Americans, African American MSM had one of the highest observed percentages of newly HIV diagnosed populations (CDC, 2015b). Furthermore, according to the CDC report (2015b), "Broader implementation of routing HIV screening and HIV testing targeted towards populations at high risk can help identify persons with undiagnosed HIV infection and link these persons to HIV medical care and prevention services. Linkage to medical care and referrals to HIV partner services and HIV prevention services among Blacks could be improved" (p. 87). Taken together, these trends need to be considered and pose critical considerations for the development and implementation of HIV-related health care delivery programs and services to strengthen systems that address unmet service needs for African American and Latino HIV gay men (e.g., comprehensive HIV testing, linkage and retention to care, health care engagement, and adherence prevention interventions (Freese et al., 2017; Friedman et al., 2017; Meanley et al., 2015).

Further, African American and Latino HIV gay men's HIV-related health care delivery needs to be considered within the broader context of the Patient Protection and Affordable Care Act (ACA), which was enacted into law in 2010 (CDC, 2015c). The ACA, including the U.S. Supreme Court ruling in the *National Federation of Independent Business v. Sebelius* legal case, established a significant milestone for health care reform in the United States (U.S. Department of Health and Human Services, n.d.). The ACA provides core provisions that address fundamental health care access inequalities (e.g., Medicaid expansion, health insurance exchanges, subsidies for people within 400% of the Federal Poverty Line, individual health insurance coverage requirement) for people in the United States (U.S. Department of Health and Human Services, n.d.). For example, one of the overall aims of Medicaid expansion involves providing insurance coverage for individuals within 133% of the Federal Poverty Line (FPL) (Robert Wood Johnson Foundation, 2013).

The Role of Health Insurance

There has been considerable discussion about the role of health insurance in the United States related to HIV care (Millett et al., 2010). Health insurance status can affect the health status of African American and Latino HIV gay men in multiple ways. For example, Alexander et al. (2014) points out that health insurance status has an impact on being able to access health care and preventative services while, at the same time, being uninsured often results in poor or negative health outcomes, increased frequencies of hospitalizations, and advanced disease diagnosis at the time of when first accessing health care services. Moreover, according to Alexander et al. (2014), current research indicates that uninsured individuals are more likely to have challenges in accessing health care and are more likely to experience sickness, injury, or premature death, than those individuals with health care insurance. Furthermore, with the Affordable Care Act, varying dimensions of HIV-related health care inequalities have been ameliorated based on provisions such as Medicaid development/expansion and subsidies for individuals associated with the Federal Poverty Line (Cahill et al., 2017).

Contextualizing Sex in African American and Latino Communities: The Role of Sexual Contexts and Networks

Current research has demonstrated that a number of sexual contexts have influenced HIV-related inequities for African American and Latino HIV positive gay men (Fields et al., 2015). Some of these contexts have related to the characteristics of sexual partners (Tieu et al., 2016), the use of the Internet in interfacing with sexual partners (e.g., sexual partners in cyberspace) (e.g., Senn et al., 2017), the use of substances (e.g., alcohol and illicit drugs before or during sex) (Martinez et al., 2016), and perceived safer sex strategies (e.g., serosorting, seropositioning, withdrawal before ejaculation) (Wilton et al., 2015). One of the strengths in conducting formative research on emerging trends and contextual factors associated with HIV sexual risk behavior in African American and Latino HIV gay men is that findings can be used to contribute to current scientific knowledge and the development and implementation of efficacious prevention and care strategies. However, one of the research challenges in this area relates to the need to incorporate culturally relevant methodologies based on strong collaborations with practitioners affiliated with community-based organizations. This represents a major component of culturally responsive prevention work as communities provide perspectives that are relevant to the experiences of MSM of Color.

HIV prevention research has posited that sexual networks have had a significant impact on the disproportionate rate of HIV prevalence in MSM of Color communities (Latkin et al., 2017). One factor that has been shown to influence sexual networks involves the influence of partner characteristics on the incidence and prevalence for African American and Latino HIV positive gay men. For example, some studies (e.g., Hickson et al., 2017) have shown that MSM of Color tend to have romantic/sexual partners reflective of their racial/ethnic backgrounds (Tieu et al., 2016). The core issue here is that HIV-related inequities heighten because research has demonstrated that African American and Latino MSM have higher frequencies of STIs, lower frequencies of consistent HIV testing, disproportionate rates of HIV infection, and higher levels of unrecognized HIV infection (Mayer et al., 2014). In terms of African American and Latino MSM, acute HIV infection has been shown to result in higher viral load and lower CD4 levels, which serve as a critical factor for HIV seroconversion (e.g., Hall et al., 2013). Therefore, African American and Latino MSM have experienced a substantially higher risk of acquiring and transmitting HIV due to the high concentration of HIV in the sexual networks of their communities.

Experiences of Violence in the Context of HIV Prevention for African American and Latino Communities

Studies have provided empirical support for examining the relationship between multiplicative forms of violence, including childhood sexual abuse (CSA), intimate partner violence (IPV), and other kinds of victimization in relation to HIV sexual risk behavior for African American and Latino HIV positive gay men (Toro-Alfonso & Rodriguez-Madera, 2004; Williams, Wilton, Magnus, et al., 2015). These areas of scholarly inquiry have been significantly understudied in MSM of Color, although some research has emerged in this area (Arreola et al., 2015). For example, in a qualitative study of childhood sexual abuse (CSA) in Black MSM, findings indicated a 32% prevalence rate in CSA, based on a sample from three geographic regions in the United States (Fields, Malebranche, & Feist-Price, 2008). Also, according to Fields et al. (2008), the contexts of CSA involved: (1) the experience of CSA from a familial individual (e.g., older male relative); (2) the attribution of "same sex desire" as a result of the experience of CSA; and (3) psychological distress (e.g., depression, suicidality) and substance use due to CSA. In another study, Black and Latino gay- and non-gay identifying MSM who reported histories of CSA, which often were connected to a history of trauma, related to HIV sexual risk behavior (Williams et al., 2004). Moreover, Toro-Alfonso & Rodriguez-Madera (2004) showed that IPV within relationships was related to HIV-related inequities in Latino MSM.

These research investigations provide empirical data for the significance of developing research studies to further examine the social contexts of how the experience of violence serves as a structural determinant to prevention and care. Moreover, the implications of these studies for both medical and mental health providers relate to the development and implementation of mechanisms to assess violence-related experiences, particularly within the context of how these dimensions relate to HIV prevention and care.

The Role of Immigration on African American and Latino HIV Positive Gay Men

The role of immigration status on the sexual health of African American and Latino HIV positive gay men has been an understudied domain in research on prevention and care (Carrillo, 2001, 2017; Mizuno, Borkowf, Ayala, Carballo-Diéguez, & Millett, 2015; Rhodes et al., 2012; Solorio, Norton-Shelpuk, Forehand, Martinez, & Aguirre, 2014). Much of the scholarly work in this area has focused on the experiences of Latino MSM (Martinez et al., 2016) with a void in studies on Caribbean (e.g., English-speaking) MSM and African MSM. Significantly, the process of immigration has been a critical factor in understanding how cultural worldviews (e.g., cultural values and beliefs) influence HIV-related inequities as well as the impact of social structures on access to health care, including prevention and care, for immigrant groups (Organista, Carrillo, & Ayala, 2004).

Ramirez et al. (2008) found that that HIV prevalence rates were significantly higher in a sample of Latino gay and bisexual men and transgender individuals in San Francisco that were born within the United States as compared to those respondents who were born outside of the United States; however, findings also demonstrated that HIV prevalence rates were higher for those respondents in Chicago whose place of birth was outside the United States as compared to individuals whose place of birth was in the United States. In a study of Latino MSM from Miami who were born outside of the United States, findings showed that higher levels of psychological distress and substance use (e.g., club drugs), greater number of sexual partners, having an HIV positive status (e.g., at the onset of immigration), and a higher level of acculturation to US culture related to HIV sexual risk behavior (e.g., condomless anal intercourse) (Akin et al., 2008).

This emerging area of research provides considerable implications for increasing the scholarly focus on the experiences and processes associated with immigration for MSM of Color that explore the complexities of the social contexts of sexuality and how these factors relate to sexual health (Carrillo, 2001, 2017; Mizuno et al., 2015). In terms of immigration, contextual factors involving identity (e.g., racial, gender, and sexual identities) as well as stigma and discrimination (e.g., based on immigration status) need to be addressed in HIV prevention research and care services for African American and Latino HIV positive gay men (Solorio et al., 2014). Indeed, a sustained emphasis on addressing how social structures have an impact on health care inequities for MSM of Color are critically significant, especially those that examine the role of discrimination based on legal status (e.g., undocumented individuals) in the United States (Arreola et al., 2015). Also, the development, implementation, and assessment of culturally congruent HIV prevention and care services, including the provision of linguistically competent services, needs to be integrated into HIV prevention and care (Solorio et al., 2014).

Psychosocial Support Needs for African American and Latino HIV Positive Gay Men

The current state of scholarly research regarding psychosocial issues for African American and Latino HIV positive gay men remains understudied (Bogart et al., 2011; Choi et al., 2013; Graham et al., 2009; Rodríguez-Díaz et al., 2015; Williams et al., 2015). According to the US Surgeon General's Report, people of color have experienced barriers in accessing quality mental health services and care and have not been adequately represented in research in the area of mental health (US DHHS, 2001). Similarly, MSM of Color have reported dissatisfaction with mental health services as a result of structural barriers including but not limited to heterosexism and homophobia (Fields et al., 2015). Further, much of the extant research on the influence of racial/ethnic discrimination on mental health for people of color utilizing population-based studies has found that the experience of racial/ethnic discrimination relates to increased psychological distress for people of color, including diagnosis of major depression, generalized anxiety disorder, and onset of substance use (e.g., Williams et al., 2003). Similarly, population-based studies of LGBT communities have shown that perceived discrimination (e.g., lifetime and daily discrimination) had a negative impact on their quality of life in addition to increases in current psychological distress and mental health disorders (Mays and Cochran, 2001; Mays et al., 2017). Other population-based studies have reported a higher prevalence of mental health disorders, suicidal ideation, and substance use among lesbian, gay, and bisexual individuals as compared to heterosexual individuals (e.g., Blosnich et al., 2016; Gilman et al., 2001; Cochran et al., 2004). In this regard, population-based studies of LGBT communities of color are needed to ascertain characteristics of mental health utilization as well as the prevalence of mental health and substance use morbidity (e.g., Cochran et al., 2004). Yet, there has been a significant void in population-based studies that have focused on MSM of Color.

Theoretical Approaches in Prevention and Care for African American and Latino HIV Positive Gay Men

A core dimension in addressing HIV-related health inequities for African American and Latino HIV positive gay men involves the development of theoretical frameworks that are nested within culturally relevant conceptualizations (Ayala et al., 2012; Bailey, 2014; Mays, Cochran, & Zamudio, 2004; Reisen, Brooks, Zea, Poppen, & Bianchi, 2013; Rodríguez-Díaz et al., 2015). In this context, a critical analytic framework for HIV prevention research—including theory, methodologies, and praxis—incorporates a connection to macro-level or socio-structural contexts (e.g., legal, political, educational, and health care systems). Thus, a major part of this work calls for a paradigm shift that links prevention and care within interdisciplinary and intersectional and interdisciplinary frameworks that are relevant to the lived experiences of African American and Latino HIV positive gay men. In particular, the concepts of stigma, marginalization, and structural inequalities provide a theoretical framework to examine the complexities of the AIDS epidemic, as situated in the everyday, lived experiences of MSM of color living with HIV.

Building on the work of Cohen (1999), these fundamental ideas provide a conceptual framework for addressing asymmetrical power relationships (i.e., power inequalities) in communities of color, including those that incorporate sociohistorical and -political experiences of "exclusion and marginalization" (e.g., axes related to race/ethnicity, gender, sexuality, social class, and immigration status). Further, according to Cohen (1999), a major component of these core concepts relate to the duality of examining macro (e.g., external processes) and micro (e.g., internal processes) structures that have an impact on communities of color in relation to the AIDS epidemic. For example, macro-level processes involve marginalization associated with larger social structures (e.g., structural inequalities based on legal, political, economic, and educational social structures such as institutionalized racism) and micro-level processes relate to "secondary marginalization" within communities of color (e.g., based on gender and sexuality) (Cohen, 1999). Therefore, the integration of transformative discourses in the area of AIDS that provide intersectional and interdisciplinary analyses serve as significant interventions in the field of public health. As such, this scholarly work must be at the center of the discourse through incorporating critical, innovative, and transformative analyses that interrogate and challenge hegemonic, Eurocentric, patriarchal, and hetero-normative discourses that pathologize communities of color.

Core theoretical paradigms in the areas of public health and social science research that relate to HIV prevention have been primarily based on Western/ Eurocentric theoretical or conceptual frameworks that focus on individual behavior (e.g., social cognitive theoretical frameworks) (Malebranche et al., 2004). As a result, the production of knowledge in HIV prevention research has often been shaped within a singular disciplinary context, thus maintaining a disconnection from transformative scholarly inquiries as well as the sociocultural realities of the lived experiences of African American and Latino HIV positive gay men's communities. Thus, building on the work of Collins (2005), as situated through an intersectional theoretical conceptualization, one of the major problematic implications of this logic is that the multiple identities of MSM of Color (e.g., racial, gender, and sexual identities) have been negatively constructed and pathologized through theoretical frameworks that have not adequately integrated the sociohistorical, -political, -economic, and -cultural contexts that have been integral to the cultural specificities of their lived experiences (Ayala et al., 2012; Bailey, 2014; Mays et al., 2004).

Building on interdisciplinary and intersectional theoretical approaches, an integral component to the study of health inequities in MSM of Color communities is the incorporation and application of epistemological/theoretical frameworks and methodologies based on cultural studies (e.g., African/African Diaspora/Caribbean Studies, Latino/a Studies), gender studies, queer/LGBT [lesbian/gay/bisexual/transgender] studies, and sexuality studies. One of the objectives in utilizing the scholarly work of these areas in the study of health inequities relates to the development of epistemological/theoretical frameworks that provide the basis for incorporating the sociohistorical, -political, -economic, and -cultural contexts that have been integral in communities of color. Theoretical and methodological approaches based on these scholarly areas work to juxtapose theory and practice that is grounded in culturally relevant conceptualizations, which are fundamental to the lived experiences of African American and Latino HIV positive gay men. These areas provide a critical approach to the work on health disparities that engage a critique of service at macro- and micro-levels with respect to the sociopolitical processes that influence structural inequalities in MSM of Color communities.

Connected to stigma, marginalization, and structural inequalities, recent research has examined the influence of sociocultural factors on HIV-related equities in MSM of Color (Ayala et al., 2012; Han et al., 2015). In one study, Diaz et al. (2004) have incorporated the concept of social oppression as a core domain to account, in part, for the disproportionate health-related disparities in HIV based on their work with a probability sample of 912 Latino gay men surveyed from three US cities. Diaz et al. (2004) provided an intersectional, tripartite model that found empirical support for the impact of sociocultural factors (e.g., racism, homophobia, and poverty) on HIV sexual risk behavior in Latino gay men. Findings demonstrated that social oppression based on racism, poverty, and homophobia related to sexual experiences that provided the context for HIV sexual risk behavior. Specifically, higher levels of social oppression (e.g., racism, poverty, and homophobia) and psychological distress were predictive of Latino gay men engaging in risky sexual situations.

Further, based on this work, social oppression influenced HIV sexual risk behavior in that Latino gay men were more likely to engage in sexual experiences that were challenging to negotiate safer sexual practices. For example, according to Diaz et al. (2004), "Men who were more discriminated and psychologically distressed were more likely to participate in sexual situations under the influence of drugs or alcohol, to engage in sex as a way to alleviate anxiety and stress, and to be with partners who resisted condom use, among others" (p. 265). Taken together, the experience of challenging "sexual situations" mediated the influence of social oppression (e.g., racism, poverty, and homophobia) on HIV sexual risk behavior (Diaz et al., 2004). These research investigations provide theoretical and empirical support in examining the impact of racism, homophobia, poverty, and immigration status as these intersectional domains manifest in the lives of MSM of Color.

Sociocultural Factors in Relation to Mental Health for MSM of Color

Building of the work of several scholars (e.g., Diaz et al., 2001), stigma has been a core critical issue for MSM of Color. Specifically, the negotiation of racial, gender, and sexual identities juxtaposed with experiences of individual and institutionalized racism and homophobia have worked as relevant culturally specific psychosocial issues for MSM of Color (Bird & Voisin, 2013; Choi et al., 2011; Quinn et al., 2017). For example, according to Wheeler (2006), Black MSM have to work through the stressors associated with being a black male (e.g., racism, unemployment, incarceration, health issues) and that of being emotionally and/or sexually attracted to the men (e.g., gender role expectations). A significant part of this work relates to the negotiation of relationships with significant others including family, friends, and sexual partners. Further, in a qualitative study of Black and Latino HIV positive MSM who reported a history of childhood sexual abuse, findings showed that the sociocultural context of the men's lives was central to their lived experiences. For example, predominant themes related to sexual identity, role of family and cultural expectations regarding children, gender role socialization, influence of substance use, religiosity and spirituality, and HIV-related stigma, marginalization, and barriers to HIV care (Williams et al., 2004).

Based on the work of Meyer (2007), the sociocultural model of minority stress in lesbian, gay, and bisexual (LGB) communities has provided a theoretical framework to examine the relationship between chronic stress and stigmatization, particularly as related to psychosocial distress. In particular, through the use of a distal-proximal domain, Meyer posited that the experiences of "minority" stressors for LGB individuals (e.g., expectations of stigma, internalized homophobia, and experiences of prejudice and discrimination) relate to mental health outcomes. As part of minority stress processes, distal refers to experiences of prejudice, discrimination and violence based on sexual identity and proximal relates to experiences associated with "expectations of rejection, concealment, and internalized homophobia" (p. 248). Additionally, with a specific focus on MSM of Color (e.g., Latino gay and bisexual men), researchers have developed theoretical models to examine the effects of social discrimination (e.g., racism, homophobia, poverty) in relation to psychological distress and resiliency (Diaz et al., 2001).

Further, the experiences of HIV-related stigma and discrimination both within and external to MSM of Color communities have served as relevant psychosocial issues for MSM of Color. For example, in a study of 301 Latino gay and bisexual men, Zea et al. (2005) found that HIV disclosure was predictive of respondents reporting higher levels of social support which had an impact on their lower depression and self-esteem. Within this context, MSM of Color living with HIV and AIDS have to negotiate their HIV positive status involving issues of disclosure to romantic and sexual partners, families, friends, health care providers, as well as other significant others (Wheeler, 2005). HIV positive MSM of Color also have to manage the stressors of stigma within MSM Communities of Color (e.g., issues of rejection and discrimination). Therefore, HIV prevention interventions need to address the stigmatization of HIV positive MSM of Color by HIV negative MSM of Color. For example, Diaz (2007) found high levels of HIV-related stigma among Latino HIV negative MSM and high levels of psychological distress associated with the experiences of HIV-related stigma for Latino HIV positive MSM.

Conclusions

African American and Latino HIV gay men have substantial HIV-related health inequities in the United States. There has been a critical void in culturally relevant conceptual frameworks utilized in research on HIV-related health inequities for African American and Latino HIV positive gay men. Traditional models used in research on HIV-related health disparities have not integrated to a substantial degree culturally relevant conceptualizations at the core of the analyses. This research poses fundamental implications regarding the development and implementation of efficacious public health strategies in addressing the AIDS epidemic for African American and Latino gay men living with HIV and AIDS in that the focus has shifted from individual behavior to include an examination of the structural factors that influence HIV-related health inequities. In this context, the next steps in ameliorating HIV-related health inequities for African American and Latino HIV positive gay men involves the development and implementation of culturally relevant HIV-related health care systems that integrate a holistic approach for prevention and care.

Effective HIV-related health care delivery systems, programs, and services are urgently needed to ameliorate the substantial HIV-related health inequities among African American and Latino gay men living with HIV and AIDS. Moreover, based on core socio-structural factors that influence HIV-related health inequities for African American and Latino HIV positive gay men (e.g., poverty, education, employment status, income, access to health care and treatment [e.g., un-/underinsured], housing and food instability, incarceration, racialized stigma and discrimination, sexuality-based stigma and discrimination, HIV stigma and discrimination; and immigration status), the strengthening of the development and implementation of HIV-related health care delivery is needed to address these substantial HIV-related health inequities for these communities that experience multiple forms of marginalization.

References

Akin, M., Fernandez, M. I., Bowen, G. S., & Warren, J. C. (2008). HIV risk behaviors of Latin American and Caribbean men who have sex with men in Miami, Florida, USA. *Pan American Journal of Public Health, 23*, 341–348.

Alexander, J. L., LaRosa, J. H., Bader, H., Garfield, S., & Alexander, W. J. (2014). *New dimensions in women's health* (6th ed.). Burlington, MA: Jones & Barlett Learning.

Arreola, S., Santos, G. M., Beck, J., Sundararaj, M., Wilson, P. A., Hebert, P., ... Ayala, G. (2015). Sexual stigma, criminalization, investment, and access to HIV services among men who have sex with men worldwide. *AIDS and Behavior, 19*(2), 227–234.

Ayala, G., Bingham, T., Kim, J., Wheeler, D. P., & Millett, G. A. (2012). Modeling the impact of social discrimination and financial hardship on the sexual risk of HIV among Latino and Black men who have sex with men. *American Journal of Public Health, 102*(Suppl 2), S242–S249.

Bailey, M. M. (2013). *Butch queens up in pumps: Gender, performance, and ballroom culture in Detroit.* Ann Arbor, MI: University of Michigan Press.

Bailey, M. M. (2014). Engendering space: Ballroom culture and the spatial practice of possibility in Detroit. *Gender, Place, and Culture, 21*(4), 489–507.

Bird, J. D., & Voisin, D. R. (2013). "You're an open target to be abused": A qualitative study of stigma and HIV self-disclosure among Black men who have sex with men. *American Journal of Public Health, 103*(12), 2193–2199.

Blosnich, J. R., Nasuti, L. J., Mays, V. M., & Cochran, S. D. (2016). Suicidality and sexual orientation: Characteristics of symptom severity, disclosure, and timing across the life course. *American Journal of Orthopsychiatry, 86*(1), 69–78.

Bogart, L. M., Landrine, H., Galvan, F. H., Wagner, G. J., & Klein, D. J. (2013). Perceived discrimination and physical health among HIV-positive Black and Latino men who have sex with men. *AIDS and Behavior, 17*(4), 1431–1441.

Bogart, L. M., Wagner, G. J., Galvan, F. H., Landrine, H., Klein, D. J., & Sticklor, L. A. (2011). Perceived discrimination and mental health symptoms among Black men with HIV. *Cultural Diversity and Ethnic Minority Psychology, 17*(3), 295–302.

Bonacci, F. A., & Holtgrave, D. R. (2016). Unmet HIV service needs among Hispanic men who have sex with men in the United States. *AIDS and Behavior, 20*(10), 2444–2451.

Bouris, A., Voisin, D., Pilloton, M., Flatt, N., Eavou, R., Hampton, K., ... Schneider J. A. (2013). Project nGage: Network supported HIV care engagement for younger Black men who have sex with men and transgender persons. *International AIDS Clinical Research, 4.* doi: 10.4172/2155-6113.1000236.

Brewer, R. A., Magnus, M., Kuo, I., Wang, L., Liu, T. Y., & Mayer, K. H. (2014). Exploring the relationship between incarceration and HIV among Black men who have sex with men in the United States. *Journal of Acquired Immune Deficiency Syndromes, 65*(2), 218–225.

Cahill, S., Trieweiler, S., Guidry, J., Rash, N., Stamper, L., Conron, K., ... Lowery, P. (2017). High rates of access to health care, disclosure of sexuality and gender identity to providers among house and ball community members in New York City. *Journal of Homosexuality.* doi: 10.1080/00918369.2017.1328221.

Carrillo, H. (2001). *The night is young: Sexuality in Mexico in the time of AIDS*. Chicago: University of Chicago Press.

Carrillo, H. (2017). *Pathways of desire: The sexual migration of Mexican gay men*. Chicago: University of Chicago Press.

Centers for Disease Control and Prevention. (2015a). Diagnoses of HIV infection in the United States and dependent areas, 2014. *HIV Surveillance Report, 26*, 1–114. Retrieved from https://www.cdc.gov/hiv/pdf/library/reports/surveillance/cdc-hiv-surveillance-report-2015-vol-27.pdf.

Centers for Disease Control and Prevention. (2015b). HIV testing and service delivery among Blacks or African Americans—61 health department jurisdictions, United States, 2013. *Morbidity and Mortality Weekly Report, 64*, 87–90.

Centers for Disease Control and Prevention. (2015c). *The Affordable Care Act helps people living with HIV/AIDS*. Retrieved from: http://www.cdc.gov/hiv/policies/aca.html.

Centers for Disease Control and Prevention. (2016). *Lifetime risk of HIV diagnosis by race/ethnicity*. Retrieved from https://www.cdc.gov/nchhstp/newsroom/images/2016/croi_lifetime_risk_msm_race_ethnicity.jpg.

Choi, K. H., Han, C. S., Paul, J., & Ayala, G. (2011). Strategies for managing racism and homophobia among U.S. ethnic and racial minority men who have sex with men. *AIDS Education and Prevention, 23*(2), 145–158.

Choi, K. H., Paul, J., Ayala, G., Boylan, R., & Gregorich, S. E. (2013). Experiences of discrimination and their impact on the mental health among African American, Asian and Pacific Islander, and Latino men who have sex with men. *American Journal of Public Health, 103*(5), 868–874.

Cochran, S. D., Ackerman, D., Mays, V. M., & Ross, M. W. (2004). Prevalence of non-medical drug use and dependence among homosexually active men and women in the US population. *Addiction, 99*, 989–998.

Cohen, C. (1999). *The boundaries of Blackness: AIDS and the breakdown of Black politics*. Chicago: University of Chicago Press.

Collins, P. H. (2005). *Black sexual politics: African Americans, gender, and the new racism*. New York, NY: Routledge Press.

Diaz, R. (2007). *In our own backyard: HIV/AIDS stigmatization in the Latino gay community. Sexual inequalities and social justice* (pp. 50–65). Berkeley: University of California Press.

Diaz, R. M., Ayala, G., & Bein, E. (2004). Sexual risk as an outcome of social oppression: Data from a probability sample of Latino gay men in three US cities. *Cultural Diversity and Ethnic Minority Psychology, 10*, 255–267.

Diaz, R. M., Ayala, G., Bein, E., & Henne, J. (2001). The impact of homophobia, poverty, and racism on the mental health of gay and bisexual Latino men: Findings from 3 US cities. *American Journal of Public Health, 91*, 927–931.

DeGroote, N. P., Korhonen, L. C., & Shouse, R. L. (2016). Unmet need for ancillary services among men who have sex with men and who are receiving HIV medical care-United States, 2013-2014. *Mortality and Morbidity Weekly Report, 65*(37), 1004–1007.

Fields, E. L., Bogart, L. M., Smith, K. C., Malebranche, D. J., Ellen, J., & Schuster, M. A. (2015). "I always felt I had to prove my manhood": Homosexuality, masculinity, gender role strain, and HIV risk among young Black men who have sex with men. *American Journal of Public Health, 105*, 122–131.

Fields, S. D., Malebranche, D., & Feist-Price, S. (2008). Childhood sexual abuse in Black men who have sex with men: Results from three qualitative studies. *Cultural Diversity and Ethnic Minority Psychology, 14*(4), 385–390.

Freese, T. E., Padwa, H., Oeser, B. T., Rutkowski, B. A., & Schulte, M. T. (2017). Real-world strategies to engage and retain racial-ethnic minority young men who have sex with men in HIV prevention services. *AIDS Patient Care and STDs, 31*(6), 275–281.

Friedman, M. R., Coulter, R. W., Silvestre, A. J., Stall, R., Teplin, L., Shoptaw, S., … Plankey, M. W. (2017). Someone to count on: Social support as an effect modifier of viral load suppression in a prospective cohort study. *AIDS Care, 29*(4), 469–480.

Galvan, F. H., Bogart, L. M., Klein, D. J., Wagner, G. J., Chen, Y.T. (2017). Medical mistrust as a key mediator in the association between perceived discrimination and adherence to antiretroviral therapy among HIV positive Latino men. *Journal of Behavioral Medicine*. doi: 10.1007/s10865-017-9843-1.

García, L. I., Lechuga, J., & Zea, M. C. (2012). Testing comprehensive models of disclosure of sexual orientation in HIV-positive Latino men who have sex with men (MSM). *AIDS Care*, *24*(9), 1087–1091.

Garcia, J., Parker, C., Parker, R. G., Wilson, P. A., Philbin, M., & Hirsch, J. S. (2016). Psychosocial implications of homophobia and HIV stigma in social support networks: Insights for high-impact HIV prevention among Black men who have sex with men. *Health Education & Behavior*, *43*(2), 217–225.

Gilman, S. E., Cochran, S. D., Mays, V. M., Hughes, M., Ostrow, D., & Kessler, R. C. (2001). Risk of psychiatric disorders among individuals reporting same-sex sexual partners in the national comobidity survey. *American Journal of Public Health*, *91*, 933–939.

Graham, L. F., Braithwaite, K., Spikes, P., Stephens, C. F., & Edu, U. F. (2009). Exploring the mental health of Black men who have sex with men. *Community Mental Health Journal*, *45*(4), 272–282.

Gwadz, M. V., Collins, L. M., Cleland, C. M., Leonard, N. R., Wilton, L., Gandhi, M., ... Ritchie, A. S. (2017). Using the multiphase optimization strategy (MOST) to optimize an HIV care continuum intervention for vulnerable populations: A study protocol. *BMC Public Health*, *17*(1), 383. doi:10.1186/s12889-017-4279-7

Hall, H. I., Holtgrave, D. R., Tang, T., & Rhodes, P. (2013). HIV transmission in the United States: Considerations of viral load, risk behavior, and health disparities. *AIDS and Behavior*, *17*(5), 1632–1636.

Han, C. S., Ayala, G., Paul, J. P., Boylan, R., Gregorich, S. E., & Choi, K. H. (2015). Stress and coping with racism and their role in sexual risk for HIV among African American, Asian/Pacific Islander, and Latino men who have sex with men. *Archives of Sexual Behavior*, *44*(2), 411–420.

Hickson, D. A., Mena, L. A., Wilton, L., Tieu, H. V., Koblin, B. A., Cummings, V., ... Mayer, K. H. (2017). Sexual networks, dyadic characteristics, and HIV acquisition and transmission behaviors among Black men who have sex with men in 6 US cities. *American Journal of Epidemiology*, *185*, 786–800.

Hussen, S. a., Andes, K., Gilliard, D., Del Rio, C., & Malebranche, D. J. (2015). Transition to adulthood and antiretroviral adherence among HIV-positive Black men who have sex with men. *American Journal of Public Health*, *105*, 725–731.

Joseph, H. A., Belcher, L., O'Donell, L., Fernandez, M. I., Spikes, P. S., & Flores, S. A. (2014). HIV testing among sexually active Hispanic/Latino MSM in Miami-Dade County and New York City: Opportunities for increasing acceptance and frequency of testing. *Health Promotion and Practice*, *15*(6), 867–880.

Latkin, C. A., Van Tieu, H., Fields, S., Hanscom, B. S., Connor, M., Hanscom, B., ... Koblin, B. A. (2017). Social network factors as correlates and predictors of high depressive symptoms among Black men who have sex with men in HPTN 061. *AIDS and Behavior*, *21*(4), 1163–1170.

Levy, M. E., Wilton, L., Phillips, G., 2nd, Glick, S. N., Kuo, I., Brewer, R. A., ... Magnus, M. (2014). Understanding structural barriers to accessing HIV testing and prevention services among Black men who have sex with men (BMSM) in the United States. *AIDS and Behavior*, *18*(5), 972–996.

Malebranche, D. J., Peterson, J. L., Fullilove, R. E., & Stackhouse, R. W. (2004). Race and sexual identity: Perceptions about medical culture and healthcare among Black men who have sex with men. *Journal of the National Medical Association*, *96*, 97–107.

Mannheimer, S. B., Wang, L., Wilton, L., Van Tieu, H., Del Rio, C., Buchbinder, S., ... Mayer, K. H. (2014). Infrequent HIV testing and late HIV diagnosis are common among a cohort of Black men who have sex with men in 6 US cities. *Journal of Acquired Immune Deficiency Syndromes*, *67*(4), 438–445.

Martinez, O., Arreola, S., Wu, E., Muñoz-Laboy, M., Levine, E. C., Rutledge, S. E., … Carballo-Diéguez, A. (2016). Syndemic factors associated with adult sexual HIV risk behaviors in a sample of Latino men who have sex with men in New York City. *Drug and Alcohol Dependence*, *166*, 258–262.

Martinez, O., Lee, J. H., Bandiera, F., Santamaria, E. K., Levine, E. C., & Operario, D. (2017). Sexual and behavioral health disparities among sexual minority Hispanics/Latinos: Findings from the National Health and Nutrition Examination Survey, 2001–2014. *American Journal of Preventive Medicine*, *53*(2), 225–231. doi:10.1016/j.amepre.2017.01.037

Mayer, K. H., Wang, L., Koblin, B., Mannheimer, S., Magnus, M., del Rio, C., … HPTN061 Protocol Team. (2014). Concomitant socioeconomic, behavioral, and biological factors associated with the disproportionate HIV infection burden among Black men who have sex with men in U.S. cities. *PLoS One*, *9*(1), e87298.

Mays, V. M., & Cochran, S. D. (2001). Mental health correlates of perceived discrimination among lesbian, gay, and bisexual adults in the United States. *American Journal of Public Health*, *91*, 1869–1876.

Mays, V. M., Cochran, S. D., & Zamudio, A. (2004). HIV prevention research: Are we meeting the needs of African American men who have sex with men? *Journal of Black Psychology*, *30*, 78–105.

Mays, V. M., Jones, A. L., Delany-Brumsey, A., Coles, C., & Cochran, S. D. (2017). Perceived discrimination in health care and mental heath/substance abuse treatment among Blacks, Latinos, and Whites. *Medical Care*, *55*(2), 173–181.

Meyer, I. (2007). Prejudice and discrimination as social stressors. In I. H. Meyer & M. E. Northridge (Eds.), *The health of sexual minorities: Public health perspectives on lesbian, gay, bisexual, and transgender populations* (pp. 242–267). New York, NY: Springer Press.

Meanley, S., Gale, A., Harmell, C., Jadwin-Cakmak, L., Pingel, E., & Bauermeister, J. A. (2015). The role of provide interactions on comprehensive sexual healthcare among young men who have sex with men. *AIDS Education and Prevention*, *27*(1), 15–26.

Mena, L., Crosby, R. A., & Geter, A. (2017). A novel measure of poverty and its association with elevated sexual risk behavior among young Black MSM. *International Journal of STDs and AIDS*, *28*(6), 602–607.

Millett, G. A., Crowley, J. S., Koh, H., Valdiserri, R. O., Frieden, T., Dieffenbach, C. W., … Fauci, A. S. (2010). A way forward: The National HIV/AIDS strategy and reducing HIV incidence in the United States. *Journal of Acquired Immune Deficiency Syndromes*, *55*, S144–S177.

Millett, G. A., Peterson, J. L., Flores, S. A., Hart, T. A., Jeffries, W. L., 4th, Wilson, P. A., … Remis, R. S. (2012). Comparisons of disparities and risks of HIV infection in black and other men who have sex with men in Canada, UK, and USA: A meta-analysis. *Lancet*, *380*(9839), 341–348.

Mizuno, Y., Borkowf, C. B., Ayala, G., Carballo-Diéguez, A., & Millett, G. A. (2015). Correlates of sexual risk for HIV among US-born and foreign-born Latino men who have sex with men (MSM): An analysis from the Brothers y Hermanos study. *Journal of Immigrant and Minority Health*, *17*(1), 47–55.

Nelson, L. E., Wilton, L., Moineddin, R., Zhang, N., Siddiqi, A., Sa, T., … HPTN 061 Study Team. (2016). Economic, legal, and social hardships associated with HIV risk among Black men who have sex with men in six US cities. *Journal of Urban Health, 93*(1), 170–88.

Newberry, J. (2017). *Racial profiling and the NYPD: The who, what, when, and why of stoop and frisk*. New York: Palgrave Macmillan.

Nieves-Lugo, K., Del Rio-Gonzalez, A. M., Reisen, C., Poppen, P., Oursler, K. K., & Zea, M. C. (2017). Greater depressive symptoms and higher viral load are associated with poor physical function among Latino men living with HIV. *International Association of Providers in AIDS Care*, *16*(1), 30–36.

Office of National AIDS Policy. (2015). *National HIV/AIDS strategy*. Retrieved from https://www.whitehouse.gov/administration/eop/onap/nhas.

Organista, K. C., Carrillo, H., & Ayala, G. (2004). HIV prevention with Mexican migrants: Review, critique, and recommendations. *Journal of Acquired Immune Deficiency Syndromes*, *37*, S227–S239.

Peek, M. E., Lopez, F. Y., Williams, H. S., Xu, L. J., McNulty, M. C., Acree, M. E., & Schneider, J. A. (2016). Development of a conceptual framework for understanding shared decision making among African American LGBT patients and their clinicians. *Journal of General Internal Medicine, 31*(6), 677–687.

Poteat, T., White, J., & van Griensven, F. (2014). The HIV care continuum in Black MSM in the USA. *Lancet, 1*(3), e97–e98.

Quinn, K., Voisin, D. R., Bouris, A., Jaffe, K., Kuhns, L., Evaou, R., & Schneider, J. (2017). Multiple dimensions of stigma and health related factors among young Black men who have sex with men. *AIDS & Behavior, 21*(1), 207–216.

Quinn, K., Voisin, D. R., Bouris, A., & Schneider, J. (2016). Psychological distress, drug use, sexual risks and medication adherence among young HIV-positive Black men who have sex with men: Exposure to community violence matters. *AIDS Care, 28*(7), 866–872.

Ramirez-Valles, J., Garcia, D., Campbell, R. T., Diaz, R. M., & Heckathorn, D. D. (2008). HIV infection, sexual risk behavior, and substance use among Latino gay and bisexual men and transgender persons. *American Journal of Public Health, 98*, 1036–1042.

Reisen, C. A., Brooks, K. D., Zea, M. C., Poppen, P. J., & Bianchi, F. T. (2013). Can additive measures add to an intersectional understanding? Experiences of gay and ethnic discrimination among HIV-positive Latino gay men. *Cultural Diversity and Ethnic Minority Psychology, 19*(2), 208–217.

Rhodes, S. D., McCoy, T. P., Hergenrather, K. C., Vissman, A. T., Wolfson, M., Alonzo, J., ... Eng, E. (2012). Prevalence estimates of health risk behaviors of immigrant Latino men who have sex with men. *The Journal of Rural Health, 28*, 73–83.

Robert Wood Johnson Foundation. (2013). *Medicaid expansion under the ACA: How states analyze the fiscal and economic trade-offs*. Retrieved from http://www.rwjf.org/content/dam/farm/reports/issue_briefs/2013/rwjf406481.

Rodríguez-Díaz, C. E., Jovet-Toledo, G. G., Ortiz-Sánchez, E. J., Rodríguez-Santiago, E. I., & Vargas-Molina, R. L. (2015). Sexual health and socioeconomic-related factors among HIV-positive men who have sex with men in Puerto Rico. *Archives of Sexual Behavior, 44*(7), 1949–1958.

Rosenberg, E. S., Millett, G. A., Sullivan, P. S., Del Rio, C., & Curran, J. W. (2014). Understanding the HIV disparities between black and white men who have sex with men in the USA using the HIV care continuum: A modeling study. *Lancet, 1*(3), e112–e118.

Scott, H. M., Irvin, R., Wilton, L., Van Tieu, H., Watson, C., Magnus, M., ... Buchbinder, S. (2015). Sexual behavior and network characteristics and their association with bacterial sexually transmitted infections among Black men who have sex with men in the United States. *PloS One, 10*(12), e0146025.

Senn, T. E., Braksmajer, A., Coury-Doniger, P., Urban, M. A., & Carey, M. P. (2017). Mobile technology use and desired technology-based intervention characteristics among HIV positive Black men who have sex with men. *AIDS Care, 29*(4), 423–427.

Seth, P., Wang, G., Collins, N. T., Belcher, L., & Centers for Disease Control and Prevention (CDC). (2015). Identifying new positives and linkage to HIV medical care—23 testing site types, United States, 2013. *Morbidity and Mortality Weekly Report, 64*(24), 663–667.

Solorio, R., Norton-Shelpuk, P., Forehand, M., Martinez, M., & Aguirre, J. (2014). HIV prevention messages targeting young Latino MSM. *AIDS Research and Treatment, 2014*, 353092. doi:10.1155/2014/353092

Spikes, P. S., Purcell, D. W., Williams, K. M., Chen, Y., Ding, H., & Sullivan, P. S. (2009). Sexual risk behaviors among HIV-positive Black men who have sex with women, with men, or with men and women: Implications for intervention development. *American Journal of Public Health, 99*(6), 1072–1078.

Tieu, H. V., Nandi, V., Hoover, D. R., Lucy, D., Stewart, K., Frye, V., ... NYC M2M Study Team. (2016). Do sexual networks of men who have sex with men in New York City differ by race/ethnicity? *AIDS Patient Care and STDs, 30*(1), 39–47.

Tieu, H. V., Nandi, V., Hoover, D. R., Lucy, D., Stewart, K., Frye, V., et al. (2016). Do sexual networks of men who have sex with men in New York City differ by race/ethnicity? *AIDS Patient Care and STDs, 17*, 102–115.

Toro-Alfonso, J., & Rodriguez-Madera, S. (2004). Domestic violence in Puerto Rican gay male couples: Perceived prevalence, intergenerational violence, addictive behaviors, and conflict resolution skills. *Journal of Interpersonal Violence, 19*, 639–654.

U.S. Department of Health and Human Services. (n.d.). *The Affordable Care Act*. Retrieved from http://www.hhs.gov/healthcare/rights/law/index.html.

U.S. Department of Health and Human Services. Office of Disease Prevention and Health Promotion. (2015). *Healthy people 2020*. Washington, DC: USDHHS. Retrieved from http://www.healthypeople.gov/2020/topics-objectives/topic/hiv.

United States Department of Health and Human Services [US DHHS]. (2001). *Mental health: Culture, race, and ethnicity—A supplement to Mental health: A report of the surgeon general*. Rockville, MD: US Department of Health and Human Services.

Vermund, S. H. (2017). The continuum of HIV care in the urban United States: Black men who have sex with men (MSM) are less likely than White MSM to receive antiretroviral therapy. *Journal of Infectious Diseases*. doi: 10.1093/infdis/jix009.

Williams, J. K., Wilton, L., Magnus, M., Wang, J., Dyer, T. P., Koblin, B. A., … HIV Prevention Trials Network 061 Study Team. (2015). Relation of childhood sexual abuse, intimate partner violence, and depression to risk factors for HIV among Black men who have sex with men n 6 US cities. *American Journal of Public Health, 105*(12), 2473–2481.

Williams, D. R., Neighbors, H. W., & Jackson, J. S. (2003). Racial/ethnic discrimination and health: Findings from community studies. *American Journal of Public Health, 93*, 200–208.

Williams, J. K., Wyatt, E., Resell, J., Peterson, J., & Asuan-O'Brien, A. (2004). Psychosocial issues among gay- and non-gay-identifying HIV-seropositive African American and Latino MSM. *Cultural Diversity and Ethnic Minority Psychology, 10*, 268–286.

Wilton, L., Koblin, B., Nandi, V., Xu, G., Latkin, C., Seal, D., … Spikes, P. (2015). Correlates of seroadaptation strategies among Black men who have sex with men (MSM) in 4 US cities. *AIDS and Behavior, 19*(12), 2333–2346.

Wheeler, D. P. (2005). Working with positive men: HIV prevention with black men who have sex with men. *AIDS Education and Prevention, 17*, 102–115.

Wheeler, D. P. (2006). Exploring HIV prevention needs for nongay-identified Black and African American men who have sex with men: A qualitative exploration. *Sexually Transmitted Diseases, 33*, S11–S16.

Zea, M. C., Reisen, C. A., Poppen, P. J., Bianchi, F. T., & Echeverry, J. J. (2005). Disclosure of HIV status and psychological well-being among Latino gay and bisexual men. *AIDS and Behavior, 9*(1), 15–26.

Chapter 11
Understanding the Developmental and Psychosocial Needs of HIV Positive Gay Adolescent Males

Jason D.P. Bird and Dexter R. Voisin

This chapter explores core developmental and psychosocial needs of gay adolescent males who are living with the human immunodeficiency virus (HIV). Adolescence represents a period of significant transition for youth who are experimenting with changing roles and responsibilities, exploring their ethnic, gender, and sexual identities, and negotiating sexual and romantic relationships (Bauermeister et al., 2010; Hussen, Harper et al., 2015; Rosario, Schrimshaw, & Hunter, 2010; Steinberg & Morris, 2001). During the developmental processes of adolescence, HIV positive gay adolescent males also experience challenges related to managing disclosure based on their sexuality and HIV status (Hightow-Weidman et al., 2013; Jeffries et al., 2015; Tharinger & Wells, 2000), and the corresponding stigma and mental health sequelae often associated with negative peer and family reactions to such disclosures (D'Augelli, Grossman, & Starks, 2006; Herek, 2002; Lam, Naar-King, & Wright, 2007; Marshal et al., 2011; Rosario, Schrimshaw, & Hunter, 2012). HIV positive gay male youth may be negotiating these challenges while they strive for academic success, which is important to their future life trajectories (Bradley & Greene, 2013; Bruce et al., 2012). Consequently, HIV positive gay adolescent males experience fundamental psychosocial needs that are not adequately understood or attended to holistically by many current HIV prevention and service delivery programs (Harper et al., 2013; Kingdon et al., 2013). It is critical that we better understand and create supportive services that address these key challenges, which, in turn, will help to raise health awareness, enhance coping skills, and improve

J.D.P. Bird (✉)
Department of Social Work, School of Arts and Sciences-Newark,
Rutgers University-Newark, Newark, NJ 07102, USA
e-mail: jason.bird@rutgers.edu

D.R. Voisin
School of Social Service Administration, University of Chicago,
Chicago, IL USA
e-mail: dvoisin@uchicago.edu

© Springer Science+Business Media LLC 2017   267
L. Wilton (ed.), *Understanding Prevention for HIV Positive Gay Men*,
DOI 10.1007/978-1-4419-0203-0_11

secondary HIV prevention for gay adolescent males living with HIV and AIDS (Bouris et al., 2013; Hussen, Chahroudi et al., 2015).

This chapter first focuses on the increasing HIV infection rates among young gay males and examines pertinent research on core issues faced by HIV-infected youth, including experiences of HIV-related stigma, family and peer relationships, mental health and substance use challenges, and psychosocial needs (e.g., basic resources such as food and shelter). While there is a larger body of research on gay youth and HIV positive adult males, less emphasis has been placed on HIV positive gay adolescent males. Thus, this chapter will draw from these related literatures and relevant empirical studies on HIV positive gay adolescent males to highlight the developmental challenges, psychosocial needs, and service delivery needs of HIV positive gay adolescent males. We will also discuss key current federal and educational policies related to protection, service provision, and treatment for this population. We begin with a review of research on the shifting demographics of HIV, which highlights the importance of focusing on HIV positive adolescent gay males.

Shifting Demographics Within the Context of HIV

Several distinct epidemics (e.g., gay men, injection drug users, hemophiliacs, and women) have emerged over the last 35 years in the United States, each impacting a specific subpopulation, which has been shaped by unique sets of predictors and prevention challenges (Amaro & Raj, 2000; Elford & Hart, 2003; Evatt, 2006; Karon, Fleming, Steketee, & De Cock, 2001; Lusher & Brownstein, 2007; Murrill et al., 2002; Pulerwitz, Amaro, Jong, Gortmaker, & Rudd, 2002). Historically, response to the HIV/AIDS epidemic focused on adult gay populations, since this group experienced the highest AIDS mortality. From the outset, the HIV epidemic tapped into a moral preoccupation that painted some people as "innocent" (e.g., hemophiliacs and children) and others as "culpable" due to their engagement in socially undesirable behaviors, such as same-sex sexuality and drug use (Mawar, Sahay, Pandit, & Mahajan, 2005; Schellenberg, Keil, & Bem, 1995). These discriminatory beliefs significantly shaped early governmental response (or non-response) to the development of HIV prevention and treatment policy in the USA (Shilts, 1988). The void in early governmental response in the HIV/AIDS epidemic also stimulated a powerful social movement within Lesbian, Gay, Bisexual, and Transgender (LGBT) communities that aimed not only to spur the government into action but also to bring a greater legitimacy to LGBT people and communities as whole, worthy, and important members of our society. Thirty-five years later, while men who have sex with men (MSM), particularly men of color, continue to bear the greatest burden of HIV/AIDS infection, the demographics of the epidemic show a gradual shift away from some populations (e.g., hemophiliacs, children infected at birth) to communities of color, young adults, and adolescents (CDC, 2015, 2016). Not surprisingly, the public and private perception of those infected with HIV continues to have a pivotal role in shaping federal and state responses to the HIV epidemic in the USA.

Currently, estimates suggest more than 1.2 million people are living with HIV in the USA (CDC, 2015). In 2015, gay men and other MSM continue to be disproportionately impacted, accounting for 67% of new HIV infections (CDC, 2015) while only comprising between 2 and 4% of the overall population (CDC, 2015; Gates, 2011). Adolescents and young adults (aged 13–24) are especially vulnerable to HIV, representing 22% of new infections in 2014 (CDC, 2015). Furthermore, Black and Latino youth are even more disproportionately impacted by HIV, accounting for 55% and 23%, respectively, of new infections among young gay males in 2014 (CDC, 2015). However, it is important to note that when statistics report on "gay youth" it is not always clear what populations fall under that broad umbrella. For example, some statistics may include gay identified youth, while others may consider MSM who do not identify as gay. In other instances, bisexual, queer, or questioning youth may be included. Nevertheless, while rates of new HIV infections have decreased or remained relatively stable among most groups (including adult gay men), new infections continue to rise among adolescent gay males, in general, and young Black gay males specifically (CDC, 2015; IOM, 2011). In fact, young Black gay males are twice as likely as other groups to be diagnosed with HIV, and both Black and Latino adolescents are more likely to become infected with HIV at younger ages than White adolescents (CDC, 2008; IOM, 2011). These factors provide evidence that the epidemic continues to disproportionately affect disenfranchised populations (e.g., communities of color and LGBT communities), mirroring other health disparities such as cancer, heart disease, and diabetes (Smedley, Stith, & Nelson, 2003).

The National HIV/AIDS Strategy

The existence of a federal HIV/AIDS policy not only sets the agenda for prevention, intervention, and service delivery, but also serves as a powerful tool for shaping how society views and responds to HIV positive individuals. The National HIV/AIDS Strategy, enacted by President Obama in 2010, identifies three primary objectives: to reduce HIV infections, increase access to care and treatment for HIV-infected individuals, and reduce HIV-related health disparities, inequities, and stigma (White House Office of National AIDS Policy, 2010). Certainly, the "on-the-ground" impact of the National HIV/AIDS Strategy once fully implemented will have some positive impact on lessening the developmental challenges for HIV positive adolescent males. However, the unfolding of this policy will take time in the midst of fiscal challenges, complex bureaucracies, and changing political landscapes. At the current moment, important adolescent developmental challenges remain.

Despite the growing rate of HIV among young gay males and a national strategy that specifically calls for more research and services directed towards populations at greatest risk, HIV positive gay male adolescents have received limited attention in the extant literature. The data from these studies was derived from diverse samples with regard to age, gender, and sexual orientation, and across a wide range of infection routes, including perinatal infection. The data was also collected at a time when HIV treatment was more limited, less HIV information was provided in schools and within broader communities, and overt HIV stigma was more socially accepted.

Adolescent Development

Adolescence is a transitional time of navigation and exploration when adolescents seek ways of becoming more autonomous while also trying to maintain security through and connectedness with supportive networks such as family and school (Spear & Kulbok, 2004). Adolescence is characterized by major changes (and potential conflict) in family and peer relationships (Lynch, Lerner, & Leventhal, 2013; Spear & Kulbok, 2004; Tillfors, Persson, Willén, & Burk, 2012); identity development, formation, and crisis (Marcia, 1980); pressures of school achievement (Lynch et al., 2013); and issues of sexuality, dating, and intimacy (Tolman & McClelland, 2011). HIV positive gay adolescent males, while experiencing these developmental processes, also have unique challenges, including recognizing and understanding their same-sex sexual attraction, learning to navigate intimate same-sex relationships, making decisions about sexual identity and HIV-related disclosure, and managing both positive and negative reactions to their disclosures to family, friends, and peers (Bauermeister et al., 2010; Hussen, Harper et al., 2015; Rosario et al., 2012; Tharinger & Wells, 2000). In the next few sections, we discuss how stigma and discrimination related to sexual minority and HIV status may influence psychosocial functioning.

LGBT Sexualities and HIV: Multiple Stigmas and Challenges

Young gay males (and other sexual minority youth) face multiple challenges, including increased risks of bullying (Austin, 2012; Roberts, Rosario, Slopen, Calzo, & Austin, 2013; Russell, Ryan, Toomey, Diaz, & Sanchez, 2011), homelessness (Corliss, Goodenow, Nichols, & Austin, 2011), substance use (Ott et al., 2013), violence (Friedman et al., 2011), incarceration, poorer school achievement (Pearson, Muller, & Wilkinson, 2007), mental health distress (e.g., depression) (Galliher, Rostosky, & Hughes, 2004; Roberts et al., 2013), and suicidal ideation (Marshal et al., 2011). These challenges are often embedded in societal stigma, discrimination, and negative treatment by others associated with their sexual identities (Wilson et al., 2010). Moreover, an HIV positive diagnosis may serve to exacerbate the more fundamental challenges experienced by young gay males. These sexuality-based and HIV-related stigmas stem from multiple macro- and microlevel sources, including family, schools, peers, religious institutions, and community organizations, and are influenced by social and community norms regarding sexuality (Bird & Voisin, 2013;

Campbell & Deacon, 2006; Cohen, 1999; Herek, 2004; Parker & Aggleton, 2003). However, examining the impact of sexuality-based stigma and discrimination on youth and the general impact of HIV-related stigma on adults with HIV may help to illuminate the potential challenges faced by HIV positive gay male adolescents.

Stigma and Discrimination Based on Sexual Minority Status

There has been substantial progress in terms of LGBTQ rights and the reduction of sexuality-based discrimination. Some of these developments have included the 2015 Supreme Court ruling in *Obergefell v. Hodges* that same-sex marriage is a constitutionally protected right, lifting of the ban on lesbian and gay US service members, the first endorsement of same-sex marriage by a sitting U.S. president, the rise of gay-straight alliances within school systems, and greater public awareness campaigns supporting young LGBTQ individuals (e.g., the "It Gets Better Campaign"). However, these advancements have been tempered by persistent negative beliefs about LGBTQ people as observed with the continued resistance to not only same-sex marriage but also to equal rights for and anti-discrimination laws protecting LGBTQ individuals (especially within highly religious and more rural communities).

Many gay youth are exposed to environmental contexts that discount their sexuality and demand silence around issues of sexual identity. This expected silence is often learned by observing how openly LGBTQ individuals are discussed and/or treated by others. Therefore, LGBTQ youth experience a sense of "otherness" around which there is a social expectation of secrecy. Additionally, some African American and Latino youth may experience increased stigma or hostility with regard to being gay or bisexual given strong familial and community norms against homosexuality in some communities of color (Lam et al., 2007). This adds more complexity and highlights the ways that multiple factors intersect to increase stress and challenge positive coping. For instance, Agronick et al. (2004) found that young Latino MSM (aged 15–25) who identified as bisexual were more likely than those individuals who identified as gay to engage in insertive condomless anal intercourse, have more than one male sex partner in the preceding 3 months, and use drugs or alcohol during their last sex act with a male partner. The researchers theorized that many Latino YMSM who primarily have sex with men might identify as bisexual due to internalized homophobia, based out of cultural and familial norms, which strongly sanction against homosexuality (Agronick et al., 2004).

In a recent qualitative study of 20 Black gay adolescents, several participants reported internal conflicts related to their identity given that immediate family members loved and accepted them, but that their sexuality or related issues were not discussed and that the topic was often ignored (Voisin & Bird, 2012). In one instance, a participant indicated that when he disclosed his sexual orientation and HIV positive status to his mother, it was made clear that he was still her son but the topic would be discussed once and never again. Participants reported that despite feeling loved by immediate family members, homophobia on the part of some family members and "their Black community," coupled with the need to avoid stigma, prevented discussions about sexuality and sexual health from taking place on a regular basis. For some respondents, societal racism and the anticipation of racism from White gay communities resulted in heightened feelings of hyper-vigilance, which led to apathy about adhering to HIV prevention messages (Voisin & Bird, 2012). In such cases, young gay males of color are challenged by the intersection of racism and racially specific norms against homosexuality, and, in the case of HIV positive youth, HIV-related stigma, and discrimination.

The need to keep emerging same-sex sexual feelings and identity secret can interfere with the connectedness LGBT youth have with family and friends and can result in increased isolation, shame, and internalized stigma and homophobia, interfering with self-confidence and feelings of self-worth (Tharinger & Wells, 2000). Moreover, it removes pathways to many of the protective social relationships that are so important to positive functioning during adolescence (Tharinger & Wells, 2000). Furthermore, this continued isolation from family and peers for LGBT youth may facilitate the search for intimate and social relationships outside of familiar social networks and, thereby, expose adolescents to increased sexual and health risks (Bird, LaSala, Hidalgo, Kuhns, & Garofalo, 2017). This may be especially true in the absence of comprehensive sex education that specifically addresses the potential risks for young gay and bisexual men.

HIV-Related Stigma and Discrimination

HIV-related stigma is based on the perception of HIV as a discrediting attribute that marks the individual as different, less desirable, and more dangerous than those who are not HIV positive (Herek, 2002). While it may be true that overt HIV-related stigma has declined somewhat over time (Flicker et al., 2005), it remains a critical issue for HIV positive youth for whom this sense of secrecy may be exacerbated (Galindo, 2013). Issues of sexuality and disease may become intertwined in ways that deepen shame and create emotional distance from family and supportive networks (Bird, LaSala et al., 2017; Lam et al., 2007). Different populations (e.g., age, race, and ethnicity, gender) experience different amounts and types of HIV-related stigma. However, evidence suggests that HIV positive adolescents widely encounter HIV-related stigma through lived negative experiences, which compound their fear of breaking the silence around their HIV positive status (Flicker et al., 2005).

While gay adolescent males represent a growing proportion of those living with HIV and AIDS, there has been limited research on their experiences of HIV-related stigma (Dowshen, Binns, & Garofalo, 2009). One study of an ethnically diverse sample of young people aged 16–24 in Chicago found associations between HIV stigma and psychological distress, lower self-esteem, and loneliness. Levels of stigma did not vary significantly based on race, age, or gender identity. Additionally, adolescent gay males in this study reported levels of HIV-related stigma comparable to other HIV positive populations in previous studies (Dowshen et al., 2009). Stigma has also been identified as a significant factor driving nonadherence to HIV medication regimens for gay adolescents (Rao, Kekwaletswe, Hosek, Martinez, & Rodriguez, 2007). Given the increased risk for stigma and discrimination that HIV positive adolescent males are likely to experience, it is not surprising that these youth are confronted with multiple psychosocial challenges.

Navigating Romantic Relationship, Family Dynamics, and Academic Success

In the following sections, we discuss family and peer dynamics and academic policy and achievement as major domains that influence positive youth outcomes and upward trajectories.

Romantic Relationships

As gay youth navigate dating and sexual exploration during adolescence, they may unknowingly place themselves or their partners at risk of HIV. A high proportion of HIV positive gay youths do not know their HIV status, and therefore may engage in sexual risk behavior that could transmit HIV to their romantic partners (Halkitis et al., 2011; Mustanski, Newcomb, Du Bois, Garcia, & Grov, 2011). If HIV positive gay adolescents who are unaware of their HIV status perceive themselves as unlikely to have HIV, they may engage in more sexual risk-taking activity, such as having condomless anal intercourse, thereby placing their partners at risk (Halkitis et al., 2013). Similarly, HIV negative youth may assume that young romantic partners are HIV negative and thereby be willing to engage in sexual risk (Mustanski et al., 2011).

One way that gay adolescents often locate potential romantic or sexual partners is through the Internet (Garofalo, Herrick, Mustanski, & Donenberg, 2007). Studies suggest that the Internet has influenced the practice of sexual risk-taking behaviors, such as condomless anal intercourse or condom misuse, with sexual partners (Garofalo, Mustanski, Johnson, & Emerson, 2010). Additionally, some gay adolescents report having older gay male sexual partners (Rind, 2001), who may be more likely to be HIV positive (Garofalo et al., 2010). While qualitative studies with young, HIV positive gay and bisexual males have indicated that older gay men can be a source of support for gay youths (Bruce, Harper, & ATN, 2011), romantic relationships with older gay men may also heighten gay adolescents' risk of HIV exposure (Bird, LaSala et al., 2017).

Gay adolescents are faced with myriad complexities as they enter their life phase of romantic and sexual exploration, which they often must negotiate on their own in the absence of peer or family support. If an adolescent is aware of their HIV positive status, this presents the additional challenge of negotiating disclosure to romantic or sexual partners—a task that requires a high level of social efficacy (Bird, Eversman, & Voisin, 2017) from youth who may already be struggling to manage various demands on their psychological and emotional resources.

Family and Peer Dynamics: Sexuality Disclosure

Due to traditional societal norms against LGBT sexualities, gay youth often face challenges related to disclosing their sexuality to and dealing with negative reactions to that disclosure from parents, family members, and friends. Furthermore, for gay adolescents, an HIV diagnosis may be perceived as providing evidence of their being gay or bisexual and the choice to disclose an HIV positive status means also disclosing their sexual identity. Therefore, the adolescent must contend with a double-disclosure to family and friends and, potentially, double stigmatization and potential "blame" for their HIV infection. A number of gay youth face parental rejection, including exposure to violence from family members and being forced to leave home due to the sexual minority disclosure (Bird, LaSala et al., 2017; Tharinger & Wells, 2000). A recent study of young HIV positive youth, aged 17–24, across four cities indicated that few of the participants reported having the support of their families as they came to terms with their sexual orientation (Bruce et al., 2011). This is especially problematic since parental rejection has been associated with negative outcomes. For example, Ryan, Huebner, Diaz, and Sanchez (2009) in a study of 224 White and Latino participants found that adolescents who had experienced family rejection on the basis of their sexual orientation were 3.4 times more likely to have engaged in condomless anal intercourse, thereby increasing their risk of contracting or transmitting HIV. This finding corroborates with a growing body of research that indicates that adolescents who lack family support may be more likely to engage in unprotected sex that places them at increased HIV risk; they are also less likely to have supportive family networks to help them come to terms with an HIV positive diagnosis (Bird, LaSala et al., 2017).

Family and Peer Dynamics: HIV Disclosure

HIV disclosure is also a primary issue with which young, HIV positive gay adolescent males must contend. This includes having to make decisions about to whom one discloses, why one might decide to disclose, and what potential reactions may occur (Bird & Voisin, 2013; Brown, Lourie, & Pao, 2000). The need to manage such sensitive and potentially stigmatizing health information can have a profound impact on relationships with family, friends, and others with or without actual disclosure. Experiences with heterosexism and HIV-related stigma during adolescence, when young gay males are coming to terms with their sexual identity, may influence HIV positive youth to remain silent about their HIV status (Flicker et al., 2005). They may also choose to keep their HIV status and/or sexuality secret in order maintain peer approval (Lam et al., 2007). Ultimately, this secrecy can result in increased social isolation and decreased access to resources. On the other hand, HIV disclosure carries the potential for negative consequences, as well, and may result in social ostracism from supportive communities and peer networks (Bird & Voisin, 2013; Hightow-Weidman et al., 2013) and potential rejection from families (Bird & Voisin, 2013), especially since an HIV disclosure may result in a broader disclosure about sexuality and sexual identity.

Few studies have specifically examined HIV disclosure outcomes among gay youth. However, based on resiliency research with other populations, we posit several factors that are likely to matter. Individual-level factors include positive intellectual functioning; the ability to form secure attachments with others; having a sociable and appealing disposition; having high levels of self-efficacy, self-confidence, and self-esteem; being goal-orientated; and feeling hopeful about the future (Tharinger & Wells, 2000). Additionally, having strong and close family relationships, being connected to extended supportive networks, and having positive school-based relationships have been shown to enhance coping for adolescents, which may make disclosure more likely. However, heterosexism and sexuality-based stigmatization and discrimination often stand as significant barriers between HIV positive gay adolescents and typical sources of support, such as family, friends, teachers or other school officials, and community or religious organizations.

Even in the case where a gay adolescent male does not "come out" to family, he may experience feelings of rejection based on how family members talk about or treat other gay and lesbian individuals (Tharinger & Wells, 2000). In the absence of parental support, Bruce et al. (2011) found that most participants spoke of feelings of loneliness and isolation. In their survey of 54 HIV positive gay adolescents and emerging adults, aged 17–24, participants were asked to describe risks and resiliencies associated with being a gay youth and many spoke of leaving home to find other males "like them," in gay communities (p. 371). Because many of these young gay males felt unsupported by their families and had moved to larger cities on their own, participants who recounted experimentation with drugs and sex often lacked a supportive network or parental guidance to help them navigate the health risks (Bruce et al., 2011). However, other participants spoke of the supportive networks or alternative families provided by others in gay communities, frequently comprised of older gay men who played a mentoring role to adolescent and emerging adult gay males. The interviews revealed that the young gay men who had left home were susceptible to a variety of risks: some reported feeling vulnerable to peer influences due to feelings of identity confusion, and others reported that deeper emotional needs led them to seek out multiple sexual partners. On the other hand, many participants reported resiliencies associated with their migration to gay communities, including feelings of increased self-reliance, strength borne out of overcoming adversity, and an open-mindedness that allowed them to encounter a rich variety of people and experiences (Bruce et al., 2011).

Furthermore, not all families reject or ill-treat their LGBTQ children, and families can provide an important protective role for LGBTQ youth by providing social support, acceptance, and security (Bouris et al., 2010). The degree and resolution of family conflict, when it occurs, is often dependent on the strength of the family relationships prior to disclosure (Tharinger & Wells, 2000), and several studies have found that young gay male participants report valuing family relationships and their families of origin (McDowell & Serovich, 2007; Serovich & Grafsky, 2011). Therefore, looking for ways to strengthen family dynamics, communication, attachment, and coping strategies has the benefit of helping families overcome negative beliefs and feelings related to sexual minorities and LGBTQ children. Furthermore, this strengthening of families could serve as a primary coping mechanism for HIV positive youth (Bird, LaSala et al., 2017; Kalichman, DiMarco, Austin, Luke, & Di-Fonzo, 2003; Serovich & Grafsky, 2011) and increase positive outcomes, such as increased adherence to HIV treatment (Murphy, Roberts, Marelich, & Hoffman, 2000).

Academic Policy and School Success

It is widely known that school achievement is associated with important future accomplishments and upward social mobility. Daily stigmatization, discrimination, or exposure to a hostile academic environment can interfere with the learning process and school achievement. Furthermore, fear about negative treatment can lead to decreased involvement in school activities and the maintenance of smaller social networks, which can increase isolation and limit access to social support and resources (Tharinger & Wells, 2000). Adolescent gay males often encounter entrenched antigay stigma and discrimination within their school settings (Solorio, Swendeman, & Rotheram-Borus, 2003), and sometimes this discrimination is institutionalized in the policies and behaviors of the school administration (Bruce et al., 2011). Additional studies have indicated that children and adolescents whose HIV status is disclosed in a school setting often face stigma and discrimination on account of their HIV status, with some children even being denied school entry (Weiner, Battles, & Heilman, 2000). Therefore, young HIV positive gay males are at risk of discrimination based on their sexual orientation and HIV status.

Regardless of the fact that HIV positive children and adolescents are vulnerable to verbal assault and discrimination in school settings, research on HIV school policies has largely focused on HIV prevention policies. In response to the potential for HIV-related stigmatization and discrimination within school systems, various organizations have created position statements for protecting HIV positive students in schools, which have often derived from federal laws. For example, the American Academy of Pediatrics (AAP) offers six recommendations: (1) that all HIV positive children and youth have equal access to high quality educational experiences; (2) that special education services be provided as needed; (3) that there be accommodation of medical needs within the school setting; (4) that continuity of education be uninterrupted by HIV management; (5) that confidentiality of HIV status be maintained; and (6) that there be coordination between the pediatrician/medical home provider and school when appropriate (AAP, 2000).

In addition to the AAP, the American Civil Liberties Union (ACLU), American Psychiatric Association (APA), American Nursing Association (ANA), and the Center for HIV Law and Policy have all released policy statements regarding the protection of HIV positive youth within schools. For example, the ACLU's AIDS Project released a report entitled "HIV & Civil Rights" (Lange, 2003), which outlines the rights of HIV positive persons to privacy and confidentiality, nondiscrimination, and accurate sexual and prevention education in schools. The ANA released "Recommendations for the School Nurse in Addressing HIV/AIDS with Adolescents" in 1996, which recommended that school nurses integrate HIV/AIDS education into their schools' health programs; take leadership in educating fellow school personnel and community members on HIV/AIDS; advocate to protect the rights of students with HIV/AIDS; and connect them and their families with community supportive resources (Uris, 1996). In its 2009 "Position Statement on HIV and Adolescents," the APA charged that HIV status should be disclosed on a "need-to-know" basis within school settings, as outlined within the framework of the law and stated that HIV positive students should not be restricted from participation in school activities (APA, 2009).

Finally, the Center for HIV Law and Policy developed the Teen SENSE (Sexual health and Education Now in State Environments) initiative to ensure that HIV positive adolescents in state custody have access to "comprehensive, scientifically accurate, LGBT-inclusive sexual health care services and education" (The Center for HIV Law & Policy, n.d.). Teen SENSE offers a federal and state legal framework that protects these rights for HIV positive adolescents, as well as model guidelines for nonjudgmental and LGBTQ-inclusive health care, education, and professional development/staff training of personnel who work with HIV positive youth in foster care and juvenile justice facilities. HIV positive students' rights are also explicitly protected by several federal laws. For example, the Rehabilitation Act of 1973, Section 504, pertains to children or adolescents with health care needs who do not require special education classes. It requires that public schools permit these students to attend regular classes and accommodate students with special support such as medical or psychological services if necessary (AAP, 2000).

Additionally, the Supreme Court's 1998 ruling in *Bragdon v. Abbott* determined that people with HIV or AIDS are protected under the Americans with Disabilities Act (ADA), as are persons who are discriminated against because they are regarded as being HIV positive, and persons who face discrimination because they have a relationship with someone who is HIV positive. The ADA prohibits state and local governments from discriminating against people with HIV, including public school systems (U.S. Department of Justice, n.d.). Finally, the Individuals with Disabilities Education Act (IDEA) applies to children and adolescents ages 3–21 with disabilities or medical concerns (including HIV/AIDS) that require special accommodation in a school setting. IDEA guarantees access to schooling and supportive services for eligible children. Schools are required to prepare an Individualized Education

Program (IEP) for each eligible child that outlines a plan to ensure that their disability or medical condition does not interfere with their education (AAP, 2000).

Various states also provide policy guidelines to assist local school districts in developing policies that protect the rights of HIV positive students. Often these guidelines include an HIV/AIDS primer to educate administrators, teachers, and families, and a host of policy recommendations, including HIV/AIDS prevention education; safeguarding students through infection control, privacy and confidentiality, and nondiscrimination; ensuring student access to communicable disease reporting and physical and psychological health services; protecting the rights of HIV positive students to participate in athletics and other student programs; and communicating policies to families. Wisconsin's School HIV/AIDS Policy Tool Kit acknowledges that "communities typically focus on the safety of children that do not have HIV infection," but suggests that "[I]n addition, messages can be developed to inform the community that policies are in place to protect the rights of all students and staff, including those infected and affected by HIV" (Cox, 2003, p. 67).

However, there is some question about the extent to which these policy guidelines are actually implemented at the local level. For example, a content analysis of HIV-related school policy in 79 school systems in North Carolina found that school boards largely failed to provide detailed HIV-related policies (Fair, Garner-Edwards, & McLees-Lane, 2005) such as the ones recommended by the state's Healthy Schools Initiative, funded by the Departments of Public Instruction and Health and Human Services. Furthermore, North Carolina passed a law in 2016 (House Bill 2) barring local ordinances protecting LGBT populations, which will likely have a negative impact on LGBTQ and HIV-infected youth in schools (House Bill 2, 2016).

A 2008 study by the CDC analyzed survey data from the 2006 School Health Profiles for public secondary schools (grades 6–12) in 36 states and 13 large urban school districts and found that approximately half of all secondary schools reported having a policy to protect the rights of staff and students infected with HIV or AIDS (CDC, 2008). The median percentage of schools with such a policy in place decreased from 71.9% in 1996 to 52.9% in 2006 among states and from 86.2 to 49.2% among school districts, when comparing results from the same 21 states and eight school districts that participated in both the 1996 and 2006 School Health Profiles surveys. While this study suffers from response bias due to self-report and non-response, it most likely overestimates the number of schools with policies to protect HIV positive high school students, suggesting that public secondary schools are falling short in providing a safe environment for HIV positive adolescents.

There are also policies that have the potential to infringe on the confidentiality of HIV positive youth. For example, a South Carolina law requires the Department of Health and Environmental Control (DHEC) to report the identities of students who are HIV positive to public school administrators (DeGroat, 2009). Besides challenging what other states have interpreted as a students' right to privacy and confidentiality, the law also potentially discourages students from getting HIV tested, in spite of the fact that the CDC recommends regular testing as an effective component of HIV prevention programs (Branson et al., 2006). Additionally, the law potentially increases the potential for HIV-related stigma and discrimination if their HIV status is shared (DeGroat, 2009).

Furthermore, in spite of legal protections for HIV positive students, various states and local governments have enacted policies that curtail the rights of HIV positive young people, leaving them vulnerable to stigmatization and substandard education quality. Whether or not the laws are enforced, the threat remains that HIV positive students may be denied equal rights within a school setting under the laws. Alabama, California, Georgia, Indiana, Louisiana, Missouri, Oklahoma, Oregon, and South Carolina have laws that devolve authority to local school boards to determine whether HIV positive students can be excluded from public school. A handful of other states do not explicitly mention HIV but permit school boards to prevent students with infectious diseases from attending school if they are deemed a health risk (National Association of State Boards of Education [NASBE], 2012). These policies exist despite the fact that the American Academy of Pediatrics asserts that HIV positive children should not be excluded from school or isolated within the school setting (AAP, 2000). Many of these states have contradictory policies—within the same state there may be one policy that grants schools the authority to suspend students due to their HIV status, and another policy that makes it compulsory to protect HIV positive students' rights to privacy, confidentiality, and accommodation within schools (NASBE, 2012).

Mental Health Concerns

Although there is a growing body of literature on the effects of sexual minority stigma and discrimination on the mental health functioning of LGBTQ youth, there has been a dearth of research exploring the unique mental health concerns experienced by young, HIV positive gay males. However, based on research involving gay youth and clinical observations, we can posit that HIV positive gay adolescent males are at an increased risk for significant mental health concerns. Given the presence of both HIV-related and sexuality-based stigma and discrimination, it is not surprising that HIV positive gay adolescents are at elevated risks of experiencing psychological distress, including decreased self-esteem (Tharinger & Wells, 2000); increased thoughts of suicide (Brown et al., 2000; Tharinger & Wells, 2000); and feelings of sadness, depression (Brown et al., 2000; Flicker et al., 2005), anxiety, hopelessness, anger (Brown et al., 2000), and isolation and loneliness (Brown et al., 2000; Flicker et al., 2005; Lam et al., 2007), especially when there is less access to others who are HIV positive (Lam et al., 2007). Furthermore, research suggests that HIV positive adolescents may be more preoccupied with mortality and fears of death (Brown et al., 2000; Flicker et al., 2005) and experience feelings of regret, shame, guilt, fear, humiliation, or anger about the circumstances of their infection (Flicker et al., 2005; Tharinger & Wells, 2000).

Benton (2010), in a review of psychiatric papers on HIV positive adolescents, posits that the rate of psychological distress appeared to be higher for HIV positive youth than HIV negative youth and that there may be a relationship between taking HAART medication and mental health concerns that should be explored in future research. Furthermore, the Youth Risk Behavior Survey (YRBS) found that the combination of LGB identity and experiencing victimization or bullying at school was associated with increased substance use, mental health problems, suicidality, and sexual risk behavior, compared to heterosexual youth. The mental health consequences of stigma for young gay males can lead to emotional distress, suicide attempts, drug use, and risky sex (Mustanski et al., 2011). Furthermore, Mustanski et al. (2011) found an association between psychological distress, depressive symptoms, and condomless anal intercourse in their urban sample of young gay males (aged 18–30), indicating that mental health concerns among HIV positive young gay men may result in sexual risk for themselves and others. Family rejection or poor familial support (e.g. being harassed by family members for being gay or being kicked out of the home) are likely to drive these negative outcomes (Bird, LaSala et al., 2017; Mustanski et al., 2011).

Substance Use

Although there is limited research specifically on substance use and HIV positive gay adolescent males, there is some data to suggest that HIV positive youth have higher levels of substance use than their HIV negative peers (Naar-King, Wright et al., 2006; Remafedi, Farrow, & Deisher, 1991). However, it is useful to explore the literature on substance use for young gay males in general, as an indicator of use among HIV positive adolescent gay males. A review of epidemiology, risk and protective factors, and interventions among young gay males found that, in comparison with their heterosexual counterparts (Brewster & Tillman, 2012; Traube, Schrager, Holloway, Weiss, & Kipke, 2012) as well as with older gay men (Salomon et al., 2009), young gay males are more likely to use a variety of different substances, including alcohol and illicit drugs, and to engage in heavy substance use. Young gay males along with other sexual minority youth also tend to begin substance use at an earlier age (Corliss et al., 2010) and to increase use more rapidly over time (Marshal, Friedman, Stall, & Thompson, 2009). Although the use of club drugs, such as stimulants and hallucinogens, is high among urban young gay men regardless of race (Mustanski et al., 2011), White young gay males are more likely than Blacks and Latinos to use club drugs (Halkitis & Palamar, 2008) notably MDMA (ecstasy) (Klitzman, Greenberg, Pollack, & Dolezal, 2002). Several studies have highlighted the correlation between club drug use and engaging in risky sexual behavior (Drumright, Patterson, & Strathdee, 2006; Garofalo, Mustanski, McKirnan, Herrick, & Donenberg, 2007; Steuve et al., 2002), which likely increases the spread of HIV and other STIs among urban young gay males. Fewer studies have examined the use of marijuana among young gay males, but findings generally show a correlation between marijuana use and sexual risk (Bryan, Schmiege, & Magnan, 2012; Outlaw et al., 2011). While there is also a correlation between alcohol and sexual risk taking, the nature of that correlation is inconsistent and merits further study (Newcomb, Clerkin, & Mustanski, 2011). Despite these correlations, the association between young gay males' drug and alcohol use and sexual risk depends on several situational variables, including partner type (primary vs. casual) and sexual role (insertive vs. receptive in anal sex) (Mustanski et al., 2011).

For many young gay males, drug and alcohol use has become a part of their sexual identity (Bruce & Harper, 2011). Urban gay culture has traditionally included drug and alcohol use, and therefore marginalized young gay males seeking to integrate into gay communities often adopt these behaviors. Several studies have found that young gay males who reported a history of forced sex were more likely to use drugs, and those with more serious levels of drug use were also more likely to report a history of having run away (Thiede et al., 2003).

Sexual Risk

Studies show that young, HIV positive gay males continue to engage in sexual risk taking—including sex with more casual sexual partners, using condoms less frequently and having survival sex more often, than their HIV negative peers (Hein & Dell, 1995; Naar-King, Wright et al., 2006; Rotheram-Borus et al., 1997). One study of 231 HIV positive gay and bisexual adolescents found that participants were younger than 15 years on average when they first had anal sex, and that their first sexual partner was generally more than 10 years older (average age 28 years) (Solorio et al., 2003, p. 86). Additionally some studies have noted a correlation between sex work, particularly street-based sex work, risky sexual behavior, and HIV. In these circumstances, young gay sex workers may lack the appropriate skills to negotiate condom use with clients, or may choose to avoid using condoms for additional money or to avoid conflicts with clients (Mustanski et al., 2011).

Some studies of adolescent and emerging adult gay and bisexual males have found that differences in HIV prevalence among various racial/ethnic groups could not be attributed to risky sexual behaviors (Garofalo et al., 2010; Solorio et al., 2003). One particular study that looked at sexual risk taking among a sample of 273 Black, Latino, and White HIV positive gay and bisexual young males found that among all three racial/ethnic groups, HIV was positively correlated with having older sexual partners, commercial sex, and sex with partners they met on the Internet (Garofalo et al., 2010). Studies have also shown that young, HIV positive gay males may generally have more difficulty negotiating safer sex or discussing HIV with sexual partners, especially within longer-term relationships (Bird, LaSala et al., 2017; Mustanski et al., 2011). These findings have implications for both the individual's health and for public health, as these risky sexual behaviors increase the possibility of transmission to others (Flicker et al., 2005; Naar-King, Wright et al., 2006).

Substance Use and Sexual Risk Behaviors

To some extent, it is not uncommon for adolescents to experiment with drugs or engage in sexual activity or some degree of risky sex (i.e., intercourse with condoms), as a normal part of adolescent development and experimentation with new social roles and scripts (Voisin & Bird, 2012). However, gay HIV positive adolescent males may engage in higher rates of risky sex compared to their heterosexual counterparts. Researchers have theorized that health disparities among adolescents and emerging adult MSM are co-occurring and mutually reinforcing (Bruce et al., 2011). This theory of "syndemic production" of health disparities among MSM youth and emerging adults suggests that high rates of drug use, depression, and HIV infection are intertwined, and result from social marginalization. This is consistent with a minority stress model inferred from several sociological and social psychological theories (e.g., critical race theory, social stigma, stress theories) and may partly explain why gay adolescent males may engage in higher rates of drug and sexual risks behaviors. In addition, it may also partially explain why these young males persist in these risk behaviors after becoming infected. According to this theory, gay youth are isolated from social structures, norms, and institutions because of their sexual minority status (Mustanski, Garofalo, Herrick, & Donenberg, 2007). Given their marginalized status, gay adolescent males are subjected to greater societal stressors because dominant culture and social structures do not typically reflect or respond to the individual's needs or realities (Meyer, 2003), which may influence drug and sexual risks.

Implications for Treatment and Intervention

Given the developmental and psychosocial needs of HIV positive gay adolescent males discussed earlier, we offer several treatment and intervention considerations. These recommendations are partly informed by the challenges addressed earlier in this chapter.

Addressing Developmental Factors Associated with Change

According to the Information-Motivation-Behavioral (IMB) model of behavior change, the pathway to creating effective behavior change is to provide information about how HIV is transmitted, raise awareness about an individual's personal vulnerability to infection, teach safer sex skills, and engender the self-efficacy to use those skills (Fisher & Fisher, 2002). In the case of young, HIV positive gay males, providing information about how HIV is transmitted and raising awareness about vulnerability is essential but not sufficient for changing sexual risk-taking behavior

(Brown et al., 2000). It is equally important to attend to adolescent-specific factors, such as cognitive immaturity, exploratory learning behavior, and impulsivity (Brooks-Gunn, Boyer, & Hein, 1988; Brown, DiClemente, & Reynolds, 1991; Brown et al., 2000; Emans, Brown, Davis, Felice, & Hein, 1991; Irwin, Igra, Eyre, & Millstein, 1997), and seek to increase empathy and a sense of responsibility so that adolescents can better understand how their actions may impact the health and lives of their sexual partners (Brown et al., 2000).

Access to Health Care and HIV Treatment

Access and adherence to HIV treatment is also a critical issue for young, HIV posi- tive gay males as adolescents have unique treatment needs and preferences for health care services (O'Byrne & Watts, 2014). Appropriate adherence to HIV treat- ment is essential to improving the long-term health of young positive men and reducing secondary transmission. Research shows that HIV positive adolescents often experience problems obtaining adequate health care services, medication, and social services (Bell et al., 2003; Brown et al., 2000; Rotheram-Borus, O'Keefe, Krackcr, & Foo, 2000). Prior research has also shown that many HIV positive ado- lescents did not receive age-specific HIV-related services (Hein & Dell, 1995), which poses implications for the provision of HIV care (Bouris et al., 2013).

Gay HIV positive adolescent males may also have unique barriers to accessing health care services and treatment (Flicker et al., 2004). First, they are a more hid- den population often disenfranchised from larger social systems and more covert about their risk behaviors and sexual identities (Bell et al., 2003). Because of this, they may be harder to identify and enroll into needed medical and social services. Secondly, many of these youth may not have access to insurance or primary care services, and those who do have access are likely covered by their parents' insur- ance plans. This may present a double barrier for young gay males who are at risk of having to both disclose their HIV status and their sexuality and sexual behavior to parents or other caregivers in order to access health care.

Effective adherence is critical not only to the individual's health but also to pub- lic health, given recent findings that viral suppression through proper treatment adherence has the added benefit of reducing the transmissibility of HIV (referred to as "Treatment as Prevention"). For adults, poor adherence to HIV treatment has been linked to lower self-efficacy, the lack of social support, and psychological distress. Naar-King, Templin et al. (2006) found in a sample of HIV positive youth that the rate of adherence was not sufficient for effectively managing the disease, and that both self-efficacy and psychological distress were associated with lower adherence. While lack of social support was not directly related to lower adherence, it was associated with lower self-efficacy (Naar-King, Templin et al., 2006) and Radcliffe, Tanney, and Rudy (2006) found that the experience of trauma among HIV positive adolescents and young adults might adversely affect adherence to HIV treatment. Moreover, Benton (2010), in a review of the literature concerning mental health issues affecting HIV positive children and adolescents, noted several studies that indicate the negative impact of mental health concerns, such as depression, on adherence. Given these barriers to access and challenges to adherence, it is important to design social service programs that help to identify HIV positive youth, increase social support, and decrease psychological distress in an effort to increase the effectiveness of treatment.

Positive Coping

Despite the fact that adolescents and young adults are disproportionately affected by the HIV epidemic, there is still limited research on the unique influences that HIV infection has on the lives of HIV positive adolescents, or the ways that they learn to cope with the disease (Brown et al., 2000). Gay adolescents living with HIV experience a variety of complications, and their ability to cope with an HIV diagnosis and the ongoing aspects of the disease is influenced by the specific psychological stressors, personality factors, and access to social support of each individual. Poor coping skills are associated with a number of negative factors, including maladjustment to HIV infection, lower fighting spirit, hopelessness, fatalism and a preoccupation with mortality, anger, and the feeling of having loss of control over life events (Brown et al., 2000). These considerations, in turn, can have a deleterious impact on an individual's relationships with family and friends, academic achievement, and risk-taking behaviors. Conversely, positive psychological coping has been associated with feelings of empowerment, and beliefs about HIV presenting an opportunity to reevaluate life goals and make positive changes that enhance relationships and health (Flicker et al., 2005).

How young, HIV positive gay males learn to respond and adapt to HIV infection is critical to their success as a basis to not only remain healthy, but also to mitigate the risk of transmitting HIV to intimate partners. Building strong social support networks with parents, family members, close friends, romantic partners, and other HIV positive youth can be an extremely valuable strategy to buffering against some of the potentially negative mental health and psychosocial challenges of being HIV positive (Flicker et al., 2005; Lam et al., 2007).

Early intervention is critical to helping navigate these stressors and increasing positive coping skills. Since adolescence is a time when youth set lifelong health and behavioral patterns, providing guidance during this important stage is essential to ensuring more healthy adulthood functioning (Flicker et al., 2004). To accomplish this, an environment that works to mitigate the negative social challenges such as HIV-related and sexuality-based stigma and discrimination is needed. One strategy is to design age-appropriate, confidential, and structured programs within schools and at community-based organizations that provide social support (both around issues of sexuality and HIV infection), enhance coping skills, increase stability (e.g., housing, education, basic needs) (Flicker et al., 2005; Hein & Dell, 1995), and address typical and age-specific adolescent challenges (e.g., impulsivity)

(Brown et al., 2000). These programs need to be multi-pronged, aiming to address the interrelated risk factors faced by HIV positive adolescents by increasing youths' motivation to decrease sexual and drug-using risk behaviors (Hein & Dell, 1995); facilitating the use of protective health behaviors such as starting and maintaining HIV treatment adherence (Naar-King, Wright et al., 2006); and providing supportive services and access to medical care to improve the immediate health and control the progression of HIV for young gay and bisexual men. It is also important that programs be implemented at the school and broader community level to increase empathy around issues of HIV and actively work against discriminatory and stigmatizing messages that isolate and silence young LGBTQ individuals and young people who are HIV infected.

Finding ways to help HIV positive gay adolescents access and stay engaged in care and social services can help provide a stable, socially supported environment and an avenue through which they can address the different psychosocial challenges that may arise throughout adolescence (Bell et al., 2003). Yet, because HIV positive gay youths are a vulnerable, disenfranchised, and often hidden population, identifying who needs access to adequate services and interventions and retaining them in care can be a primary barrier (Bell et al., 2003; Hein & Dell, 1995). Intervening at the moment of testing may be a critical strategy to engage young, HIV positive gay males, and has the potential for shaping future health and risk behaviors. Project Engage is one example of an innovative network support intervention designed to link and keep newly diagnosed HIV positive Black male adolescent engaged in care (Bouris et al., 2013). Currently, we know that HIV treatment is another form of prevention, given that keeping viral loads undetectable can reduce the rates of transmission to sexual partners (Bell et al., 2003).

However, voluntary counseling and immediately referring to treatment may become more difficult as home HIV testing becomes standard and pre- and post-test counseling is de-emphasized in favor of increased speed and access to testing. These technological developments around home testing elevate the importance of embracing the use of new technologies to find HIV positive adolescents, provide supportive communities, and transmit health information. HIV positive youth increasingly feel comfortable with and rely upon the Internet to access a wide variety of resources specific to their needs (Flicker et al., 2004). The Internet appears to be an important tool regardless of socioeconomic status or other demographic factors such as age, gender, and race ethnicity (Flicker et al., 2004). However, while the Internet has proven useful for building supportive communities, it is not currently used as a primary source of information about health or ways to access information on HIV prevention (Voisin, Bird, Shi Shiu, & Kreiger, 2013). Leveraging the Internet to be a tool for advocacy, information seeking, and health promotion for young HIV positive gay and bisexual men may be essential, as it holds potential as a source where HIV positive gay adolescents could anonymously and comfortably access information and support with reduced fear of stigma and discrimination.

Finally, given the significance of education in the lives of all adolescents it is important to address the largely unmet sexual health education needs of gay male youth, especially given that an increasing number of these teens are becoming HIV infected. A recent qualitative study of Black gay male youth illustrated the short-comings of HIV education in school settings, with participants indicating that schools were not a significant source of HIV prevention information because sex education classes were primarily focused on pregnancy prevention, not STIs or HIV prevention. As a result, the sex education content received by these participants and their peers was mostly irrelevant to the needs and special challenges of gay youth (Voisin & Bird, 2012). This finding corroborates with prior results that document the inadequacy of school-based sexual health education in addressing the needs of gay youth (Kubicek, Beyer, Weiss, Iverson, & Kipke, 2010). In fact, the exclusion of same sex content in many sexual health curricula may reinforce a sense of alien-ation and "otherness," which may foster feelings of negative self-regard for some gay male youth and add to minority stress (Voisin et al., 2013).

Comprehensive sex education is critical to destigmatizing gay and HIV positive youth and decreasing rising HIV rates for this vulnerable population. Despite this need, there is a scarcity of LGBTQ-inclusive curricular content and a general lack of political will at the state level to enact such policies. Furthermore, even in school districts that promote HIV education, the curriculum is not often written for adoles-cents who are already living with HIV. This oversight represents a missed opportu-nity to provide a hard-to-reach population with health information and social support and dispel misinformation about HIV that leads to fear and stigma. Given this, it is time for the federal government to enact a comprehensive, national sex education policy that provides critical health information for all youth, including those who are gay and HIV positive. Such progressive actions at the federal level would send a strong message of support to gay adolescents living with HIV, affirm-ing a national commitment to their health, inclusion, and well-being.

Acknowledgments The authors will like to thank Brooke Fisher and Rachel Narrow for their invaluable assistance with the preparation of this chapter.

References

Agronick, G., O'Donnell, L., Stueve, A., San Doval, A., Duran, R., & Vargo, S. (2004). Sexual behaviors and risks among bisexually- and gay-identified young Latino men. *AIDS and Behavior*, *8*(2), 185–197.

Amaro, H., & Raj, A. (2000). On the margin: Power and women's HIV risk reduction strategies. *Sex Roles*, *42*(7/8), 723–749.

American Academy of Pediatrics (AAP). (2000). Education of children with human immunodefi-ciency virus infection. *Pediatrics*, *105*(6), 1358–1360.

American Psychiatric Association (APA). (2009). *Position statement on HIV and adolescents*. Retrieved from https://docs.google.com/viewer?a=v&q=cache:LQaqJz49L0EJ:www.psychia-try.org/File%2520Library/Advocacy%2520and%2520Newsroom/Position%2520Statements/ps2009_HIVadolescents.pdf+&hl=en&gl=us&pid=bl&srcid=ADGEESieyitZX9O_we7B7FJe8WJsqnQkhuyFl9RwVOEhr349X66I9iL15WfUz_6iwfMhXb79PubDu_5Ft6ycDeuBE4AIIsMS_WNQcKnvuBxWDMUDT3fKmnUIeC0mMp6iKRiKKK_V3w_r&sig=AHIEtbQRf_pZh5SJPUfgh0VNdg6mUqXllA.

Austin, S. B. (2012). Elevated risk of posttraumatic stress in sexual minority youths: Mediation by childhood abuse and gender nonconformity. *American Journal of Public Health, 102*(8), 1587–1593.

Bauermeister, J. A., Johns, M. M., Sandfort, T. G., Eisenberg, A., Grossman, A. H., & D'Augelli, A. R. (2010). Relationship trajectories and psychological well-being among sexual minority youth. *Journal of Youth and Adolescence, 39*(10), 1148–1163.

Bell, D., Martinez, J., Botwinick, G., Shaw, K., Walker, L., Dodds, S., & Siciliano, C. (2003). Case finding for HIV-positive youth: A special type of hidden population. *Journal of Adolescent Health, 33*(2), 10–22.

Benton, T. D. (2010). Psychiatric considerations in children and adolescents with HIV/AIDS. *Child & Adolescent Psychiatric Clinics of North America, 19*(2), 387–400.

Bird, J. D., Eversman, M., & Voisin, D. R. (2017). "You just can't trust everybody": the impact of sexual risk, partner type and perceived partner trustworthiness on HIV-status disclosure decisions among HIV-positive black gay and bisexual men. Culture, *health & sexuality, 19*(8), 829–843. DOI: 10.1080/13691058.2016.1267408

Bird, J. D. P., LaSala, M., Hidalgo, M., Kuhns, L., & Garofalo, R. (2017). "I had to go to the streets to get love": Pathways from parental rejection to HIV risk among young gay men. *Journal of Homosexuality, 64*(3), 321–342.

Bird, J. D. P., & Voisin, D. (2013). "You're an open target to be abused": A qualitative study of stigma and HIV self-disclosure among black men who have sex with men. *American Journal of Public Health, 103*(12), 2193–2199.

Bouris, A., Guilamo-Ramos, V., Pickard, A., Shiu, C., Loosier, P. S., Dittus, P., ... Waldmiller, M. J. (2010). A systematic review of parental influences on the health and well-being of lesbian, gay, and bisexual youth: Time for a new public health research and practice agenda. *Journal of Primary Prevention, 31*(5-6), 273–309.

Bouris, A., Voisin, D., Pilloton, M., Flatt, N., Eavou, R., Hampton, K.,... John A Schneider (2013). Project nGage: Network supported HIV care engagement for younger black men who have sex with men and transgender persons. *Journal of AIDS & Clinical Research, 4*. doi:10.4172/2155-6113.1000236, 04.

Bradley, B. J., & Greene, A. C. (2013). Do health and education agencies in the United States share responsibility for academic achievement and health? A review of 25 years of evidence about the relationship of adolescents' academic achievement and health behaviors. *Journal of Adolescent Health, 52*, 523–532.

Branson, B., Handsfield, H., Lampe, M., Janssen, R., Taylor, A., Lyss, S., & Clark, J. (2006). Revised recommendations for HIV testing of adults, adolescents, and pregnant women in health-care settings. *Morbidity & Mortality Weekly Report, 55*, 752–783.

Brewster, K. L., & Tillman, K. H. (2012). Sexual orientation and substance use among adolescents and young adults. *American Journal of Public Health, 102*(6), 1168–1176.

Brooks-Gunn, J., Boyer, C. B., & Hein, K. (1988). Preventing HIV infection and AIDS in children and adolescents: Behavioral research and intervention strategies. *American Psychologist, 43*(11), 958–964.

Brown, L. K., DiClemente, R. J., & Reynolds, L. A. (1991). HIV prevention for adolescents: Utility of the health belief model. *AIDS Education and Prevention, 3*(1), 50–59.

Brown, L. K., Lourie, K. J., & Pao, M. (2000). Children and adolescents living with HIV and AIDS: A review. *Journal of Child Psychology and Psychiatry, 41*(1), 81–96.

Bruce, D., Harper, G. W., & Adolescent Medicine Trials Network for HIV/AIDS Interventions (ATN). (2011). Operating without a safety net: Gay male adolescents and emerging adults' experiences of marginalization and migration, and implications for theory of syndemic production of health disparities. *Health Education & Behavior, 38*(4), 367–378.

Bruce, D., Harper, G. W., & Adolescent Medicine Trials Network for HIV/AIDS Interventions (ATN). (2012). Future life goals of HIV-positive gay and bisexual male emerging adults. *Journal of Adolescent Research, 27*(4), 449–470.

Bryan, A. D., Schmiege, S. J., & Magnan, R. E. (2012). Marijuana use and risky sexual behavior among high-risk adolescents: Trajectories, risk factors, and event-level relationships. *Developmental Psychology, 48*(5), 1429–1442.

Campbell, C., & Deacon, H. (2006). Unraveling the contexts of stigma: From internalization to resistance to change. *Journal of Community & Applied Social Psychology, 16*(6), 411–417.

Centers for Disease Control and Prevention (CDC). (2008). HIV prevention education and HIV-related policies in secondary schools—selected sites, United States, 2006. *MMWR: Morbidity & Mortality Weekly Report, 57*(30), 822–825.

Centers for Disease Control and Prevention (CDC). (2015). *HIV in the United States: At a glance.* Retrieved from http://www.cdc.gov/hiv/resources/factsheets/PDF/stats_basics_factsheet.pdf.

Centers for Disease Control and Prevention (CDC). (2016). *HIV among youth.* Retrieved from https://www.cdc.gov/hiv/group/age/youth/index.html.

Cohen, C. J. (1999). *The boundaries of blackness: AIDS and the breakdown of black politics.* Chicago, IL: University of Chicago Press.

Corliss, H. L., Goodenow, C. S., Nichols, L., & Austin, S. B. (2011). High burden of homelessness among sexual-minority adolescents: Findings from a representative Massachusetts high school sample. *American Journal of Public Health, 101*(9), 1683–1689.

Corliss, H. L., Rosario, M., Wypij, D., Wylie, S. A., Frazier, A. L., & Austin, S. B. (2010). Sexual orientation and drug use in a longitudinal cohort study of U.S. adolescents. *Addictive Behaviors, 35*(5), 517–521.

Cox, N. S. (2003). *School HIV/AIDS policy toolkit.* Madison, WI: Wisconsin Department of Public Instruction.

D'Augelli, A. R., Grossman, A. H., & Starks, M. T. (2006). Childhood gender a typicality, victimization, and PTSD among lesbian, gay, and bisexual youth. *Journal of Interpersonal Violence, 21*(11), 1462–1482.

DeGroat, D. M. (2009). When students test positive, their privacy fails: The unconstitutionality of South Carolina's HIV/AIDS reporting requirement. *American University Journal of Gender, Social Policy & the Law, 17*, 751–785.

Dowshen, N., Binns, H., & Garofalo, R. (2009). Experiences of HIV-related stigma among young men who have sex with men. *AIDS Patient Care and STDs, 23*(5), 371.

Drumright, L. N., Patterson, T. L., & Strathdee, S. A. (2006). Club drugs as causal risk factors for HIV acquisition among men who have sex with men: A review. *Substance Use & Misuse, 41*(10-12), 1551–1601.

Elford, J., & Hart, G. (2003). If HIV prevention works, why are rates of high-risk sexual behavior increasing among MSM? *AIDS Education and Prevention, 15*(4), 294–308.

Emans, S. J., Brown, R. T., Davis, A., Felice, M., & Hein, K. (1991). Society for adolescent medicine position paper on reproductive health care for adolescents. *Journal of Adolescent Health, 12*(8), 649–661.

Evatt, B. L. (2006). The tragic history of AIDS in the hemophilia population, 1982–1984. *Journal of Thrombosis and Haemostasis, 4*(11), 2295–2301.

Fair, C., Garner-Edwards, D., & McLees-Lane, M. (2005). Assessment of HIV-related school policy in North Carolina. *Journal of HIV/AIDS & Social Services, 4*(4), 47–63.

Fisher, J. D., & Fisher, W. A. (2002). The information-motivation-behavioral skills model. In R. J. DiClemente, R. A. Crosby, & M. C. Kegler (Eds.), *Emerging theories in health promotion practice and research: Strategies for improving public health* (pp. 40–70). San Francisco: Jossey-Bass.

Flicker, S., Goldberg, E., Read, S., Veinot, T., McClelland, A., Saulnier, P., & Skinner, H. (2004). HIV-positive youth's perspectives on the internet and ehealth. *Journal of Medical Internet Research, 6*(3), e32.

Flicker, S., Skinner, H., Read, S., Veinot, T., McClelland, A., Saulnier, P., & Goldberg, E. (2005). Falling through the cracks of the big cities: Who is meeting the needs of HIV-positive youth? *Canadian Journal of Public Health, 96*(4), 308–312.

Friedman, M. S., Marshal, M. P., Guadamuz, T. E., Wei, C., Wong, C. F., Saewyc, E. M., & Stall, R. (2011). A meta-analysis of disparities in childhood sexual abuse, parental physical abuse, and peer victimization among sexual minority and sexual nonminority individuals. *American Journal of Public Health*, *101*(8), 1481–1494.

Galindo, G. R. (2013). A loss of moral experience: Understanding HIV-related stigma in the New York City house and ball community. *American Journal of Public Health*, *103*(2), 293–299.

Galliher, R. V., Rostosky, S. S., & Hughes, H. K. (2004). School belonging, self-esteem, and depressive symptoms in adolescents: An examination of sex, sexual attraction status, and urbanicity. *Journal of Youth and Adolescence*, *33*(3), 235–245.

Garofalo, R., Herrick, A., Mustanski, B., & Donenberg, G. R. (2007). Tip of the iceberg: Young men who have sex with men, the internet, and HIV risk. *American Journal of Public Health*, *97*, 1113–1117.

Garofalo, R., Mustanski, B., Johnson, A., & Emerson, E. (2010). Exploring factors that underlie racial/ethnic disparities in HIV risk among young men who have sex with men. *Journal of Urban Health*, *87*(2), 318–323.

Garofalo, R., Mustanski, B., McKirnan, D., Herrick, A., & Donenberg, G. (2007). Methamphetamine and young men who have sex with men: Understanding patterns and correlates of use and the association with HIV-related sexual risk. *Archives of Pediatrics & Adolescent Medicine*, *161*(6), 591–596.

Gates, G. J. (2011, April). *How many people are lesbian, gay, bisexual, and transgender?* Retrieved from http://williamsinstitute.law.ucla.edu/wp-content/uploads/Gates-How-Many-People-LGBT-Apr-2011.pdf.

Halkitis, P. N., Brockwell, S., Siconolfi, D. E., Moeller, R. W., Sussman, R. D., Mougues, P. J., … Sweeney, M. M. (2011). Sexual behaviors of adolescent emerging and young adult men who have sex with men ages 13-29 in New York City. *Journal of Acquired Immune Deficiency Syndromes*, *56*, 285–291.

Halkitis, P. N., Kapadia, F., Siconolfi, D. E., Moeller, R. W., Figueroa, R. P., Barton, S. C., & Blachman-Forshay, J. (2013). Individual, psychosocial, and social correlates of unprotected anal intercourse in a new generation of young men who have sex with men in New York City. *American Journal of Public Health*, *103*, 889–895.

Halkitis, P. N., & Palamar, J. J. (2008). Club drug initiation: Multivariate modeling of club drug use initiation among gay and bisexual men. *Substance Use & Misuse*, *43*, 871–879.

Harper, G. W., Fernandez, I. M., Bruce, D., Hosek, S. G., Jacobs, R. J., & Adolescent Medicine Trials Network for HIV/AIDS Interventions (ATN). (2013). The role of multiple identities in adherence to medical appointments among gay/bisexual male adolescents living with HIV. *AIDS and Behavior*, *17*(1), 213–223.

Hein, K., & Dell, R. (1995). Comparison of HIV+ and HIV- adolescents: Risks factors and psychosocial determinants. *Pediatrics*, *95*(1), 96–104.

Herek, G. M. (2002). Thinking about AIDS and stigma: A psychologist's perspective. *Journal of Law, Medicine, and Ethics*, *30*, 594–607.

Herek, G. M. (2004). Beyond "homophobia": Thinking about sexual prejudice and stigma in the twenty-first century. *Sexuality Research & Social Policy*, *1*(2), 6–24.

Hightow-Weidman, L. B., Phillips, G., II, Outlaw, A. Y., Wohl, A. R., Fields, S., Hildalgo, J., & LeGrand, S. (2013). Patterns of HIV disclosure and condom use among HIV-infected young racial/ethnic minority men who have sex with men. *AIDS and Behavior*, *17*(1), 360–368.

House Bill 2. (2016). Retrieved from http://www.ncleg.net/sessions/2015e2/bills/house/pdf/h2v4.pdf.

Hussen, S. A., Chahroudi, A., Boylan, A., Camacho-Gonzalez, A. F., Hackett, S., & Chakraborty, R. (2015). Transition of youth living with HIV infection pediatric to adult-centered healthcare: A review of the literature. *Future Virology*, *9*, 921–929.

Hussen, S. A., Harper, G. W., Bauermeister, J. A., Hightow-Weidman, L. B., & Adolescent Medicine Trials Network for HIV/AIDS Interventions. (2015). Psychosocial influences on engagement in care among HIV-positive young black gay/bisexual and other men who have sex with men. *AIDS Patient Care & STDs*, *29*, 77–85.

Institute of Medicine of the National Academies (IOM). (2011). Childhood/adolescence. In *The health of lesbian, gay, bisexual, and transgender people: Building a foundation for better understanding* (pp. 141–184). Washington, DC: The National Academies Press.

Irwin, C. E., Igra, V., Eyre, S., & Millstein, S. (1997). Risk-taking behavior in adolescents: The paradigm. *Annals of New York Academy of Sciences, 817,* 1–35.

Jeffries, W. L., 4th, Townsend, E. S., Gelaude, D. J., Torrone, E. A., Gasiorowicz, M., & Bertolli, J. (2015). HIV stigma experienced by young men who have sex with men (MSM) living with HIV infection. *AIDS Education and Prevention, 27,* 58–71.

Kalichman, S. C., DiMarco, M., Austin, J., Luke, W., & Di-Fonzo, K. (2003). Stress, social support, and HIV-status disclosure to family and friends among HIV-positive men and women. *Journal of Behavioral Medicine, 26,* 315–332.

Karon, J., Fleming, P., Steketee, R., & De Cock, K. (2001). HIV in the united states at the turn of the century: An epidemic in transition. *American Journal of Public Health, 91*(7), 1060–1068.

Kingdon, M. J., Storholm, E. D., Halkitis, P. N., Jones, D. C., Moeller, R. W., Siconolfi, D., & Solomon, T. M. (2013). Targeting HIV prevention messaging to a new generation of gay, bisexual, and other young men who have sex with men. *Journal of Health Communication, 18,* 325–342.

Klitzman, R. L., Greenberg, J. D., Pollack, L. M., & Dolezal, C. (2002). MDMA ('ecstasy') use, and its association with high risk behaviors, mental health, and other factors among gay/bisexual men in New York city. *Drug and Alcohol Dependence, 66,* 115–125.

Kubicek, K., Beyer, W. J., Weiss, G., Iverson, E., & Kipke, M. D. (2010). In the dark: Young men's stories of sexual initiation in the absence of relevant sexual health information. *Health Education & Behavior, 37*(2), 243–263.

Lam, P. K., Naar-King, S., & Wright, K. (2007). Social support and disclosure as predictors of mental health in HIV-positive youth. *AIDS Patient Care and STDs, 21*(1), 20–29.

Lange, T. (2003). *HIV and civil rights.* New York: ACLU AIDS Project. Retrieved from http://www.aclu.org/pdfs/hivaids/hiv_civilrights.pdf.

Lusher, J. M., & Brownstein, A. P. (2007). HIV and hemophilia. *Journal of Thrombosis and Haemostasis, 5*(3), 609–610.

Lynch, A. D., Lerner, R. M., & Leventhal, T. (2013). Adolescent academic achievement and school engagement: An examination of the role of school-wide peer culture. *Journal of Youth and Adolescence, 42*(1), 6–19.

Marcia, J. (1980). Identity in adolescence. In J. Adelson (Ed.), *Handbook of adolescent psychology* (pp. 159–187). Hoboken, NJ: Wiley & Sons.

Marshal, M. P., Dietz, L. J., Friedman, M. S., Stall, R., Smith, H. A., McGinley, J., ... Brent, D. A. (2011). Suicidality and depression disparities between sexual minority and heterosexual youth: A meta-analytic review. *Journal of Adolescent Health, 49*(2), 115–123.

Marshal, M. P., Friedman, M. S., Stall, R., & Thompson, A. L. (2009). Individual trajectories of substance use in lesbian, gay, and bisexual youth and heterosexual youth. *Addiction, 104,* 974–981.

Mawar, N., Sahay, S., Pandit, A., & Mahajan, U. (2005). The third phase of HIV pandemic: Social consequences of HIV/AIDS stigma & discrimination & future needs. *Indian Journal of Medical Research, 122*(6), 471–484.

McDowell, T. L., & Serovich, J. M. (2007). The effect of perceived and actual social support on the mental health of HIV+ individuals. *AIDS Care, 19,* 1223–1229.

Meyer, I. H. (2003). Prejudice, social stress, and mental health in lesbian, gay, and bisexual populations: Conceptual issues and research evidence. *Psychological Bulletin, 129*(5), 674–697.

Murphy, D., Roberts, K., Marelich, W., & Hoffman, D. (2000). Barriers to antiretroviral adherence among HIV-infected adults. *AIDS Patient Care, 14,* 47–58.

Murrill, C. S., Weeks, H., Castrucci, B. C., Weinstock, H. S., Bell, B. P., Spruill, C., & Gwinn, M. (2002). Age-specific seroprevalence of HIV, hepatitis B virus, and hepatitis C virus infection among injection drug users admitted to drug treatment in 6 US cities. *The American Journal of Public Health, 92*(3), 385–387.

Mustanski, B., Garofalo, R., Herrick, A., & Donenberg, G. (2007). Psychosocial health problems increase risk for HIV among urban young men who have sex with men: Preliminary evidence of a syndemic in need of attention. *Annals of Behavioral Medicine, 34*(1), 37–45.

Mustanski, B., Newcomb, M., Du Bois, S., Garcia, S., & Grov, C. (2011). HIV in young men who have sex with men: A review of epidemiology, risk and protective factors, and interventions. *Journal of Sex Research, 48*(2-3), 218–253.

Naar-King, S., Templin, T., Wright, K., Frey, M., Parsons, J., & Lam, P. (2006). Psychosocial factors and medication adherence in HIV-positive youth. *AIDS Patient Care and STDs, 20*(1), 44–47.

Naar-King, S., Wright, K., Parsons, J., Frey, M., Templin, T., Lam, P., & Murphy, D. (2006). Healthy choices: Motivational enhancement therapy for health risk behaviors in HIV-positive youth. *AIDS Education & Prevention, 18*(1), 1–11.

National Association of State Boards of Education (NASBE). (2012). *State school healthy policy database.* Retrieved from http://nasbe.org/healthy_schools/hs/bytopics.php?topicid=5110&ca tExpand=acdnbtm_catE.

Newcomb, M. E., Clerkin, E. M., & Mustanski, B. (2011). Sensation seeking moderates the effects of alcohol and drug use prior to sex on sexual risk in young men who have sex with men. *AIDS and Behavior, 15*, 565–575.

O'Byrne, P., & Watts, J. (2014). Include, differentiate and manage: Gay male youth, stigma and healthcare utilization. *Nursing Inquiry, 21*(1), 20–29. doi:10.1111/nin. 12014

Ott, M. Q., Wypij, D., Corliss, H. L., Rosario, M., Reisner, S. L., Gordon, A. R., & Austin, S. B. (2013). Repeated changes in reported sexual orientation identity linked to substance use behaviors in youth. *Journal of Adolescent Health, 52*(4), 465–472.

Outlaw, A. Y., Phillips, G., Hightow-Weidman, L. B., Fields, S. D., Hidalgo, J., Halpern-Felsher, B., & Green-Jones, A. (2011). Age of MSM sexual debut and risk factors: Results from a multisite study of racial/ethnic minority YMSM living with HIV. *AIDS Patient Care & STDs, 25*, S23–S29.

Parker, R., & Aggleton, P. (2003). HIV and AIDS-related stigma and discrimination: A conceptual framework and implications for action. *Social Science & Medicine, 57*(1), 13–24.

Pearson, J., Muller, C., & Wilkinson, L. (2007). Adolescent same-sex attraction and academic outcomes: The role of school attachment and engagement. *Social Problems, 54*(4), 523–542.

Pulerwitz, J., Amaro, H., Jong, W. D., Gortmaker, S. L., & Rudd, R. (2002). Relationship power, condom use and HIV risk among women in the USA. *AIDS Care, 14*(6), 789–800.

Radcliffe, J., Tanney, M., & Rudy, B. J. (2006). Post-traumatic stress and adherence to medical treatment among youth with HIV. *Journal of Adolescent Health, 38*(2), 110–111.

Rao, D., Kekwaletswe, T., Hosek, S., Martinez, J., & Rodriguez, F. (2007). Stigma and social barriers to medication adherence with urban youth living with HIV. *AIDS Care, 19*(1), 28–33.

Remafedi, G., Farrow, J. A., & Deisher, R. W. (1991). Risk factors for attempted suicide in gay and bisexual youth. *Pediatrics, 87*(6), 869–875. Retrieved from http://www.psych.org/ advocacy--newsroom/position-statements.

Rind, B. (2001). Gay and bisexual adolescent boys' sexual experiences with men: An empirical examination of psychological correlates in a nonclinical sample. *Archives of Sexual Behavior, 50*(4), 345–368.

Roberts, A. L., Rosario, M., Slopen, N., Calzo, J. P., & Austin, S. B. (2013). Childhood gender nonconformity, bullying victimization, and depressive symptoms across adolescence and early adulthood: An 11-year longitudinal study. *Journal of the American Academy of Child and Adolescent Psychiatry, 52*(2), 143–152.

Rosario, M., Schrimshaw, E. W., & Hunter, J. (2010). Different patterns of sexual identity development over time: Implications for the psychological adjustment of lesbian, gay, and bisexual youths. *Journal of Sex Research, 48*(1), 3–15.

Rosario, M., Schrimshaw, E. W., & Hunter, J. (2012). Homelessness among lesbian, gay, and bisexual youth: Implications for subsequent internalizing and externalizing symptoms. *Journal of Youth and Adolescence, 41*(5), 544–560.

Rotheram-Borus, M. J., Murphy, D. A., Coleman, C. L., Kennedy, M., Reid, H. M., Cline, T. R., ... Kipke, M. (1997). Risk acts, health care, and medical adherence among HIV+ youths in care over time. *AIDS and Behavior, 1*(1), 43–52.

Rotheram-Borus, M. J., O'Keefe, Z., Kracker, R., & Foo, H. (2000). Prevention of HIV among adolescents. *Prevention Science, 1*(1), 15–30.

Russell, S. T., Ryan, C., Toomey, R. B., Diaz, R. M., & Sanchez, J. (2011). Lesbian, gay, bisexual, and transgender adolescent school victimization: Implications for young adult health and adjustment. *Journal of School Health, 81*(5), 223–230.

Ryan, C., Huebner, D., Diaz, R. M., & Sanchez, J. (2009). Family rejection as a predictor of negative health outcomes in white and Latino lesbian, gay, and bisexual young adults. *Pediatrics, 123*(1), 346–352.

Salomon, E., Mimiaga, M., Husnik, M., Welles, S., Manseau, M., Montenegro, A., ... Mayer, K. (2009). Depressive symptoms, utilization of mental health care, substance use and sexual risk among young men who have sex with men in EXPLORE: Implications for age-specific interventions. *AIDS and Behavior, 13*(4), 811–821.

Schellenberg, E. G., Keil, J. M., & Bem, S. L. (1995). "innocent victims" of AIDS: Identifying the subtext. *Journal of Applied Social Psychology, 25*(20), 1790–1800.

Serovich, J. M., & Grafsky, E. L. (2011). Does family matter to HIV-positive men who have sex with men? *Journal of Marital and Family Therapy, 37*(3), 290–298.

Shilts, R. (1988). *And the band played on: Politics, people, and the AIDS epidemic.* New York, NY: Penguin Books.

Smedley, B. D., Stith, A. Y., & Nelson, A. R. (Eds.). (2003). *Unequal treatment: Confronting racial and ethnic disparities in health care.* Washington, DC: The National Academy of Sciences Press.

Solorio, R., Swendeman, D., & Rotheram-Borus, M. J. (2003). Risk among young gay and bisexual men living with HIV. *AIDS Education and Prevention, 15*(1_supplement), 80–89.

Spear, H. J., & Kulbok, P. (2004). Autonomy and adolescence: A concept analysis. *Public Health Nursing, 21*(2), 144–152.

Steinberg, L., & Morris, S. A. (2001). Adolescent development. *Annual Review of Psychology, 52,* 83–110.

Stueve, A. A., O'Donnell, L. L., Duran, R. R., Doval, A. S., Geier, J. J., & Community Intervention Trial for Youth Study. (2002). Being high and taking sexual risks: Findings from a multisite survey of urban young men who have sex with men. *AIDS Education and Prevention, 14,* 482–495.

Tharinger, D., & Wells, G. (2000). An attachment perspective on the developmental challenges of gay and lesbian adolescents: The needs for continuity of caregiving from family and schools. *School Psychology Review, 29*(2), 158–172.

The Center for HIV Law & Policy. (n.d.). *Teen SENSE: Model sexual health education standards for youth in state custody.* Retrieved from http://www.hivlawandpolicy.org/public/initiatives/teensense.

Thiede, H., Valleroy, L., MacKellar, D., Celentano, D., Ford, W., Hagan, H., & Torian, L. (2003). Regional patterns and correlates of substance use among young men who have sex with men in 7 U.S. urban areas. *American Journal of Public Health, 93*(11), 1915–1921.

Tillfors, M., Persson, S., Willén, M., & Burk, W. J. (2012). Prospective links between social anxiety and adolescent peer relations. *Journal of Adolescence, 35*(5), 1255–1263.

Tolman, D. L., & McClelland, S. I. (2011). Normative sexuality development in adolescence: A decade in review, 2000–2009. *Journal of Research on Adolescence, 21*(1), 242–255.

Traube, D. E., Schrager, S. M., Holloway, I. W., Weiss, G., & Kipke, M. D. (2012). *Environmental risk, social cognition, and drug use among young men who have sex with men: Longitudinal effects of minority status on health processes and outcomes.* Drug and Alcohol Dependence. Retrieved from http://www.sciencedirect.com/science/article/pii/S0376871612002244.

U.S. Department of Justice (n.d.). *Questions and answers: The Americans with disabilities act and persons with HIV/AIDS.* Retrieved from http://www.ada.gov/archive/hivqanda.txt.

Uris, P. (1996). *Recommendations for the school health nurse in addressing HIV/AIDS with adolescents. (nurses campaign for public health)*. Washington, DC: American Nurses Association.

Voisin, D., & Bird, D. (2012). "you get more respect," reasons for sex among African American youth. *Journal of Social Service Research*, *38*(3), 392–401.

Voisin, D., Bird, J., Shi Shiu, C., & Kreiger, C. (2013). "It's crazy being a black and gay youth." getting information about HIV prevention: A pilot study. *Journal of Adolescence*, *36*(1), 111–119.

Weiner, L. S., Battles, H. B., & Heilman, N. (2000). Public disclosure of a child's HIV infection: Impact on children and families. *AIDS Patient Care and STDs*, *14*(9), 485–497.

White House Office of National AIDS Policy. (2010). *National HIV/AIDS strategy for the United States*. Retrieved from http://www.whitehouse.gov/sites/default/files/uploads/NHAS.pdf.

Wilson, B. D., Harper, G. W., Hidalgo, M. A., Jamil, O. B., Torres, R. S., & Fernandez, M. I. (2010). Negotiating dominant masculinity ideology: Strategies used by gay, bisexual and questioning male adolescents. *American Journal of Community Psychology*, *45*(1-2), 169–185.

Chapter 12
HIV Within the House Ball Community and the Promise of Community-Based Social Structures for Intervention and Support

Emily A. Arnold and Marlon M. Bailey

Introduction

The House Ball Community is an underground community that has its roots in the drag balls of Harlem from the 1920s (Bailey, 2013; Chauncey, 1994). The House Ball Community, made up of houses and the elaborate balls they organize and perform in, exists in a number of metropolitan centers across the United States (US) and increasingly in various countries such as Canada, the United Kingdom, Russia, and Sweden. Members of the House Ball Community come predominantly from Black and Latino/a communities of gay, lesbian, bisexual, and transgender (GLBT) youth, with a variety of gender presentations. For example, an entire range of gender and sexual identities are revered and celebrated in the context of ballroom performances and institutionalized within the houses, including butch queens, butch queens up in drag, butches, and femme queens. These social activities and alliances represent safe subaltern spaces for young people to give and receive affirmation for non-heteronormative gender and sexual identities, as well as to take part in a community that celebrates gender fluidity and a cornucopia of sexual desires (Bailey, 2014). Most crucial to HIV prevention is that Ballroom members expand gender and sexual possibilities by taking up multiple articulations and performances of both masculinity and femininity.

E.A. Arnold (✉)
Center for AIDS Prevention Studies, Department of Medicine,
University of California, San Francisco (UCSF), San Francisco, CA 94143, USA
e-mail: Emily.Arnold@ucsf.edu

M.M. Bailey
Women and Gender Studies Program, School of Social Transformation,
Arizona State University, Tempe, AZ, USA

© Springer Science+Business Media LLC 2017
L. Wilton (ed.), *Understanding Prevention for HIV Positive Gay Men*,
DOI 10.1007/978-1-4419-0203-0_12

The House Ball Community has been largely unknown in the public health literature until relatively recently, when a handful of investigators have begun to publish findings from studies with the population (Alio et al., 2014; Arnold & Bailey, 2009; Bailey, 2009, 2013; Galindo, 2013; Kipke, Kubicek, Supan, Weiss, & Schrager, 2013; Kubicek, et al., 2013; Murrill et al., 2008; Rowan, DeSousa, Randall, White, & Holley, 2014; Wong, Schrager, Holloway, Meyer, & Kipke, 2014; Young et al., 2017). The House Ball Community first appeared in popular media in Jennie Livingston's documentary *Paris is Burning*, and, subsequently, in Wolfgang Busch's documentary *How do I look*, Madonna's *Vogue*, as well as the featuring of the dance group "Vogue Evolution" in "Do you think you can dance." Although there have been a number of depictions of the House Ball Community within popular media, these mostly cinematic representations fail to capture the full dimensions of the House Ball Community, such as the gender system and the complex kinship structure upon which the community depends. Notwithstanding this exposure in popular media, albeit limited, this community is still relatively unknown in academic circles (Bailey, 2013). The ball event is the central means through which members of the community affirm, celebrate, and constructively critique its fellow members. Houses organize and invite the larger House Ball Community to compete in particular categories listed on flyers or call sheets. Balls are festive affairs, usually held in older dance halls, community centers, bars/clubs, or rented hotel event rooms, in the middle of the night. Recent funding for HIV prevention activities, in conjunction with a policy of test and treat, has started to put the community on the radar in public health circles as departments of health and community-based organizations begin to use balls as a way to capture young men who have sex with men (MSM) and transgender women of color in particular for HIV testing and case detection (van Doorn, 2012).

HIV Prevalence and Cofactors Driving the Epidemic in the House Ball Community

A limited number of studies have also been conducted with the House Ball Community to determine HIV prevalence rates, HIV-related risk activities, as well as potential avenues for intervention (Young et al., 2017). A groundbreaking study, known as the House Ball Survey, was conducted with the NYC House Ball Community in 2004, and utilized venue-based time day sampling as well as biological determinants of HIV status to examine prevalence and risk behavior. This study reported that 17% of participants tested were HIV positive, and 73% of those who were HIV positive were unaware of their HIV positive status (Murrill et al., 2008). This study also reported high levels of HIV-related risk behavior, with 24% of the sample having had more than five sexual partners in the past 12 months, 40% reporting condomless anal intercourse with a male partner within the same time period, and 37% exchanging sex for money, drugs, or shelter in the past 12 months.

Murrill et al. also found that 42% of the sample had symptoms of depression, measured by a CES-D (Center for Epidemiologic Studies Depression Scale) score over 16 in the past 7 days, and a majority of the sample had experienced at least one stressful life event in the past 12 months. In a more recent study conducted with the House Ball Community in Los Angeles, California, Kipke et al. used venue-based day time sampling and found an overall rate of 6% self-reported HIV prevalence among the 263 participants in their study, which was much lower than that found in the NYC House Ball Community (Kipke et al., 2013). Kipke et al. also reported high use of alcohol (72%) and other drugs including marijuana (53%), ecstasy (12%), and cocaine (4%) in the past 3 months. More disconcerting, findings indicated that 25% of participants used other drugs in conjunction with sexual activity in the past 3 months. In a study conducted from 2011 to 2012 with the House Ball Community in the San Francisco Bay Area, Arnold et al. found HIV prevalence, measured by self-report, to be 27% in a sample of 274 participants attending ballroom events in the San Francisco Bay Area (Arnold, Sterrett-Hong, Jonas, & Pollack, 2016).

Because transgender members assume an important role in the community, including occupying positions of leadership in many houses, they must be considered in any discussion of HIV prevalence in the House Ball Community. Several investigators have reported high rates of exchange sex among gay men and transgender members of the House Ball Community. Sanchez, Finlayson, Murrill, Guilin, and Dean (2010) examined the NYC House Ball Community survey data looking specifically at exchange sex, stigmatization, stressful life events and high risk related behavior and comparing findings between MSM and transgender female respondents (Sanchez et al., 2010). Transgender members were especially vulnerable, with findings indicating significantly higher rates of exchange sex, 7% compared to 39%, respectively. In a study conducted among male-to-female (MTF) transgender House Ball Community participants in New York, Hwahng and Nuttbrock found that engaging in sex work along with drug use as a way to cope with sex work, was a "rite of passage" for many young MTF transgender people entering the scene (Hwahng & Nuttbrock, 2007). Sex work, in many cases survival sex, was employed to help pay for basic necessities such as food, clothing, and shelter, as well as body modification through silicone injections, surgery, and hormones. Hwahng and Nuttbrock point out that it was difficult for their transgender informants to find other forms of employment in the formal economy due to gender and sexual discrimination. Importantly, the authors examined the salience of belonging within particular ethnocultural communities, and how marginalization plays out for communities positioned differently within the larger graded power structure within the US context. Several investigators, including Hwahng and Nuttbrock, have recommended the development of prevention strategies to improve public acceptance of gender variation and increasing opportunities for transgender and gay youth of color in the more traditional workforce.

Much of the research on young MSM and transgender women of color has found that they are difficult to engage in care, and these findings that have been supported in studies with House Ball Community participants. Holloway et al. (2012) indicated that while services exist for young MSM, House Ball Community members did not access service programs in the Los Angeles study (Holloway et al., 2012). Although 80% of the sample reported testing for HIV, only 26% used HIV prevention programs. In a literature review, Phillips, Peterson, Binson, Hidalgo, and Magnus (2011) identified several opportunities within the structure of the House Ball Community to engage with participants to encourage more regular testing, prevention activities, and treatment adherence, citing programs such as the House of Latex program conducted by the Gay Men's Health Crisis (GMHC) in New York City as a model for successful engagement with the House Ball Community (Phillips et al., 2011). Painter, Ngalame, Lucas, Lauby, and Herbst (2010) described working with People of Color in Crisis (POCC), a community-based organization (CBO) in Brooklyn, New York, to engage with the New York City-based House Ball Community to recruit young MSM of color for their Many Men, Many Voices (3MV) program when recruitment initially lagged (Painter et al., 2010). POCC worked with house leaders to recruit and retain participants, tapping into the membership networks of House Ball Communities. Eventually 338 men were enrolled in their evaluation of 3MV, one of the only HIV prevention interventions that has been found to significantly reduce HIV-related risk behavior among Black MSM (Wilton et al., 2009).

Some social scientists have been more critical of the recent reliance on the House Ball Community to engage young people in HIV prevention strategies. Van Doorn (2012) conducted ethnographic research with the House Ball Community in Baltimore as "Test and Treat" became the new paradigm for HIV prevention (van Doorn, 2012). Van Doorn argued that using the "affective labor performed by members of the House Ball Community attracts a host of optimistic investments in collective and individual prosperity that have yet to be realized." In what he calls the "labour of cruel optimism," van Doorn contends that while employing members of the House Ball Community to help bring in their peers for HIV testing and treatment serves public health, the larger systemic production of inequality will not change, because the language of viral containment depoliticizes the struggle against HIV. While testing assists the Department of Health in achieving their numbers and creates a professional workforce among disenfranchised communities, health, as articulated by van Doorn, is too narrowly defined and does not address the root causes of HIV and other syndemics affecting the House Ball Community. Homelessness, crime, racism, and homophobia remain more immediate threats to the health and well-being of young people involved in the House Ball Community (van Doorn, 2012). Other social scientists suggest that in addition to the aforementioned factors, racial discrimination, incarceration, poverty, and overall social dispossession are also primary drivers of high HIV prevalence among African American GLBT individuals (Harris, 2010; Lemelle, 2010; Watkins-Hayes, Patterson, & Armour, 2011)—who constitute the majority of the membership of House Ball Communities. Although perhaps unintended, the abandonment of HIV negative men, with a refocus of federal resources on treatment adherence and medical care, leaves these more immediate causes of inequality and poor health among members of the House Ball Community in place.

Researchers have also pointed to the need to address HIV-related stigma operating within the House Ball Community, a particularly intractable issue since achieving ballroom status is one of the key organizing principles of the community (Arnold et al., 2012; Bailey, 2013, Galindo, 2013). Using qualitative interviews with 20 members of the House Ball Community in New York City, Galindo (2013) reported that the hierarchical structure of the community, and its emphasis on competition, in conjunction with HIV-related stigma, could impede efforts for HIV prevention among HIV positive members (Galindo, 2013). Galindo points out that HIV-related stigma leads to a loss of moral experience among those in House Ball Community identified as HIV positive, losing ball status as well as a loss of social and emotional support for community members. Thus, Galindo's participants reported carefully guarding their HIV positive serostatus for fear of undermining their standing in the community as individuals and house members. Similarly, Arnold et al. found that HIV-related stigma created barriers for engaging in HIV prevention activities, based on 67 in-depth interviews with House Ball Community members in the San Francisco Bay Area (Arnold, Williams, Blount, & Pierceson, 2012). HIV-related stigma undermined disclosure, testing, and seeking support for living with HIV. Consistent with Galindo's findings, HIV status was rarely disclosed to sexual partners or friends, partly due to the fact that many members engaged in sex work to support themselves. Although support existed for HIV testing from house mothers, members took pains not to seek out testing in front of other house siblings should a positive diagnosis be made and the information used against them. HIV treatment adherence was impacted due to an unwillingness to take medications regularly and attend HIV clinics for fear of being outed with their HIV status.

In order to ground recommendations for promoting HIV prevention and treatment with the House Ball Community, it is necessary to describe two core dimensions of the community: the gender system and the balls/houses.

The House Ball Community: Gender System

The gender system, the kinship structure (houses), and ball events (particularly prevention balls) are three inextricable core dimensions of the House Ball Community and these components are important considerations for developing more effective HIV prevention strategies for this community. First, what members refer to as the "gender system" is a collection of gender and sexual subjectivities that extend beyond the binary/ternary categories in dominant society such as male/female, man/woman and gay/lesbian/bisexual, and straight (Bailey, 2011). This system is the basis of all House Ball Community subjectivities, familial roles, and the competitive performance categories at ball events. In this system, categories of sex, gender, and sexuality are linked but not always conflated.[1]

To be clear, the genders and sexualities found in the House Ball Community are subjectivities, insofar as members identify and fashion themselves by and through the convergent notions of sex, gender and sexuality within the community *and* as those meanings are imposed on them by society (Bailey, 2011). Thus, House Ball Community members do not reject dominant gender norms entirely, nor do they desire doing so; rather, by revealing and exploiting the unstable and fluid nature of socially produced and performed gender categories, members forge more creative and expansive ways of living their gender and sexual lives. Ultimately, as Enoch Page and Matt U. Richardson (Page & Richardson, 2010) suggest, queer gender subjectivities reflect the multitude of experiences of creatively non-conforming gender identities, sexualities, and bodily configurations, both anatomic and performative (Page & Richardson, 2010). The gender system in the House Ball Community consists of six categories, which we delineate here with brief descriptions[2]:

1. *Butch Queens up in Drag* (gay men who perform in drag but do not take hormones and do not live as women).
2. *Femme Queens* (transgender women or MTF at various stages of gender transition involving hormonal or surgical processes, such as breast implants).
3. *Butches* (transgender men or FTM at various stages of gender transition involving hormonal therapy, breast wrapping or removal, etc., or masculine lesbians or females appearing as men irrespective of sexuality).
4. *Women* (cisgender women who are lesbian or straight identified or queer).
5. *Men/Trade* (cisgender men who are usually very masculine, and straight identified or non-gay identified).
6. *Butch Queens* (cisgender men who live and identify as gay or bisexual men and who can be masculine, hyper-masculine—performing thug masculinity—or very feminine).

The gender system is integral to the House Ball Community's performative gender and sexual identities, kinship structure, and ball events. Regarding the former, each member of the community identifies as or is assigned one of the six categories in the gender system. Because gender performance is central to self-identification and can imply a whole range of sexual identities in the House Ball Community, the system reflects how the members define themselves largely based on the categories they

---

[1] What we call the gender identity system is typically called the "gender system" within Ballroom culture. The outline of the six subjectivities within the system is based on ethnographic data including attendance/participation in balls, analysis of numerous ball flyers, and interviews with members from all over the country over a 9 year period. Despite a few discrepancies among different sectors of the community, the general components of the system are standard throughout the Ballroom scene. The gender system is separate but inextricably linked to the competitive categories that appear on ball flyers. At balls, competitive performance categories abound, but the gender system serves as the basis upon which the competitive categories are created.

[2] In *Paris is Burning* and in the debates that the film generated, there is limited engagement with the gender system, even though the gender subjectivities existed.

walk/perform. It is important to note that some of the categories in the system are strictly gender categories, such as Femme Queens (Bailey, 2011). Hence, Femme Queens can be heterosexual, lesbian, bisexual, and queer, etc. Another example is the category "Women," consisting of cisgender women (with few exceptions), demarcates gender, while implying a range of sexualities (Schilt & Westbrook, 2009). Those in the Women category are primarily heterosexual, feminine lesbians, or queer. However, other categories in the House Ball Community conflate gender and sexuality; for example, the Butch Queen, who is at once a cisgender man and gay. This gender system does not totally break from hegemonic norms of sex, gender, and sexuality, but it offers more gender and sexual identities to adopt and express than are available to members in larger society.

The House Ball Community: House Structure and Ball Events

The second core dimension of the House Ball Community is houses—the kinship structure. The gender system defines the roles that members serve in the house. Houses are socially, rather than biologically, configured kinship structures. Although houses are primarily social configurations, at times, they serve as literal homes or gathering places for their members (Arnold & Bailey, 2009). Houses are typically named after *haute couture* designers, but some are named after mottos and symbols that express qualities and attributes with which the leaders want a house to be associated. These alternative families are led by "mothers" and "fathers," house parents who provide guidance for their "children" of various ages, races/ethnicities, genders, and sexualities.

> The most conspicuous function of houses is organizing and competing in ball events. The gender system and kin labor system create a close-knit community and this community expresses its essence at these events. House parents recruit, socialize, and prepare their protégés to compete successfully in performative identity and performance categories. When one "walks a ball," the participant competes in the categories that coincide with their gender identity within the House Ball Community. For instance, a Femme Queen can only "walk" (perform) in categories that are listed under the Femme Queen heading. These intensely competitive performances at the ball events are a part of communal gender practice that occurs and is enhanced within the Black GLBT affirming spaces that House Ball Community members produce.

In the House Ball scene, competitive categories abound, for example, "realness" categories such as "schoolboy realness," call for a performance in which partici- pants are judged on how effectively they act, dress, and walk, in ways that are indis- tinguishable from any other working class man or woman in everyday society, as in the case of schoolboy or schoolgirl realness, a working class young man or woman going to school.[3] Participants compete vigorously against one another on behalf of

---

[3] For a video example of this category, please see: http://www.youtube.com/watch?v=Xws6bQTYFFo.

their respective houses, and, at times, as individuals, in which case they are "free agents," or "007s." The ball event is the central means through which members of the community affirm, celebrate, and constructively critique its fellow members. Thus, the gender system—gender and sexual identities—and the ball events combined with the social relations that underpin and exist within the houses (both within and outside the ball space) are mutually constitutive and, taken together, make up the social world of the House Ball Community. Most importantly, these dimensions constituted the spaces in which effective HIV/AIDS prevention and social support for both HIV negative and positive members can be developed and implemented.

Avenues for Intervention

Based on ethnographic work in both the Detroit and San Francisco Bay Area House Ball Communities, Arnold and Bailey (2009) were the first published investigators to discuss the importance of house structures and gender roles within the House Ball Community in informing HIV-related interventions for MSM and transgender youth of color (Arnold & Bailey, 2009). Our study of the Ballroom community documented several forms of intravention (Friedman et al., 2004), or forms of intervention or strategies that occur organically within community settings, and the importance of the gender system, houses, and balls in organizing these practices. Since houses are metaphorical homes for Black gay youth, they are prime configurations for providing various forms of support for HIV prevention. As a house mother and HIV prevention worker in Detroit explained, "The structure of the Ballroom community already allows for prevention work, you know, just in the fact that someone can say to you, 'Now you know you need to wear a condom' and it be from someone that you have built that trust factor with. People in the community do prevention work all of the time." We offered recommendations for community-based organizations to make use of existing social structures within the community and the salient concepts of home and family, to provide HIV-related services and support. We argued that HIV prevention interventions necessarily required a more culturally appropriate, nuanced approach to reaching Black youth at risk.

More recently, Kubicek, McNeeley, Holloway, Weiss, and Kipke (2012) have put forth a resiliency model that could also strengthen HIV prevention programming with the House Ball Community (Kubicek et al., 2012). Based on the data collected with the House Ball Community in Los Angeles, this model taps into culturally appropriate themes around competition and resilience. "Resiliency" in this articulation includes four manifestations—shamelessness, social creativity, volunteerism, and social support. Shameless, in this case, correlates with a sense of pride and celebration of oneself in the context of Ball competitions, and serves as a counterpoint to internalized homophobia. Social creativity is deployed to counter a lack of social support that young people encounter in their communities of origin, thus the House Ball Community becomes a source of support, with the affiliation with fictive kin within houses. Volunteerism is a reaction to violence, victimization, and homophobia, and takes the form of house parents giving back to their communities. Finally, social support, which counters unhealthy relationships and loneliness, is observed in the sense of camaraderie participants described at the Balls and within their houses.

Prevention Houses

It is important to bring into focus the ways in which HIV prevention support is developed and facilitated within the inextricable relationship between balls and the community-fashioned kinship system in the House Ball Community. This linkage constitutes what House Ball Community members refer to as *prevention houses*. A prevention house may have either a formal or an informal relationship with a community-based organization. Besides organizing prevention balls, which is explained below, a core mission of a prevention house is to develop and implement strategies for the prevention of HIV and other sexually transmitted infections by fostering open and informed discussions about sex and advocating "safer sex" practices. Prevention houses also provide social support for those members who are HIV positive, which is a critical aspect of the HIV prevention and treatment dyad. Generally, in theory, the prevention house is a safe and supportive space, providing social and, at times, material support and care that House Ball Community members, both HIV negative and positive, often do not get from their families of origin nor elsewhere among the larger Black GLBT community, particularly youth.

House mothers and house fathers in particular provide daily parental guidance for House Ball Community members regarding intimate/romantic relationships, sex, gender and sexual identities, health, hormonal therapy, and body presentation, among other issues. Yet, in prevention houses, HIV prevention is another crucial role that house parents assume as leaders of houses. We refer to their unique role as *prevention parenting*. In the Detroit chapter of The House of Prestige, for example, the late Noir Prestige, a Butch Queen, explained how prevention parenting works in houses: "Even in the traditional sense, if I'm supposed to be the matriarch or the patriarch of the family, the head, if I see one of my kids is just out there being a whore, then it's my duty to go, 'Are you protecting yourself?'" This aspect of parenting—nurturing and caring for the members—is typically undertaken by house mothers, indeed HIV prevention parenting is mostly a house mother endeavor (Arnold & Bailey, 2009; Bailey, 2013). Prevention parenting is especially important for Femme Queens who are taking hormones. Because members of the House Ball Community have limited or no access to safe hormone injections, some Femme Queen mothers ensure their kids use clean needles, and they draw from their own experience or knowledge they have gained to guide their children through their hormonal therapy (Bailey, 2013). In many cases, Femme Queen house mothers can keep their kids from getting hormone shots through shady and unsafe sources on the street.

House parents also were in positions to challenge HIV-related stigma and gossip that could occur in the House Ball Community, should a house member's status be disclosed. They understood the meaning associated with living as an HIV positive person within the community, and offered support in a culturally appropriate way that also recognized the complex realities of the lives of their children. Says one Bay Area house father, "You may lose your livelihood if someone finds out you're HIV positive...there's a lot of competition for [sex work] clients, for status, for looks, for this, for that...street survival is that if you find someone has got it you're going to use that information to your advantage... And so no I don't blame the kids for not disclosing. I give them props if they go get tested. I give them props if they seek treatment." Within the houses, members consult with their parents and their house siblings on issues that, either by choice or by necessity, they cannot discuss with their biological parents. This is not always an issue related to fear of exclusion or retribution; rather, it is often just more feasible and practical to rely on one's house parents in the House Ball Community who generally have more knowledge and experience with issues confronting marginalized Black GLBT people and communities.

Prevention Balls

Aside from HIV-related prevention and support within the houses, HIV prevention education takes place at "Prevention Balls," which were typically sponsored by HIV prevention programs, often held in CBOs, and featured categories specifically developed with a safer sex or HIV-related theme in mind. Prevention balls are designed to educate community members about healthy sexual practices and to promote sexual responsibility, through the competitive performances at the balls. By incorporating safer sex awareness and practice, the balls themselves are a means of intervention for House Ball Community members. Having young people "walk" the runway displaying their knowledge of HIV transmission, showcasing safer sex paraphernalia, and, in some cases, actually wearing this paraphernalia in front of the crowd allows these norms to not only be disseminated throughout the community, but allows for the practice and expectations of safer sex to be inscribed on the bodies of those who compete in the balls. One of the most famous prevention houses is GMHC's The House of Latex in New York City. For almost 20 years, GMHC has organized The House of Latex ball, one of the most popular HIV/AIDS prevention balls in the country, drawing between 2500 and 3000 audience members/participants. Prevention balls are designed to educate House Ball Community members about healthy sexual practices and awareness, through the competitive performances at the balls.

It is worth reiterating here that the Ballroom community is a place in which Black GLBT youth, especially, look for guidance, nurturing, care, and support. Given the absence of youth voices on community-based organization staffs and boards, the House Ball Community embrace of Black GLBT youth is essential to

HIV prevention and social support for HIV positive youth. According to House Ball Community members and HIV prevention workers, the members are getting younger and younger. "These 'kids,' literally, are more prone to high-risk sexual behavior," said Tino, a Butch Queen. He further suggested that, "A lot of people who are involved in the community are dealing with being put out of the home 'cause of their parents and maybe they are out at an early age and they get involved with sex and substance abuse at an early age." At the time of the interview, Tino was an HIV prevention and treatment advocate at The Horizons Project and a member of The House of Prestige in Detroit. Consequently, for young Black GLBT youth, the House Ball Community becomes a space that counters the social conditions that produce these risk factors. As Tino observes:

> The main reason why I got involved in Ballroom was to deal with my own biases and mis-information by observing. But also to connect with people who were infected that others in the scene didn't know. I was able to connect with people at the balls. During a Ninja ball, I ran into a guy who was HIV positive who had missed his appointment. I encouraged him to come to his appointment to follow up on his health. He came but still has problems with adherence with his appointments. He is 18 years old and probably hasn't come to grips with it and is afraid.

Since balls have major drawing power, they offer a space in which to engage younger members in unique ways. People such as Tino's client will not go to a community-based organization to access treatment resources, nor is he able to discuss his status with his biological family. But the young HIV positive man participates in balls, and he may or may not be a member of a house. House Ball Community prevention workers such as Tino encourage their clients to take better care of their overall health and to remember to take their HIV medication. Especially for Black GLBT youth in urban spaces like Detroit and the San Francisco Bay Area, depressed social conditions for them contribute to diminished health and increases their likelihood of infecting someone else. Tino's movement between the House Ball Community and HIV prevention is evidence of his understanding of the magnitude of the problem of HIV infection rates among Black GLBT youth. These critical issues should be considered in any prevention program.

Research Priorities with the House Ball Community

Given the complexity of the House Ball Community, and the need to position any quantitative findings within the intricate social and contextual realities of the lives of community members, we recommend that investigators develop interdisciplinary research teams that use both qualitative and quantitative approaches (Creswell & Plano Clark, 2007). Scholars who have the ability to collaborate with multidisciplinary teams, which should include social scientists such as sociologists, anthropologists, human geographers, and gender, sexuality and cultural theorists, will be especially relevant to furthering research agendas with the House Ball Community.

Likewise, research that utilizes a community-based participatory research paradigm and involves members of the community must be prioritized (Minkler & Wallerstein, 2008). This can take many forms, including consulting members of a community advisory board, hiring and training House Ball Community members to participate in the research process, or partnering with ballroom alliances and houses to design research studies and interpret findings. Finally, researchers should acknowledge, take seriously, and draw from forms of intravention already taking place within House Ball Communities. Recognizing the ingenuity of this community will be crucial in developing programmatic strategies for reducing HIV prevalence among House Ball Communities in particular and larger Black GLBT communities in general.

Conclusions

Although the House Ball Community offers great promise for reaching Black GLBT youth with HIV-related information, support, and interventions, it is also a very dynamic and somewhat ever-changing community. The economic resources that House Ball Community leaders can access are limited and constrained, and many members engage in informal and unstable work and experience periods of unemployment. Thus, linkages to more formal services, employment programs, job training, housing, and other economic resources offered through community-based organizations and social service agencies would be of great benefit to House Ball Community members, and must not be overlooked in the recent "Test and Treat" paradigm. Indeed, it is essential that members of the House Ball Community who are both HIV positive and negative to come together to advocate for public forms of funding to continue to cover substance use treatment programs, mental health services, housing, and job training, and educational opportunities to benefit the community. Community-based organizations should also make sure that house parents, particularly house fathers, are informed about broader programs to increase well-being and economic opportunities for young HIV positive people involved in the House Ball Community, as well as offering them support for continuing to promote lower risk behavior and treatment adherence.

References

Alio, A. P., Fields, S. D., Humes, D. L., Bunce, C. A., Wallace, S. E., Lewis, C., … for the NIAID HIV Vaccine Trials Network (2014). Project VOGUE: A partnership for increasing HIV knowledge and HIV vaccine trial awareness among house ball leaders in Western New York. *Journal of Gay & Lesbian Social Services, 26*, 336–354.

Arnold, E. A., & Bailey, M. M. (2009). Constructing home and family: How the ballroom community supports African American GLBTQ Youth in the Face of HIV/AIDS. *Journal of Gay & Lesbian Social Services, 21*(2-3), 171–188.

Arnold, E., Sterrett-Hong, E., Jonas, A., & Pollack, L.M. (2016). Social networks and social support among ball-attending African American men who have sex with men and transgender women are associated with HIV-related outcomes. *Global Public Health*, 1–15.

Arnold, E. A., Williams, D., Blount, E., & Pierceson, D. (2012). *HIV-related stigma and its impact on disclosure, testing and treatment adherence among Young African American Gay Bisexual and Transgender (GBT) individuals.* Paper presented at the International AIDS Conference.

Bailey, M. M. (2009). Performance as Intravention: Ballroom culture and the politics of HIV/AIDS in Detroit. *Souls, 11*(3), 253–274.

Bailey, M. M. (2011). Gender/racial realness: Theorizing the gender system in ballroom culture. *Feminist Studies, 37*(2), 365–384.

Bailey, M. M. (2013). *Butch queens up in pumps: Gender, performance, and ballroom culture in Detroit.* Ann Arbor: University of Michigan Press.

Bailey, M. M. (2014). Engendering space: Ballroom culture and the spatial practice of possibility in Detroit. *Gender, Place and Culture: The Journal of Feminist Geography, 21*, 489–507.

Chauncey, G. (1994). *Gay New York: Gender, urban culture, and the makings of the gay male world, 1890–1940.* New York: BasicBooks.

Creswell, J. W., & Plano Clark, V. L. (2007). *Designing and conducting mixed methods research.* Thousand Oaks, CA: Sage Publishers.

Friedman, S. R., Maslow, C., Bolyard, M., Sandoval, M., Mateu-Gelabert, P., & Neaigus, A. (2004). Urging others to be healthy: "intravention" by injection drug users as a community prevention goal. *AIDS Education and Prevention: Official Publication of the International Society for AIDS Education, 16*(3), 250–263.

Galindo, G. R. (2013). A loss of moral experience: Understanding HIV related stigma in the New York City House and Ball Community. *American Journal of Public Health, 103*(2), 293–299.

Harris, A. (2010). Sex, stigma, and the holy ghost: The black church and the construction of AIDS in New York City. *Journal of African American Studies, 14*, 21–43.

Holloway, I. W., Traube, D. E., Kubicek, K., Supan, J., Weiss, G., & Kipke, M. D. (2012). HIV prevention service utilization in the Los Angeles House and Ball communities: Past experiences and recommendations for the future. *AIDS Education and Prevention: Official Publication of the International Society for AIDS Education, 24*(5), 431–444.

Hwahng, S. J., & Nuttbrock, L. (2007). Sex workers, fem queens, and cross-dressers: Differential Marginalizations and HIV vulnerabilities among three ethnocultural male-to-female transgender communities in New York City. *Sexuality Research & Social Policy, 4*(4), 36–59.

Kipke, M. D., Kubicek, K., Supan, J., Weiss, G., & Schrager, S. (2013). Laying the groundwork for an HIV prevention intervention: A descriptive profile of the Los Angeles House and Ball communities. *AIDS & Behavior, 17*, 1068–1081.

Kubicek, K., Beyer, W. H., McNeeley, M., Weiss, G., Ultra Omni, L. F., & Kipke, M. D. (2013). Community-engaged research to identify house parent perspectives on support and risk within the house and ball scene. *Journal of Sex Research, 50*(2), 178–189.

Kubicek, K., McNeeley, M., Holloway, I. W., Weiss, G., & Kipke, M. D. (2012). "It's like our own little world": Resilience as a factor in participating in the ballroom community subculture. *AIDS & Behavior.* doi: 10.1007/s10461-012-0205-2, 17, 1524.

Lemelle, A. J. (2010). Racialized justice spreads HIV/AIDS among blacks. In J. Battle & S. L. Barnes (Eds.), *Black sexualities: Probing powers, passions, practices, and policies.* New Brunswick: Rutgers University Press.

Minkler, M., & Wallerstein, N. (Eds.). (2008). *Community-based participatory research for health.* San Francisco: Jossey-Bass.

Murrill, C. S., Liu, K. L., Guilin, V., Colon, E. R., Dean, L., Buckley, L. A., … Torian, L. V. (2008). HIV prevalence and associated risk behaviors in New York City's house ball community. *American Journal of Public Health, 98*(6), 1074–1080.

Page, E., & Richardson, M. U. (2010). On the fear of small numbers. In J. Battle & S. L. Barnes (Eds.), *Black sexualities: Probing powers, passions, practices, and policies* (p. 61). New Brunswick: Rutgers University Press.

Painter, T. M., Ngalame, P. M., Lucas, B., Lauby, J. L., & Herbst, J. H. (2010). Strategies used by community-based organizations to evaluate their locally developed HIV prevention interventions: Lessons learned from the CDC's innovative interventions project. *AIDS Education and Prevention: Official Publication of the International Society for AIDS Education, 22*(5), 387–401.

Phillips, G., 2nd, Peterson, J., Binson, D., Hidalgo, J., & Magnus, M. (2011). House/ball culture and adolescent African-American transgender persons and men who have sex with men: A synthesis of the literature. *AIDS Care, 23*(4), 515–520.

Rowan, D., DeSousa, M., Randall, E. M., White, C., & Holley, L. (2014). "We're just targeted as the flock that has HIV": Health care experiences of members of the house/ball culture. *Social Work in Health Care, 53*, 460–477.

Sanchez, T., Finlayson, T., Murrill, C., Guilin, V., & Dean, L. (2010). Risk behaviors and psychosocial stressors in the New York City House Ball Community: A comparison of men and transgender women who have sex with men. *AIDS and Behavior, 14*(2), 351–358.

Schilt, K., & Westbrook, L. (2009). Doing gender, doing heteronormativity: 'Gender Normals,' transgender people, and the social maintenance of heterosexuality. *Gender & Society, 23*(4), 440–464.

van Doorn, N. (2012). Between hope and abandonment: Black queer collectivity and the affective labour of biomedicalised HIV prevention. *Culture, Health & Sexuality, 14*(7), 827–840.

Watkins-Hayes, C., Patterson, C. J., & Armour, A. R. (2011). Precious: Black women, neighborhood HIV/AIDS risk, and institutional buffers. *Du Bois Review, 8*(01), 229–240.

Wilton, L., Herbst, J. H., Coury-Doniger, P., Painter, T. M., English, G., Alvarez, M. E., … Carey, J. W. (2009). Efficacy of an HIV/STI prevention intervention for black men who have sex with men: Findings from the Many Men, Many Voices (3MV) project. *AIDS and Behavior, 13*(3), 532–544.

Wong, C. F., Schrager, S. M., Holloway, I. W., Meyer, I. H., & Kipke, M. D. (2014). Minority stress experiences and psychological well-being: The impact of support from and connection to social networks within the Los Angeles House and Ball communities. *Prevention Science, 15*, 44–55.

Young, L. E., Jonas, A. B., Michaels, S., Jackson, J. D., Pierce, M. L., Schneider, J. A., & uConnect Study Team. (2017). Social-structural properties and HIV prevention among young men who have sex with men in the ballroom house and independent gay family communities. *Social Science and Medicine, 174*, 26–34.

Chapter 13
Religiousness, Spirituality, and Well-Being Among HIV Positive Gay Men

Ja'Nina J. Garrett-Walker and John E. Pérez

Introduction

Religiousness and spirituality have the ability to enhance cognitive and affective well-being and quality of life among diverse populations (Cotton, Tsevat et al., 2006; Ellison, 1991; Lassiter et al., 2017, Lee, 2007; Meanley, Pingel, & Bauermeister, 2016; Pargament, Koenig, Tarakeshwar, & Hahn, 2004; Simoni & Ortiz, 2003). However, the intersection of religiousness, spirituality, sexuality, and health for HIV positive gay men may not be as positive (Nelson et al., 2016; Quinn, Dickson-Gomez, & Young, 2016). Due to the stigmatizing role that organized religion often plays in the lives of gay men living with HIV, the ability to utilize religion to deal with stress and depression may become increasingly difficult. However, spirituality may provide HIV positive gay men with a personal connection to their Higher Power that does not require organized religion (Foster, Arnold, Rebchook, & Kegeles, 2011; Lassiter et al., 2017; Lee, 2007). Researchers have begun to more closely assess the role of religion and spirituality in the lives of lesbian, gay, bisexual, and transgender (LGBT) individuals in addition to people living with HIV/AIDS (PLWHA) (Etergoff, 2017; Jeffries Iv, Sutton, & Eke, 2017). While a wide body of research has illuminated the positive association between religiousness, spirituality, and well-being among HIV positive populations (Szaflarski, 2013), fewer studies have focused specifically on HIV positive gay men (Hampton, Halkitis, & Mattis, 2010; Jeffries et al., 2014). In this chapter, we examine the role of religiousness and spirituality in the lives of HIV positive gay men by (1) exploring current definitions of religiousness and spirituality; (2) discussing the positive influences of religiousness and spirituality on physical and mental health of people living with HIV; (3) examining the potential negative impact of organized religion in

J.J. Garrett-Walker (✉) • J.E. Pérez
Department of Psychology, College of Arts and Sciences,
University of San Francisco (USF), San Francisco, CA, USA
e-mail: jgarrettwalker@usfca.edu

© Springer Science+Business Media LLC 2017
L. Wilton (ed.), *Understanding Prevention for HIV Positive Gay Men*,
DOI 10.1007/978-1-4419-0203-0_13

the lives of HIV positive gay men; and (4) assessing the ways in which religiousness and spirituality can be and have been utilized in HIV prevention efforts.

Defining Religiousness and Spirituality

Religiousness and spirituality are broad, complex, and often overlapping constructs. Despite academic attempts to provide singular definitions of religiousness and spirituality, these concepts are considered latent and multidimensional (Miller & Thoresen, 2003). Religiousness has traditionally been referred to as shared beliefs, values, and practices governed by a faith-based organization. Various dimensions of religiousness in the research literature include religious affiliation, religious service attendance, religious beliefs, private religious practices, organizational religiousness, religious support, and religious coping (Fetzer & NIA, 2003). Advances in the measurement of this construct has led to a better understanding of how specific variables have varying associations with health and well-being outcomes (Hill & Pargament, 2008). While religion is defined by its boundaries, spirituality has been demarcated by its ability to transcend boundaries.

Spirituality is a multifaceted construct that holds different meanings to different people. Some refer to spirituality as one's personal relationship with God, the divine, or a Higher Power (Emmons, 1999; Miller & Thoresen, 2003). Others have defined spirituality as a search for the sacred (Hill & Pargament, 2008; Pargament, 2013). Spirituality has been operationalized in many different ways including but not limited to general spirituality, daily spiritual experiences, spiritual striving/growth, spiritual coping, spiritual modeling, spiritual transcendence, spiritual needs, and spiritual well-being (Fetzer & NIA, 2003; Monod et al., 2011; Oman, 2013; Pérez et al., 2009; Piedmont, Ciarrochi, Dy-Liacco, & Williams, 2009). While multiple definitions[1] pose as a challenge to empirical science of spirituality and health (Koenig, 2008; Salander, 2006), the flexible definition of spirituality may be beneficial to people who may opt to define their spirituality outside of the boundaries of religious organizations. This flexibility becomes increasingly important for gay men and PLWHA given the stigma they often endure within the confines of traditional religion.

Religiousness, Spirituality, and Well-Being Among PLWHA

Many PLWHA report being raised in an organized religious community. In a national sample of gay, lesbian, or bisexual respondents ($N = 1604$), 59% reported a religious affiliation (predominantly Protestant and Roman Catholic) (Pew Research Center, 2015). In a sample of 450 HIV positive adults, 80% identified with a specific religious affiliation (predominantly Roman Catholic and Southern Baptist) (Cotton, Puchalski

---

[1] Throughout this chapter, we refer to the specific religious and spiritual constructs as they are operationalized in the research literature.

et al., 2006). While some HIV positive gay men are connected to a specific religion, others may develop a more spiritual connection to their High Power. Below, we review the empirical evidence linking various dimensions of religiousness and spirituality to both physical and mental health among PLWHA.

HIV Diagnosis and Quality of Life

A significant percentage of PLWHA have reported an increase in spirituality after their diagnosis (Cotton, Tsevat et al., 2006; Kremer, Ironson, & Kaplan, 2009; Lutz, Kremer, & Ironson, 2011). For many, HIV diagnosis facilitated a stronger relationship with their God/Higher Power and with family members (Tarakeshwar, Khan, & Sikkema, 2006). In a longitudinal study of 450 PLWHA, 75% of participants expressed the ways in which their HIV diagnosis strengthened their faith and spiritual beliefs. Participants were also more likely to utilize positive religious coping mechanisms (e.g., sought God's love and care) as opposed to negative religious coping mechanisms (e.g., decided the devil made this happen; Cotton, Puchalski et al., 2006). In a study of 347 adults with HIV/AIDS, 24% of participants said they felt more alienated by a religious group since their HIV/AIDS diagnosis and 10% said they changed their place of worship because of HIV/AIDS. Yet, 41% reported becoming more spiritual since their HIV/AIDS diagnosis (Cotton, Tsevat et al., 2006). Foster et al. (2011) found that Black HIV positive gay men conveyed the importance of spirituality in their ability to cope with the challenges they faced in daily life, one of them being living with HIV. Although many have expressed a strengthening of their spiritual beliefs, some HIV positive gay men have expressed that religious practices are more meaningful than practices defined as spiritual but not religious. This may be particularly true for African American gay men as family and social life are often embedded in Black churches (Jeffries Iv et al., 2017; Seegers, 2007; Garrett-Walker, 2016; Watkins et al., 2016; Wilson, Wittlin, Munoz-Lavoy, & Parker, 2011). Both quantitative and qualitative studies suggest that greater positive religious coping and lower spiritual struggle are associated with perceived improvements in quality of life among PLWHA (Cotton, Puchalski et al., 2006; Cotton, Tsevat et al., 2006; Kremer & Ironson, 2009; Seegers, 2007: Siegel & Schrimshaw, 2002; Szaflarski et al., 2006; Trevino et al., 2010; Tsevat et al., 2009).

In contrast to perceived changes in quality of life, greater spiritual beliefs have been inconclusively linked to perceived pain among PLWHA. In a longitudinal study of 226 HIV positive men, spiritual growth—defined as existential feelings of connection with a force greater than oneself—was not associated with pain management (Frame, Uphold, Shehan, & Reid, 2005). In a sample of 158 low-income, ethnically diverse participants (45% gay men), endorsement of spiritual beliefs (e.g., belief in God/Higher Power) was greater among PLWHA who experienced constant pain in the past 6 months compared to PLWHA who did not experience constant pain in the past 6 months (Pérez et al., 2008). In a sample of 420 predominantly Latino (79%) and male (82%) PLWHA, higher levels of spirituality were associated with lower levels of pain (Ramer, Johnson, Chan, & Barrett, 2006). In the latter study, spirituality was measured by items assessing overall satisfaction with life, peace of mind, and personal faith in God, confounding spirituality with well-being. These mixed findings coincide with broader literature on the link between religiousness/spirituality and chronic pain (Koenig, King, & Carson, 2012). The relationship between spirituality and pain may depend on the operational definitions of both spirituality and pain selected by the researchers. Moreover, the cross-sectional design of many of these studies fails to rule out the possibility that pain levels may influence the level of spirituality reported by participants. Whereas more research is needed to better understand the relationships among spirituality, quality of life, and pain for PLWHA, research on the link between depressive symptoms and religiousness/spirituality is clearer.

Depressive Symptoms

Empirical evidence suggests that depressive symptoms are linked to more rapid disease progression and higher mortality rates among PLWHA (Ickovics et al., 2001; Leserman et al., 2007; Mayne, Vittinghoff, Chesney, Barett, & Coates, 1996). While depression has been shown to accelerate disease progression, religiousness/spirituality may buffer against this process. Several studies have shown that religiousness and spirituality are associated with lower levels of depressive symptoms among PLWHA (Simoni & Ortiz, 2003; Woods, Antoni, Ironson, & Kling, 1999; Yi et al., 2006). Some researchers have attempted to uncover possible mechanisms for linking religiousness and spirituality with lower depressive symptoms. For example, in a cross-sectional study with 264 HIV positive individuals (49% gay men) on highly active antiretroviral therapy (HAART), Carrico et al. (2006) found a link between spirituality, depressive symptoms, and 24-h cortisol output. The authors used the Ironson-Woods Spirituality/Religiousness Index, which includes four spirituality factors: sense of peace, faith in God, religious behavior, and compassionate view of others (Ironson et al., 2002). Using path modeling, Carrico et al. (2006) found that spirituality was associated with greater positive reappraisal (using positive reinterpretation of one's HIV concerns or problems) and greater benefit finding (positive benefits or life changes resulting from living with HIV). In turn, positive reappraisal and benefit finding were both associated with lower depressive symptoms. In addition, greater benefit finding was associated with decreased 24-h cortisol output—a biological marker linked to stress and depression (Carrico et al., 2006).

Additionally, Pérez et al. (2009) examined the longitudinal association between spiritual striving (i.e., process of trying to grow spiritually and pursuing a meaningful and fulfilling daily life) and depressive symptoms among 180 culturally diverse adults living with HIV/AIDS. After controlling for covariates (treatment status, HIV-related symptoms, and baseline depressive symptoms), greater spiritual striving predicted decreases in depressive symptoms over 6 months. This link was partially mediated by acceptance coping. The authors suggested that the peace of mind associated with spiritual striving may decrease depressive symptoms by increasing the use of acceptance coping in situations that are out of the control of the individual (Pérez et al., 2009). Given the connection between depressive symptoms and poor health outcomes among PLWHA, it is important to understand the mechanisms that link religious and spiritual factors to lower depressive symptoms. Moreover, there is some evidence to suggest that depressive symptoms are associated with lower HAART adherence and higher mortality among PLWHA (Lima et al., 2007).

Treatment Adherence

Understanding the relationship between religiousness/spirituality and HIV treatment adherence (e.g., entering or remaining in medical treatment, keeping appointments, taking medications) is important because treatment nonadherence has been associated with drug resistance, greater disease progression, and higher mortality among PLWHA (Bangsberg, Moss, & Deeks, 2004; Bangsberg et al., 2001). When compared to non-church-attending MSM, research has recently shown that MSM who attended church were more likely to present with lower CD4 counts at the onset of HIV treatment (Van Wagoner et al., 2014). In a mixed methods study of 79 PLWHA, participants who believed that God/Higher Power controls one's health were 4.75 times more likely to refuse antiretroviral treatment; conversely, those who believed that spirituality helps coping with side effects reported better treatment adherence and fewer symptoms and side effects (Kremer, Ironson, & Porr, 2009). In a cross-sectional study of 18 prenatally HIV positive youth aged 14–22 years, religious factors were associated with adherence to HAART. Participants with excellent adherence reported greater religious beliefs and practices than those who had poor adherence (Park & Nachman, 2010). In an intervention study with HIV positive adolescents aged 14–21 years, participants who believed that HIV was a punishment from God scored lower on spiritual well-being and lower on adherence to HAART (Lyon et al., 2011). In a cross-sectional study of HIV positive adults ($N = 306$), the men in the study who were currently in medical care were less likely to believe that HIV is a sin compared to those who were not in medical care. In addition, men who kept an appointment in the past 3 months reported a higher frequency of church attendance and were less likely to believe that HIV is a sin (Parsons, Cruise, Davenport, & Jones, 2006).

These findings indicate that increases in passive (e.g., God/Higher Power controls one's health) and negative (e.g., HIV is a sin/punishment from God) religious beliefs may be associated with poorer treatment adherence, whereas positive religious beliefs (e.g., intrinsic religious motivation) and practices (e.g., prayer, religious service attendance) may be associated with greater treatment adherence. More research needs to examine the possible link between passive religious beliefs, negative religious coping, and adherence to HAART among HIV positive gay men, as treatment adherence greatly impacts HIV disease progression.

HIV Disease Progression

Few studies have examined the longitudinal relationship between religiousness, spirituality, and HIV disease progression. A recent literature review identified 15 studies that addressed the association between religiousness, spirituality, and clinical outcomes in HIV positive individuals. Ten (67%) studies demonstrated a positive association between religiousness or spirituality and a clinical HIV outcome, two (13%) studies demonstrated a negative association, two (13%) studies failed to detect an association, and one (7%) study found both positive and negative associations with clinical HIV outcomes (Doolittle, Justice, & Fiellin, 2016). Here, we highlight results from some notable longitudinal studies. Ironson, Stuetzle, and Fletcher (2006) studied changes in religiousness/spirituality and disease progression among 100 PLWHA over a 4-year period. Change in religiousness/spirituality was assessed with a single item indicating the degree to which the participants became more or less religious/spiritual after learning of their HIV serostatus. Results showed that many participants (45%) reported an increase in religiousness/spirituality after their HIV diagnosis. More importantly, participants reporting an increase in religiousness/spirituality after their HIV diagnosis maintained significantly higher levels of CD4 cells and better control of viral load over the 4-year period. On the other hand, participants who reported a decrease in religiousness/spirituality lost CD4 cells 4.5 times faster than those who showed an increase in religiousness/spirituality (Ironson et al., 2006). In a secondary analysis with the same sample, Ironson et al. (2011) found that a positive view of God also predicted better preservation of CD4 cells and better control of viral load, whereas a negative view of God predicted faster disease progression over 4 years. Specifically, participants who viewed God as merciful/benevolent/forgiving had five times better preservation of CD4 cells than those who did not have a positive view of God. Conversely, participants who had a harsh/judgmental/punishing view of God lost CD4 cells at more than twice the rate of those who had a positive view of God (Ironson et al., 2011).

In subsequent studies, researchers examined the longitudinal association between HIV disease progression and more specific spiritual constructs. In a study with 177 people living with HIV, spiritual coping predicted sustained undetectable viral load and CD4-cell preservation over 4 years; moreover, when controlling for the effect of viral load suppression, CD4-cell decline was 2.25 times faster among those engaged in negative versus positive spiritual coping (Kremer et al., 2015). In a long-term follow-up analysis with the same sample, researchers examined the association between mortality and several specific spiritual constructs. Participants who used spiritual practices, spiritual reframing, overcoming spiritual guilt, spiritual gratitude, and spiritual empowerment were 2–4 times more likely to survive over a 17-year period (Ironson, Kremer, & Lucette, 2016). The few longitudinal studies examining the link between religiousness/spirituality and HIV disease progression are promising. More research is needed on valid, reliable, and specific religious and spiritual constructs that predict the course of HIV disease progression, as well as mechanisms that may explain their relationship. While the positive relations between religiousness, spirituality, HIV, and health have been examined, it is important to reflect on the ways in which the confines of religious organizations may marginalize HIV positive gay men (Garrett-Walker & Torres, 2016; Wilson et al., 2011). Due to the stigma attached to being gay and living with HIV/AIDS in mainstream organized religions, many HIV positive gay men have sought to define their personal spirituality outside of the context of organized religion (Jeffries et al., 2014; Miller, 2005, 2007; Nelson et al., 2016; Siegel & Schrimshaw, 2002).

Sexuality and Religion

Religion, and the negative images of same-sex behavior often portrayed by religious institutions, may have an adverse effect on mental and physical health of LGBT individuals and PLWHA. The Bible and the Torah state that a man shall not lay with another man, as it is an abomination (Leviticus, 18:22). This verse has been used as the basis for many of the negative attitudes regarding same-sex behavior and has been used in sermons and religious teachings to defile same-sex behavior for LGBT individuals. LGBT individuals are often raised hearing such messages in their respective religious communities. The obstacles religious and/or spiritual gay and lesbian individuals may experience have been explored in theoretical articulations and empirical research (Buchanan, Dzelme, Harris, & Hecker, 2001; Coyle & Rafalin, 2000; Jeffries Iv et al., 2017; Lassiter et al., 2017; Meladze & Brown, 2015; Miller, 2007). Research has shown that gay men reporting higher levels of intrinsic religious faith also reported higher levels of internalized homonegativity. Additionally, gay men of Jewish, Christian, and Muslim faith reported higher levels of internalized homonegativity when compared to individuals with no religious affiliation (Meladze & Brown, 2015).

Coyle and Rafalin (2000) found that Jewish gay men felt a sense of identity conflict between their religious and sexual identities. Men expressed the turmoil they often experienced due to their seemingly conflicting identities and its impact on their psychological well-being (Coyle & Rafalin, 2000). Schnoor (2006) articulated the ways in which Jewish men manage their identities. While some men may be able to successfully integrate their religious and sexual identities, some may feel their identities are mutually exclusive, and others may feel the need to choose between their religious and sexual identities (Schnoor, 2006). Christian participants have shown similar experiences of identity negotiation as Jewish samples (Miller, 2007; Pitt, 2010). Pitt (2010) found that Christian Black men who have sex with men (BMSM) exhibited different strategies to neutralize anti-gay messages they received from their pastors. Men expressed their ability to contextualize religious text and teachings from clergy who they felt did not have a vast knowledge of psychological and biological processes regarding sexual behavior. Men were also adamant in their belief that many clergy members lacked the moral authority to condemn people based on their sexual behavior (Pitt, 2010). While it seems that some people are effective at navigating the religious messages they hear in their church homes, others have not been as successful. Golub, Walker, Longmire-Avital, Bimbi, and Parsons (2010) found that transgender women (51% HIV positive) who reported high religious behaviors and beliefs reported increased incidence of unprotected sexual behavior (Golub et al., 2010). Although the experiences of transgender women are not synonymous with those of HIV positive gay men, both groups represent marginalized and stigmatized populations whose multiple identities may lead to similar behavior patterns. It seems that engagement in organized religious practices, which may increase one's chances of hearing negative religious rhetoric, may adversely impact individual behavior.

Miller (2007) found that some Black MSM have had negative experiences with their church in relation to their sexual behavior. They felt that their church condemned their behavior and gave homophobic sermons, which forced some men to leave the church (Miller, 2007). Men reported that they stopped attending church services and opted for a personal relationship with God where they did not feel the social oppression that they often felt from organized religion. Moreover, HIV positive gay men have expressed that they continue to pray daily despite no longer attending religious services (Foster et al., 2011; Miller, 2007). Thus, a personalized spiritual relationship with God often supersedes the need for a religious community to fulfill spiritual needs. Similar to the teachings of Christianity and Judaism, Islamic text also prohibits same-sex behavior (Quran, Sura IV: 19–21). However, limited research has been conducted on the experiences of individuals who are gay and Muslim (Boellstorff, 2005; Jaspal, 2010). In a qualitative assessment of British Muslim gay men, Jaspal and Cinnirella (2010) found that some Muslim gay men were unable to integrate their religious and sexual identities. Men discussed the ways in which Islamic law prohibits same-sex behavior and the struggle they experienced in trying to suppress their same-sex desires. Some men felt their same-sex desire was a temptation presented by Shaitan (Satan) to deter them from Allah. While some felt their same-sex desire was a sin, other men articulated the ways in which Allah created them, so their sexuality was of his making (Jaspal & Cinnirella, 2010). Regardless of one's organized religion, the negative experiences do not diminish the importance and relevance that religiousness or spirituality has in the lives of many LGBT individuals including PLWHA (Arnett, 2004; Miller, 2007).

Among Black lesbian, gay, and bisexual emerging adults, Walker and Longmire-Avital (2012) found that participants reporting increases in religious faith were more resilient when simultaneously reporting higher levels of internalized homonegativity than their counterparts reporting lower levels of religious faith. While some churches serve as a source of oppression, other churches have sought to serve as a refuge for LGBT individuals and PLWHA. *Open and affirming* churches have actively provided traditionally marginalized populations with a religious and spiritual place of worship (Rodriguez & Ouellette, 2000; Scheitle, Merino, & Moore, 2010). Given the positive role of religiousness and spirituality in the lives of LGBT individuals and PLWHA, in addition to the great influence that churches have in communities, churches should take an active stance in the fight against HIV (Wilson et al., 2011).

Role of Church in HIV Prevention Efforts

It is imperative that churches take a proactive approach toward HIV awareness and treatment. Using a conservative estimate, Frenk and Chaves (2012) suggest that roughly 14,564 congregations in the United States have congregants who are living with HIV. Churches have great influence especially in communities of color and within socially and economically under-resourced areas (Fullilove & Fullilove, 1999; Griffin, 2006; Kaufman & Raphel, 1996; Miller, 2007; Taylor, Mattis, & Chatters, 1999). It is estimated that churches provide sermons and messages to 53,603,588 people weekly (Frenk & Chaves, 2012). Given the numbers of people reached by clergy, churches can be instrumental in primary (i.e., to reduce HIV incidence rates) and secondary (i.e., maintenance of ideal health for PLWHA) HIV prevention efforts in addition to decreasing HIV stigma (Wilson et al., 2011). Clergy have utilized their religious leadership authority to advocate for many health screenings among their parishioners (e.g., diabetes, hypertension, cancer) (Lumpkins, Greiner, Daley, Mabachi, & Neuhaus, 2011). Similar efforts should also be made regarding HIV. Unfortunately, many congregations conceptualize HIV as a consequence of sinful behavior (i.e., same-sex behavior, intravenous drug use). This articulation makes discussions around HIV risk behaviors less likely to happen within the confines of a religious setting.

Some churches have expressed a reluctance to have discussions regarding sexual behavior and risk reduction (Cunningham, Kerrigan, McNeely, & Ellen, 2011). The primary conversations some churches are willing to have regarding sexual behavior come from a heteronormative abstinence framework. Other churches have conceptualized HIV transmission as a consequence of same-sex behavior, which is considered going against the word of God (Cunningham et al., 2011). Neither articulation is conducive to raising awareness among congregants regarding HIV transmission and reducing HIV stigma. Although gay men have the highest incidence rates of HIV in the United States, others (heterosexual women and men) are not exempt from possible HIV transmission (Center for Disease Control [CDC], 2007). While discussions around sexuality, sex, and HIV may be difficult for some churches to have, some traditionally Black churches have made a concerted effort to have open dialogues regarding HIV (Cunningham et al., 2011; Francis & Liverpool, 2009).

Using a sample of diverse church congregations in Baltimore City, Maryland, Cunningham et al. (2011) found that churches varied greatly in their investment in HIV awareness and dissemination of HIV information to their congregants. Some pastors conveyed their responsibility by passing harm-reduction messages to their parishioners even if their denomination's policies dictated conversations regarding abstinence only. Pastors were clear that discussions and programs regarding HIV were greatly dependent on the complex intersection of church ideology and community demographics (Cunningham et al., 2011). Churches in North Carolina have demonstrated the multifaceted ways in which clergy disseminate information regarding HIV/AIDS. Using multiple interpersonal outlets such as health fairs, wearing HIV ribbons, and providing HIV information in church bulletins, pastors have communicated an awareness of HIV and HIV stigma to congregants (Moore, Onsomu, Timmons, Abuya, & Moore, 2012).

In regard to faith-based HIV prevention interventions, churches in the USA have implemented programs to address the HIV epidemic, including interventions targeted specifically to African American communities (Sutton & Parks, 2013). Francis and Liverpool (2009) conducted a meta-analysis of faith-based HIV prevention programs evaluated in peer-reviewed journals. The target audience of the programs ranged from faith-based leaders to adolescents. Although the programs provided people with effective HIV risk reduction information and connected congregants to community resources, none of the programs focused specifically on the needs of LGBT individuals (Francis & Liverpool, 2009). The programs were also all primary HIV prevention efforts. Currently, there is a critical void in secondary HIV prevention (maintenance of ideal health for PLWHA) programs that are currently being implemented. Secondary HIV prevention efforts are needed to ensure that PLWHA are supported in the management of their HIV treatment, viral load, and CD4 counts, which greatly decreases disease transmission and progression (CDC, 2013; Van Wagoner, 2014). Additionally, the Centers for Disease Control and Prevention (CDC's) compendium of HIV prevention interventions does not include an evidence-based intervention that focuses on religion or spirituality.

Conclusions

It is clear that religiousness and spirituality play an intricate role in the lives of HIV positive gay men. Although religious institutions may be a source of social marginalization for HIV positive gay men, many men have been able to filter out the oppression they may have received while maintaining the positive components that religiousness and spirituality can contribute to their lives. While some churches may be a source of marginalization, open and affirming churches have been a safe space for many LGBT individuals in addition to PLWHA (Rodriguez & Ouellette, 2000; Scheitle et al., 2010). Such churches may serve as a source of peace for HIV positive gay men who do not always feel comfortable or welcomed in traditional churches. Although some HIV positive gay men have made the decision to remove themselves from organized religion, religious communities can still play an instrumental role in the dissemination of HIV risk reduction information and help diminish HIV stigma among congregants. Although the intersection of religiousness and sexuality may place some clergy in a paradoxical situation, the fight to educate and protect others should provide clergy with a sense of responsibility to provide their followers with as much information as possible to protect their physical and mental well-being (Cunningham et al., 2011; Moore et al., 2012).

Limitations and Future Directions

There are several limitations regarding research on religiousness/spirituality and health among PLWHA. One of the core limitations involves the lack of construct validity of the measures used to assess religiousness and particularly spirituality. For example, several studies utilized a single item to assess change in religiousness and/or spirituality (Cotton, Tsevat et al., 2006; Ironson et al., 2006). In addition, participants were often asked to rate changes in religiousness/spirituality retrospectively, which may have led to recall bias. Another challenge is the multitude of definitions for spirituality, making it difficult to compare findings across studies. Next, the majority of studies were cross-sectional, restricting our ability to infer causal relationships between different measures of religiousness/spirituality, health, and the potential mechanisms linking them among PLWHA. In particular, very few studies have focused on religiousness, spirituality, and HIV disease progression using longitudinal designs (Ironson et al., 2006). Further, current HIV interventions have all been implemented within a Christian framework, with a specific focus on Black churches. Other religious groups may want to consider their position on HIV and take a stance in the fight against HIV. Finally, few authors have used a theoretical framework to guide their hypotheses, which is needed to advance scientific knowledge about the role of religiousness and spirituality in the lives of HIV positive gay men.

Future research on religiousness, spirituality, HIV/AIDS, and health should be theory-driven and include reliable and valid operational definitions of religiousness and spirituality. Research is particularly needed on religious and spiritual factors that predict HIV disease progression. In addition, research is needed to explore interacting risk factors and specific psychosocial mechanisms that link religiousness and spirituality to the health and well-being of HIV positive gay men, while controlling for potential confounds such as HIV-related symptoms (Lassiter & Parsons, 2016). Understanding such mechanisms will facilitate the development of effective psychosocial interventions that promote well-being among HIV positive gay men.

While churches vary greatly in the ways in which they approach the topic of HIV, Hill and McNeely (2013) provide researchers and community-based organizations with seven components to the implementation of effective faith-based HIV prevention efforts: "(1) include community-based participatory research and social marketing strategies, (2) engage the faith community through data sharing, (3) specifically target and equip church leaders in addition to laity, (4) involve effective collaboration and compromise between public health practitioners and faith leaders, (5) emphasize spirituality and compassion, (6) utilize popular opinion leaders, and (7) be intergenerational" (Hill & McNeely, 2013, p. 484). These steps can greatly transform the ways in which researchers, community-based organizations, and religious leaders discuss HIV transmission and help minimize HIV stigma within their communities. Given our understanding of the positive role of religiousness and spirituality in the lives of HIV positive gay men, churches would be remiss to not utilize their platform as a means to educate people about HIV and serve as a positive resource in the lives of HIV positive gay men.

References

Arnett, J. (2004). *Emerging adulthood: The winding road from the late teens through the twenties.* Oxford: New York.

Bangsberg, D. R., Moss, A. R., & Deeks, S. G. (2004). Paradoxes of adherence and drug resistance to HIV antiretroviral therapy. *Journal of Antimicrobial Chemotherapy, 53,* 696–699. doi:10.1093/jac/dkh162

Bangsberg, D. R., Perry, S., Charlebois, E. D., Clark, R. A., Roberston, M., Zolopa, A. R., & Moss, A. (2001). Non-adherence to highly active antiretroviral therapy predicts progression to AIDS. *AIDS, 15,* 1181–1183.

Boellstorff, T. (2005). Between religion and desire: Being Muslim and gay in Indonesia. *American Anthropologist, 107,* 575–585. doi:10.1525/aa.2005.107.4.575

Buchanan, M., Dzelme, K., Harris, D., & Hecker, L. (2001). Challenges of being simultaneously gay or lesbian and spiritual and/or religious: A narrative perspective. *American Journal of Family Therapy, 29,* 435–449. doi:10.1080/01926180127629

Carrico, A. W., Ironson, G., Antoni, M. H., Lechner, S. C., Duran, R. E., Kumar, M., & Schneiderman, N. (2006). A path model of the effects of spirituality on depressive symptoms and 24-h urinary-free cortisol in HIV-positive persons. *Journal of Psychosomatic Research, 61,* 51–58. doi:10.1016/j.jpsychores.2006.04.005

Center for Disease Control. (2007, July). *HIV and AIDS: Are you at risk?* Retrieved June 11, 2013 from http://www.cdc.gov/hiv/resources/brochures/pdf/at-risk.pdf.

Center for Disease Control. (2013, January. *Background brief on the prevention benefits of HIV treatment.* Retrieved June 15, 2013 from http://www.cdc.gov/hiv/pdf/prevention_tap_benefits_of_HIV_treatement.pdf.

Cotton, S., Puchalski, C. M., Sherman, S. N., Mrus, J. M., Peterman, A. H., Feinberg, J., ... Tsevat, J. (2006). Spirituality and religion in patients with HIV/AIDS. *Journal of General Internal Medicine, 21,* S5–S13. doi:10.1111/j.1525-1497.2006.00642.x

Cotton, S., Tsevat, J., Szaflarski, M., Kudel, I., Sherman, S. N., Feinberg, J., ... Holmes, W. C. (2006). Changes in religiousness and spirituality attributed to HIV/AIDS: Are there sex and races differences? *Journal of General Internal Medicine, 21,* S14–S20. doi:10.1111/j.1525-1497.2006.00641.x

Coyle, A., & Rafalin, D. (2000). Jewish gay men's accounts of negotiating cultural, religious, and sexual identity: A qualitative study. *Journal of Psychology & Human Sexuality, 12,* 21–48. doi:10.1300/J056v12n04_02

Cunningham, S. D., Kerrigan, D. L., McNeely, C. A., & Ellen, J. M. (2011). The role of structure versus individual agency in churches' responses to HIV/AIDS: A case study of Baltimore City churches. *Journal of Religion and Health, 50,* 407–421. doi:10.1007/s10943-009-9281-7

Doolittle, B. R., Justice, A. C., & Fiellin, D. A. (2016). Religion, spirituality, and HIV clinical outcomes: A systematic review of the literature. *AIDS and Behavior.* doi:10.1007/s10461-016-1651-z

Ellison, C. G. (1991). Religious involvement and subjective well-being. *Journal of Health and Social Behavior, 32,* 80–99. doi:10.2307/2136801

Emmons, R. (1999). *The psychology of ultimate concerns.* New York: Guilford.

Etergoff, C. (2017). Petitioning for social change: Letters to religious leaders from gay men and their family allies. *Journal of Homosexuality, 64,* 166–194.

Fetzer Institute & National Institute on Aging (NIA) Working Group. (2003). *Multidimensional measurement of religiousness/spirituality for use in health research: A report of the Fetzer Institute/National Institute on Aging working group.* Kalamazoo, MI: Fetzer Institute.

Foster, M. L., Arnold, E., Rebchook, G., & Kegeles, S. M. (2011). 'It's my inner strength': Spirituality, religion and HIV in the lives of young African American men who have sex with men. *Culture, Health & Sexuality, 13,* 1103–1117. doi:10.1080/13691058.2011.600460

Frame, M. W., Uphold, C. R., Shehan, C. L., & Reid, K. J. (2005). Effects of spirituality on health-related quality of life in men with HIV/AIDS: Implications for counseling. *Counseling and Values, 50,* 5–19. doi:10.1002/j.2161-007X.2005.tb00037.x

Francis, S. A., & Liverpool, J. (2009). A review of faith-based HIV prevention programs. *Journal of Religion and Health, 48*, 6–15. doi:10.1007/s10943-008-9171-4

Frenk, S. M., & Chaves, M. (2012). Proportion of US congregations that have people living with HIV. *Journal of Religion and Health, 51*, 371–380. doi:10.1007/s10943-010-9379-y

Fullilove, M., & Fullilove, R. (1999). Stigma as an obstacle to AIDS action: The case of the African American community. *American Behavioral Scientist, 42*, 1117–1129. doi:10.1177/00027649921954796

Garrett-Walker, J. J., & Torres, V. (2016). Personal and social consequences of negative religious rhetoric in the lives of Black gay and bisexual emerging adult men. *Journal of Homosexuality*. Advance online publication. http://dx.doi.org/10.1080/00918369.2016.1267465

Golub, S. A., Walker, J. J., Longmire-Avital, B., Bimbi, D. S., & Parsons, J. T. (2010). The role of religiosity, social support, and stress-related growth in protecting against HIV risk among transgender women. *Journal of Health Psychology, 15*, 1135–1144. doi:10.1177/1359105310364169

Griffin, H. (2006). *Their own receive them not: African American lesbian and gays in black churches*. Cleveland, OH: Pilgrim Press.

Hampton, M. C., Halkitis, P. N., & Mattis, J. S. (2010). Coping, drug use, and religiosity/spirituality in relation to HIV serostatus among gay and bisexual men. *AIDS Education & Prevention, 22*, 417–429.

Hill, P. C., & Pargament, K. I. (2008). Advances in the conceptualization and measurement of religion and spirituality: Implications for physical and mental health research. *Psychology of Religion and Spirituality, S*, 3–17. doi:10.1037/1941-1022.S.1.3

Hill, W. A., & McNeely, C. (2013). HIV/AIDS disparity between African-American and Caucasian men who have sex with men: Intervention strategies for the black church. *Journal of Religion and Health, 52*, 475 487. doi:10.1007/s10943 011 9496 2

Ickovics, J. R., Hamburger, M. E., Vlahov, D., Schoenbaum, E. E., Schuman, P., Boland, R. J., & Moore, J. (2001). Mortality, CD4 cell count decline, and depressive symptoms among HIV-seropositive women: Longitudinal analysis from the HIV epidemiology research study. *Journal of the American Medical Association, 285*, 1466–1474. doi:10.1001/jama.285.11.1466

Ironson, G., Kremer, H., & Lucette, A. (2016). Relationship between spiritual coping and survival in patients with HIV. *Journal of General Internal Medicine, 31*, 1068–1076. doi:10.1007/s11606-016-3668-4

Ironson, G., Solomon, G. F., Balbin, E. G., O'Cleirigh, C. O., George, A., Kumar, M., … Woods, T. E. (2002). The Ironson–woods spirituality/religiousness index is associated with long survival, health behaviors, less distress, and low cortisol in people with HIV/AIDS. *Annals of Behavioral Medicine, 24*, 34–48. doi:10.1207/S15324796ABM2401_05

Ironson, G., Stuetzle, R., & Fletcher, M. A. (2006). An increase in religiousness/spirituality occurs after HIV diagnosis and predicts slower disease progression over 4 years in people with HIV. *Journal of General Internal Medicine, 21*, S62–S68. doi:10.1111/j.1525-1497.2006.00648.x

Ironson, G., Stuetzle, R., Ironson, D., Balbin, E., Kremer, H., George, A., … Fletcher, M. A. (2011). View of god as benevolent and forgiving or punishing and judgmental predicts HIV disease progression. *Journal of Behavioral Medicine, 34*, 414–425. doi:10.1007/s10865-011-9314-z

Jaspal, R. (2010). Identity threat among British Muslim gay men. *The Psychologist, 23*, 639–641.

Jaspal, R., & Cinnirella, M. (2010). Coping with potentially incompatible identities: Accounts of religious, ethnic, and sexual identities from British Pakistani men who identify as Muslim and gay. *British Journal of Social Psychology, 49*, 849–870. doi:10.1348/014466609X485025

Jeffries Iv, W. L., Sutton, M. Y., & Eke, A. N. (2017). On the battlefield: The black church, public health, and the fight against HIV among African American gay and bisexual men. Journal of Urban Health. 94(3):384-398. (Epub ahead of print).

Jeffries, W. L., IV, Okeke, J. O., Gelaude, D. J., Torrone, E. A., Gasiorowicz, M., Oster, A. M., … Bertolli, J. (2014). An exploration of religion and spirituality among young, HIV-infected gay and bisexual men in the USA. *Culture, Health, and Sexuality, 16*, 1070–1083. doi:10.1080/13691058.2014.928370

Kaufman, G., & Raphel, L. (1996). *Coming out of shame: Transforming gay and lesbian lives*. New York: Doubleday.

Koenig, H. G. (2008). Concerns about measuring "spirituality" in research. *Journal of Nervous and Mental Disease, 196*, 349–355. doi:10.1097/NMD.0b013e31816ff796

Koenig, H. G., King, D. E., & Carson, V. B. (2012). *The handbook of religion and health* (2nd ed.). New York: Oxford University Press.

Kremer, H., & Ironson, G. (2009). Everything changed: Spiritual transformation in people with HIV. *International Journal of Psychiatry in Medicine, 39*, 243–262. doi:10.2190/PM.39.3.c

Kremer, H., Ironson, G., & Kaplan, L. (2009). The fork in the road: HIV as a potential positive turning point and the role of spirituality. *AIDS Care, 21*, 368–377. doi:10.1080/09540120802183479

Kremer, H., Ironson, G., Kaplan, L., Stuetzele, R., Baker, N., & Fletcher, M. A. (2015). Spiritual coping predicts CD4-cell preservation and undetectable viral load over four years. *AIDS Care, 27*, 71–79. doi:10.1080/09540121.2014.952220

Kremer, H., Ironson, G., & Porr, M. (2009). Spiritual and mind-body beliefs as barriers and motivators to HIV-treatment decision-making and medication adherence? A qualitative study. *AIDS Patient Care and STDs, 23*, 127–134. doi:10.1089/apc.2008.0131

Lassiter, J. M., & Parsons, J. T. (2016). Religion and spirituality's influences on HIV syndemics among MSM: A systematic review and conceptual model. *AIDS and Behavior, 20*, 461–472. doi:10.1007/s10461-015-1173-0

Lassiter, J. M., Saleh, L., Starks, T., Grov, C., Ventuneac, A., & Parsons, J. T. (2017). Race, ethnicity, religious affiliation, and education are associated with gay and bisexual men's religious and spiritual participation and beliefs: Results from the one thousand strong cohort. *Cultural Diversity and Ethnic Minority Psychology*. doi:10.1037/cdp0000143. (Epub ahead of print).

Lee, B. (2007). Moderating effects of religious/spiritual coping in the relation between perceived stress and psychological well-being. *Pastoral Psychology, 55*, 751–759. doi:10.1007/s11089-007-0080-3

Leserman, J., Pence, B. W., Whetten, K., Mugavero, M. J., Thielman, N. M., Swartz, M. S., & Stangl, D. (2007). Relation of lifetime trauma and depressive symptoms to mortality in HIV. *American Journal of Psychiatry, 164*, 1707–1713. doi:10.1176/appi.ajp.2007.06111775

Lima, V. D., Geller, J., Bangsberg, D. R., Patterson, T. L., Daniel, M., Kerr, T., … Hogg, R. S. (2007). The effect of adherence on the association between depressive symptoms and mortality among HIV-infected individuals first initiating HAART. *AIDS, 21*, 1175–1183. doi:10.1097/QAD.0b013e32811ebf57

Lumpkins, C. Y., Greiner, K. A., Daley, C., Mabachi, N. M., & Neuhaus, K. (2011). Promoting healthy behavior from the pulpit: Clergy share their perspectives on effective health communication in the African American church. *Journal of Religion and Health, 52*(4), 1093–1107. doi:10.1007/s10943-011-9533-1

Lutz, F., Kremer, H., & Ironson, G. (2011). Being diagnosed with HIV as a trigger for spiritual transformation. *Religions, 2*, 398–409. doi:10.3390/rel2030398

Lyon, M. E., Garvie, P. A., Kao, E., Briggs, L., He, J., Malow, R., … McCarter, R. (2011). Spirituality in HIV-infected adolescents and their families: FAmily CEntered (FACE) advance care planning and medication adherence. *Journal of Adolescent Health, 48*, 633–636. doi:10.1016/j.jadohealth.2010.09.006

Mayne, T. J., Vittinghoff, E., Chesney, M. A., Barett, D. C., & Coates, T. J. (1996). Depressive affect and survival among gay and bisexual men infected with HIV. *Archives of Internal Medicine, 156*, 2233–2238. doi:10.1001/archinte.1996.00440180095012

Meanley, S., Pingel, E. S., & Bauermeister, J. A. (2016). Psychological well-being among religious and spiritual-identified young gay and bisexual men. *Sexuality Research and Social Policy, 13*, 35–45.

Meladze, P., & Brown, J. (2015). Religion, sexuality, and internalized homonegativity: Confronting cognitive dissonance in the Abrahamic religions. *Journal of Religion and Health, 54*, 1950–1962. doi:10.1007/s10943-015-0018-5

Miller, R. L., Jr. (2005). An appointment with god: AIDS, place, and spirituality. *Journal of Sex Research, 42*, 35–45. doi:10.1080/00224490509552255

Miller, R. L., Jr. (2007). Legacy denied: African American gay men, AIDS and the black church. *Social Work, 52*, 51–61. doi:10.1093/sw/52.1.51

Miller, W. R., & Thoresen, C. E. (2003). Spirituality, religion, and health: An emerging research field. *American Psychologist, 58*, 24–35. doi:10.1037/0003-066X.58.1.24

Monod, S., Brennan, M., Rochat, E., Martin, E., Rochat, S., & Büla, C. J. (2011). Instruments measuring spirituality in clinical research: A systematic review. *Journal of General Internal Medicine, 26*, 1345–1357. doi:10.1007/s11606-011-1769-7

Moore, D., Onsomu, E. O., Timmons, S. M., Abuya, B. A., & Moore, C. (2012). Communicating HIV/AIDS through African American churches in North Carolina: Implications and recommendations for HIV/AIDS faith-based programs. *Journal of Religion and Health, 51*, 865–878. doi:10.1007/s10943-010-9396-x

Nelson, L. E., Wilton, L., Zhang, N., Regan, R., Thach, C. T., Dyer, T. V. et al. (2016). Childhood exposure to religions with high prevalence of members who discourage homosexuality is associated with adult HIV risk behaviors and HIV infection in Black men who have sex with men. *American Journal of Men's Health*. pii: 1557988315626264.

Oman, D. (2013). Spiritual modeling and the social learning of spirituality and religion. In K. I. Pargament, J. J. Exline, & J. W. Jones (Eds.), *APA handbook of psychology, religion, and spirituality (Vol. 1): Context, theory, and research* (pp. 187–204). Washington, DC: American Psychological Association.

Pargament, K., Koenig, H., Tarakeshwar, N., & Hahn, J. (2004). Religious coping methods as predictors of psychological, physical and spiritual outcomes among medically ill elderly patients: A two year longitudinal study. *Journal of Health Psychology, 9*, 713–730. doi:10.1177/1359105304045366

Pargament, K. I. (2013). Searching for the sacred: Toward a nonreductionistic theory of spirituality. In K. I. Pargament, J. J. Exline, & J. W. Jones (Eds.), *APA handbook of psychology, religion, and spirituality (Vol. 1): Context, theory, and research* (pp. 257–273). Washington, DC: American Psychological Association.

Park, J., & Nachman, S. (2010). The link between religion and HAART adherence in pediatric HIV patients. *AIDS Care, 22*, 556–561. doi:10.1080/09540120903254013

Parsons, S. K., Cruise, P. L., Davenport, W. M., & Jones, V. (2006). Religious beliefs, practices and treatment adherence among individuals with HIV in the southern United States. *AIDS Patient Care and STDs, 20*, 97–111. doi:10.1089/apc.2006.20.97

Pérez, J. E., Chartier, M., Koopman, C., Vosvick, M., Gore-Felton, C., & Spiegel, D. (2009). Spiritual striving, acceptance coping, and depressive symptoms among adults living with HIV/AIDS. *Journal of Health Psychology, 14*, 88–97. doi:10.1177/1359105308097949

Pérez, J. E., Forero-Puerta, T., Palesh, O., Lubega, S., Thoresen, C., Bowman, E., … Spiegel, D. (2008). Pain, distress, and social support in relation to spiritual beliefs and experiences among persons living with HIV/AIDS. In J. C. Upton (Ed.), *Religion and psychology: New research* (pp. 1–25). New York: Nova Science.

Pew Research Center. (2015). America's changing religious landscape: Chapter 4: *The shifting religious identity of demographic groups*. Retrieved from http://www.pewforum.org/2015/05/12/chapter-4-the-shifting-religious-identity-of-demographic-groups/.

Piedmont, R. L., Ciarrochi, J. W., Dy-Liacco, G. S., & Williams, J. E. G. (2009). The empirical and conceptual value of spiritual transcendence and religious involvement scales for personality research. *Psychology of Religion and Spirituality, 1*, 162–179. doi:10.1037/a0015883

Pitt, R. N. (2010). "killing the messenger": Religious black gay men's neutralization of anti-gay religious messages. *Journal for the Scientific Study of Religion, 49*, 56–72. doi:10.1111/j.1468-5906.2009.01492.x

Quinn, K., Dickson-Gomez, J., & Young, S. (2016). The influence of pastors' ideologies of homosexuality on HIV prevention in the black church. *Journal of Religion and Health, 55*, 1700–1716.

Ramer, L., Johnson, D., Chan, L., & Barrett, M. T. (2006). The effect of HIV/AIDS disease progression on spirituality and self-transcendence in a multicultural population. *Journal of Transcultural Nursing, 17*, 280–289. doi:10.1177/1043659606288373

Rodriguez, E. M., & Ouellette, S. C. (2000). Gay and lesbian Christians: Homosexual and religious identity integration in the members and participants of a gay-positive church. *Journal for the Scientific Study of Religion, 39*, 333–347. doi:10.1111/0021-8294.00028

Salander, P. (2006). Who needs the concept of 'spirituality'? *Psycho-Oncology, 15*, 647–649. doi:10.1002/pon.1060

Scheitle, C. P., Merino, S. M., & Moore, A. (2010). On the varying meaning of "open and affirming". *Journal of Homosexuality, 57*, 1223–1236. doi:10.1080/00918369.2010.517064

Schnoor, R. F. (2006). Being gay and Jewish: Negotiating intersecting identities. *Sociology of Religion, 67*, 43–60.

Seegers, D. L. (2007). Spiritual and religious experiences of gay men with HIV illness. *Journal of the Association of Nurses in AIDS Care, 18*, 5–12. doi:10.1016/j.jana.2007.03.001

Siegel, K., & Schrimshaw, E. W. (2002). The perceived benefits of religious and spiritual coping among older adults living with HIV/AIDS. *Journal for the Scientific Study of Religion, 41*, 91–102. doi:10.1111/1468-5906.00103

Simoni, J. M., & Ortiz, M. Z. (2003). Mediational models of spirituality and depressive symptomatology among HIV-positive Puerto Rican women. *Cultural Diversity and Ethnic Minority Psychology, 9*, 3–15. doi:10.1037/1099-9809.9.1.3

Sutton, M. Y., & Parks, C. P. (2013). HIV/AIDS prevention, faith, and spirituality among black/African American and Latino communities in the United States: Strengthening scientific faith-based efforts to shift the course of the epidemic and reduce HIV-related health disparities. *Journal of Religion and Health, 52*, 514–530. doi:10.1007/s10943-011-9499-z

Szaflarski, M. (2013). Spirituality and religion among HIV-infected individuals. *Current HIV/AIDS Reports, 10*, 324–332. doi:10.1007/s11904-013-0175-7

Szaflarski, M., Ritchey, P. N., Leonard, A. C., Mrus, J. M., Peterman, A. H., Ellison, C. G., ... Tsevat, J. (2006). Modeling the effects of spirituality/religion on patients' perceptions of living with HIV/AIDS. *Journal of General Internal Medicine, 21*, S28–S38. doi:10.1111/j.1525-1497.2006.00646.x

Tarakeshwar, N., Khan, N., & Sikkema, K. J. (2006). A relationship-based framework of spirituality for individuals with HIV. *AIDS and Behavior, 10*, 59–70. doi:10.1007/s10461-005-9052-8

Taylor, R., Mattis, J., & Chatters, L. (1999). Subjective religiosity among African Americans: A synthesis of findings from five national samples. *Journal of Black Psychology, 25*, 524–543. doi:10.1177/0095798499025004004

Trevino, K. M., Pargament, K. I., Cotton, S., Leonard, A. C., Hahn, J., Caprini-Faigin, C. A., & Tsevat, J. (2010). Religious coping and physiological, psychological, social, and spiritual outcomes in patients with HIV/AIDS: Cross-sectional and longitudinal findings. *AIDS and Behavior, 14*, 379–389. doi:10.1007/s10461-007-9332-6

Tsevat, J., Leonard, A. C., Szaflarski, M., Sherman, S. N., Cotton, S., Mrus, J. M., & Feinberg, J. (2009). Change in quality of life after being diagnosed with HIV: A multicenter longitudinal study. *AIDS Patient Care and STDs, 23*, 931–937. doi:10.1089/apc.2009.0026

Van Wagoner, N., Mugavero, M., Westfall, A., Hollimon, J., Slater, L. Z., Burkholder, G., Raper, J. L., & Hook, E. W. (2014). Church attendance in men who have sex with men diagnosed with HIV is associated with later presentation for HIV care. *Clinical Infectious Diseases, 58*, 295–299.

Walker, J. J., & Longmire-Avital, B. (2012). The impact of religious faith and internalized homonegativity on resiliency for black lesbian, gay, and bisexual emerging adults. *Developmental Psychology, 49*(9), 1723–1731. doi:10.1037/a0031059

Watkins, T. L., Jr., Simpson, C., Cofield, S. S., Davies, S., Kohler, C., & Usdan, S. (2016). The relationship between HIV risk, high-risk behavior, religiosity, and spirituality among black men who have sex with men (MSM): An exploratory study. *Journal of Religion and Health, 55*, 535–548. doi:10.1007/s10943-015-0142-2

Wilson, P. A., Wittlin, N. M., Munoz-Lavoy, M., & Parker, R. (2011). Ideologies of black churches in New York and the public health crisis of HIV among black men who have sex with men. *Global Public Health, 6*, S227–S242.

Woods, T. E., Antoni, M. H., Ironson, G. H., & Kling, D. W. (1999). Religiosity is associated with affective and immune status in symptomatic HIV-infected gay men. *Journal of Psychosomatic Research, 46*, 165–176. doi:10.1016/S0022-3999(98)00078-6

Yi, M. S., Mrus, J. M., Wade, T. J., Ho, M. L., Hornung, R. W., Cotton, S., ... Tsevat, J. (2006). Religion, spirituality, and depressive symptoms in patients with HIV/AIDS. *Journal of General Internal Medicine, 21*, S21–S27. doi:10.1111/j.1525-1497.2006.00643.x

Part IV
Structural Contexts

Chapter 14
Addressing Social Determinants of Health Among HIV Positive Men Who Have Sex with Men (MSM): The Need for Synergy

Y. Omar Whiteside, Jordan J. White, and Kenneth T. Jones

Introduction

From 2008 to 2010, the estimated number of new HIV infections remained stable in the USA (Centers for Disease Control and Prevention [CDC], 2012a, 2012b, 2012c). However, men who have sex with men (MSM) continue to represent a disproportionate burden of new HIV infections. While MSM are estimated to comprise from 3.9% (Purcell et al., 2012) to 6.8% (Lieb et al., 2009) of the US population, they accounted for 63% of all new HIV infections in 2010 (CDC, 2012a, 2012b, 2012c). Comparatively, the number of new infections among MSM increased by 12% from 2008 to 2010, while among women, the number of new HIV infections attributed to heterosexual contact decreased during the same time period (CDC, 2012a, 2012b, 2012c). There was a statistically significant increase ($p < 0.05$) in the number of new HIV infections among MSM in 2010 compared to the same group in 2008 (CDC, 2012a, 2012b, 2012c). These findings were largely due to the statistically significant increase in new HIV infections among MSM 13–24 years of age compared to the previous 2 years (CDC, 2012a, 2012b, 2012c).

The findings and conclusions in this book chapter are those of the authors and do not necessarily represent the views of the Centers for Disease Control and Prevention.

Y.O. Whiteside (✉)
Division of HIV/AIDS Prevention, National Center for HIV/AIDS, Viral Hepatitis, STD, and TB Prevention, Centers for Disease Control and Prevention, Atlanta, GA, USA
e-mail: yowhiteside@gmail.com

J.J. White
Desmond M. Tutu Fellow of Public Health and Human Rights, Johns Hopkins Bloomberg School of Public Health, Johns Hopkins University, Baltimore, MD, USA

K.T. Jones
Office of Health Equity, U.S. Department of Veterans Affairs, Washington, DC, USA

Division of HIV/AIDS Prevention, National Center for HIV/AIDS, Viral Hepatitis, STD, and TB Prevention, Centers for Disease Control and Prevention (CDC), Atlanta, GA, USA

© Springer Science+Business Media LLC 2017 327
L. Wilton (ed.), *Understanding Prevention for HIV Positive Gay Men*,
DOI 10.1007/978-1-4419-0203-0_14

The incongruence between HIV rates and the estimated population size of MSM highlights the need to consider other factors—beyond individual risk taking—that may be driving HIV infections for MSM. Much of the HIV prevention and treatment research has examined individual-level factors such as an individual's self-reports of unprotected anal sex (CDC, 2011; Politch et al., 2012; Stein, Silivera, Hagerty, & Marmor, 2012). However, investigators have recently begun to explore the relationship between structural-level factors such as social determinants of health and sexual decision-making (Dale et al., 2016; Frye et al., 2006, 2010, 2016; Jones, 2012; Mayer, Bekker et al., 2012; Mayer, Pape et al., 2012; Phillips et al., 2015; White et al., 2013). Though sexual decision-making occurs on the individual level, individuals make these decisions within a larger social context (Frye et al., 2006, 2010). Consequently, researchers are broadening their efforts to not only identify direct (individual-level) causes for sexual decision-making but also indirect (structural-level) causes (Frye et al., 2006, 2010, 2016). In an effort to explore this relationship among MSM, we will first examine why it is important to consider social determinants of health (not just individual behavior) when discussing health behaviors, particularly risk behaviors for HIV infection. Next, we will review the pertinent current research on the role of structural-level factors in the lives of MSM. Then, we will highlight two federal-level programs which are currently underway to help overcome these structural-level factors. Finally, we will end our discussion with actions that can be taken on two emerging structural-level factors to improve the health of HIV positive MSM.

Why Social Determinants of Health?

Biology, individual behavior, social environment, physical environment, and health services have been accepted as determinants of population health (Beltran, Harrison, Hall, & Dean, 2011). Social environment, physical environment, and health services fall under the category of social determinants of health (Beltran et al., 2011). In 2008, the World Health Organization's (WHO) Commission on Social Determinants of Health (CSDH) called on governments across the world to address social determinants of health as a means of achieving health equity in a disparate world (CSDH, 2008). Consequently, national public health agencies in the USA began emphasizing the need to address those structural-level factors that influence disease acquisition. In conveying this importance, Frieden (2010) noted that social determinants of health form the foundation of society and that seeking to address these factors has significant potential to improve health in the USA. In 2010, the National Center for HIV/AIDS, Viral Hepatitis, STD, and TB Prevention (NCHHSTP) released a white paper in which it urged the use of individual-level interventions in tandem with approaches that addressed interpersonal, institutional, and community-level factors (CDC, 2010). NCHHSTP recommended community partners to advance this systems approach (CDC, 2010). The NCHHSTP's stance highlighted the need to reduce the impact that social determinants of health such as poverty, incarceration, and racism have in HIV, viral hepatitis, sexually transmitted infections (STIs), and other infectious diseases (CDC, 2010).

Strides have been made in applying social determinants of health to HIV behavioral research. Social determinants of health can influence the potential for HIV infection through individual decision-making, access to prevention services, and HIV care (Aral, Adimora, & Fenton, 2008; Raphael, 2006). For example, among heterosexual Black women in Syracuse, New York, researchers determined that community-level factors such as increased STI rates due to socially or geographically isolated individuals choosing sexual partners from within their own constrained networks and barriers to accessing STI care may contribute to disproportionate HIV in this population (Lane, Rubinstein, Keefe, & Webster, 2004). These factors alone may not be social determinants of health but they resulted from factors which include: disproportionate incarceration rates in Black men, residential segregation (Lane et al., 2004). Other community-level factors such as income inequality and the proportion of unmarried persons living in a county may also be associated with increased rates of HIV infection (Gant et al., 2012). However, there is a dearth of research on how social determinants of health may influence the HIV risk behaviors of MSM, particularly HIV positive MSM. Of the few studies identified, a few structural-level factors have emerged as potentially contributing to the risk of HIV acquisition in MSM. Of the few studies identified, a few structural-level factors have emerged as potentially contributing to the risk of HIV acquisition in MSM. Using key words relevant to exploring the role of social determinants of health in the lives of MSM and the subsequent citation lists that resulted from those searches, the authors summarized relevant literature and derived themes that were used to outline this chapter. This chapter is not meant to be a formal synthesis or an exhaustive exploration of the role of social determinants of health in the health of MSM but instead is conceptual in nature and is meant to amalgamate some of the most prominent factors seen in the literature.

Structural Barriers to Health Among MSM

Stigma

Today, an HIV diagnosis is not the death sentence it once was in the USA. In many cases it is a manageable chronic disease. Research shows that the life expectancy for individuals at age 20 who are on antiretroviral therapy (ART) has increased from 36.1 years in 1996–1999 to 49.4 in 2003–2005 (The Antiretroviral Therapy Cohort Collaboration, 2008). In addition, ART) also helps reduce the likelihood that an HIV positive heterosexual person will infect a sexual partner by up to 96% (Cohen, McCauley, & Gamble, 2012). Nonetheless, stigmas (e.g., HIV stigma, sexual orientation stigma) may act as barriers to HIV prevention (Hatzenbuehler, O'Cleirigh, Mayer, Mimiaga, & Safren, 2011), testing (Lorenc et al., 2010), and treatment (Wohl et al., 2012) for MSM, discouraging some men at risk from getting tested or those with HIV from receiving treatment. Stigma may "out" them to their communities, social networks, and families (Wohl et al., 2012). Stigma may also lead to active social discrimination, fear, and shame, particularly for those living with HIV infection.

Stigma may affect individuals within the MSM communities differently. Due to cultural differences stigma may be experienced differently based on an MSM's race/ethnicity which may, in turn, lead to behaviors that play a role in increasing the risk of HIV infection (Rao, Pryor, Gaddhist, & Mayer, 2008; Wilson & Yoshikawa, 2006; Wohl et al., 2012). For example, a nationally representative study examining attitudes towards homosexuality (Glick & Golden, 2010) compared changes over time among persons who believed that homosexuality was "always wrong." Findings showed that 72% of Black respondents endorsed this belief which indicated very little change since the 1970s. White respondents showed a decline from 70.8% in the 1970s to 51.6% in 2008. Among MSM, 57.1% of Blacks reported homosexuality as "always wrong" compared to 26.8% of whites. For Black MSM especially, these beliefs may diminish any sense of personal obligation to protect themselves or their sexual partners (Jones, Wilton, Millett, & Johnson, 2010; Peterson & Jones, 2009; Stokes & Peterson, 1998; Woodyard, Peterson, & Stokes, 2000). HIV stigma may be experienced differently among Hispanic or Latino MSM. Wohl et al. (2012) determined that HIV positive Hispanic or Latino MSM experienced more stigma related to their HIV status and less related to their sexual orientation than their Black counterparts. The implications may be that it is more difficult for some Hispanic or Latino MSM to disclose their HIV status. Additionally, the HIV stigma that Hispanic/Latino MSM experienced was significant enough to prevent them from seeking HIV care, although this was not observed among black MSM. The experience with stigma may also be different for whites. HIV positive Whites described feeling greater stigma related to HIV status which resulted in keeping their status secret for fear of interpersonal rejection (Rao, Pryor, Gaddhist, & Mayer, 2008). The implications may be that it is more difficult for some Whites, including MSM, to disclose their HIV status. Understanding how HIV stigma and sexual orientation stigma operate at the intersections of gender, place, sexuality, race, and power can assist in elucidating the social inequalities that result in negative outcomes for the most affected groups. Although national communication and education campaigns have attempted to destigmatize HIV and homosexuality, stigmatization continues to be far-reaching and can affect many aspects of life (e.g., employment, housing, access to care) and consequently health (Center for AIDS Prevention Studies [CAPS], 2006).

Housing

The importance of housing in positive health outcomes has been well documented in public health (Lennon et al., 2013; Massey & Denton, 1993; Matte & Jacobs, 2000; Ruel, Oakley, Wilson, & Maddox, 2010), but stable housing represents an even greater challenge for people living with HIV (Holtgrave et al., 2012; Wolitski et al., 2010). The transiency associated with homelessness or being unstably housed disconnects individuals from health care services. When these individuals are finally stable enough to access HIV care, it is often at a later point in the progression of the disease leading to poorer HIV treatment outcomes. Furthermore, they are also less likely to be adherent to antiretrovirals (Milloy, Marshall, Montaner, & Wood, 2012), and more likely to have a detectable viral load (Wolitski et al., 2010). Moreover, homeless individuals may be more likely to experience depression, which has been associated with both poor health status and poor HIV treatment outcomes (Riley et al., 2003; Weiser et al., 2006).

Homeless individuals may also be more likely to participate in high-risk sexual behaviors (Aidala, Cross, Stall, Harre, & Sumartojo, 2005; Mimiaga et al., 2009) such as sexual risk taking (Clatts, Goldsamt, & Yi, 2005), sex exchange (Aidala et al., 2005; Kidder, Wolitski, Pals, & Campsmith, 2008), and have a greater number of sex partners (Kidder et al., 2008). The effects of homelessness may be especially striking for MSM. Halkitis et al. (2013) determined that homeless MSM, or those with unstable housing, may have increased risks of recent unprotected anal inter- course (UAI) and of engaging in at least one episode of UAI within the past year (Mimiaga et al., 2009). Perhaps one of the keys to improving the health of HIV posi- tive MSM is helping those who are homeless to secure stable housing; this not only has implications for HIV prevention but also for improving health outcomes (Aidala et al., 2005; Kidder et al., 2008; Milloy et al., 2012).

Neighborhood Composition

Research also suggests that the neighborhood where a person lives affects their health (Cubbin & Winkleby, 2005; Diez-Roux et al., 1999; Diez-Roux et al., 2001; Kawachi & Berkman, 2003; Latkin & Curry, 2003; Ross & Mirowsky, 2001; Stafford & Marmot, 2003; Williams & Collins, 2001; Yen & Kaplan, 1999a, 1999b). Studies assessing the neighborhood composition and HIV acquisition are limited (Fuller et al., 2005; Latkin & Curry, 2003). Nevertheless, investigators have deter- mined that neighborhood composition has been associated with adolescent initia- tion of injection drug use (Fuller et al., 2005), depression in current and former drug users at high risk for HIV infection (Latkin & Curry, 2003), and high prevalence of sexually transmitted infections (STI) (Semaan, Sternberg, Zaidi, & Aral, 2007).

Frye et al. (2006) proposed several pathways through which the urban environ- ment might influence the sexual risk behaviors of MSM. In one of the pathways, sexual risk behavior was associated with psychological distress resulting from physical disorder (e.g., blighted neighborhoods, high crime, and a large number of liquor stores). This finding was also supported in a recent publication by the authors (2016).

Another focus of research has been on determining the effect of living in pre- dominantly gay neighborhoods. Buttram and Kurtz (2012) found its protective effect against cocaine use and substance dependence, which differed from the findings of Carpiano, Kelly, Easterbrook, and Parsons (2011) who determined that MSM who lived in gay neighborhoods were at an increased risk for drug use. Other contradictory findings abound concerning the effect of MSM living in gay neighborhoods. For example, Frye et al. (2010) examined neighborhood characteristics of MSM who were between the ages of 23 and 29 in New York City (NYC), and gay presence was a protective factor for UAI. However, in their study of MSM age 18 and older in New York City, Kelly, Carpiano, Easterbrook, and Parsons (2012) found that living in a gay enclave was associated with UAI. Given these mixed findings, further investigations of the impact of neighborhood composition and HIV risk for MSM may be needed. In addition, studies focusing on identifying neighborhood characteristics (e.g., residential segregation, poverty) associated with multiple health concerns (e.g., HIV and hypertension) and similar at-risk groups (e.g., black men) to determine effective and cost-efficient public health approaches would be warranted as well.

Incarceration

Since 2002, the USA has had the highest incarceration rate in the world (Pettit, 2012). One in every 107 people in the USA was in prison or jail in 2011 (US Department of Justice, 2012). The race/ethnicity composition of the incarcerated population differs from the US population during this timeframe, where Whites comprised 61% of the US population but only 31% of the incarcerated population; Blacks made up 14% of the US population but 36% of the prison population; and Hispanics or Latinos comprised 16% of the US population but 24% of the US prison population (U.S Department of Justice, 2012). Over 1% of state and federal prisoners were reported to be living with HIV infection (CDC, 2012a, 2012b, 2012c). High HIV prevalence rates have been reported among incarcerated MSM (Adams et al., 2011; Chen, Bovée, & Kerndt, 2003) although studies have found that those who had HIV were already infected prior to incarceration (CDC, 2006). A recent study found overrepresentation of sexual minorities (Meyer et al., 2016). Nearly one out of ten men either identified as gay or bisexual or reported prior sex with another man. Investigators in a six-city study multicomponent intervention study reported a 35% incidence of incarceration for Black MSM. Nearly a quarter of these men (24%) reported recent incarceration (Brewer et al., 2014).

HIV testing is not compulsory in all correctional settings. At the end of 2006, less than half of State prisons tested all inmates for HIV infection at admission, while in prison, or upon release (CDC, 2009). Prisons and jails could play a key role in facilitating HIV testing through routine opt-out HIV testing opportunities (Westergaard, Spaulding, & Flanigan, 2013). For example, in the Washington DC City jail, all inmates are offered a voluntary HIV test upon entry and as a result the jail has become one of the leading facilities for identifying undiagnosed HIV infections in the city (DC Appleseed Center, 2012).

Sex is illegal in most correctional facilities and prisoners are not allowed to have condoms (U.S. Department of Justice, 1999). Inmates who are sexually active, whether willingly or unwillingly, while incarcerated oftentimes cannot benefit from correctional facility-based HIV interventions, as many of them focus on case management for HIV care upon release (Draine, McTighe, & Bourgois, 2011).

Because the median State prison sentence for a felony was 17 months in 2006 (U.S. Bureau of Justice Statistics, 2009), most inmates will quickly return to the communities in which they lived. When individuals are released from prison, they are at greater risk for HIV transmission and acquisition based on social determinants of health such as limited employment or housing opportunities. For example, incarceration increases an individual's risk of being homeless or marginally housed (Dumont, Brockmann, Dickman, Alexander, & Rich, 2012). Those with felony or misdemeanor convictions have fewer opportunities for federal public assistance than individuals without a criminal history. In some instances, felons are barred from receiving federal public assistance (i.e., housing, food), federal financial aid for college, and voting privileges. Felons also have limited employment options which may directly affect their ability to repay debt. Consequently, a history of incarceration often relegates former prisoners to a life of poverty (Dumont et al., 2012). Once HIV positive inmates are released, many of them lack health insurance to continue receiving the routine HIV care they received while incarcerated (Westergaard et al., 2013). No matter the circumstances which may have delivered these men to prison, their felony status may limit their ability to improve their circumstances. These results may be even more troubling for felons who are HIV positive and MSM because they bear the burden of three identities (criminal history, positive HIV serostatus, and sexual orientation) which are all stigmatized. Public health and the criminal justice system may need to work collaboratively to meet the needs of these individuals not only when they are incarcerated but also when they are released (Adams et al., 2011; Chen et al., 2003; Dumont et al., 2012; Westergaard et al., 2013).

HIV Care

Access to and retention in HIV care can improve the health of HIV positive MSM and potentially reduce HIV transmission. Previous research has highlighted that a high level of engagement in HIV care has been associated with reduced sexual risk behaviors (Metsch et al., 2008). Having a high level of HIV care can also provide MSM with access to HAART which can improve survival and make life with HIV more manageable, similar to many chronic diseases (Giordano et al., 2007). Treatment is also important because it can reduce an HIV positive individual's viral load thus reducing the risk of transmission to others (Friedman et al., 2013; Hall, Holtgrave, Tang, & Rhodes, 2013). Despite these benefits, however, some individuals do not readily access HIV care. For example, Giordano et al. (2005) reported that 48% of individuals who enrolled in intake at an HIV clinic in Houston were either not established in HIV care or poorly established 6 months after enrolment. Research has also determined that less than two-thirds of individuals with an HIV diagnosis in 2008 were involved in HIV care a year following diagnosis (Hall et al., 2012). Equally important, of those living with an HIV diagnosis in 2009, only 45% met the criteria for retention in care (Hall et al., 2012). Blacks and Hispanics/Latinos were less likely to be retained in care compared to Whites (Hall et al., 2012), and Black MSM had the lowest levels of HIV care among each step of the continuum compared to other MSM (Singh et al., 2014). Undocumented Hispanics/Latinos may have even more barriers to HIV care. Dennis et al. (2013) reported that Hispanic/Latino immigrants in their study were significantly more likely to enter HIV care with advanced HIV disease and less likely to have health insurance than US-born Hispanics/Latinos.

There are myriad reasons why individuals are not engaged in HIV care: lack of health insurance (Muthulingham, Chin, Hsu, Scheer, & Schwarcz, 2013), international migration (Taylor et al., 2011), immigrant status (Dennis et al., 2013), unstable housing, relocation, stigma, and/or forgetfulness (Pecoraro et al., 2013). More specifically, MSM have a unique set of circumstances that serve as barriers to HIV care, which may also include lack of culturally competent health care facilities and providers (Beyer et al., 2012; Mayer, Bekker et al., 2012; Mayer, Pape et al., 2012). For some MSM, the HIV care that is provided has been described as inadequate and in some instances even discriminatory (Mayer, Bekker et al., 2012; Mayer, Pape et al., 2012). Factors that put MSM at risk for HIV also delay their entry into the health care system and consequently contribute to HIV complications and AIDS mortality among those infected. Accessing services is a key factor to addressing HIV among MSM.

Low Socioeconomic Status

Although the link between low socioeconomic status and health disparities has been well documented (Adler et al., 1994; Feldman & Steptoe, 2004; McLaughlin & Stokes, 2002; Phuong, 2009; Steptoe & Feldman, 2001; Williams, 1999; Williams, Mohammed, Leavell, & Collins, 2010), there are limited studies looking at this phenomenon from the perspective of HIV-infected persons. Joy et al. (2008) investigated the effect of neighborhood socioeconomic status and the uptake of HIV treatment in an international setting where universal health care was being offered and found that low socioeconomic status was associated with treatment delay. Compared to those of higher socioeconomic status, persons of lower socioeconomic status may be less likely to be prescribed HAART (WHO, 2013; Wood et al., 2002). Jones (2012) found MSM living in neighborhoods characterized by lower socioeconomic status were less likely to be knowledgeable about HAART. These findings may elucidate the poor outlook for survival for individuals with HIV infection with low socioeconomic status. For example, McFarland, Chen, Hsu, Schwarcz, and Katz (2003) determined that the percentage of neighborhood residents living below the poverty level was associated with increased AIDS mortality (McFarland et al., 2003). Individual and concentrated levels of low socioeconomic status are important risk factors for HIV infection for heterosexuals in the USA (Adimora et al., 2001; Denning & DiNenno, 2010; Hixson, Omer, del Rio, & Frew, 2011; LaLota et al., 2011; Raj & Bowleg, 2011). Growing research has begun examining this relationship for MSM. Gayles, Kuhns, Kwon, Mustanski, and Garofalo (2016) found that not working or being in school (termed socioeconomic disconnection) was associated with HIV status in young MSM. Mays, Cochran, and Zamudio (2004) reported associations between unsafe sex and low individual socioeconomic status among Black MSM. For some MSM, even the perception of being of lower socioeconomic status (SES) may influence their sexual behaviors. Halkitis and Figueroa (2013) found that young MSM who perceived themselves to be of lower SES were more likely to engage in high-risk sexual behaviors in the previous 30 days compared to those who did not. Because Halkitis and Figueroa (2013) did not objectively define lower SES, they did not provide an explanation of whether participants' perceptions were correct. Nonetheless, removing real or even perceived socioeconomic barriers for MSM may help to improve the health of this community and may be done in concert with programs that seek to change individual-level risks. An example could include an HIV prevention intervention designed for MSM that not only seeks to change behavior on the individual level but that also includes a component that provides access to educational or job opportunities or job training.

Federal and Local Efforts to Address Structural Barriers

More than three decades after the first cases of HIV were diagnosed in the USA, MSM continue to be disproportionately infected with the disease. Several individual-level and structural-level factors are potential contributors to this situation. Therefore, it is important to use a two-prong approach which addresses individual-level factors and social determinants of health to improve the health of individuals. This approach will have to be further developed to address those unique structural-level barriers and policies that threaten the physical, mental, or social well-being (WHO, 1948) of HIV positive MSM.

Increasing Access to Care and Preventive Services

One effort to increase access to care and prevention services is the Care and Prevention in the US (CAPUS) Demonstration Project. CAPUS is a collaborative effort among the CDC; Office of the Assistant Secretary for Health (Office of HIV/AIDS and Infectious Disease Policy, Office of Minority Health, Office on Women's Health); the Health Resources and Services Administration (both the HIV/AIDS

Bureau and the Bureau of Primary Health Care); and the Substance Abuse and Mental Health Services Administration (CDC, 2012a). The project provides 3 years of funding to eight health departments (Georgia Department of Public Health, Illinois Department of Public Health, Louisiana State Department of Health and Hospitals, Mississippi State Department of Health, Missouri Department of Health and Senior Services, North Carolina State Department of Health and Human Services, Tennessee State Department of Health, and Virginia State Department of Health) to bolster their efforts to develop innovative methods to increase linkage to, retention in, and return to care for all HIV-infected persons, especially racial and ethnic minorities. The purpose of the project is to reduce HIV-related morbidity and mortality by addressing social, economic, clinical, and structural factors influencing HIV health outcomes (CDC, 2012a). Each health department is required to create a work plan which includes several required components: (1) increase HIV testing, linkage to, retention in, and reengagement with care, treatment, and prevention; (2) enhance navigation services; (3) use surveillance data and data systems to improve care and prevention; and (4) address social and structural factors directly affecting HIV testing, linkage to, retention in, and reengagement with care, treatment, and prevention (CDC, 2012a). In order to reach its goal, CAPUS grantees also fund community-based organizations within each jurisdiction (CDC, 2012a). Because of the high burden of HIV disease morbidity among MSM, MSM are poised to benefit from these efforts. Project successes will be compiled and shared with health departments across the nation (CDC, 2012a).

Another effort to increase access to care and prevention services is the Affordable Care Act. Provisions of the Affordable Care Act provide opportunities for health coverage and reduce barriers to obtaining preventive services for those living with HIV and AIDS. On March 23, 2010, President Barack Obama signed the Affordable Care Act, which contains several components that will make health insurance more available to HIV positive individuals by (1) promoting the expansion of Medicaid programs in states; and (2) making reforms to the insurance market rules, such as eliminating denial of coverage for preexisting conditions (Health Resources and Services Administration, 2013a, 2013b). The Affordable Care Act also seeks to ensure the quality of health care by ensuring that most health plans cover preventive screenings, which may include free HIV screening for everyone aged 15–65 years and other ages at increased risk (U.S. Centers for Medicaid & Medicaid Services, 2013). The law also seeks to address the lack of cultural competence that has arisen as a deterrent for engagement in HIV care among MSM (CDC, 2012a, 2012b, 2012c; Lieb et al., 2011). It bolsters cultural competency through the National LGBT Health Education Center which will provide free trainings for health care centers in an attempt to ensure that there is equality in medical treatment for lesbian, gay, bisexual, and transgender individuals (AIDS.gov, 2012) Public health officials may want to consider investigating whether the advent of the Affordable Care Act increases the number of HIV positive MSM who are not only engaged in HIV care but are also receiving the culturally competent HIV care.

The Ryan White HIV/AIDS Treatment Extension Act preceded the Affordable Care Act and was enacted to provide funding for HIV care to individuals who did not have health care coverage or who were inadequately covered. Today, Ryan White is one of the top three largest federal providers of funding for HIV care and treatment and has helped to provide HIV-related services for more than half a million individuals (Health Resources and Services Administration, 2013a, 2013b). Through its five components (Part A, Part B, Part C, Part D, and Part F), Ryan White provides funding for a variety of HIV-related health care services ranging from direct funding for HIV care to eligible metropolitan areas with high HIV morbidity (Part A), to providing funding for medications for people who are HIV positive (Part B), to special projects of national significance which provides funding for research projects related to addressing client needs (Part F) (Health Resources and Services Administration, 2013a, 2013b). In 2008, 66% of the individuals who were served through AIDS Drug Assistance Programs (ADAP) were male and 47% of ADAP recipients were Black (Health Resources and Services Administration, 2010). The Ryan White program has emerged as one of the most important federal programs for HIV positive individuals. With the Affordable Care Act poised to be fully implemented, future research could investigate the impact that these two programs will have on the health of HIV positive MSM and whether their combined efforts translate into fewer new HIV infections among MSM. In addition, public health agencies will be interested to learn what changes to Ryan White funding will occur as a result of the implementation of the Affordable Care Act.

Finally, in an effort to increase access to and the use of Pre-Exposure Prophylaxis (PrEP), in 2014, the CDC–U.S. Public Health Service released guidelines for the use of PrEP to prevent HIV infection. The guidelines recommend the use of PrEP among adult MSM, heterosexuals, and injection drug users who may be at high risk for HIV infection in tandem with other prevention services (U.S. Public Health Service, 2014). Consistent use of PrEP has been shown to be effective in preventing HIV infection across risk populations (Fonner et al., 2016) and in combination with other HIV prevention strategies, like HIV testing, it could help to reduce new HIV infections by as much as 95% (Zablotska, 2016). Clinicians' awareness of PrEP has also increased (Smith, Mendoza, Stryker, & Rose, 2016). Increasing access to and retention in HIV care among HIV positive MSM and increasing access to and consistent use of PrEP and prevention services among high-risk HIV negative MSM could decrease HIV infections among MSM.

Increasing Awareness and Access to Testing

CDC supports several national HIV/AIDS Awareness Days, which are collaborative efforts between the CDC, local health agencies, and community-based organizations to increase dialogue about HIV (CDC, 2012b). One of these is National Gay Men's HIV/AIDS Awareness Day (NGMHAAD). NGMHAAD occurs annually on September 27th. NGMAAD is described as an opportunity to reflect on the toll of HIV/AIDS on MSM and the opportunity to acknowledge the contributions of MSM in the fight against HIV/AIDS (CDC, 2012b).

There are also several testing initiatives underway to increase HIV testing among MSM. *Testing Together* is a testing initiative that focuses on MSM and is available in some US cities. *Testing Together* makes it possible for MSM to be tested for HIV with their partner at local health departments or community-based organizations (CDC, 2012b). The dyadic approach enables couples to develop risk reduction plans based on the HIV status of both partners (CDC, 2012b).

Testing Makes Us Stronger is the CDC's nation-wide HIV testing campaign that targets MSM, particularly Black/African American MSM 18–44 years of age for HIV testing (CDC, 2012c). The goal of the program is twofold: (1) to increase testing among Black/African American MSM 18–44 years of age, and (2) to change social norms among this demographic so that HIV testing stops being feared but becomes a source of strength (CDC, 2012c).

HIV Criminalization

People living with HIV infection (PLWH) can be criminally prosecuted for nondisclosure of their HIV status even when the sex is not forced but is consensual. Currently 33 states have HIV-specific laws and statutes (CDC, 2012a, 2012b, 2012c). Many of the laws and statutes were enacted in the 1980s and early 1990s when most Americans had very little knowledge about HIV and no effective treatment was available. These laws may not even reduce HIV transmission (Galletly, Glasman, Pinkerton, & DiFranceisco, 2012).

The National HIV/AIDS Strategy for the USA was released by the White House in July 2010 and calls for HIV criminalization laws to be re-examined (White House Office of National AIDS Policy, 2010). When HIV criminal cases are prosecuted, one of the main factors brought to bear is the defendant's knowledge of his or her HIV status.

Same-Sex Marriage

Same-sex marriage was illegal in most of the USA until the Supreme Court ruled otherwise on June 25, 2015. The effects of the recent ruling are still unknown. Longitudinal studies are needed to examine any impact of marriage on HIV for Black MSM. Research on marriage has been shown to positively impact an individual's health (Burman & Margolin, 1992; Choi & Marks, 2011; Homish & Leonard, 2005; Umberson, Williams, Powers, Liu, & Needham, 2006; Waite & Gallagher, 2000), although the benefit may vary in heterosexual marriages according to an individual's sex (Williams & Umberson, 2004). Researchers have also suggested that it is not just marriage itself but the quality of the marriage that has the biggest effect on a married individual's health (Umberson et al., 2006; Williams, 2003).

Limited research has been conducted to determine the health benefits of same-sex marriages. Badgett (2011) showed that same-sex marriages were associated with an increased feeling of social inclusion. This raises the question of whether the legacy of state-level bans on same-sex marriage results in deleterious effects. Francis, Mialon, and Peng (2011) linked bans on same-sex marriage to increasing HIV rates in the USA, and Hatzenbuehler, McLaughlin, Keyes, and Hasin (2010) found an association between living in a state with a constitutional ban on same-sex marriage and an increased rate of psychiatric disorders among lesbians, gays, and bisexuals (LGB). Herek (2011) asserts that exposure to anti-gay messages cause gays and lesbians to devalue their relationships and make them believe that neighbors and other members of their community hold anti-gay sentiments. Future research could examine whether recognition of same-sex marriages has had a positive effect on the health of MSM in same-sex marriages whether health outcomes differ between MSM who live in states that were the early adopters of same-sex marriage and those that resulted from the Supreme Court decision in 2015.

Shifting the Paradigm

Despite some advances in the war against HIV infection, the disease continues to be a threat to the health of Americans, especially for MSM, who bear a disproportionate burden of the disease. Public health is broadening its focus to include social determinants of health and other structural-level factors. Stigma, lack of housing, lack of access to appropriate HIV care and services, neighborhood characteristics, and low socioeconomic status may contribute to the risk for HIV acquisition in MSM. Although public health agencies may be unable to single-handedly improve these factors for MSM, engaging other government agencies which may be able to better address these issues may be beneficial. The barriers discussed in this chapter are not an exhaustive list of all the structural-level factors that may impede the health of MSM but are only a small part of a conversation that may improve the health of this population.

References

Adams, L., Kendall, S., Smith, A., Quigley, E., Stuewig, J. B., & Tangney, J. P. (2011). HIV risk behaviors of male and female jail inmates prior to incarceration and one year post-release. *AIDS and Behavior, 17*(8), 2685–2694. doi:10.1007/s10461-011-9990-2

Adimora, A. A., Schoenbach, V. J., Martinson, F. A., Donaldson, K., Fullilove, R. E., & Aral, S. O. (2001). Social context of sexual relationships among rural African Americans. *Sexually Transmitted Diseases, 28*(2), 69–76.

Adler, N. E., Boyce, T., Chesney, M. A., Cohen, S., Folkman, S., Kahn, R. L., & Syme, S. L. (1994). Socioeconomic status and health: The challenge of the gradient. *American Psychologist, 49*(1), 15–24.

Aidala, A., Cross, J. E., Stall, R., Harre, D., & Sumartojo, E. (2005). Housing status and HIV risk behaviors: Implications for prevention and policy. *AIDS and Behavior, 9*(3), 251–265.

Aral, S. O., Adimora, A. A., & Fenton, K. A. (2008). Understanding and responding to disparities in HIV and other sexually transmitted infections in African Americans. *Lancet, 372*(9635), 337–340.

AIDS.gov- AIDS.gov (2012). The Affordable Care Act Helps People Living with HIV/AIDS. Available: http://aids.gov/federal-resources/policies/health-care-reform/. Accessed January 7, 2013.

Badgett, M. V. L. (2011). Social inclusion and the value of marriage equality in Massachusetts and the Netherlands. *Journal of Social Issues, 67*, 316–334.

Beltran, V. M., Harrison, K. M., Hall, I. H., & Dean, H. D. (2011). Collection of social determinant of health measures in U.S. National Surveillance Systems for HIV, viral hepatitis, STDs, and TB. *Public Health Reports, 6*(Suppl. 3), 41–53.

Beyer, C., Sullivan, P. S., Sanchez, J., Dowdy, D., Altman, D., Trapence, G., … Mayer, K. H. (2012). A call to action for comprehensive HIV services for men who have sex with men. *The Lancet, 380*, 424–438.

Brewer, R. A., Magnus, M., Kuo, I., Wang, L., Liu, T. Y., & Mayer, K. H. (2014). Exploring the relationship between incarceration and HIV among black men who have sex with men in the United States. *Journal of Acquired Immune Deficiency Syndromes (1999), 65*(2), 218.

Burman, B., & Margolin, G. (1992). Analysis of the association between marital relationships and health problems: An interactional perspective. *Psychological Bulletin, 112*, 39–63.

Buttram, M. E., & Kurtz, S. P. (2012). Risk and protective factors associated with gay neighborhood residence. *American Journal of Men's Health, 7*(2), 110–118. doi:10.1177/1557988312458793

Carpiano, R. M., Kelly, B. C., Easterbrook, A., & Parsons, J. T. (2011). Community and drug use among gay men: The role of neighborhoods and networks. *Journal of Health and Social Behavior, 52*(1), 74–90.

CDC. (2006). HIV transmission among male inmates in a state prison system --- Georgia, 1992— 2005. *Morbidity and Mortality Weekly Report, 55*(15), 421–426.

CDC. (2009). *HIV testing implementation guidance for correctional settings*. Retrieved from http://www.cdc.gov/hiv/topics/testing/guideline.htm.

CDC. (2010). *Establishing a holistic framework to reduce inequities in HIV, viral hepatitis, STDs, and tuberculosis in the United States*. Atlanta, GA: U.S. Department of Health and Human Services, Centers for Disease Control and Prevention.

CDC. (2011). HIV risk, prevention, and testing behaviors among men who have sex with men— National HIV behavioral surveillance system, 21 U.S. cities, United States, 2008. *Morbidity and Mortality Weekly Report, 60*(14), 1–40.

CDC. (2012a). Estimated HIV incidence in the United States, 2007–2010. *HIV Surveillance Supplemental Report, 17*(4), 1–25. Retrieved from http://www.cdc.gov/hiv/topics/surveillance/resources/reports/#supplemental.

CDC. (2012b). *HIV among gay and bisexual men*. Retrieved from http://www.cdc.gov/hiv/topics/msm/.

CDC. (2012c). *HIV in correctional settings*. Retrieved from http://www.cdc.gov/hiv/topics/correctiona/.

Center for AIDS Prevention Studies (CAPS). (2006). *CAPS Fact Sheet 60E: How does stigma affect HIV prevention and treatment?* Retrieved from http://caps.ucsf.edu/uploads/pubs/FS/pdf/stigmaFS.pdf.

Chen, J. L., Bovée, M. C., & Kerndt, P. R. (2003). Sexually transmitted diseases surveillance among incarcerated men who have sex with men—An opportunity for HIV prevention. *AIDS Education and Prevention, 15*., HIV prevention for men of color who have sex with men (MSM) and men of color who have sex with men and women (MSM/W), 117–126.

Choi, H., & Marks, N. F. (2011). Socioeconomic status, marital status continuity and change, marital conflict, and mortality. *Journal of Aging and Health, 23*(4), 714–742.

Clatts, M. C., Goldsamt, L. A., & Yi, H. (2005). Drug and sexual risk in four men who have sex with men populations: Evidence for a sustained HIV epidemic in New York City. *Journal of Urban Health: Bulletin of the New York Academy of Medicine, 82*(1_suppl_1), i9–i17.

Cohen, M. S., McCauley, M., & Gamble, T. R. (2012). HIV treatment as prevention and HPTN 052. *Current Opinion in HIV and AIDS, 7*(2), 99–105.

CSDH. (2008). Closing the gap in a generation: Health equity through action on the social determinants of health. In *Final report of the commission on social determinants of health*. Geneva, Switzerland: World Health Organization.

Cubbin, C., & Winkleby, M. A. (2005). Protective and harmful effects of neighborhood-level deprivation on individual-level health knowledge, behavior changes, and risk of coronary heart disease. *American Journal of Epidemiology, 162*(6), 559–568. doi:10.1093/aje/kwi250

Dale, S. K., Bogart, L. M., Galvan, F. H., Wagner, G. J., Pantalone, D. W., & Klein, D. J. (2016). Discrimination and hate crimes in the context of neighborhood poverty and stressors among HIV-positive African-American men who have sex with men. *Journal of Community Health, 41*(3), 574–583.

DC Appleseed Center. (2012). *HIV/AIDS in the Nation's capital – Report card 7*. Washington, DC. Retrieved April 7, 2013, from http://www.dcappleseed.org/library/ReportCard7.pdf.

Denning, P., & DiNenno, E. (2010, July 21). *Community in crisis: Is there a generalized HIV epidemic in impoverished urban areas of the United States?* Vienna: Paper presented at the International AIDS Conference.

Dennis, A. M., Wheeler, J. B., Valer, E., Hightow-Wideman, L., Napravnik, S., Swygard, H., ... Eron, J. J. (2013). HIV risk behaviors and sociodemographic features of HIV-infected Latinos residing in a new Latino settlement area in the southeastern United States. *AIDS Care, 25*(10), 1298–1307.

Diez-Roux, A. V., Merkin, S. S., Arnett, D., Chambless, L., Massing, M., Nieto, F. J., ... Watson, R. L. (2001). Neighborhood of residence and incidence of coronary heart disease. *New England Journal of Medicine, 345*(2), 99–106. doi:10.1056/NEJM200107123450205

Diez-Roux, A. V., Nieto, F. J., Caulfield, L., Tyroler, H. A., Watson, R. L., & Szklo, M. (1999). Neighborhood differences in diet: The atherosclerosis risk in communities (ARIC) study. *Journal of Epidemiology & Community Health, 53*(1), 55–63.

Draine, J., McTighe, L., & Bourgois, P. (2011). Education, empowerment and community based structural reinforcement: An HIV prevention response to mass incarceration and removal. *International Journal of Law and Psychiatry, 34*(4), 295–302. doi:10.1016/j.ijlp.2011.07.009

Dumont, D. M., Brockmann, B., Dickman, S., Alexander, N., & Rich, J. D. (2012). Public health and the epidemic of incarceration. *Annual Review of Public Health, 33*, 325–339.

Feldman, P. J., & Steptoe, A. (2004). How neighborhoods and physical functioning are related: The roles of neighborhood socioeconomic status, perceived neighborhood strain, and individual health risk factors. *Annals of Behavior Medicine, 27*(2), 91–99. doi:10.1207/s15324796abm2702_3

Fonner, V. A., Dalglish, S. L., Kennedy, C. E., Baggaley, R., O'Reilly, K. R., Koechlin, F. M., ... Grant, R. M. (2016). Effectiveness and safety of oral HIV preexposure prophylaxis for all populations. *AIDS, 30*, 1973–1983. doi:10.1097/QAD.0000000000001145

Francis, A. M., Mialon, H. M., & Peng, H. (2011). *In sickness and in health: Same-sex marriage bans and sexually transmitted infections*. Emory law and economics research paper no. 11–97. Retrieved from SSRN http://Ssrn.Com/Abstract=1773144 or http://dx.doi.org/10.2139/ssrn.1773144.

Frieden, T. R. (2010). A framework for public health action: The health impact pyramid. *American Journal of Public Health, 100*, 590–595.

Friedman, S. R., West, B. S., Pouget, E. R., Hall, H. I., Cantrell, J., Tempalski, B., ... Des Jarlais, D. C. (2013). Metropolitan social environments and pre-HAART/HAART era changes in mortality rates (per 10,000 adult residents) among injection drug users living with AIDS. *PLoS One, 8*(2), e57201. doi:10.1371/journal

Frye, V., Koblin, B., Chin, J., Beard, J., Blaney, S., Halkitis, P., ... Galea, S. (2010). Neighborhood-level correlates of consistent condom use among men who have sex with men: A multi-level analysis. *AIDS and Behavior, 14*(4), 974–985. doi:10.1007/s10461-008-9438-5

Frye, V., Latka, M., Koblin, B., Halkitis, P., Putnam, S., Galea, S., & Vlahov, D. (2006). The urban environment and sexual risk behavior among men who have sex with men. *Journal of Urban Health, 83*(2), 308–324. doi:10.1007/s11524-006-9033-x

Frye, V., Nandi, V., Egan, J. E., Cerda, M., Rundle, A., Quinn, J. W., … Koblin, B. (2016). Associations among neighborhood characteristics and sexual risk behavior among black and white MSM living in a major urban area. *AIDS and Behavior*, 1–21.

Fuller, C. M., Borrell, L. N., Latkin, C. A., Galea, S., Ompad, D. C., Strathdee, S. A., & Vlahov, D. (2005). Effects of race, neighborhood, and social network on age at initiation of injection drug use. *American Journal of Public Health, 95*(4), 689–695. doi:10.2105/AJPH.2003.02178

Galletly, C. L., Glasman, L. R., Pinkerton, S. D., & DiFranceisco, W. (2012). New Jersey's HIV-related attitudes, beliefs, and sexual and seropositive status disclosure behaviors of persons living with HIV. *American Journal of Public Health, 102*(11), 2135–2140.

Gant, Z., Lomotey, M., Hall, H. I., Hu, X., Guo, X., & Song, R. (2012). A county-level examination of the relationship between HIV and social determinants of health: 40 states, 2006–2008. *Open AIDS Journal, 6*, 1–7.

Gayles, T. A., Kuhns, L. M., Kwon, S., Mustanski, B., & Garofalo, R. (2016). Socioeconomic disconnection as a risk factor for increased HIV infection in young men who have sex with men. *LGBT health, 3*(3), 219–224.

Giordano, T. P., Gifford, A. L., White, A. C., Suarez-Almazor, M. E., Rabeneck, L., Hartman, C., … Morgan, R. O. (2007). Retention in care: A challenge to survival with HIV infection. *Clinical Infectious Diseases, 44*, 1493–1499.

Giordano, T. P., Visnegarwala, F., White, A. C., Jr., Troisi, C. L., Frankowski, R. F., Hartman, C. M., & Grimes, R. M. (2005). Patients referred to an urban HIV clinic frequently fail to establish care: Factors predicting failure. *AIDS Care, 17*(6), 773–783.

Glick, S. N., & Golden, M. R. (2010). Persistence of racial differences in attitudes toward homosexuality in the United States. *Journal of Acquired Immune Deficiency Syndromes, 55*(4), 516–523. doi:10.1097/QAI.0b013e3181f275e0

Halkitis, P. N., & Figueroa, R. P. (2013). Sociodemographic characteristics explain differences in unprotected sexual behavior among young HIV-negative gay, bisexual, and other Y MSM in New York City. *AIDS Patient Care and STDs, 27*(3), 181–190.

Halkitis, P. N., Kapadia, F., Siconolfi, D. E., Moeller, R. W., Figueroa, R. P., Barton, S. C., & Blachman-Forshay, J. (2013). Individual, psychosocial, and social correlates of unprotected anal intercourse in a new generation of young men who have sex with men in New York City. *American Journal of Public Health, 103*(5), 889–895. doi:10.2105/AJPH.2012.300963

Hall, H. I., Gray, K. M., Tang, T., Li, J., Shouse, L., & Mermin, J. (2012). Retention in care of adults and adolescents living with HIV in 13 US areas. *Journal of Acquired Immune Deficiency Syndromes, 60*, 77–82.

Hall, H. I., Holtgrave, D. R., Tang, T., & Rhodes, P. (2013). HIV transmission in the United States: considerations of viral load, risk behavior, and health disparities. *AIDS and Behavior, 17*(5), 1632–1636. doi:10.1007/s10461-013-0426-z

Hatzenbuehler, M. L., McLaughlin, K. A., Keyes, K. M., & Hasin, D. S. (2010). The impact of institutional discrimination on psychiatric disorders in lesbian, gay, and bisexual populations: A prospective study. *American Journal of Public Health, 100*(3), 452–459.

Hatzenbuehler, M. L., O'Cleirigh, C., Mayer, K. H., Mimiaga, M. J., & Safren, S. A. (2011). Prospective associations between HIV-related stigma, transmission risk behaviors, and adverse mental health outcomes in men who have sex with men. *Annals of Behavioral Medicine, 42*(2), 227–234. doi:10.1007/s12160-011-9275-z

Health Resources and Services Administration. (2010). *Going the distance: The Ryan White HIV/AIDS program*. Retrieved from http://www.impactmc.net/downloads/samples/writing/Going-the-Distance-20-years-of-the-Ryan-White-HIV-AIDS-Program.pdf.

Health Resources and Services Administration. (2013a). *Key provisions of the affordable care act for the Ryan White HIV/AIDS Programs*. Retrieved from http://hab.hrsa.gov/affordablecareact/keyprovisions.pdf.

Health Resources and Services Administration. (2013b). *About the Ryan White HIV/AIDS Program*. Retrieved from http://hab.hrsa.gov/abouthab/aboutprogram.html.

Herek, G. M. (2011). Anti-equality marriage amendments and sexual stigma. *Journal of Social Issues*, *67*(2), 413–426.

Hixson, B., Omer, S., del Rio, C., & Frew, P. (2011). Spatial clustering of HIV prevalence in Atlanta, Georgia and population characteristics associated with case concentrations. *Journal of Urban Health*, *88*(1), 129–141. doi:10.1007/s11524-010-9510-0

Holtgrave, D. R., Wolitski, R. J., Pals, S. L., Aidala, A., Kidder, D. P., Vos, D., ... Bendixen, A. V. (2012). Cost-utility analysis of the housing and health intervention for homeless and unstably housed persons living with HIV. *AIDS and Behavior*, *17*(5), 1626–1631. doi:10.1007/s10461-012-0204-3

Homish, G. G., & Leonard, K. E. (2005). Spousal influence on smoking behaviors in a US community sample of newly married couples. *Social Science & Medicine*, *61*, 2557–2567.

Jones, K., Wilton, L., Millett, G., & Johnson, W. D. (2010). Formulating the stress and severity model of minority social stress for black men who have sex with men. In D. H. McCree, K. T. Jones, & A. O'Leary (Eds.), *African Americans and HIV/AIDS* (pp. 223–238). New York: Springer.

Jones, K. T. (2012, August). A focus on neighborhood composition to better understand racial HIV disparities among black and white men who have sex with men (MSM). Retrieved from http://www.iasociety.org/.

Joy, R., Druyts, E. F., Brandson, E. K., Lima, V. D., Rustad, C. A., McPhil, R., ... Hogg, R. S. (2008). Impact of neighborhood-level socioeconomic status on HIV disease progression in a universal health care setting. *Journal of Acquired Immune Deficiency Syndromes*, *47*, 500–505.

Kawachi, I., & Berkman, L. F. (2003). *Neighborhoods and health*. Oxford; New York: Oxford University Press.

Kelly, B. C., Carpiano, R. M., Easterbrook, A., & Parsons, J. T. (2012). Sex and the community: The implications of neighborhoods and social networks for sexual risk behaviors among urban gay men. *Sociology of Health & Illness*, *34*(7), 1085–1102. doi:10.1111/j.1467-9566.2011.01446.x

Kidder, D. P., Wolitski, R. J., Pals, S. L., & Campsmith, M. L. (2008). Housing status and HIV risk behaviors among homeless and housed persons with HIV. *Journal of Acquired Immune Deficiency Syndromes*, *49*(4), 451–455.

LaLota, M., Beck, D., Metsch, L., Brewer, T., Forrest, D., Cardenas, G., & Liberti, T. (2011). HIV seropositivity and correlates of infection among heterosexually active adults in high-risk areas in South Florida. *AIDS and Behavior*, *15*(6), 1259–1263. doi:10.1007/s10461-010-9856-z

Lane, S. D., Rubinstein, R. A., Keefe, R. H., & Webster, N. (2004). Structural violence and racial disparity in HIV transmission. *Journal of Healthcare for the Poor and Underserved*, *15*(3), 319–335.

Latkin, C. A., & Curry, A. D. (2003). Stressful neighborhoods and depression: A prospective study of the impact of neighborhood disorder. *Journal of Health & Social Behavior*, *44*(1), 34–44.

Lennon, C. A., Pellowski, J. A., White, A. C., Kalichman, S. C., Finitsis, D. J., Turcios-Cotto, V., ... Lanouette, G. A. (2013). Service priorities and unmet service needs among people living with HIV/AIDS: Results from a nationwide interview of HIV/AIDS housing organizations. *AIDS Care: Psychological and Socio-Medical Aspects of AIDS/HIV*, *25*(9), 1083–1091. doi:10.1080/09540121.2012.7493371-9

Lieb, S., Prejean, J., Thompson, D. R., Fallon, S. J., Cooper, H., & Gates, J. G. (2011). HIV prevalence rates among men who have sex with men in the southern United States: Population-based estimates by race/ethnicity. *AIDS and Behavior*, *15*, 596–606.

Lieb, S., Thompson, D. R., Misra, S., Gates, G. J., Duffus, W. A., Fallon, S. J., ... Southern AIDS Coalition MSM Project Team, Southern AIDS Coalition MSM Project Team. (2009). Estimating populations of men who have sex with men in the southern United States. *Journal of Urban Health: Bulletin of the New York Academy of Medicine*, *86*(6), 887–901. doi:10.1007/s11524-009-9401-4

Lorenc, T., Marrero-Guillamon, I., Llewellyn, A., Aggleton, P., Cooper, C., Lehmann, A., & Lindsay, C. (2010). HIV testing among men who have sex with men (MSM): Systematic review of qualitative evidence. *Health Education Research*, *26*(5), 834–846.

Massey, D. S., & Denton, N. A. (1993). *American apartheid: Segregation and the making of the underclass*. Cambridge, MA: Harvard University Press.

Matte, T., & Jacobs, D. E. (2000). Housing and health: Current issues and implications for research and programs. *Journal of Urban Health, 77,* 7–25.

Mayer, K. H., Bekker, L., Stall, R., Grulich, A. E., Colfax, G., & Lama, J. R. (2012). Comprehensive clinical Care for men who have sex with men: An integrated approach. *The Lancet, 380,* 378–387.

Mayer, K. H., Pape, J. W., Wilson, P., Diallo, D. D., Saavedra, J., Mimiaga, M. J., … Farmer, P. (2012). Multiple determinants, common vulnerabilities, and creative responses: Addressing the AIDS epidemic in diverse populations globally. *Journal of Acquired Immune Deficiency Syndromes, 60*(Suppl 2), S31–S34. doi:10.1097/QAI.0b013e31825c16d9

Mays, V. M., Cochran, S. D., & Zamudio, A. (2004). HIV prevention research: Are we meeting the needs of African-American men who have sex with men? *Journal of Black Psychology, 30*(1), 78–105.

McFarland, W., Chen, S., Hsu, L., Schwarcz, S., & Katz, M. (2003). Low socioeconomic status is associated with a higher rate of death in the era of highly active antiretroviral therapy, San Francisco. *Journal of Acquired Immune Deficiency Syndromes, 33*(1), 96–103.

McLaughlin, D. K., & Stokes, C. S. (2002). Income inequality and mortality in US counties: Does minority racial concentration matter? *American Journal of Public Health, 92*(1), 99–104. doi:10.2105/ajph.92.1.99

Metsch, L. R., Pereyra, M., Messinger, S., del Rio, C., Strathdee, S. A., & Anderson-Mahoney, P. (2008). HIV transmission risk behaviors among HIV-infected persons who are successfully linked to care. *Clinical Infectious Diseases, 47,* 577–584.

Meyer, I. H., Flores, A. R., Stemple, L., Romero, A. P., Wilson, B. D., & Herman, J. L. (2016). Incarceration rates and traits of sexual minorities in the United States: National Inmate Survey, 2011–2012. *American Journal of Public Health, 107*(2), 234–240.

Milloy, M. J., Marshall, B. D. L., Montaner, J., & Wood, E. (2012). Housing status and the health of people living with HIV/AIDS. *Current HIV/AIDS Reports, 9,* 364–374.

Mimiaga, M. J., Reisner, S. L., Cranston, K., Isenberg, D., Bright, D., Daffin, G., … Mayer, K. H. (2009). Sexual mixing patterns and partner characteristics of black MSM in Massachusetts at increased risk for HIV infection and transmission. *Journal of Urban Research: Bulletin of the New York Academy of Medicine, 86*(4), 602–623. doi:10.1007/s11524-009-9363-6

Muthulingham, D., Chin, J., Hsu, L., Scheer, S., & Schwarcz, S. (2013). Disparities in engagement in care and viral suppression among persons with HIV. *Journal of Acquired Immune Deficiency Syndromes, 63*(1), 112–119.

Pecoraro, A., Royer-Malvestuto, C., Rosenwasser, B., Moore, K., Howell, A., Ma, M., & Woody, G. E. (2013). Factors contributing to dropping out from and returning to HIV treatment in an inner city primary care HIV clinic in the United States. *AIDS Care: Psychological and Socio-Medical Aspects of AIDS/HIV, 25*(11), 1399–1406. doi:10.1080/09540121.2013.772273

Peterson, J. L., & Jones, K. T. (2009). HIV prevention for black men who have sex with men in the United States. *American Journal of Public Health, 99*(6), 976–980.

Pettit, B. (2012). *Invisible men: Mass incarceration and the myth of black progress.* New York: Russell Sage Foundation.

Phillips, G., II, Birkett, M., Kuhns, L., Hatchel, T., Garofalo, R., & Mustanski, B. (2015). Neighborhood-level associations with HIV infection among young men who have sex with men in Chicago. *Archives of Sexual Behavior, 44*(7), 1773–1786.

Phuong, D. (2009). The dynamics of income and neighborhood context for population health: Do long-term measures of socioeconomic status explain more of the black/white health disparity than single-point-in-time measures? *Social Science & Medicine, 68*(8), 1368–1375. doi:10.1016/j.socscimed.2009.01.028

Politch, J. A., Mayer, K. H., Welles, S. L., O'Brien, W. H., Xu, C., & Bowman, F. P. (2012). Highly active antiretroviral therapy does not completely suppress HIV in semen of sexually active HIV-infected men who have sex with men. *AIDS, 26,* 1535–1543.

Purcell, D. W., Johnson, C. H., Lansky, A., Prejean, J., Stein, R., Denning, P., … Crepaz, N. (2012). Estimating the population size of men who have sex with men in the United States to obtain HIV and syphilis rates. *The Open AIDS Journal, 6*(1), 98–107.

Raj, A., & Bowleg, L. (2011). Heterosexual risk for HIV among black men in the United States: A call to action against a neglected crisis in Black Communities. *American Journal of Men's Health, 6*(3), 178–181. doi:10.1177/1557988311416496

Raphael, D. (2006). Social determinants of health: Present status, unanswered questions, and future directions. *International Journal of Health Services, 36*(4), 651–677.

Rao, D., Pryor, J.B., Gaddist, B., & Mayer R. (2008). Stigma, secrecy, and discrimination: ethnic/racial differences in the concerns of people living with HIV/AIDS. *AIDS and Behavior, 12,* 265–271.

Riley, E. D., Wu, A. W., Perry, S., Clark, R. A., Moss, A. R., Crane, J., & Bangsberg, D. R. (2003). Depression and drug use impact health status among marginally housed HIV-infected individuals. *AIDS Patient Care and STDs, 17,* 401–406.

Ross, C. E., & Mirowsky, J. (2001). Neighborhood disadvantage, disorder, and health. *Journal of Health and Social Behavior, 42*(3), 258–276.

Ruel, E., Oakley, D., Wilson, G. E., & Maddox, R. (2010). Is public housing the cause of poor health or a safety net for the unhealthy poor? *Journal of Urban Health, 87*(5), 827–838.

Semaan, S., Sternberg, M., Zaidi, A., & Aral, S. O. (2007). Social capital and rates of gonorrhea and syphilis in the United States: Spatial regression analyses of state-level associations. *Social Science & Medicine, 64*(11), 2324–2341. doi:10.1016/j.socscimed.2007.02.023

Singh, S., Bradley, H., Hu, X., Skarbinski, J., Hall, H. I., & Lansky, A. (2014). Men living with diagnosed HIV who have sex with men: Progress along the continuum of HIV care — United States, 2010. *MMWR, 63,* 829–833.

Smith, D. K., Mendoza, M. C. B., Stryker, J. L., & Rose, C. E. (2016). PrEP awareness and attitudes in a national survey of primary care clinicians in the United States, 2009–2015. *PLoS One, 11*(6), e0156592. doi:10.1371/journal.pone.0156592

Stafford, M., & Marmot, M. (2003). Neighborhood deprivation and health: Does it affect us all equally? *International Journal of Epidemiology, 32*(3), 357–366.

Stein, D., Silivera, R., Hagerty, R., & Marmor, M. (2012). Viewing pornography depicting unprotected anal intercourse: Are there implications for HIV prevention among men who have sex with men? *Archives of Sexual Behavior, 41*(2), 411–419.

Steptoe, A., & Feldman, P. (2001). Neighborhood problems as sources of chronic stress: Development of a measure of neighborhood problems, and associations with socioeconomic status and health. *Annals of Behavioral Medicine, 23*(3), 177–185. doi:10.1207/s15324796abm2303_5

Stokes, J. P., & Peterson, J. L. (1998). Homophobia, self-esteem, and risk for HIV among African American men who have sex with men. *AIDS Education and Prevention, 10*(3), 278–292.

Taylor, B. S., Garduno, L. S., Reyes, E. V., Valino, R., Rojas, R., Donastorg, Y., ... Hirsch, J. (2011). HIV care for geographically mobile populations. *Mount Sinai Journal of Medicine, 78*(3), 342–351. doi:10.1002/msj.20255

The Antiretroviral Therapy Cohort Collaboration. (2008). Life expectancy of individuals on combination therapy in high-income countries: A collaborative analysis of 14 cohort studies. *The Lancet, 372,* 293–299.

U. S. Bureau of Justice Statistics. (2009). *Felony sentences in state courts, 2006-statistical tables.* Retrieved from http://bjs.gov/index.cfm?ty=pbdetail&iid=1747.

U. S. Department of Justice. (1999). *1996–1997 update: HIV, STDs, and TB in correctional facilities.* Washington, DC: National Institute of Justice.

U.S. Centers for Medicaid & Medicaid Services. (2013). *What are my preventive care benefits?* Retrieved from https://www.healthcare.gov/what-are-my-preventive-care-benefits/.

U.S. Department of Justice. (2012). *Prisoners in 2011.* Washington, DC: Carson, Anne & Sabol, William.

U.S. Public Health Service. 2014, May 14. Preexposure prophylaxis for the prevention of HIV infection in the United States: A clinical practice guideline.

Umberson, D., Williams, K., Powers, D. A., Liu, H., & Needham, B. (2006). You make me sick: Marital quality and health over the life course. *Journal of Health and Social Behavior, 47*(1), 1–16.

Waite, L., & Gallagher, M. (2000). *The case for marriage: Why married people are happier, healthier, and better off financially*. New York: Broadway Books.

Weiser, S. D., Riley, E. D., Ragland, K., Hammer, G., Clark, R., & Bangsberg, D. R. (2006). Brief report: Factors associated with depression among homeless and marginally housed HIV-infected men in San Francisco. *Journal of General Internal Medicine, 21*, 61–64.

Westergaard, R. P., Spaulding, A. C., & Flanigan, T. P. (2013). HIV among persons incarcerated in the USA: A review of evolving concepts in testing, treatment, and linkage to community care. *Current Opinion in Infectious Diseases, 26*(1), 10–16.

White House Office of National AIDS Policy. (2010, July 13). National HIV/AIDS Strategy for the United States. Washington, DC: The White House. Retrieved August 28, 2012 from http://www.whitehouse.gov/sites/default/files/uploads/NHAS.pdf2.

White, K., Rudolph, A. E., Jones, K. C., Latkin, C., Benjamin, E. O., Crawford, N. D., & Fuller, C. M. (2013). Social and individuals risk determinants of HIV testing practices among noninjection drug users at high risk for HIV/AIDS. *AIDS Care: Psychological and Socio- medical Aspects of AIDS/HIV, 25*(2), 230–238.

WHO. (1948). Preamble to the Constitution of the World Health Organization as adopted by the International Health Conference, New York, 19–22 June, 1946; signed on 22 July 1946 by the representatives of 61 States (Official Records of the World Health Organization, no. 2, p. 100) and entered into force on 7 April 1948.

WHO. (2013). HIV/AIDS antiretrovial therapy. Retrieved from http://www.who.int/hiv/topics/treatment/en/index.html.

Williams, D. R. (1999). Race, socioeconomic status, and health: The added effects of racism and discrimination. *Annals of the New York Academy of Sciences, 896*(1), 173–188. doi:10.1111/j.1749-6632.1999.tb08114.x

Williams, D. R., & Collins, C. (2001). Racial residential segregation: A fundamental cause of racial disparities in health. *Public Health Reports, 116*(5), 404–416.

Williams, D. R., Mohammed, S. A., Leavell, J., & Collins, C. (2010). Race, socioeconomic status, and health: Complexities, ongoing challenges, and research opportunities. *Annals of the New York Academy of Sciences, 1186*, 69–101. doi:10.1111/j.1749-6632.2009.05339.x

Williams, K. (2003). Has the future of marriage arrived? A contemporary examination of gender, marriage, and psychological well-being. *Journal of Health and Social Behavior, 44*, 470–487.

Williams, K., & Umberson, D. (2004). Marital status, marital transitions, and health: A gendered life course perspective. *Journal of Health and Social Behavior, 45*(1), 81–98.

Wilson, P. A., & Yoshikawa, H. (2006). Improving access to quality healthcare among African-American, Asian & Pacific islander, and Latino lesbian, gay and bisexual populations. In I. Meyer & M. E. Northridge (Eds.), *The health of sexual minorities: Public health perspectives on lesbian, gay, bisexual, and transgender populations* (pp. 607–637). New York: Springer.

Wohl, A. R., Galvan, F. H., Carlos, J., Myers, H. F., Garland, W., Witt, M. D., … George, S. (2012). A comparison of MSM stigma, HIV stigma and depression in HIV-positive Latino and African American men who have sex with men (MSM). *AIDS and Behavior, 17*(4), 1454–1464. doi:10.1007/s10461-012-0385-9

Wolitski, R. J., Kidder, D. P., Pals, S. L., Royal, S., Aidala, A., Stall, R., … House and Health Study Team, House and Health Study Team. (2010). Randomized trial of the effects of housing assistance on the health and risk behaviors of homeless and unstably housed people living with HIV. *AIDS and Behavior, 14*(3), 493–503.

Wood, E., Montaner, J. S., Chan, K., Tyndall, M. W., Schechter, M. T., Bangsberg, D., … Hogg, R. S. (2002). Socioeconomic status, access to triple therapy, and survival from HIV-disease since 1996. *AIDS, 16*(15), 2065–2072.

Woodyard, J. L., Peterson, J. L., & Stokes, J. P. (2000). Let us go into the house of the Lord: Participation in African American churches among young African American men who have sex with men. *Journal of Pastoral Care, 54*(4), 451–460.

Yen, I. H., & Kaplan, G. A. (1999a). Neighborhood social environment and risk of death: Multilevel evidence from the Alameda County study. *American Journal of Epidemiology, 149*(10), 898–907.

Yen, I. H., & Kaplan, G. A. (1999b). Poverty area residence and changes in depression and perceived health status: Evidence from the Alameda County study. *International Journal of Epidemiology, 28*(1), 90–94.

Zablotska, I. B. (2016). Likely impact of pre-exposure prophylaxis on HIV epidemics among men who have sex with men. *Sexual Health.* doi:10.1071/sh16153.

Chapter 15
Social Networks of HIV Positive Gay Men: Their Role and Importance in HIV Prevention

Karin E. Tobin and Carl A. Latkin

Introduction

HIV positive gay men are embedded within diverse and rich social networks consisting of family, friends, romantic partners, medical providers, HIV negative gay men, persons living with HIV/AIDS (PLWHA), and others (Frye et al., 2017; Holloway et al., 2017; Tieu et al., 2016). These social connections and interactions play significant roles in numerous aspects of their physical and mental health (Latkin et al., 2017). In the beginning of the AIDS epidemic, before the advent of highly active antiretroviral therapy (HAART), social networks were the primary source of care, aiding in managing the illness, navigating end of life issues, and encouraging activism to demand research for treatment and prevention (Hart, Fitzpatrick, McLean, Dawson, & Boulton, 1990; Latkin et al., 2012; Tieu et al., 2016). As research advanced and medical treatments improved (e.g., HAART), attention was increased on the role that social networks could have for improving adherence to medical care through peer-navigator based programs (Broadhead et al., 2002; Gardenier, Andrews, Thomas, Bookhardt-Murray, & Fitzpatrick, 2010; Horvath et al., 2013). Finally, with the dramatic rise of Internet-based social media and sex partner venues, social networks of HIV positive gay men have reached virtual capacities, no longer constrained by geography (Holloway et al., 2017). Websites designed for meeting sexual partners and web-based applications (e.g., grindr) have proliferated and have added a new dimension to the role that social networks have in HIV risk.

The unique set of issues faced by HIV positive gay men (e.g., receiving regular medical care, overlapping stigma and disclosure of HIV positive status

K.E. Tobin (✉) • C.A. Latkin
Department of Health, Behavior and Society, Johns Hopkins Bloomberg School of Public Health, Johns Hopkins University, Baltimore, MD, USA
e-mail: ktobin2@jhu.edu

© Springer Science+Business Media LLC 2017
L. Wilton (ed.), *Understanding Prevention for HIV Positive Gay Men*,
DOI 10.1007/978-1-4419-0203-0_15

and sexual orientation, as well as concerns about re-infection, medication resistant strains of HIV and re-emergent sexually transmitted infection [STI] trends)
exist in a larger social context (Ayala, Bingham, Kim, Wheeler, & Millett, 2012;
Buseh et al., 2006; Hickson et al., 2017; Holloway et al., 2017; Peterson &
Jones, 2009; Tobin, Cutchin, Latkin, & Takahashi, 2013). The individuals with
whom a person interacts can have a large impact on how HIV positive gay men
understand and cope with these issues. As such, expanding scientific frameworks
to include the social network is critical in designing more effective primary and
secondary prevention interventions. In this chapter, we aim to (1) discuss the
state of the evidence on social networks and health for HIV positive gay men
and HIV positive men who have sex with men (MSM), (2) provide an overview
of network-oriented intervention approaches that have been used with HIV
positive gay men and MSM, and (3) conclude with recommendations for future
research and practice.

Social Network Structure

A social network can be defined as an actor or set of actors, usually comprised of
individuals but can include organizations, such as AIDS Service Organizations,
HIV medical care facilities, or other entities, who are linked to a focal person by a
behavior or interaction (e.g., sexual contact, drug sharing) (Friedman & Aral, 2001;
Frye et al., 2017; Miller, Klotz, & Eckholdt, 1998). Networks influence behavior
through processes such as information sharing, role modeling, as well as through
social rewards and sanctions (Latkin & Knowlton, 2005). There are two types of
social networks that have been the focus of research: personal (i.e., ego-centric)
and sociometric. Personal social networks focus on one individual and his or her
connections with various others. Sociometric networks focus on how groups of
individuals are connected.

Structures of personal networks have been found to have implications for risk
behavior and HIV and STI primary and secondary prevention (Adimora &
Schoenbach, 2005; Aral et al., 1999; Jennings et al., 2010). However, there is a paucity of empirical evidence in the scientific literature that describes the structures of
HIV positive gay men's networks. Much of what has been published has narrowly
focused on the role of support networks or risk networks. Nevertheless, there are a
number of structural components of personal networks that are specifically relevant
to HIV positive gay men's health:

- *Total network size*: the number of network members identified by the ego who
  are important to them or fill specific roles. Among HIV positive gay men, the
  proportion of the total network size (especially the social support network) to
  whom the ego has disclosed HIV status and/or sexual identity may have implications for the ego's mental and physical well-being. In one study, of a sample of
  76 HIV positive gay men, the median social network size was 22 members, 80%

of whom were aware of the ego's HIV positive status (Serovich, Mason, Bautista, & Toviessi, 2006).

- *Types, intensity, and direction of the relationships*: The social networks of HIV positive gay men are varied and can include sex partners, kin, friends, professionals, and religious professionals. In addition to assessing the types of relationships within a social network, attention to the direction of the relationship, unidirectional or bidirectional, can be important. The degree of reciprocity between an ego and network members has been found to be associated with stress and feelings of social isolation. Intensity of relationship can be measured subjectively, such as emotional closeness, or objectively such as frequency of contact.
- *Centrality:* There are several types of network centrality. The general concept of centrality is based on the numbers of direct and indirect ties. It has been hypothesized that individuals who have a greater degree centrality in their network also have the greatest potential to influence network members' behaviors through diffusing information, resources, and changing norms of behavior.
- *Density*: can be assessed at the network level as the proportion of individuals within a network who are linked to each other or an individual can be assessed by their density relative to others in the network. Dense social networks may be more efficient in social monitoring of individuals behaviors and may be more efficient for diffusion of social norms; however, dense social networks may be more resistant to behavior change.
- *Network turnover:* the movement of people into and out of the social network. Turnover has been associated with HIV risk behaviors and serostatus (Costenbader, Astone, & Latkin, 2006; Friedman & Aral, 2001). Disclosure of sexual orientation and HIV status and loss of network members due to HIV-related deaths have been prominent factors that contribute to network composition and turnover for HIV positive gay men. HIV positive gay men and other stigmatized populations may experience numerous disruptions to social networks through housing instability, discrimination, household and community violence, and incarceration. Disruptions to sexual networks may lead not only to seeking new sexual partnerships but also to depression and contribute to substance use and sex under the influence (Takahashi & Magalong, 2008).

Social Network Function

Support

Despite over two decades of public health campaigns to educate and raise awareness in communities, HIV positive gay men continue to face stigma and discrimination related to both their HIV status and their sexual behavior. There is strong and consistent evidence that social support reduces depression through a main effect and by buffering the effects of stress from stigma and discrimination (Britton, Zarski, & Hobfoll, 1993; Holloway et al., 2017). Social support is a multi-dimensional construct that is often used interchangeably with the term social network. However, there is no accepted definition of social support or how to measure it. Types of social support include:

- Emotional support (e.g., providing advice, perceive to be accepting); material support (e.g., providing money, housing, food)
- Social participation (e.g., engage in social activities, such as parties, clubs, dining); instrumental support (e.g., providing transportation, informal health care)
- Information support (e.g., information on HIV and STI treatment, risk reduction techniques)

A network approach can focus on engaging specific individuals who provide specific types of support as well as the structure of these relationships. One of the advantages of a network approach to social support is that it does not assume that specific individuals, such as family or friends, provide specific types of support. In addition to specifying the types of support of interest, studies have also focused on the sources of support, such as family, friends, other HIV positive individuals, and the gay community (Peterson, Rintamaki, Brashers, Goldsmith, & Neidig, 2012). An early study that focused on the impact of HIV on the lives of gay men in Hollywood, California, highlighted the role of a "strong social network" (page 75) to provide camaraderie, support, assistance with medical care and daily activities (Wilton, 1996).

Studies of HIV positive MSM in predominately White samples have shown that friends are a greater source of support as compared to family (Hall, 1999; Kimberly & Serovich, 1999). One key study (Hays, Catania, McKusick, & Coates, 1990) of an urban sample of HIV positive MSM found that psychological well-being was associated with the number of close ties in a network as opposed to the size of the network. Another study of a small sample of HIV positive MSM found that density of the network was correlated with daily emotional support, yet size correlated with problem-oriented instrumental support (White & Cant, 2003). Results from one study of a sample of HIV positive MSM with a weak social network and weak social support had lower levels of CD4 (Persson, Ostergren, Hanson, Lindgren, & Naucler, 2002).

Accessing HIV-Related Care

Networks provide support for accessing and maintaining medical care. Social support has been conceptualized as an enabling factor for access and adherence to HIV-related formal and informal medical care. Observational and intervention studies indicate that social network members, particularly main partners, have among the most robust and lasting effects on health behavior change (Christakis & Fowler, 2008; El-Bassel, Gilbert et al., 2010; El-Bassel, Jemmott et al., 2010; Holloway et al., 2017). There is a strong body of evidence that specific types of social support from network members lead to lower level of depression, and that depression is linked to a range of poor health outcomes among MSM (Parsons, Halkitis, Wolitski, Gomez,, & Seropositive Urban Men's Study Team, 2003; Reisner et al., 2010; Tucker et al., 2012). Peer-support, in the form of support groups or through peer-navigation or buddy based programs, has been shown to complement medical care through information sharing about treatment and medication regimens, side effects, and symptoms of HIV. A study by George and colleagues (George et al., 2009) eloquently delineates the types of support mechanisms delivered by various social network members ranging from health care providers, HIV-related organizations, friends, and family. Another study which assessed network characteristics and network helping behavior found that the social networks of HIV positive gay men included other PLWHA, friends, and family whose behavior were described as both helpful and unhelpful (Hays, Magee, & Chauncey, 1994). Helpful behaviors of the network members included expressions of love, serving as a confidant, providing assistance, information, advice, and encouragement. Alternatively, some social network members were also described as being overly protective, excluding them from social activities, and breaking confidentiality. These unhelpful behaviors were a source of stress and frustration for the individual. These findings highlight the important implications that social networks are not always supportive and network member can be simultaneously helpful and stressful. In a sample with a majority of HIV gay positive men, unsupportive social interactions such as insensitivity, blaming, forces optimism, and disconnecting were found to be linked to depression (Ingram, Jones, Fass, Neidig, & Song, 1999). Studies of HIV positive low-income African Americans indicate that network support is strongly linked to medication adherence and viral load (Knowlton et al., 2011), yet these studies have not been replicated in gay populations.

There is a gap in the literature that focuses on social support among HIV positive gay men of color (e.g., Asian/Pacific Islander, African American, Latino), many of whom may not identify as gay and have female sexual partners, as well as HIV positive gay men who use drugs. As support has been found to function differently in a variety of populations, it is important to assess the dynamics of network support for variability in key outcomes among HIV positive gay men of color.

Disclosure

Disclosure of one's HIV status is a complex social process that can have significant consequences for relationships, health, and well-being of the individual disclosing (Tobin, Cutchin et al., 2013; Tobin, Kuramoto et al., 2013; Waddell & Messeri, 2006; Wohl et al., 2011). These consequences can be both negative and positive. Rejection, loss of employment or housing, and psychological distress have been reported as negative outcomes from disclosure. Alternatively, gains in social support as well as increased intimacy and self-esteem have also been documented (Simoni, Demas, Mason, Drossman, & Davis, 2000; Zea, Reisen, Poppen, Bianchi, & Echeverry, 2005). For HIV positive individuals, disclosure may also facilitate support with obtaining medical care as well as medication adherence. Moreover, not disclosing to network members may be stressful due to anticipation of negative reactions when the network members discover an individual's HIV positive status.

Research focused on social networks of HIV positive gay men has shown that disclosure varies by type of network member. Disclosure tends to be greatest with close friends versus family and gay friends as opposed to heterosexual friends (Kalichman, DiMarco, Austin, Luke, & DiFonzo, 2003; Mansergh, Marks, & Simoni, 1995; Marks et al., 1992; Serovich, Esbensen, & Mason, 2007; Zea, Reisen, Poppen, Echeverry, & Bianchi, 2004). Degree of emotional closeness with family in the network is a factor that determines disclosure of HIV status (Zea et al., 2004). In a study of HIV positive mixed race gay men in Ohio, the social network members who were the least likely to know the HIV status of the participants were network members from the workplace. The level of regret associated with disclosure was the greatest among those participants who had coworkers who knew their HIV status (Serovich et al., 2006). A study of HIV positive African American MSM found that disclosure of HIV positive status was associated with the network member also being HIV positive, older, providing emotional and financial support, and not being a male sex partner (Latkin et al., 2012). Disclosure of status has also been found to vary by type of sexual relationship, where disclosure is greatest in committed or noncasual relationships compared to anonymous relationships and relationships in the beginning stages (Bairan et al., 2007; Hart et al., 2005).

Disclosure of HIV status is also necessary for purposeful seroadaptation practices (e.g., sero-sorting and strategic positioning). Sero-sorting and strategic positioning have emerged as HIV risk reduction strategies that are utilized by gay men and other MSM (McConnell, Bragg, Shiboski, & Grant, 2010; McFarland et al., 2011; Murphy, Gorbach, Weiss, Hucks-Ortiz, & Shoptaw, 2013). Sero-sorting is a practice where MSM purposively choose sexual partners with the same or perceived HIV status as a HIV risk reduction strategy. For example, HIV positive gay men may limit their sex partners to HIV positive individuals. Strategic positioning, in a HIV serodiscordant (e.g., HIV positive/HIV negative) sexual relationship, often involves condomless anal intercourse where the HIV negative partner assumes the insertive role during anal intercourse as a method to limit HIV transmission to the negative or unknown status partner. For sero-sorting and strategic positioning, both partners must disclose accurate HIV status information. This disclosure may occur directly through face-to-face conversations, indirectly by providing cues to serostatus, or overtly on websites for meeting partners.

Disclosure of MSM Behavior

Due to issues of stigma and identity, many African American MSM are reluctant to disclose their sexual behavior to others (Jimenez, 2003; Kraft, Beeker, Stokes, & Peterson, 2000; Wheeler, 2006). Non-disclosure of sexual orientation and/or same sex sexual behaviors has also been associated with risk (Bingham, Harawa, & Williams, 2013). Recent research has also examined men who have sex with men and women (MSMW) (Bingham et al., 2013; Harawa et al., 2008; Harawa, McCuller, Chavers, & Janson, 2013; Latkin et al., 2011; Tieu et al., 2012; Wheeler, Lauby, Liu, Van Sluytman, & Murrill, 2008). Comparing MSM who have and have not disclosed, non-disclosers appear more likely to report sex with a woman (Centers for Disease Control and Prevention, 2003) and less likely to attend "gay" identified venues, such as clubs, bars, or parks where they could be associated with same sex sexual activities (Centers for Disease Control and Prevention, 2003; Kraft et al., 2000).

Addressing different social norms of behavior for both non-gay and gay identified men is important when discussing HIV prevention needs of HIV positive men. One such approach to disclosure of male-to-male sexual behavior may be a more detailed method of examining variations in disclosure to social network members. For example, some men may not disclose MSM behavior to most or all close network members, whereas others may have many network members who are aware of their same sex behaviors.

Social Norms

Social networks have been found to have powerful influences on individuals' behaviors, through processes of norm formation and maintenance (Hickson et al., 2017; Neighbors, Lee, Lewis, Fossos, & Larimer, 2007; Real & Rimal, 2007; Rosenquist, Murabito, Fowler, & Christakis, 2010; Teunissen et al., 2012; Tieu et al., 2016). There are two types of norms: descriptive norms which are perceptions of the prevalence of other's behaviors and injunctive norms which are perceptions of behaviors that are appropriate by others. One example of social norms relevant to HIV positive gay men is that of condom use. A recent study by Peterson and colleagues reported that African American men perceived that their friends endorsed the injunctive norm of approval of condom use but that the descriptive norm of perception of friends' actual condom use was low (Bakeman, Peterson,, & Community Intervention Trial for Youth Study Team, 2007; Peterson, Rothenberg, Kraft, Beeker, & Trotter, 2009).

Norms on drug and alcohol use have also been studied in samples of HIV positive gay men and suggest that increased individual use of drugs and alcohol was associated with perceptions of greater use by peers. A study with a multi-ethnic sample of young MSM found that binge drinking was associated with a greater number of peers who engaged in drug, alcohol, or sex risk behavior (Wong, Kipke, & Weiss, 2008).

A key consideration when examining social norms among HIV positive gay men is the reference group or source of social influence, which may vary according to relationship and similarity between the individual and his network. Considering the heterogeneity within communities of HIV positive gay men by sexual identity, socioeconomic status, race, etc., determining the source of social influence is critical to developing interventions that aim to alter norms. For example, having a public service announcement that focuses on changing perceptions about norms of alcohol use may be limited in effectiveness if the actor is not perceived to be a similar other.

Types of Social Networks to Consider

The *sexual network* is comprised of the number of different people with whom the individual has had sexual contact. The sexual network has been a central focus of HIV prevention research. Sexual mixing patterns, by race, age, and serostatus, within sexual networks have been studied to explain epidemiologic trends in HIV prevalence and transmission dynamics among gay men (Aral et al., 1999; Berry, Raymond, & McFarland, 2007; Eaton, Kalichman, & Cherry, 2010; Laumann & Youm, 1999). Evidence suggests that patterns of sexual networks differ between African Americans and Whites (Aral et al., 1999; Bingham et al., 2003; Laumann & Youm, 1999). Studies comparing African American MSM to White MSM have found that African American MSM are more likely to choose partners who are coming from a network of higher prevalence and incidence of STIs (Berry et al., 2007; Raymond & McFarland, 2009). Consequently, condomless anal intercourse within these networks is more likely to lead to disease transmission and infection (Eaton et al., 2010), which may be amplified in networks of HIV positive gay men. *Concurrency*, sexual partnerships that overlap during the same time period (Doherty, Schoenbach, & Adimora, 2009), is hypothesized to explain racial disparities in HIV. In a sample of MSM from San Francisco, African American MSM were significantly more likely to have concurrent partnerships compared to their White counterparts (Bohl, Raymond, Arnold, & McFarland, 2009).

The *drug network* is comprised of the number of drug users in the personal egocentric network and has been found to prospectively increase sexual risk (Latkin, Mandell, & Vlahov, 1996; Tobin, Cutchin et al., 2013; Tobin, Kuramoto et al., 2013). Studies of HIV positive gay men have consistently demonstrated a strong association between HIV risk and drug use. In a sample of HIV positive MSM and HIV negative MSM, those that engaged in methamphetamine use were significantly more likely to report a higher level of sex related HIV risk regardless of HIV status (Forrest et al., 2010). Carpiano and colleagues (Carpiano, Kelly, Easterbrook, & Parsons, 2011) found that having a network composed of predominately gay-identified social network members was directly associated with drug use as compared to men who had fewer gay-identified network members. In a sample of African American MSM in Baltimore, of whom 46% were HIV positive, crack-using African American MSM networks were composed of higher risk individuals, namely drug users, exchange partners, and partners who were both drug and sex partners compared to non-crack users (Tobin, German, Spikes, Patterson, & Latkin, 2011). In examining the drug use among network members, it is important to assess the frequency and type of drug use of network members as it may differ by geographic region, social class, ethnicity of network members, as well as local drug use trends.

Older HIV Positive Gay Men

With the advancement in HIV treatment and improved access to HIV care, individuals who are infected with HIV are living longer (Rosenfeld, Bartlam, & Smith, 2012; Shippy & Karpiak, 2005). The aging population of HIV positive gay men has received limited attention in the research, and therefore little is known about their social networks. One study conducted in New York City of men and women living with HIV and aged 50 years or older found that the majority lived alone and experienced isolation from family and less than half disclosed their status to friends and coworkers (Shippy & Karpiak, 2005). As discussed previously, older HIV positive gay men are likely to experience numerous disruptions to their social networks due to deaths. There are opportunities to leverage the social network to facilitate support through the grieving process and to foster resilience.

HIV Positive MSM of Color

HIV positive MSM of color, namely Latino and African American, continue to experience racial disparities in HIV infection, not attributable to individual-level factors (Holloway et al., 2017; Lieb et al., 2011; Magnus et al., 2010; Millett, Flores, Peterson, & Bakeman, 2007; Sifakis et al., 2007, 2010). MSM of color experience multiple stigmas and discrimination based on their sexual identity, race, and HIV status (Jimenez, 2003). To date, there have been limited studies that have examined the social network differences between HIV positive gay men of color compared to HIV positive gay White men. For example, it is unclear whether the social networks of African American HIV positive MSM who do not identify as gay are similar in composition to African American gay-identified HIV positive men. However, two recent studies conducted in Baltimore with a sample of adult African American MSM have shown that the networks of African American men who had sex with men only (MSMO) compared to men who had sex with men and women (MSMW) had less risky sex partners (Latkin et al., 2011) and that crack-using African American MSM networks were composed of higher risk individuals, namely drug users, exchange partners and partners who were both drug and sex partners (Tobin et al., 2011; Tobin, Kuramoto, Davey-Rothwell, & Latkin, 2011).

Social Network-Oriented Interventions for HIV Positive Gay Men

The Centers for Disease Control and Prevention (CDC) DEBI (Diffusing Effective Behavioral Interventions) offers a compendium of evidence-based interventions that are available for use (Effective interventions: HIV prevention that works, n.d.). There are five prevention interventions that are designed to address the HIV prevention needs of men who have sex with men. However, there are none that are specific to HIV positive gay men and none that target their social networks.

It is well established that social network and peer-based approaches are effective in reducing risk behaviors among adult populations (Davey-Rothwell, Tobin, Yang, Sun, & Latkin, 2011; Latkin, Sherman, & Knowlton, 2003; Tobin, Kuramoto et al., 2011). Informed by a number of social influence and network-oriented theories such as Social Learning Theory, Social Identity Theory, Exchange Theory, and Diffusion of Innovation, these types of interventions focus on introducing or altering social norms related to health, role-modeling behaviors, and promoting healthy social identities. Through social diffusion processes, indigenous peer outreach has the potential to impact community level risk behaviors (Friedman, Curtis, Neaigus, Jose, & Des Jarlais, 1999; Kelly, 1999; Peterson, Bakeman, Blackshear, & Stokes, 2003). Peer outreach may also be a means of self- and community empowerment, and serve as an important step in organizing HIV positive gay men of color (Friedman et al., 1987).

One approach that has been used with gay men is to train opinion leaders to educate peers on HIV and risk reduction. Community Popular Opinion Leader (CPOL) is an intervention that identified gay men who had a high degree of centrality in the social network and therefore had the most potential to influence other members of the social network, thus these individuals were considered community popular opinion leaders. In CPOL, individuals who were nominated as popular were invited to be trained to be opinion leaders and promote HIV prevention and condom use in gay bars with other patrons. In these studies, often the CPOLs are promoting HIV prevention with members of their social networks. CPOL is an example of an approach to norm change and demonstrates the long-term sustainability of community-level, norm altering approaches to behavior change. Effectiveness of CPOL has been demonstrated in numerous countries (Kelly, 2004), however, CPOL has not been implemented exclusively with HIV positive gay men to address issues related to access to HIV care or disclosure. Moreover, some studies using the CPOL approach with gay men and other populations have not found evidence of risk reduction (Hart, Williamson, & Flowers, 2004).

With high HIV prevalence among African American MSM, there has been increased attention and effort to develop and test rigorous culturally tailored behavioral interventions. D-Up (Jones et al., 2008) is based on the CPOL Model (Kelly et al., 1991, 1992), which identified key opinion leaders at local night clubs and then trained them to promote sexual risk reduction. Condom use and condom-less anal intercourse were assessed with sample of nightclub patrons over a 12-month period. POL strategies need to consider the role of sociocultural contexts of HIV- or MSM-related stigma, such as in communities of color or in faith-based institutions in order to be effective. For example, individuals may believe that advocating risk reduction to peers may lead to disclosure about their HIV status or sexual orientation, which may result in discrimination. Other interventions have been tailored to address the unique needs of young African American gay and bisexual men (Kegeles, Hays, & Coates, 1996; Wilton et al., 2009) and men who have sex with men and women (Operario, Smith, Arnold, & Kegeles, 2010; Williams, Ramamurthi, Manago, & Harawa, 2009). Unity in Diversity was a group-level, network-oriented HIV prevention intervention tailored for African American MSM (Tobin, Cutchin et al., 2013; Tobin, Kuramoto et al., 2013). This intervention was based on a framework of taking care of self, relationships, and community and encouraged study participants to diffuse information and skills from the program to social network members.

There has been a growing body of pilot studies and formative research using social network media via the Internet with computers and mobile based technologies to deliver HIV prevention messages and interventions primarily to young adults (Bull, McFarlane, & King, 2001; Noar, 2011). Studies have shown that computer-based interventions delivered through social network sites are efficacious (Bowen, Horvath, & Williams, 2007). Recently, Jaganath and colleagues (Jaganath, Gill, Cohen, & Young, 2012) trained opinion leaders to use Facebook to promote HIV prevention. Hightow-Weidman (Hightow-Weidman et al., 2011) developed an interactive and multicomponent website specifically for African American MSM aged 18–30 and Rice and colleagues (Rice, Tulbert, Cederbaum, Barman Adhikari, & Milburn, 2012) trained homeless youth to recruit peers and develop HIV prevention promotion videos that were shared via social networking sites (e.g., Facebook). These pilot studies have demonstrated acceptability of these methods with young MSM. Other studies have shown feasibility and acceptability of using electronic network and text messaging to deliver health information (Levine, McCright, Dobkin, Woodruff, & Klausner, 2008), reminders for STI testing (Bourne et al., 2011), and to encourage condom use (Cornelius & St Lawrence, 2009; Juzang, Fortune, Black, Wright, & Bull, 2011; Wright, Fortune, Juzang, & Bull, 2011).

Future Research Agenda

HIV positive gay men are not a monolithic population. Instead, there is heterogeneity in race, sexual identity, age, socioeconomic status, drug use, and sexual behaviors within this group. HIV positive gay men often live in communities with markedly different levels of support. By understanding pathways and processes of social network influences on health behaviors, researchers and public health practitioners may be able to identify key structural characteristics and specific network members to target for prevention and care interventions. Network approaches have the potential to be more effective at reaching HIV positive MSM, especially non-gay identified, substance-using and men of color. There remains a need for research focused on elucidating the structure and functions of social networks of HIV positive gay men, including men of color and older gay men. Studies that focus on the role of the social network to facilitate resilience can inform development of interventions that aim to leverage the social networks to sustain health-promoting norms and behaviors.

References

Adimora, A. A., & Schoenbach, V. J. (2005). Social context, sexual networks, and racial disparities in rates of sexually transmitted infections. *The Journal of Infectious Diseases, 191*(s1), S115–S122.

Aral, S. O., Hughes, J. P., Stoner, B., Whittington, W., Handsfield, H. H., Anderson, R. M., & Holmes, K. K. (1999). Sexual mixing patterns in the spread of gonococcal and chlamydial infections. *American Journal of Public Health, 89*(6), 825–833.

Ayala, G., Bingham, T., Kim, J., Wheeler, D. P., & Millett, G. A. (2012). Modeling the impact of social discrimination and financial hardship on the sexual risk of HIV among Latino and black men who have sex with men. *American Journal of Public Health, 102*(S2), S242–S249.

Bairan, A., Taylor, G. A. J., Blake, B. J., Akers, T., Sowell, R., & Mendiola, R., Jr. (2007). A model of HIV disclosure: Disclosure and types of social relationships. *Journal of the American Academy of Nurse Practitioners, 19*(5), 242–250.

Bakeman, R., Peterson, J. L., & Community Intervention Trial for Youth Study Team. (2007). Do beliefs about HIV treatments affect peer norms and risky sexual behaviour among African-American men who have sex with men? *International Journal of STD & AIDS, 18*(2), 105–108.

Berry, M., Raymond, H. F., & McFarland, W. (2007). Same race and older partner selection may explain higher HIV prevalence among black men who have sex with men. *AIDS (London, England), 21*(17), 2349–2350.

Bingham, T. A., Harawa, N. T., Johnson, D. F., Secura, G. M., MacKellar, D. A., & Valleroy, L. A. (2003). The effect of partner characteristics on HIV infection among African American men who have sex with men in the young men's survey, Los Angeles, 1999–2000. *AIDS Education and Prevention: Official Publication of the International Society for AIDS Education, 15*(1_ supplement), 39–52.

Bingham, T. A., Harawa, N. T., & Williams, J. K. (2013). Gender role conflict among African American men who have sex with men and women: Associations with mental health and sexual risk and disclosure behaviors. *American Journal of Public Health, 103*(1), 127–133.

Bohl, D. D., Raymond, H. F., Arnold, M., & McFarland, W. (2009). Concurrent sexual partnerships and racial disparities in HIV infection among men who have sex with men. *Sexually Transmitted Infections, 85*(5), 367–369.

Bourne, C., Knight, V., Guy, R., Wand, H., Lu, H., & McNulty, A. (2011). Short message service reminder intervention doubles sexually transmitted infection/HIV re-testing rates among men who have sex with men. *Sexually Transmitted Infections, 87*(3), 229–231.

Bowen, A. M., Horvath, K., & Williams, M. L. (2007). A randomized control trial of internet-delivered HIV prevention targeting rural MSM. *Health Education Research, 22*(1), 120–127.

Britton, P. J., Zarski, J. J., & Hobfoll, S. E. (1993). Psychological distress and the role of significant others in a population of gay/bisexual men in the era of HIV. *AIDS Care, 5*(1), 43–54.

Broadhead, R. S., Heckathorn, D. D., Altice, F. L., van Hulst, Y., Carbone, M., Friedland, G. H., & Selwyn, P. A. (2002). Increasing drug users' adherence to HIV treatment: Results of a peer-driven intervention feasibility study. *Social Science & Medicine (1982), 55*(2), 235–246.

Bull, S. S., McFarlane, M., & King, D. (2001). Barriers to STD/HIV prevention on the internet. *Health Education Research, 16*(6), 661–670.

Buseh, A. G., Stevens, P. E., McManus, P., Addison, R. J., Morgan, S., & Millon-Underwood, S. (2006). Challenges and opportunities for HIV prevention and care: Insights from focus groups of HIV-infected African American men. *The Journal of the Association of Nurses in AIDS Care: JANAC, 17*(4), 3–15.

Carpiano, R. M., Kelly, B. C., Easterbrook, A., & Parsons, J. T. (2011). Community and drug use among gay men: The role of neighborhoods and networks. *Journal of Health and Social Behavior, 52*(1), 74–90.

Centers for Disease Control and Prevention. (2003). From the centers for disease control and prevention. HIV/STD risks in young men who have sex with men who do not disclose their sexual orientation--six U.S. cities, 1994–2000. *JAMA: The Journal of the American Medical Association, 289*(8), 975–977.

Christakis, N. A., & Fowler, J. H. (2008). The collective dynamics of smoking in a large social network. *The New England Journal of Medicine, 358*(21), 2249–2258.

Cornelius, J. B., & St Lawrence, J. S. (2009). Receptivity of African American adolescents to an HIV-prevention curriculum enhanced by text messaging. *Journal for Specialists in Pediatric Nursing: JSPN, 14*(2), 123–131.

Costenbader, E. C., Astone, N. M., & Latkin, C. A. (2006). The dynamics of injection drug users' personal networks and HIV risk behaviors. *Addiction (Abingdon, England), 101*(7), 1003–1013.

Davey-Rothwell, M. A., Tobin, K., Yang, C., Sun, C. J., & Latkin, C. A. (2011). Results of a randomized controlled trial of a peer mentor HIV/STI prevention intervention for women over an 18 month follow-up. *AIDS and Behavior, 15*(8), 1654–1663.

Doherty, I. A., Schoenbach, V. J., & Adimora, A. A. (2009). Condom use and duration of concurrent partnerships among men in the United States. *Sexually Transmitted Diseases, 36*(5), 265–272.

Eaton, L. A., Kalichman, S. C., & Cherry, C. (2010). Sexual partner selection and HIV risk reduction among black and white men who have sex with men. *American Journal of Public Health, 100*(3), 503–509.

Effective interventions: HIV prevention that works. (n.d.). Retrieved from https://www.effectiveinterventions.org/en/Home.aspx.

El-Bassel, N., Gilbert, L., Witte, S., Wu, E., Hunt, T., & Remien, R. H. (2010). Couple-based HIV prevention in the United States: Advantages, gaps, and future directions. *Journal of Acquired Immune Deficiency Syndromes, 55*(Suppl 2), S98–S101.

El-Bassel, N., Jemmott, J. B., Landis, J. R., Pequegnat, W., Wingood, G. M., Wyatt, G. E., ... for the NIMH Multisite HIV/STD Prevention Trial for African American Couples Group. (2010). National institute of mental health multisite eban HIV/STD prevention intervention for African American HIV serodiscordant couples: A cluster randomized trial. *Archives of Internal Medicine, 170*(17), 1594–1601.

Forrest, D. W., Metsch, L. R., LaLota, M., Cardenas, G., Beck, D. W., & Jeanty, Y. (2010). Crystal methamphetamine use and sexual risk behaviors among HIV-positive and HIV-negative men who have sex with men in south Florida. *Journal of Urban Health: Bulletin of the New York Academy of Medicine, 87*(3), 480–485.

Friedman, S. R., & Aral, S. (2001). Social networks, risk-potential networks, health, and disease. *Journal of Urban Health: Bulletin of the New York Academy of Medicine, 78*(3), 411–418.

Friedman, S. R., Curtis, R., Neaigus, A., Jose, B., & Des Jarlais, D. C. (1999). *Social networks, drug injectors' lives, and HIV/AIDS*. New York: Kluwer Academic/Plenum Publishers.

Friedman, S. R., Des Jarlais, D. C., Sotheran, J. L., Garber, J., Cohen, H., & Smith, D. (1987). AIDS and self-organization among intravenous drug users. *The International Journal of the Addictions, 22*(3), 201–219.

Frye, V., Nandi, V., Egan, J. E., Cerda, M., Rundle, A., Quinn, J. W., ... Koblin, B. (2017). Associations among neighborhood characteristics and sexual risk behavior among black and white MSM living in a major urban area. *AIDS and Behavior, 21*, 870–890.

Gardenier, D., Andrews, C. M., Thomas, D. C., Bookhardt-Murray, L. J., & Fitzpatrick, J. J. (2010). Social support and adherence: Differences among clients in an AIDS day health care program. *The Journal of the Association of Nurses in AIDS Care: JANAC, 21*(1), 75–85.

George, S., Garth, B., Wohl, A. R., Galvan, F. H., Garland, W., & Myers, H. F. (2009). Sources and types of social support that influence engagement in HIV care among Latinos and African Americans. *Journal of Health Care for the Poor and Underserved, 20*(4), 1012–1035.

Hall, V. P. (1999). The relationship between social support and health in gay men with HIV/AIDS: An integrative review. *The Journal of the Association of Nurses in AIDS Care: JANAC, 10*(3), 74–86.

Harawa, N. T., McCuller, W. J., Chavers, C., & Janson, M. (2013). HIV risk behaviors among black/African American and Hispanic/Latina female partners of men who have sex with men and women. *AIDS and Behavior, 17*(3), 848–855.

Harawa, N. T., Williams, J. K., Ramamurthi, H. C., Manago, C., Avina, S., & Jones, M. (2008). Sexual behavior, sexual identity, and substance abuse among low-income bisexual and non-gay-identifying African American men who have sex with men. *Archives of Sexual Behavior*, *37*(5), 748–762.

Hart, G., Fitzpatrick, R., McLean, J., Dawson, J., & Boulton, M. (1990). Gay men, social support and HIV disease: A study of social integration in the gay community. *AIDS Care*, *2*(2), 163–170.

Hart, G. J., Williamson, L. M., & Flowers, P. (2004). Good in parts: The gay men's task force in Glasgow - a response to Kelly. *AIDS Care - Psychological and Socio-Medical Aspects of AIDS/HIV*, *16*(2), 159–165.

Hart, T. A., Wolitski, R. J., Purcell, D. W., Parsons, J. T., Gomez, C. A., & Seropositive Urban Men's Study Team. (2005). Partner awareness of the serostatus of HIV-seropositive men who have sex with men: Impact on unprotected sexual behavior. *AIDS and Behavior*, *9*(2), 155–166.

Hays, R. B., Catania, J. A., McKusick, L., & Coates, T. J. (1990). Help-seeking for AIDS-related concerns: A comparison of gay men with various HIV diagnoses. *American Journal of Community Psychology*, *18*(5), 743–755.

Hays, R. B., Magee, R. H., & Chauncey, S. (1994). Identifying helpful and unhelpful behaviours of loved ones: The PWA's perspective. *AIDS Care*, *6*(4), 379–392.

Hickson, D. A., Mena, L. A., Wilton, L., Tieu, V. H., Koblin, B. A., Latkin, C., … Mayer, K. H. (2017). Sexual networks, dyadic characteristics, and HIV acquisition and transmission behaviors among black men who have sex with men in 6 US cities. *American Journal of Epidemiology*, *185*, 786–800.

Hightow-Weidman, L. B., Fowler, B., Kibe, J., McCoy, R., Pike, E., Calabria, M., & Adimora, A. (2011). HealthMpowerment.Org: Development of a theory-based HIV/STI website for young black MSM. *AIDS Education and Prevention:Official Publication of the International Society for AIDS Education*, *23*(1), 1–12.

Holloway, I. W., Tan, D., Dunlap, S. L., Palmer, L., Beougher, S., & Cederbaum, J. A. (2017). Network support, technology use, depression, and ART adherence among HIV-positive MSM of color. AIDS Care. 29(9):1153-1161. [Epub ahead of print].

Horvath, K. J., Michael Oakes, J., Simon Rosser, B. R., Danilenko, G., Vezina, H., Rivet Amico, K., … Simoni, J. (2013). Feasibility, acceptability and preliminary efficacy of an online peer-to-peer social support ART adherence intervention. *AIDS and Behavior*, *17*(6), 2031–2044.

Ingram, K. M., Jones, D. A., Fass, R. J., Neidig, J. L., & Song, Y. S. (1999). Social support and unsupportive social interactions: Their association with depression among people living with HIV. *AIDS Care - Psychological and Socio-Medical Aspects of AIDS/HIV*, *11*(3), 313–329.

Jaganath, D., Gill, H. K., Cohen, A. C., & Young, S. D. (2012). Harnessing online peer education (HOPE): Integrating C-POL and social media to train peer leaders in HIV prevention. *AIDS Care*, *24*(5), 593–600.

Jennings, J. M., Taylor, R., Iannacchione, V. G., Rogers, S. M., Chung, S. E., Huettner, S., & Ellen, J. M. (2010). The available pool of sex partners and risk for a current bacterial sexually transmitted infection. *Annals of Epidemiology*, *20*(7), 532–538.

Jimenez, A. D. (2003). Triple jeopardy: Targeting older men of color who have sex with men. *Journal of Acquired Immune Deficiency Syndromes (1999)*, *33*(Sup 2), S222–S225.

Jones, K. T., Gray, P., Whiteside, Y. O., Wang, T., Bost, D., Dunbar, E., … Johnson, W. D. (2008). Evaluation of an HIV prevention intervention adapted for black men who have sex with men. *American Journal of Public Health*, *98*(6), 1043–1050.

Juzang, I., Fortune, T., Black, S., Wright, E., & Bull, S. (2011). A pilot programme using mobile phones for HIV prevention. *Journal of Telemedicine and Telecare*, *17*(3), 150–153.

Kalichman, S. C., DiMarco, M., Austin, J., Luke, W., & DiFonzo, K. (2003). Stress, social support, and HIV-status disclosure to family and friends among HIV-positive men and women. *Journal of Behavioral Medicine*, *26*(4), 315–332.

Kegeles, S. M., Hays, R. B., & Coates, T. J. (1996). The Mpowerment project: A community-level HIV prevention intervention for young gay men. *American Journal of Public Health*, *86*(8_Pt_1), 1129–1136.

Kelly, J. A. (1999). Community-level interventions are needed to prevent new HIV infections. *American Journal of Public Health, 89*(3), 299–301.

Kelly, J. A. (2004). Popular opinion leaders and HIV prevention peer education: Resolving discrepant findings, and implications for the development of effective community programmes. *AIDS Care, 16*(2), 139–150.

Kelly, J. A., St Lawrence, J. S., Diaz, Y. E., Stevenson, L. Y., Hauth, A. C., Brasfield, T. L., ... Andrew, M. E. (1991). HIV risk behavior reduction following intervention with key opinion leaders of population: An experimental analysis. *American Journal of Public Health, 81*(2), 168–171.

Kelly, J. A., St Lawrence, J. S., Stevenson, L. Y., Hauth, A. C., Kalichman, S. C., Diaz, Y. E., ... Morgan, M. G. (1992). Community AIDS/HIV risk reduction: The effects of endorsements by popular people in three cities. *American Journal of Public Health, 82*(11), 1483–1489.

Kimberly, J. A., & Serovich, J. M. (1999). The role of family and friend social support in reducing risk behaviors among HIV-positive gay men. *AIDS Education and Prevention, 11*(6), 465–475.

Knowlton, A. R., Yang, C., Bohnert, A., Wissow, L., Chander, G., & Arnsten, J. A. (2011). Informal care and reciprocity of support are associated with HAART adherence among men in Baltimore, MD, USA. *AIDS and Behavior, 15*(7), 1429–1436.

Kraft, J. M., Beeker, C., Stokes, J. P., & Peterson, J. L. (2000). Finding the "community" in community-level HIV/AIDS interventions: Formative research with young African American men who have sex with men. *Health Education & Behavior: The Official Publication of the Society for Public Health Education, 27*(4), 430–441.

Latkin, C., Yang, C., Tobin, K., Roebuck, G., Spikes, P., & Patterson, J. (2012). Social network predictors of disclosure of MSM behavior and HIV-positive serostatus among African American MSM in Baltimore, Maryland. *AIDS and Behavior, 16*(3), 535–542.

Latkin, C. A., & Knowlton, A. R. (2005). Micro-social structural approaches to HIV prevention: A social ecological perspective. *AIDS Care, 17*(Suppl 1), S102–S113.

Latkin, C. A., Mandell, W., & Vlahov, D. (1996). The relationship between risk networks' patterns of crack cocaine and alcohol consumption and HIV-related sexual behaviors among adult injection drug users: A prospective study. *Drug and Alcohol Dependence, 42*(3), 175–181.

Latkin, C. A., Sherman, S., & Knowlton, A. (2003). HIV prevention among drug users: Outcome of a network-oriented peer outreach intervention. *Health Psychology:Official Journal of the Division of Health Psychology, American Psychological Association, 22*(4), 332–339.

Latkin, C. A., Van Tieu, H., Fields, S., Hanscom, B. S., Connor, M., Hascom, B., ... Koblin, B. A. (2017). Social network factors as correlates and predictors of high depressive symptoms among black men who have sex with men in HPTN 061. *AIDS and Behavior, 21*, 113–1170.

Latkin, C. A., Yang, C., Tobin, K., Penniman, T., Patterson, J., & Spikes, P. (2011). Differences in the social networks of African American men who have sex with men only and those who have sex with men and women. *American Journal of Public Health, 101*(10), e18–e23.

Laumann, E. O., & Youm, Y. (1999). Racial/ethnic group differences in the prevalence of sexually transmitted diseases in the United States: A network explanation. *Sexually Transmitted Diseases, 26*(5), 250–261.

Levine, D., McCright, J., Dobkin, L., Woodruff, A. J., & Klausner, J. D. (2008). SEXINFO: A sexual health text messaging service for San Francisco youth. *American Journal of Public Health, 98*(3), 393–395.

Lieb, S., Prejean, J., Thompson, D. R., Fallon, S. J., Cooper, H., Gates, G. J., ... Malow, R. M. (2011). HIV prevalence rates among men who have sex with men in the southern United States: Population-based estimates by race/ethnicity. *AIDS and Behavior, 15*(3), 596–606.

Magnus, M., Kuo, I., Phillips, G., Shelley, K., Rawls, A., Montanez, L., ... Greenberg, A. E. (2010). Elevated HIV prevalence despite lower rates of sexual risk behaviors among black men in the District of Columbia who have sex with men. *AIDS Patient Care and STDs, 24*(10), 615–622.

Mansergh, G., Marks, G., & Simoni, J. M. (1995). Self-disclosure of HIV infection among men who vary in time since seropositive diagnosis and symptomatic status. *AIDS, 9*(6), 639–644.

Marks, G., Bundek, N. I., Richardson, J. L., Ruiz, M. S., Maldonado, N., & Mason, H. R. (1992). Self-disclosure of HIV infection: Preliminary results from a sample of Hispanic men. *Health*

Psychology: Official Journal of the Division of Health Psychology, American Psychological Association, 11(5), 300–306.

McConnell, J. J., Bragg, L., Shiboski, S., & Grant, R. M. (2010). Sexual seroadaptation: Lessons for prevention and sex research from a cohort of HIV-positive men who have sex with men. *PLoS One, 5*(1), e8831.

McFarland, W., Chen, Y. H., Raymond, H. F., Nguyen, B., Colfax, G., Mehrtens, J., … Truong, H. M. (2011). HIV seroadaptation among individuals, within sexual dyads, and by sexual episodes, men who have sex with men, San Francisco, 2008. *AIDS Care, 23*(3), 261–268.

Miller, R. L., Klotz, D., & Eckholdt, H. M. (1998). HIV prevention with male prostitutes and patrons of hustler bars: Replication of an HIV preventive intervention. *American Journal of Community Psychology, 26*(1), 97–131.

Millett, G. A., Flores, S. A., Peterson, J. L., & Bakeman, R. (2007). Explaining disparities in HIV infection among black and white men who have sex with men: A meta-analysis of HIV risk behaviors. *AIDS (London, England), 21*(15), 2083–2091.

Murphy, R. D., Gorbach, P. M., Weiss, R. E., Hucks-Ortiz, C., & Shoptaw, S. J. (2013). Seroadaptation in a sample of very poor Los Angeles area men who have sex with men. *AIDS and Behavior, 17*(5), 1862–1872.

Neighbors, C., Lee, C. M., Lewis, M. A., Fossos, N., & Larimer, M. E. (2007). Are social norms the best predictor of outcomes among heavy-drinking college students? *Journal of Studies on Alcohol and Drugs, 68*(4), 556–565.

Noar, S. M. (2011). Computer technology-based interventions in HIV prevention: State of the evidence and future directions for research. *AIDS Care, 23*(5), 525–533.

Operario, D., Smith, C. D., Arnold, E., & Kegeles, S. (2010). The bruthas project: Evaluation of a community-based HIV prevention intervention for African American men who have sex with men and women. *AIDS Education and Prevention: Official Publication of the International Society for AIDS Education, 22*(1), 37–48.

Parsons, J. T., Halkitis, P. N., Wolitski, R. J., Gomez, C. A., & Seropositive Urban Men's Study Team. (2003). Correlates of sexual risk behaviors among HIV-positive men who have sex with men. *AIDS Education and Prevention: Official Publication of the International Society for AIDS Education, 15*(5), 383–400.

Persson, L., Ostergren, P. O., Hanson, B. S., Lindgren, A., & Naucler, A. (2002). Social network, social support and the rate of decline of CD4 lymphocytes in asymptomatic HIV-positive homosexual men. *Scandinavian Journal of Public Health, 30*(3), 184–190.

Peterson, J. L., Bakeman, R., Blackshear, J. H., Jr., & Stokes, J. P. (2003). Perceptions of condom use among African American men who have sex with men. *Culture, Health and Sexuality, 5*(5), 409–424.

Peterson, J. L., & Jones, K. T. (2009). HIV prevention for black men who have sex with men in the United States. *American Journal of Public Health, 99*(6), 976–980.

Peterson, J. L., Rintamaki, L. S., Brashers, D. E., Goldsmith, D. J., & Neidig, J. L. (2012). The forms and functions of peer social support for people living with HIV. *The Journal of the Association of Nurses in AIDS Care: JANAC, 23*(4), 294–305.

Peterson, J. L., Rothenberg, R., Kraft, J. M., Beeker, C., & Trotter, R. (2009). Perceived condom norms and HIV risks among social and sexual networks of young African American men who have sex with men. *Health Education Research, 24*(1), 119–127.

Raymond, H. F., & McFarland, W. (2009). Racial mixing and HIV risk among men who have sex with men. *AIDS and Behavior, 13*(4), 630–637. doi:10.1007/s10461-009-9574-6

Real, K., & Rimal, R. N. (2007). Friends talk to friends about drinking: Exploring the role of peer communication in the theory of normative social behavior. *Health Communication, 22*(2), 169–180.

Reisner, S. L., Mimiaga, M. J., Bland, S., Skeer, M., Cranston, K., Isenberg, D., … Mayer, K. H. (2010). Problematic alcohol use and HIV risk among black men who have sex with men in Massachusetts. *AIDS Care, 22*(5), 577–587.

Rice, E., Tulbert, E., Cederbaum, J., Barman Adhikari, A., & Milburn, N. G. (2012). Mobilizing homeless youth for HIV prevention: A social network analysis of the acceptability of a face-to-face and online social networking intervention. *Health Education Research, 27*(2), 226–236.

Rosenfeld, D., Bartlam, B., & Smith, R. D. (2012). Out of the closet and into the trenches: Gay male baby boomers, aging, and HIV/AIDS. *The Gerontologist, 52*(2), 255–264.

Rosenquist, J. N., Murabito, J., Fowler, J. H., & Christakis, N. A. (2010). The spread of alcohol consumption behavior in a large social network. Annals of Internal Medicine, 152(7), 426–33, W141., W141.

Serovich, J. M., Esbensen, A. J., & Mason, T. L. (2007). Disclosure of positive HIV serostatus by men who have sex with men to family and friends over time. *AIDS Patient Care and STDs, 21*(7), 492–500.

Serovich, J. M., Mason, T. L., Bautista, D., & Toviessi, P. (2006). Gay men's report of regret of HIV disclosure to family, friends, and sex partners. *AIDS Education and Prevention: Official Publication of the International Society for AIDS Education, 18*(2), 132–138.

Shippy, R. A., & Karpiak, S. E. (2005). The aging HIV/AIDS population: Fragile social networks. *Aging & Mental Health, 9*(3), 246–254.

Sifakis, F., Hylton, J. B., Flynn, C., Solomon, L., Mackellar, D. A., Valleroy, L. A., & Celentano, D. D. (2007). Racial disparities in HIV incidence among young men who have sex with men: The Baltimore young men's survey. *Journal of Acquired Immune Deficiency Syndromes (1999), 46*(3), 343–348.

Sifakis, F., Hylton, J. B., Flynn, C., Solomon, L., MacKellar, D. A., Valleroy, L. A., & Celentano, D. D. (2010). Prevalence of HIV infection and prior HIV testing among young men who have sex with men. The Baltimore young men's survey. *AIDS and Behavior, 14*(4), 904–912.

Simoni, J. M., Demas, P., Mason, H. R. C., Drossman, J. A., & Davis, M. L. (2000). HIV disclosure among women of African descent: Associations with coping, social support, and psychological adaptation. *AIDS and Behavior, 4*(2), 147–158.

Takahashi, L. M., & Magalong, M. G. (2008). Disruptive social capital: (un)healthy socio-spatial interactions among Filipino men living with HIV/AIDS. *Health & Place, 14*(2), 182–197.

Teunissen, H. A., Spijkerman, R., Prinstein, M. J., Cohen, G. L., Engels, R. C. M. E., & Scholte, R. H. J. (2012). Adolescents' conformity to their peers' pro-alcohol and anti-alcohol norms: The power of popularity. *Alcoholism: Clinical and Experimental Research, 36*(7), 1257–1267.

Tieu, H. V., Nandi, V., Hoover, D. R., Lucy, D., Stewart, K., Frye, V. ... NYC M2M Study Team. (2016). Do sexual networks of men who have sex with men in New York City differ by race/ethnicity? *AIDS Patient Care and STDs, 30*, 39–47.

Tieu, H. V., Spikes, P., Patterson, J., Bonner, S., Egan, J. E., Goodman, K., ... Koblin, B. A. (2012). Sociodemographic and risk behavior characteristics associated with unprotected sex with women among black men who have sex with men and women in New York City. *AIDS Care, 24*(9), 1111–1119.

Tobin, K. E., Cutchin, M., Latkin, C. A., & Takahashi, L. M. (2013). Social geographies of African American men who have sex with men (MSM): A qualitative exploration of the social, spatial and temporal context of HIV risk in Baltimore, Maryland. *Health & Place, 22C*, 1–6.

Tobin, K. E., German, D., Spikes, P., Patterson, J., & Latkin, C. (2011). A comparison of the social and sexual networks of crack-using and non-crack using African American men who have sex with men. *Journal of Urban Health, 88*(6), 1052–1062.

Tobin, K. E., Kuramoto, S. J., Davey-Rothwell, M. A., & Latkin, C. A. (2011). The STEP into action study: A peer-based, personal risk network-focused HIV prevention intervention with injection drug users in Baltimore, Maryland. *Addiction (Abingdon, England), 106*(2), 366–375.

Tobin, K. E., Kuramoto, S. J., German, D., Fields, E., Spikes, P., Patterson, J., & Latkin, C. (2013). Unity in diversity: Results of a randomized clinical culturally tailored pilot HIV prevention intervention trial in Baltimore, MD, for African American men who have sex with men. *Health Education and Behavior, 40*(3), 286–295.

Tucker, J. S., Hu, J., Golinelli, D., Kennedy, D. P., Green, H. D., Jr., & Wenzel, S. L. (2012). Social network and individual correlates of sexual risk behavior among homeless young men who have sex with men. *Journal of Adolescent Health, 51*(4), 386–392.

Waddell, E. N., & Messeri, P. A. (2006). Social support, disclosure, and use of antiretroviral therapy. *AIDS and Behavior, 10*(3), 263–272.

Wheeler, D. P. (2006). Exploring HIV prevention needs for nongay-identified black and African American men who have sex with men: A qualitative exploration. *Sexually Transmitted Diseases, 33*(Supplement), S11–S16.

Wheeler, D. P., Lauby, J. L., Liu, K. L., Van Sluytman, L. G., & Murrill, C. (2008). A comparative analysis of sexual risk characteristics of black men who have sex with men or with men and women. *Archives of Sexual Behavior, 37*(5), 697–707.

White, L., & Cant, B. (2003). Social networks, social support, health and HIV-positive gay men. *Health & Social Care in the Community, 11*(4), 329–334.

Williams, J. K., Ramamurthi, H. C., Manago, C., & Harawa, N. T. (2009). Learning from successful interventions: A culturally congruent HIV risk-reduction intervention for African American men who have sex with men and women. *American Journal of Public Health, 99*(6), 1008–1012.

Wilton, L., Herbst, J. H., Coury-Doniger, P., Painter, T. M., English, G., Alvarez, M. E., ... Carey, J. W. (2009). Efficacy of an HIV/STI prevention intervention for black men who have sex with men: Findings from the many men, many voices (3MV) project. *AIDS and Behavior, 13*(3), 532–544.

Wilton, R. D. (1996). Diminished worlds? The geography of everyday life with HIV/AIDS. *Health & Place, 2*(2), 69–83.

Wohl, A. R., Galvan, F. H., Myers, H. F., Garland, W., George, S., Witt, M., ... Lee, M. L. (2011). Do social support, stress, disclosure and stigma influence retention in HIV care for Latino and African American men who have sex with men and women? *AIDS and Behavior, 15*(6), 1098–1110.

Wong, C. F., Kipke, M. D., & Weiss, G. (2008). Risk factors for alcohol use, frequent use, and binge drinking among young men who have sex with men. *Addictive Behaviors, 33*(8), 1012–1020.

Wright, E., Fortune, T., Juzang, I., & Bull, S. (2011). Text messaging for HIV prevention with young black men: Formative research and campaign development. *AIDS Care, 23*(5), 534–541.

Zea, M. C., Reisen, C. A., Poppen, P. J., Bianchi, F. T., & Echeverry, J. J. (2005). Disclosure of HIV status and psychological well-being among Latino gay and bisexual men. *AIDS and Behavior, 9*(1), 15–26.

Zea, M. C., Reisen, C. A., Poppen, P. J., Echeverry, J. J., & Bianchi, F. T. (2004). Disclosure of HIV-positive status to Latino gay men's social networks. *American Journal of Community Psychology, 33*(1-2), 107–116.

Chapter 16
"Poz" in the Age of Technology: Technology, Sex, and Interventions to Reduce Risk for HIV Positive Men Who Have Sex with Men

Keith J. Horvath and Sabina Hirshfield

Introduction

The resurgence of HIV among men who have sex with men (MSM) in the USA and Western Europe has been attributed to a number of factors, including increased rates of condomless anal sex (CAS), higher rates of sexually transmitted infections (STIs), reduced concern about the severity of HIV, and the lack of regular HIV testing (Stahlman et al., 2016; Sullivan et al., 2009; Wolitski, Vadiserri, Denning, & Levine, 2001). Moreover, with improved survival due to early diagnosis and more effective antiretroviral therapies, there are increasing numbers of people in need of treatment and with the potential to transmit HIV, which presents a continued public health challenge (Kilmarx & Mermin, 2012). Among MSM who are aware of their HIV diagnosis, Black MSM are the most likely to be virally unsuppressed (71.8%), followed by Latino MSM (63%) and White MSM (53.2%) (Hall, Holtgrave, Tang, & Rhodes, 2013). Although many HIV positive MSM modify their sexual behaviors to reduce possible transmission after receiving an HIV positive diagnosis, some continue to engage in sexual risk (Crepaz & Marks, 2002; Gorbach, Drumright, Daar, & Little, 2006; Kalichman, Rompa, & Cage, 2000; Scheer, Chu, Klausner, Katz, & Schwarcz, 2001; Schwarcz et al., 2007).

In addition to changing perceptions of the risks associated with CAS among MSM, the dramatic increase in the use of the Internet to facilitate partner seeking may partially explain increasing rates of HIV (Chiasson et al., 2006; Halkitis, Parsons, & Wilton, 2003; Hirshfield, Grov, Parsons, Anderson, & Chiasson, 2015;

K.J. Horvath (✉)
Division of Epidemiology & Community Health, University of Minnesota,
Minneapolis, MN, USA
e-mail: horva018@umn.edu

S. Hirshfield
Division of Research and Evaluation, Public Health Solutions, New York, NY, USA
e-mail: shirshfield@healthsolutions.org

© Springer Science+Business Media LLC 2017
L. Wilton (ed.), *Understanding Prevention for HIV Positive Gay Men*,
DOI 10.1007/978-1-4419-0203-0_16

Hirshfield et al., 2015; McFarlane, Bull, & Reitmeijer, 2000; Pennise et al., 2015). In this chapter, we describe the current state of research on technology use for sex seeking among HIV positive MSM, and technology-based interventions to address sexual risk taking among this population. The chapter opens with a brief history of research about online sex seeking, followed by a discussion of the methodological considerations in technology-based research. Next, we review online sex seeking and the risks associated with this behavior, with a focus on the psychological and social factors associated with online sexual encounters. We conclude with considering ways that technology has been used to provide prevention interventions to people living with HIV (PLWH) and provide critical areas for future research.

Two points are needed to put the discussion that follows into greater context. First, while the focus of this chapter is on the relationship between technology use and the risk for HIV and other STIs—particularly among HIV positive MSM—the benefits of technology for many people should not be overlooked. The Internet offers unprecedented access to health and medical resources (Young, Holloway, Jaganath, Westmoreland, & Coates, 2014). Eighty-seven percent of the US adult population in 2014 went online (Pew Research Center, 2014a) and 80% of Internet users in 2010 (the most recent data available) have searched for health information (Pew Research Center, 2011). With roughly 1.2 million PLWH in the USA, studies show that many such persons are turning to the Internet for health-seeking purposes (Horvath, Carrico et al., 2013; Horvath, Michael Oakes et al., 2013). For example, an early study of how PLWH use the Internet showed that 46% of respondents searched online for information about antiretroviral therapy treatment (Kremer & Ironson, 2007). Therefore, this review should not be viewed as a one-sided depiction of the dangers of the Internet or other forms of technology.

Second, we and others (Lewis, Uhrig, Ayala, & Stryker, 2011; Weiss & Samenow, 2010) recognize that the use of the Internet in its traditional form (e.g., sitting at a desktop computer at home) to seek sex partners is now augmented by mobile- and global positioning system (GPS) -facilitated sex-seeking tools. However, research on these newer modes of technology-based sex-seeking tools is relatively recent (e.g., Goedel & Duncan, 2015, 2016; Hirshfield et al., 2012; Landovitz et al., 2012). Thus, we primarily focus on existing literature related to use of the Internet to meet sexual partners among HIV positive MSM and factors that may facilitate CAS with partners met online.

Early Research on Online Sex Seeking

Earliest reports of the association between HIV/STI risk and online sex seeking emerged at the beginning of this millennium. In the first study to receive widespread attention, McFarlane et al., (2000) reported that among a sample of 856 male and female clients receiving services at a Denver HIV clinic, persons who had sought sex partners online reported significantly more STIs, higher numbers of sex partners, higher rates of anal sex, more sex with men, and more partners known to be

HIV positive than those who did not seek sex online. This early study demonstrated that a higher percentage of MSM went online to seek sex partners more than their heterosexual counterparts (59 vs. 32%), and that online sex seeking more often than offline sex seeking resulted in in-person sexual encounters (67 vs. 23%). A series of studies followed that demonstrated increased rates of actual or possible risk for HIV and other STIs among online sex-seeking persons, particularly among MSM (Bull, McFarlane, & King, 2001; Bull, McFarlane, & Reitmeijer, 2001; Rietmeijer, Bull, & McFarlane, 2001).

At the same time, several studies showed evidence directly linking online sex seeking with STI or HIV diagnoses. A syphilis outbreak among MSM in San Francisco was traced to users of a particular chat room to meet men for sex (Klausner, Wolf, Fischer-Ponce, Zolt, & Katz, 2000). In a second study, two cases of acute HIV infection were linked to sex with partners met in online chat rooms, prompting the call for physicians to discuss the risks of online sex seeking among their patients (Tashima, Alt, Harwell, Fiebich-Perez, & Flanigan, 2003). Taken together, these studies not only confirmed that risk for HIV and STIs is higher among persons who use the Internet for partner seeking, but that infections could be directly traced to online sex seeking.

Findings from these early studies were largely confirmed in a subsequent meta analysis of online sex-seeking behavior among MSM, showing high rates of CAS among Internet-using MSM (Lewnard & Berrang-Ford, 2014). For these reasons, and the continued growth of the Internet to meet sexual partners among MSM (Rosser, West, & Weinmeyer 2008), interest remains high in how MSM use the Internet and other forms of technology (e.g., sex-seeking mobile applications) to facilitate partner selection and the possible risks inherent in such activities (Landovitz et al., 2012; Rendina, Jimenez, Grov, Ventuneac, & Parsons, 2014; Rosenberg, Khosropour, & Sullivan, 2012).

Methodological Considerations of Technology-Based Research

It is important to acknowledge the strengths and limitations of technology-based research and of studies on the association between technology use and risk behavior. A recognized strength of computer-based surveys is that they tend to elicit higher reporting of sexual risk and substance-using behaviors than mail, phone, and in-person surveys (Elford, Bolding, Davis, Sherr, & Hart, 2003; Link & Mokdad, 2005; Newman et al., 2002; Perlis, Des Jarlais, Friedman, Arasteh, & Turner, 2004). In addition, several large-scale studies comparing online to mail survey modes have found that online surveys have lower overall response rates but yield higher item response rates on both open- and close-ended questions, suggesting higher data quality (Bech & Kristensen, 2009; Denscombe, 2009; Kwak & Radler, 2002; Shin, Johnson, & Rao, 2012). These strengths and others (e.g., the potential to reach a wider segment of the target population; Pequegnat et al., 2007) are primary reasons why technology-based data collection is widely used in HIV-related research.

Limitations of technology-based research have been widely discussed (Chiasson et al., 2006; Pequegnat et al., 2007) and, therefore, interested readers are referred to these resources. We highlight two challenges that are particularly salient to the discussion below: generalizability and attrition. With respect to generalizability, it is common for studies examining the association between online sex seeking and risky sexual behavior among HIV positive MSM to recruit from online sex-seeking websites. Such websites facilitate identifying men with specific partner characteristics (e.g., men of a specific race or ethnicity), and may also facilitate locating sexual partners who seek particular sexual experiences (e.g., condomless sexual encounters). Thus, we suggest caution in extrapolating the results of these studies of online sex seeking and CAS among HIV positive MSM to the larger population of HIV positive MSM or those who do not use the Internet as a sex-seeking tool, as the recruitment source itself may attract high-risk HIV positive MSM (Mustanski, 2007).

A second identified challenge for online studies—particularly those that require multiple data collection points—is attrition. Online research studies tend to report higher attrition than offline research as there are fewer social constraints to retain participants in studies (Birnbaum, 2004). High attrition can threaten internal and external validity especially when attrition is associated with the main outcome variable (Johnson et al., 2008). Attrition is often associated with younger age and higher psychological distress (Johnson et al., 2008; Kalichman & Hunter, 1992; Orellana, Picciano, Roffman, Swanson, & Kalichman, 2006; Roffman, Klepsch, Wertz, Simpson, & Stephens, 1993; Vanable, Carey, Carey, & Maisto, 2002) and, depending on the study, reported as high as 85% (Bull, Lloyd, Rietmeijer, & McFarlane 2004) and as low as 13% (Horvath, Nygaard et al., 2012) in longitudinal online HIV prevention trials. However, attrition-related nonresponse alone does not mean that the data are inherently biased or invalid (Groves & Peytcheva, 2008). Recent advances in online retention protocols and technology are greatly improving online retention rates in HIV prevention trials, reporting similar rates to offline studies (Hirshfield et al., 2016; Khosropour, 2011; Rosser et al., 2010). These two limitations (generalizability and attrition) are important to recognize and should be considered when interpreting findings presented below.

Reasons for Seeking Sexual Partners Online

MSM were early adopters of technology and social media (Bolding, Davis, Sherr, Hart, & Elford, 2004; Wong, Gullo, & Stafford 2004), in part because the Internet holds a number of advantages in seeking sex partners over more traditional offline venues (Margolis et al., 2014). Ross and colleagues (2007) examined the responses of 1017 Latino MSM (5% of whom self-reported as HIV positive) to the question of whether they preferred to meet online or in person. The primary advantages that men reported for seeking sex partners online include the ability to seek partners anonymously, increased excitement with online sex seeking, ease and selection of sex partners, avoidance of interpersonal contact (i.e., being shy), the ability to get to know someone better, and the ability to present oneself positively, among others. In contrast, men in the study reported that advantages of meeting partners in person were to get a feel for the "real presence" of the person and to build a relationship.

The Internet and other forms of technology (e.g., global positioning system or GPS) are efficient for sex-seeking purposes in that they can allow seekers to choose partners based on certain characteristics (e.g., HIV status), sexual preferences (e.g., a preference for condomless sex), or geography (e.g., same city, same block). These features may confer benefits or risks on users depending on the accuracy of information posted in these venues and whether such information informs subsequent sexual activity. Studies suggest that online partner seeking may facilitate seroadaptative practices to reduce HIV risk, such as serosorting (i.e., selecting a sexual partner based on an identical HIV status) or strategic positioning (i.e., assuming a sexual role based on the HIV status of the sexual partner). A meta-analysis of the sexual practices of HIV positive MSM in the US showed that the prevalence of CAS with seroconcordant partners (i.e., partners who were also HIV positive) was higher (30%) than with serodiscordant partners (16% for unknown HIV status and 13% for HIV negative partners; Crepaz et al., 2009). In a study of nearly 400 PLWH attending a medical clinic in Seattle, WA, approximately one-quarter reported that they decided not to have sex with a potential partner because the partner was HIV negative (Golden, Wood, Buskin, Fleming, & Harrington, 2007). In the same study, 31% of HIV positive men reported that a potential sex partner declined sex because of the HIV positive partner's serostatus. In contrast, a study of Internet-using MSM in San Francisco found that while HIV negative men who went online to seek sex partners were at higher risk for having sex with a potentially serodiscordant partner, there was a trend toward seroconcordant partnerships among Internet-using HIV positive MSM (Berry, Raymond, Kellogg, & McFarland, 2008).

Regarding sexual negotiation with partners met online versus offline, it also appears that MSM report different reasons for not using condoms. In an analysis of written responses of the reasons for not using condoms with online and offline partners, MSM (9% self-reported HIV positive) who had CAS with online partners were more likely to cite an individual preference for sex without condoms (often referring to greater physical pleasure) and mutually agreeing to forgo condoms prior to the sexual encounter compared to reasons for CAS with their offline partners (Ostergren, Rosser, & Horvath, 2010). In the same study, CAS with offline partners was more likely attributed to contextual (e.g., alcohol and drugs) and relationship (e.g., in a monogamous relationship) factors.

Finally, in a study of condomless sex and the Internet, a high percentage of MSM (all of whom were familiar with the term "barebacking" and 20% of whom were HIV positive) agreed with the following statements: "Barebackers can find others like them to communicate with on [the] Internet" (75.7%); "[The] Internet makes it easy to find other men who bareback" (73.4%); and "Because [the] Internet is anonymous, gay men are more likely to use it to look for other barebackers" (70.0%) (Halkitis et al., 2003). Although these studies were not exclusively restricted to PLWH, the results demonstrate the complex relationships between the technological features afforded by the Internet, individual preferences for partner selection, sexual negotiation, and sexual practices. Whether or not the Internet and other technology-based venues for sex seeking heightens or reduces sexual risk depends on the personal characteristics of individuals who use these technologies (e.g., individual level of risk taking or risk aversion), the social norms about HIV disclosure and risk taking on the particular venue (i.e., whether the site caters to persons seeking condomless sex or not) appears to translate into tangible sexual practices when partners meet offline. The dynamic interplay between these factors often results in findings from research studies that do not consistently align with each other, and call for continued efforts to understand these associations as the relationship between the individual and technologies change over time.

Online Sex Seeking and Risk Behavior

The Internet is a common venue for MSM to seek sex partners (Lewnard & Berrang-Ford, 2014). A meta-analysis of online sex-seeking and sexual risk showed that approximately 40% of MSM had used the Internet to seek sex partners (Liau et al., 2006). In a separate study of 1683 MSM (11% self-reporting as HIV positive) who completed an online survey, results showed that the majority (82%) had sex with someone they met online, and 66% stated that they had more sex once they started meeting partners online (Chiasson et al., 2007). A study in which MSM were intercepted at gay community events in Los Angeles and New York showed that over half (53.5%) of MSM (12.5% of whom self-reported as HIV positive) reported meeting sex partners online in the past 3 months, compared to 55% who met sex partners at the bar and 40% who met sex partners at bathhouses (Grov, Parsons, & Bimbi, 2007).

In general, online studies of MSM find that men who meet men on the Internet report a greater number of sex partners (Benotsch, Kalichman, & Cage, 2002; Horvath, Rosser, & Remafedi, 2008; Margolis et al., 2014; McFarlane, Bull, & Rietmeijer, 2000; Rosser, Miner et al., 2009; Rosser, Oakes et al., 2009; Rosser et al., 2008; Taylor et al., 2004), having sex with casual partners (Horvath et al., 2008; Kim, Kent, McFarland, & Klausner, 2001; Rosser, Miner et al., 2009; Rosser, Oakes et al., 2009; Rosser et al., 2008; Taylor et al., 2004; Tikkanen & Ross, 2003), and higher rates of CAS (Benotsch et al., 2002; for a recent review see Lewnard & Berrang-Ford, 2014). However, some studies did not find a higher reporting of CAS among men who met sex partners online versus offline (Chiasson et al., 2007). A possible explanation for these contradictory findings is a difference in study measures to assess CAS. Studies that use the frequency of CAS in a given time period as the main outcome show that men who meet sex partners on the Internet appear to be at higher risk because of the heightened availability of sex partners found through online venues. However, when CAS is calculated as a *proportion* of sex partners met either online or offline, several studies have shown less risk behavior with online partners (Horvath et al., 2008; Mustanski, 2007). Therefore, in addition to the methodological considerations of technology-based research described earlier, close attention to issues of measurement is needed to understand the complexity of findings regarding sexual risk.

HIV positive gay men and other MSM appear to utilize the Internet more often and have greater levels of CAS with online partners, than MSM who have not been diagnosed with HIV (Lewnard & Berrang-Ford, 2014). The meta-analysis by Liau and his colleagues (Liau et al., 2006) showed that nearly one-half of HIV positive MSM went online seeking sex partners, compared to 41% of MSM who had not been diagnosed with HIV. The odds of CAS with sex partners met online was 1.68 times higher than for sex partners not met online, and this was particularly true for HIV positive MSM. The results of another study suggested that differences in risk behavior by venue are magnified among very highly sexually active MSM. In a study of 50 MSM who reported nine or more sex partners in the past 90 days, HIV positive men were more likely than HIV negative men to use the Internet to meet men for sex (95 vs. 68%), and were more likely to report CAS with online partners than HIV negative men (63 vs. 20%) (Grov, Golub, & Parsons, 2010). Online sex seeking is high among samples of HIV positive youth. In a recent qualitative study of 68 HIV positive (68% of the sample) and HIV negative youth (ages 18–24), 71% of HIV positive participants spent 5 or more hours on dating applications (or apps) a day (Camacho-Gonzalez et al., 2016).

Studies that focus on serodiscordant CAS (i.e., HIV positive persons reporting CAS with a HIV negative or HIV status unknown partner) as the outcome also reveal concerning rates of risk behavior among a substantial minority of HIV positive MSM. For example, the prevalence of serodiscordant CAS among samples of HIV positive MSM recruited online ranged from 23 to 51% (Chiasson, Hirshfield, Humberstone, DiFilippi et al., 2005; Chiasson, Hirshfield, Humberstone, Remien et al., 2005; Chiasson et al., 2007; Grov, Hirshfield, Remien, Humberstone, & Chiasson, 2011; Hirshfield, Remien, Humberstone et al., 2004a). These results are comparable to those in a community-based venue study in New York and California in which 47% of HIV positive men with non-main partners reported serodiscordant CAS in the previous 3 months (Parsons et al., 2005). The findings of these and other studies (Halkitis & Parsons, 2003; Halkitis et al., 2003) are reflected in a recent meta-analysis (Lewnard & Berrang-Ford, 2014) of the sexual behavior among MSM with online and offline partners across 11 studies. Findings showed that online partner seeking was associated with higher odds of CAS, seroconcordant CAS, and seroconcordant CAS with strategic positioning compared to offline partner seeking, with higher effect sizes noted among HIV positive compared to HIV negative groups across these outcomes. Therefore, there is a clear need to target HIV positive MSM who seek online partners with effective interventions.

Online sex seeking may be driven by a number of factors that are particularly salient to MSM living with HIV, including HIV disclosure, personal beliefs about responsibility to reduce the risk for transmission to sex partners, and mental health and substance use issues. Each of these is discussed in more detail below.

Contextual Issues Affecting Online Sex Seeking and HIV Transmission

HIV Disclosure Online and Offline. Disclosure of HIV status has been identified as a critical—although an imperfect (Horvath, Oakes, & Rosser, 2008)—component of sexual negotiation for MSM that has been cited in empirical studies (Carballo-Dieguez, Miner, Dolezal, Rosser, & Jacoby, 2006; Klitzman et al., 2007; Rietmeijer, Bull, McFarlane, Patnaik, & Douglas, 2002) and by the CDC (Centers for Disease Control and Prevention, 2003). Belief among PLWH that HIV positive individuals should disclose their status to sex partners has been associated with more frequent disclosure to sex partners (Duru et al., 2006). HIV positive men who do not disclose their serostatus and engage in condomless sex may be more likely to report using drugs before sex and less likely to know their partner's serostatus (Marks & Crepaz, 2001).

A study by Rosser and colleagues showed that approximately equal proportions of HIV positive MSM disclosed their HIV status to none (30%), some (31%), or all (39%) of their secondary sexual partners (Rosser, Horvath et al., 2008). The same study found that higher disclosure was associated with having fewer sex partners, being extremely out as a gay or bisexual man, more years of living with HIV, knowledge of CD4 count, having a detectable viral load, and White race. Biomedical advances in HIV prevention (i.e., treatment as prevention; Cohen et al., 2011) suggest that disclosure may include sharing one's health status in addition to HIV status. Evidence that effective HIV treatment greatly reduces the likelihood of HIV transmission among those who are virally suppressed—especially for early ART initiators (i.e., those who begin treatment immediately after receiving an HIV diagnosis, regardless of CD4 count)—provides strong support for the disclosure of whether antiretroviral therapy is being taken and current viral load status (Cohen et al., 2016). In a study of 304 HIV negative and 22 HIV positive MSM recruited online, CAS was reported in 75% of sexual encounters in which viral load was not discussed compared to 56% of sexual encounters in which viral load was discussed (Horvath, Smolenski, Iantaff et al., 2012).

Many reasons exist for why PLWH may not disclose their HIV status to potential sex partners, such as fear of a stigmatizing response with each new disclosure (Berger, Ferrans, & Lashley, 2001). To complicate matters, disclosure to sexual partners and its relationship to sexual risk can vary by partner type and venue (Grov, 2011; Grov et al., 2011; Simoni & Pantalone, 2004). Some studies show that men may be more likely to disclose to sex partners met online (Carballo-Dieguez et al., 2006; Chiasson et al., 2007). HIV status disclosure may be facilitated online through synchronous discussions in Internet chat rooms or mobile GPS apps and by disclosing HIV status through online profiles. In November 2016, Grindr, a popular GPS smartphone app used by MSM to meet other men, added two optional fields to user profiles to assist in the HIV disclosure process: HIV status (HIV positive; HIV positive, Undetectable; HIV negative; HIV negative, On PrEP [pre-exposure prophy-laxis]) and last HIV test date (Corbett, 2016).

Studies show mixed results regarding the use of online profiles as an HIV status disclosure tool. A study of whether MSM report their HIV status on their online profiles showed that 72% of MSM who had never tested for HIV and 75% of HIV negative men reported that they were HIV negative in all of their online profiles (Horvath et al., 2008). In contrast, the same study found that 16.8% of HIV positive MSM reported their status as HIV negative in all of their online profiles, while only 25% reported their status as HIV positive in all of their online profiles. Nodin and colleagues examined 199 online sex-seeking profiles of MSM on six of the most popular websites for men seeking condomless sex in New York City (Nodin, Valera, Ventuneac, Maynard, & Carballo-Diéguez, 2011). Profiles indicating that the user was HIV positive were more likely to contain full body pictures (50 vs. 22%), face pictures (77 vs. 51%), and multiple pictures (89 vs. 67%). Together, these results suggest that HIV positive MSM may be less likely to accurately disclose their HIV status in online profiles; however, among those that do, HIV positive MSM may be more inclined to reveal other physical attributes of themselves than HIV negative or serostatus unknown men. Revealing these attributes may be a way that some HIV positive MSM manage stigma surrounding their HIV status by projecting to poten tial sex partners that they have desirable characteristics rather than solely being identified with their HIV status.

Personal Responsibility to Reduce Risk for Transmission. Most HIV positive men feel a personal responsibility to protect their sex partners, via disclosure and/or condom use (O'Leary & Wolitski, 2009). Some PLWH, however, report having lower feelings of personal responsibility to not transmit HIV, which they may justify by minimizing potential consequences (Bandura, 1999, 2002) and based on uncon-firmed assumptions about a sex partner's serostatus (Parsons et al., 2006). Studies using quantitative measures of personal responsibility among HIV positive MSM show that higher personal responsibility ratings are correlated with less sexual transmission risk behavior (Parsons, Halkitis, Wolitski, & Gomez, 2003; Wolitski, Flores, O'Leary, Bimbi, & Gomez, 2007).

Personal responsibility appears to vary by venue in which HIV positive MSM meet their sex partners. One study showed that HIV positive MSM had highest lev-els of personal responsibility to protect their sexual partners from HIV or other STIs when they met those partners through friends or family (O'Leary, Horvath, & Rosser, 2012). Personal responsibility was next highest for partners met at a bar, followed by the Internet and finally for sex partners met in public sex venues. Among the 98 men who reported meeting sex partners in multiple venues, those who reported inconsistent responsibility beliefs across venues where sex partners were met or had lower personality beliefs across all venues reported higher risk behavior than those who reported consistently very high personal responsibility beliefs across venues. Collectively, these studies demonstrate that personal respon-sibility beliefs may be critical targets for prevention, and that addressing beliefs by venue may be important since responsibility beliefs appear to differ with partners met online and offline.

Mental Health Depression is common in men with, or at risk for, HIV (Dew et al., 1997). Rates of depression among MSM participating in research studies are higher than that of the general population (Rabkin, McElhiney, & Ferrando, 2004). Several nationally representative US surveys have found that 1–3% of men report same-sex partners or self-identify as gay or bisexual; among these men, past-year major depression ranged from 10 to 31%, compared to men who report sex with women, with past year ranges from 5 to 10% (Cochran & Mays, 2000; Cochran, Sullivan, & Mays, 2003; Gilman et al., 2001). In a US-based household probability sample of MSM (Mills et al., 2004), 17% screened positive for depression and 12% for distress (subthreshold for depression). Characteristics associated with depression included not having a domestic partner and not identifying as gay/homosexual. In another study of young MSM (Kipke et al., 2007), 21% screened positive for depression and 18% for distress, with 12% of men from the sample reporting no access to care when ill or in need of health advice. Using the two-item Patient Health Questionnaire (PHQ-2), 18% screened positive for current depressives symptoms in an online study among MSM from the USA and Canada (Hirshfield et al., 2008); characteristics associated with a positive screen included having low education, being HIV positive, not having a main same-sex partner, being married to a woman, and not reporting recent sex. Another online study among US MSM found a 17% prevalence of current depressive symptoms, which were associated with a recent STI diagnosis (Downing, Chiasson, & Hirshfield, 2016).

Many individuals with depressed mood report decreased sexual interest and activity (Casper et al., 1985; Kennedy, Dickens, Eisfeld, & Bagby, 1999; Mathew & Weinman, 1982). However, in a study of mood and sexual interest among 662 MSM, a minority (16%) of men reported increased sexual interest when depressed and nearly one-quarter reported heightened sexual interest when anxious (Bancroft, Janssen, Strong, & Vukadinovic, 2003). The relationship between mood, sexual interest, and sexual behavior is complex among PLWH. In a study of the relationship between negative affective states (e.g., depression-dejection, tension-anxiety, confusion-bewilderment) and risk behavior among 155 sexually active HIV positive men, negative affective states were associated with CAS with male partners, but not female partners (Marks, Bingman, & Duval, 1998). Other studies have confirmed an increase in sexual risk behavior among HIV positive MSM with high levels of depressive symptoms (Beck, McNally, & Petrak, 2003; Kelly et al., 1993; Parsons et al., 2003). HIV positive men who experience depression may feel disconnected from others and may consequently be less likely to enact risk-reduction strategies with sexual partners (Poppen, Reisen, Zea, Bianchi, & Echeverry, 2004).

Findings on the association between Internet use and depression are not uniform. Some studies show that Internet use is associated with high depressive symptomatology (Kraut et al., 1998), while other studies have found that online activities in which people interact with one another (e-mail, chat rooms) was associated with lower levels of loneliness and depression (Morgan & Cotten, 2003; Shaw & Gant, 2002).

Kalichman and colleagues examined levels of depressive symptoms among HIV positive men who seek sex partners online compared to those who only seek sex partners offline (Kalichman, Cherry, Cain, Pope, & Kalichman, 2005). Unadjusted models showed that depression scores were higher among men who sought sex partners online compared to men who did not (Centers for Epidemiologic Studies Depression Scale [CES-D] = 17.5 vs. 13.2). However, CES-D scores were not significantly associated with online sex seeking in the multivariate model. In sum, there is modest evidence that online sex seeking is associated with depression, although this relationship may be attenuated by other factors (e.g., levels of social support or adaptive coping). Persons who report high levels of depressive symptoms and are either at risk for HIV or are currently living with HIV should be assessed for partner-seeking behaviors to address possible depression-related risk activity in need of intervention.

Drug Use Drug use has been consistently linked to HIV transmission risk, particularly among MSM (Carey et al., 2009; Harawa et al., 2008). Certain drugs such as poppers (nitrite inhalants), ecstasy (MDMA), and crystal methamphetamine may be used specifically to enhance sexual experiences (Lewis & Ross, 1995). Ecstasy, crystal methamphetamine, gamma hydroxybutyrate (G or GHB), cocaine, and other substances have been associated with increased sexual risk behaviors, including CAS and group sex with anonymous, HIV negative or unknown status partners (Beck & Rosenbaum, 1994; Carey et al., 2009; Chiasson, Hirshfield, Humberstone, DiFilippi et al., 2005; Chiasson, Hirshfield, Humberstone, Remien et al., 2005; Chiasson, Shuchat Shaw, Humberstone, Hirshfield, & Hartel, 2009; Chiasson et al., 2006; Frosch, Shoptaw, Huber, Rawson, & Ling, 1996; Hirshfield, Grov et al., 2015; Hirshfield, Schrimshaw et al., 2015; Hirshfield, Remien, & Chiasson, 2006; Hirshfield, Remien, Humberstone et al., 2004a; Phillips, Grov, & Mustanski, 2015; Hirshfield, Remien, Walavalkar et al., 2004b; Semple, Zians, Strathdee, & Patterson, 2008; Thiede et al., 2008; Topp, Hando, & Dillon, 1999; Yu, Wall, Chiasson, & Hirshfield, 2015).

Substance use and its relationship to high-risk sexual behavior among MSM is of particular concern, as drugs and alcohol may help men to avoid feelings of anxiety associated with same-sex behavior and self-awareness of HIV (Mckirnan, Ostrow, & Hope, 1996; McKirnan, Vanable, Ostrow, & Hope, 2001). Impaired judgment due to drug use may lead to condomless sex, increasing the risk of HIV/STI transmission (Colfax & Guzman, 2006; Halkitis, Parsons, & Stirratt, 2001). Polydrug use and frequent drug use have been associated with HIV seropositivity or unknown HIV serostatus (Greenwood et al., 2001). For these reasons, it is not surprising that a high proportion (70%) of MSM who report engaging in CAS attribute increasing acceptance and practice of "barebacking" to the use of club drugs, including methamphetamines, ecstasy, and GHB (Halkitis et al., 2003).

High levels of substance use have been shown among MSM who seek sex partners online. In a study of MSM recruited at a gay pride event in Atlanta, Georgia, those who reported meeting sex partners via the Internet (*n* = 201) were more likely to report using methamphetamines and in the previous 6 months than men who did not meet sex partners online (10 vs. 5%) (Benotsch et al., 2002). Another study showed that MSM (of which one-sixth were HIV positive) who reported online sex seeking were significantly more likely to report ecstasy use during sex (Mettey, Crosby, DiClemente, & Holtgrave, 2003). Moreover, among men diagnosed with early stage syphilis infection, online sex seeking was associated with non-intravenous drug use after controlling for other factors (Taylor et al., 2004).

Recent HIV seroconversion is significantly associated with drug use during sex (Carey et al., 2009) and substance use is high among HIV positive MSM recruited both online and offline. One study showed that a high proportion of HIV positive White MSM reported recent stimulant (30%), methamphetamine (27%), and amyl nitrite (46%) use, while crack and cocaine use were high among Black MSM (38%) (Hatfield et al., 2009). In a study of MSM recruited to participate in an online survey, HIV positive men were significantly more likely to use two or more drugs before or during sex than their HIV negative or HIV status unknown counterparts (Hirshfield, Remien, Humberstone et al., 2004a). Other studies have similarly found associations between drug use and seroconversion (Plankey et al., 2007), particularly among MSM who use methamphetamine (Colfax, Shoptaw, Colfax, & Shoptaw, 2005; Hirshfield, Remien, Walavalkar et al., 2004b; Mimiaga et al., 2008).

Locating sex partners who may want to use drugs to enhance their sexual experiences may be facilitated by online profile options. Horvath and colleagues found that 12.5% of HIV positive MSM reported that all or some of their online profiles reported a preference for drug use during sex ("Party and Play"), compared to 6.9% of profiles of men who have only tested HIV negative and 4.5% of profiles of men who have never been tested for HIV (Horvath et al., 2008). Thus, although drug use may not necessarily be more common among HIV positive MSM who use the Internet to seek sex partners, the Internet may facilitate locating sex partners who wish to use drugs to enhance the sexual experience.

Overall, there is a consistent association between drug use, online sex seeking, and HIV risk. Addressing drug use as a risk factor for HIV and other STIs remains an important avenue to address high HIV/STI rates among MSM. However, as noted in a review of treatment outcome studies of HIV positive MSM who abuse methamphetamines (Rajasingham et al., 2012), effective interventions to reduce rates of drug use among this group remain sparse. Thus, greater emphasis should be placed on developing novel and culturally tailored interventions to address drug use among HIV-infected MSM to improve their own health outcomes and reduce risk for HIV transmission to sexual partners (Horvath, Carrico et al., 2013; Horvath, Michael Oakes et al., 2013).

Internet Use Among MSM of Color and Sexual Risk Taking

Although Black and Latino MSM are at a significant increased risk for HIV, few HIV risk reduction interventions—and even fewer that use technology—have been designed to target these groups (Young et al., 2014). The lack of technology-based interventions focusing on gay and MSM of color at risk or infected with HIV may stem in part from the belief that communities of color have not adopted technology as widely as White MSM or other non-minority groups. However, the US population online now has similar proportions of White (85%), Black (81%), and Latino/a adults (83%) (Pew Research Center, 2014a; Smith, 2010b). Black (90%) and English-speaking Latino/a (92%) adults are as or more likely to own a mobile phone than Whites (90%; Pew Research Center, 2014b), and are also more likely to use their mobile devices to send text messages, use social networking sites, watch videos, and e-mail (Smith, 2010a).

Although most studies examining Internet use and sexual risk taking do not exclusively focus on MSM of color, there are several notable exceptions. A series of published studies from the MINTS trial led by Rosser and a team of investigators focused on Internet use and sexual risk among Latino MSM (Carballo-Dieguez et al., 2006; Ross, Rosser, & Stanton, 2004; Ross, Rosser, Stanton, & Konstan, 2004; Rosser, Miner et al., 2009; Rosser, Oakes et al., 2009). In one of those studies, sexual negotiation and serostatus disclosure were more likely to occur with online than offline sexual partners among both HIV positive and HIV negative MSM; however, HIV positive participants were less likely to disclose their status than HIV negative MSM (Carballo-Dieguez et al., 2006). The same study showed that HIV positive Latino MSM reported lower intentions to use condoms than HIV negative Latino MSM, citing greater pleasure with condomless intercourse. In another study by this research team, Latino MSM—5% who self-identified as HIV positive (as reported in Rosser, Miner et al., 2009; Rosser, Oakes et al., 2009)—who reported a high preference for using the Internet to facilitate face-to-face interactions also reported relatively low levels of HIV status disclosure and discussions about safer sex with prospective partners and reported high rates of receptive oral and anal sex during Internet-mediated sexual liaisons (Ross, Rosser, & Stanton, 2004).

A study of online sex seeking among Black MSM (18% of who were living with HIV) showed that 20% reported meeting a sexual partner in the past 12 months (White, Mimiaga, Reisner, & Mayer, 2012). Findings also showed that Black MSM who met partners online reported more male sex partners and higher rates of condomless sex than Black MSM who did not report meeting sex partners online. Online sex seeking was significantly associated with condomless sex in multivariate models. In a second online study of serodisclosure in partnerships among men of varying races and ethnicities, HIV positive Black men were 60% less likely than White men to discuss their serostatus with sexual partnerships (Winter, Sullivan, Khosropour, & Rosenberg, 2012). In the same study, discussion of serostatus were more likely to occur with CAS partners than among non-CAS partner for HIV negative and HIV positive White MSM and HIV negative Latino and Black MSM; however, serostatus discussions were less likely among CAS partners than non-CAS partners for HIV positive Black and Latino MSM.

Low rates of serostatus disclosure among Internet-recruited Black and Latino HIV positive MSM has been attributed to both minority stress and high rates of homophobia experienced by these groups (Mays, Cochran, & Zamudio, 2004; Radcliffe et al., 2010; Stein et al., 1998; Winter et al., 2012). Thus, calls for interventions that address stigma and experiences of minority stress have been made (Winter et al., 2012), with a need to promote serostatus disclosure as normative behavior prior to sexual activity. Such intervention may benefit from addressing issues of sexual stereotyping in online partner selection that may increase possible risk behavior. Sexual stereotyping was investigated in a study by Wilson and colleagues that showed that online sex-seeking MSM of varying races and ethnicities used race-based sexual stereotypes that both directly and indirectly affected sexual partnering choices (Wilson et al., 2009). For example, Black MSM reported feeling a deeper connection with sexual partners who were Black, and feeling objectified by White sexual partners. The study by Wilson and colleagues shows the complex ways that MSM may be using the Internet to locate sex partners based on a variety of existing racial and ethnic stereotypes, which may be facilitated by online profiles (providing visual cues indicating race and ethnicity) or technology-mediated discussions (via supporting sexual stereotypes through conversational cues).

HIV Positive Perspectives on Technology-Based HIV Resources

Technology-based intervention approaches may benefit from research examining the perspectives of PLWH about technology-supported HIV-related resources. In a mixed method study of gay men, heterosexual women and men, and transgender women who were recently (<1 year) diagnosed with HIV, participants were asked about their perceptions of HIV-related websites (Courtenay-Quirk et al., 2010). The most appealing aspects of highly rated websites included websites that: provided relevant information on topics that were important to participants' health and well-being, were easy to navigate, were perceived as trustworthy, and represented a diversity of perspectives that represented a broad spectrum of PLWH. Participants in this study reported greatest interest in online resources that addressed HIV treatment issues, strategies for coping with depression and fear about living with HIV, and ways to learn how others have coped with HIV.

A study of technology use among PLWH in the USA demonstrated the widespread use of social networking websites and mobile phones among this population (Horvath, Danilenko et al., 2012; Horvath, Nygaard et al., 2012). When asked to describe their ideal social networking health website for PLWH, participants overall described it as one that would facilitate social interactions between people, contain relevant HIV-related information, and address privacy issues. In a more recent study, HIV positive MSM attending focus groups were asked about features and functions of mobile applications (apps) they believed keep them engaged with the apps on their smartphones (Horvath, Alemu, Danh, Baker, & Carrico, 2016). Consistent with theories of technology acceptance (Venkatesh & Bala, 2008), men in the study reported that the apps they used most often and for long periods of time were useful, easy to use, engaging (i.e., fun, visually engaging), credible, secure, and ones that they had control over (e.g., could easily change notifications or other features). Taken together, the results of these studies draw attention to two important points. First, that technology use is common among some PLWH, and therefore technology-based environments may be important venues to deliver interventions. Second, providing intervention in a technology-based environment will require considerations of both the advantages that such mediums provide (e.g., the ability to connect with other PLWH) as well as the potential concerns that PLWH have regarding technology (e.g., privacy concerns).

Technology-Based HIV Prevention Strategies: Promising Evidence and Clear Gaps

Meta-analyses of the efficacy of computer technology-based HIV prevention interventions showed a statistically significant impact of these interventions on sexual health knowledge, safer sex self-efficacy, safer-sex intentions, and condom use, suggesting that technology-based HIV prevention interventions have similar or higher efficacy than more traditional, face-to-face interventions (Bailey et al., 2012, Noar, Black, & Pierce, 2009). Technology-based HIV prevention approaches include computer and Internet-based, mobile app, chat room, text messaging, and social media interventions (for reviews see Noar & Willoughby, 2012; Simoni, Kutner, & Horvath, 2015; Sullivan, Jones, Kishore, & Stephenson, 2015). However, relatively few *face-to-face* interventions have been developed and evaluated for HIV positive MSM. For example, out of the nearly 100 evidence-based interventions for best practices for HIV prevention compiled by the CDC, only 15 target HIV positive persons; of those, 13 are delivered face to face (Centers for Disease Control and Prevention, 2016). With few notable exceptions (see below), most existing online or other technology-delivered HIV prevention interventions that have been rigorously tested do not specifically target PLWH (Bailey et al., 2010). Published randomized control trials (RCTs) of online HIV behavioral interventions targeting HIV negative MSM have shown reductions in one or more HIV risk behaviors (Bull, Pratte, Whitesell, Rietmeijer, & McFarlane, 2008; Carpenter, Stoner, Mikko, Dhanak, & Parsons, 2009; Hirshfield et al., 2012; Lelutiu-Weinberger et al., 2015; Mustanski, Garofalo, Monahan, Gratzer, & Andrews, 2013; Rosser et al., 2010), increases in HIV testing (Bauermeister et al., 2015; Blas et al., 2010), or short-term increases in knowledge, self-efficacy, and outcome expectancies (Bowen, Horvath, & Williams, 2007). However, other trials reported no changes in behavior (Bull, Lloyd, Rietmeijer, & McFarlane, 2004; Lau, Lau, Cheung, & Tsui, 2008).

In addition to Internet-based studies, reaching and engaging MSM of color for HIV prevention through mobile technology has also shown promise (Young et al., 2014). Preliminary data show that text messaging is an acceptable and viable method for reaching young Black men with prevention messages (Wright, Fortune, Juzang, & Bull, 2011) and that a sufficient proportion of this population can be retained in a text message intervention over at least 3 months (77%, although retention at 6 months was 65%; Fortune, Wright, Juzang, & Bull, 2010). Approaches that leverage commonly used social media platforms, such as Facebook, to deliver peer-delivered HIV information have been shown to be associated with a higher likelihood of getting tested for HIV and discussions of sexual behaviors online among mostly Black and Latino MSM (Huang, Marlin, Young, Medline, & Klausner, 2016; Young et al., 2014). These results indicate that technology-based approaches to HIV prevention intervention are promising, however, there continues to be a gap in extending these approaches to address the needs of PLWH (Noar & Willoughby, 2012). These gaps may be addressed through closer coordination of efforts between researchers and community-based organizations to develop and test technology-delivered interventions to address risk reduction strategies among PLWH, and through the prioritization of funding mechanisms by federal and state agencies to support technology-based approaches to prevention among high-risk PLWH.

Despite the dearth of research in this area, a few notable technology-based interventions have emerged that may address the prevention and healthcare needs of PLWH. These include interventions to teach HIV positive persons Internet information consumer skills (Kalichman et al., 2006); online, texting, and pager interventions to assist people living with HIV manage their health and adherence to antiretroviral medication (Gamage et al., 2011; Harris et al., 2010; Horvath, Carrico et al., 2013; Horvath, Oakes et al., 2013; Lester et al., 2010; for a review see Amico, 2015); and an Internet-based intervention to reduce HIV-related stigma (Adam et al., 2011). Thus, most technology-based interventions focus on helping PLWH to manage their HIV illness, rather than on reducing sexual risk.

There are recent efforts to include HIV positive MSM in technology-based sexual risk reduction interventions that also include HIV negative or unknown serostatus MSM. For example, although not exclusively targeted to PLWH, Hightow-Weidman and colleagues recently developed and reported the feasibility and acceptability of an online intervention to reduce sexual risk among young Black MSM, of whom 42% reported living with HIV (Hightow-Weidman et al., 2012). As described by the authors: "Key interactive features of the site include live chats with an HIV expert, interactive quizzes of varying levels of difficulty, personalized health and 'hook-up/sex' journals, and decision support tools for assessing and modifying risk behaviors (p. 911)." At the conclusion of the pilot study (50 men, half of whom were randomized to the intervention and the other half to control), high levels of 1- (90%) and 3-month (78%) follow-up assessment retention were attained, and intervention assigned participants reported high satisfaction and interest in the website and low levels of frustration with website features. Another technology-delivered online RCT study compared the effect of two videos and a HIV prevention webpage to a control condition to lower sexual risk taking among MSM, 25% of whom were either HIV positive or did not know their serostatus (Hirshfield et al., 2012). At follow-up, HIV positive men who received the videos reported significantly lower CAS and serodiscordant CAS compared to those in the control condition. Both the study by Hightow-Weidman et al., (2012), and a new online video RCT for suboptimally adherent HIV positive MSM (Hirshfield et al., 2016), are currently being tested in large-scale efficacy trials. In sum, studies that recruit HIV positive MSM in addition to men of other serostatus show evidence that technology-delivered interventions may reduce sexual risk, and should be explored in future research.

Several technology-facilitated interventions that focus exclusively on PLWH have been published, with encouraging findings. HIV positive MSM were asked to complete a computerized sexual risk assessment prior to their next HIV medical appointment (Chen et al., 2008). The results of the assessment were given to the provider to prompt discussions about sexual risk with their patients. Positive ratings were given by the majority of providers (79%) and patients (84%) regarding the quality of prevention services during the appointment, and providers reported feeling more confident in communicating prevention strategies with their patients. However, no information was collected on whether men reduced their sexual risk behavior as a result of the intervention. In a similar study (Bachmann et al., 2013), a printed hand-out from a computer-based assessment of HIV positive MSM's intention to change in one of three risk behaviors (condom use, reduction in sex partners, and HIV disclosure) were given to providers during the healthcare encounter to guide discussion about sexual risk reduction. In this single-condition trial, reductions in CAS with seroconcordant and serodiscordant sex partners and in the number of male sex partners in the prior 6 months were shown at post-intervention follow up. The "Positive Choice: Interactive Video Doctor intervention" (Gilbert et al., 2008) is administered to PLWH while they wait for their healthcare appointment. PLWH complete a computerized risk assessment, which is followed by a virtual doctor delivering tailored risk reduction messages. A printout of these messages was available to patients and provided to their healthcare provider to guide discussion about risk reduction. Among 471 PLWH randomized to intervention or control arm, 51% were MSM and most were Black or Hispanic/Latino. Significant reductions in CAS and condomless vaginal intercourse were shown at 3- and 6-month assessment time points compared to the control condition, as well as fewer casual sex partners at the 6-month follow-up assessment. Finally, "CARE+" is an individually delivered, computer-based counseling intervention with the goal of improving medication adherence and reducing sexual risk behavior among 239 PLWH (Kurth et al., 2014). Nearly three-quarters of the sample identified as a gay, bisexual or other MSM, and just over half were white. Compared to the control group, those receiving the CARE+ intervention demonstrated greater reductions in sexual risk (i.e., CAS or condom use with errors) at the 6- and 9-month assessment time points, as well as improved self-reported ART adherence.

Conclusions and Recommendations

Addressing the sexual, physical, and mental health needs of people living with HIV has received increasing attention in recent years, recognizing that reducing risk for transmission among persons already infected with the virus can have a larger impact on overall rates of HIV than focusing efforts on low or moderate risk uninfected individuals (Lasry, Sansom, Hicks, & Uzunangelov, 2012). Despite evidence that technology-mediated HIV risk reduction approaches are efficacious (Bailey et al., 2012), limited prevention interventions have been developed and rigorously tested exclusively for HIV positive populations (Horvath, Carrico et al., 2013; Horvath, Oakes et al., 2013).

Three conclusions are reached from this review of technology use, risk associated with online sex seeking, and current technology-based interventions for persons living with HIV. First, technology use is widespread among HIV positive populations who (much like other people living with chronic health conditions) are using technology as a resource to inform their medical care and connect with others who are living with HIV. Their experiences with, and beliefs about, technology provide invaluable information about best practices for designing interventions with a focus on HIV positive persons. However, people living with HIV are not a single homogenous group; rather, HIV status intersects with one or more identities (sexual orientation; gender; age; race and ethnicity; geographic residency) that will impact needs, preferences, and response to interventions. Therefore, inclusion of the target population in the development and testing of technology-based intervention approaches for PLWH is critical to design and implement effective interventions. This may take the form of community-based participatory research (Cashman et al., 2008; Rhodes et al., 2007), establishing a community advisory board, or conducting formative research prior to intervention development.

Second, even considering substantial methodological limitations of current studies of HIV risk behavior among HIV positive samples, studies consistently demonstrate high rates of HIV risk behavior among PLWH, particularly MSM. This may be in large part the result of broader social and cultural factors that influence PLWH at an individual level. Developing interventions that can reach and engage at-risk PLWH in their routine contexts and in a cost-effective manner are advantages of technology-based prevention approaches, and should be further developed. This review suggests that technology-mediated approaches targeting at-risk HIV positive persons may be enhanced by addressing issues of stigma, HIV status disclosure, personal responsibility, mental health problems, and substance use factors associated with increased risk for transmission. These complex issues may have more credibility and acceptability if they are rolled into interventions that also address the medical and social support needs of persons living with HIV.

Third, substantially more financial resources and institutional support are needed to develop and rigorously evaluate technology-based risk reduction approaches for PLWH, particularly those that target Black and Latino MSM, and to address critical questions that remain about these approaches (Noar, 2011; Sullivan et al., 2015). MSM of color are greatly underrepresented in intervention efforts, in contrast to the overrepresentation of MSM of color living with HIV (Wolitski et al., 2001). Failing to provide such support will result in a notable missed opportunity to improve the physical and mental well-being of PLWH through technology-based communication channels, as well as to reduce overall high rates of HIV infection among these populations (Simoni et al., 2015).

Numerous reviews of technology-based interventions note the vast opportunities that these approaches open for the HIV prevention field to address core needs of groups most affected and infected with HIV (Bailey et al., 2010; Chiasson et al., 2006; Noar & Willoughby, 2012; Sullivan et al., 2015). Despite this promise and evidence that PLWH are appropriate targets for intervention, we have collectively failed to take full advantage of technology-based approaches to HIV intervention. Despite the challenges that remain ahead, the time is right to invest in this future.

References

Adam, B. D., Murray, J., Ross, S., Oliver, J., Lincoln, S. G., & Rynard, V. (2011). ivstigma.com, an innovative web-supported stigma reduction intervention for gay and bisexual men. *Health Education Research, 26*(5), 795–807.

Amico, K. R. (2015). Evidence for technology interventions to promote ART adherence in adult populations: A review of the literature 2012–2015. *Current HIV/AIDS Reports*, 1–10. doi:10.1007/s11904-015-0286-4

Bachmann, L. H., Grimley, D. M., Gao, H., Aban, I., Chen, H., Raper, J. L., ... Hook, E. W. (2013). Impact of a computer-assisted, provider-delivered intervention on sexual risk behaviors in HIV-positive men who have sex with men (MSM) in a primary care setting. *AIDS Education and Prevention, 25*(2), 87–101. doi:10.1521/aeap.2013.25.2.87

Bailey, J. V., Murray, E., Rait, G., Mercer, C. H., Morris, R. W., Peacock, R., ... Nazareth, I. (2010). Interactive computer-based interventions for sexual health promotion. *Cochrane Database of Systematic Reviews, 9*, CD006483.

Bailey, J. V., Murray, E., Rait, G., Mercer, C. H., Morris, R. W., Peacock, R., ... Nazareth, I. (2012). Computer-based interventions for sexual health promotion: Systematic review and meta-analyses. *International Journal of STD & AIDS, 23*(6), 408–413.

Bancroft, J., Janssen, E., Strong, D., & Vukadinovic, Z. (2003). The relation between mood and sexuality in gay men. *Archives of Sexual Behavior, 32*(3), 231–242.

Bandura, A. (1999). Moral disengagement in the perpetration of inhumanities. *Personality and Social Psychology Review, 3*, 193–209.

Bandura, A. (2002). Selective moral disengagement in the exercise of moral agency. *Journal of Moral Education, 31*, 101–119.

Bauermeister, J. A., Pingel, E. S., Jadwin-Cakmak, L., Harper, G. W., Horvath, K., Weiss, G., & Dittus, P. (2015). Acceptability and preliminary efficacy of a tailored online HIV/STI testing intervention for young men who have sex with men: The get connected! Program. *AIDS and Behavior*. doi:10.1007/s10461-015-1009-y

Bech, M., & Kristensen, M. B. (2009). Differential response rates in postal and web-based surveys among older respondents. *Survey Research Methods, 3*, 1–6.

Beck, A., McNally, I., & Petrak, J. (2003). Psychosocial predictors of HIV/STI risk behaviours in a sample of homosexual men. *Sexually Transmitted Infections, 79*(2), 142–146.

Beck, J., & Rosenbaum, M. (1994). *Pursuit of ecstasy: The MDMA experience*. New York: State University of New York Press.

Benotsch, E., Kalichman, S., & Cage, M. (2002). Men who have met sex partners via the internet: Prevalence, predictors, and implications for HIV prevention. *Archives of Sexual Behavior, 31*(2), 177–183.

Berger, B. E., Ferrans, C. E., & Lashley, F. R. (2001). Measuring stigma in people with HIV: Psychometric assessment of the HIV stigma scale. *Research in Nursing & Health, 24*(6), 518–529.

Berry, M., Raymond, H. F., Kellogg, T., & McFarland, W. (2008). The internet, HIV serosorting and transmission risk among men who have sex with men, San Francisco. *AIDS, 22*(6), 787–789.

Birnbaum, M. (2004). Human research and data collection via the internet. *Annual Review of Psychology, 55*, 803–832.

Blas, M. M., Alva, I. E., Carcamo, C. P., Cabello, R., Goodreau, S. M., Kimball, A. M., & Kurth, A. E. (2010). Effect of an online video-based intervention to increase HIV testing in men who have sex with men in Peru. *PLoS One, 5*(5), e10448.

Bolding, G., Davis, M., Sherr, L., Hart, G., & Elford, J. (2004). Use of gay internet sites and views about online health promotion among men who have sex with men. *AIDS Care, 16*, 993–1001.

Bowen, A. M., Horvath, K., & Williams, M. L. (2007). A randomized control trial of internet-delivered HIV prevention targeting rural MSM. *Health Education Research, 22*(1), 120–127.

Bull, S., Lloyd, L., Rietmeijer, C., & McFarlane, M. (2004). Recruitment and retention of an online sample for an HIV prevention intervention targeting men who have sex with men: The smart sex quest project. *AIDS Care, 16*(8), 931–943.

Bull, S., McFarlane, M., & King, D. (2001). Barriers to STD/HIV prevention on the internet. *Health Education Research, 16*(6), 661–670.

Bull, S., Pratte, K., Whitesell, N., Rietmeijer, C., & McFarlane, M. (2008). Effects of an internet-based intervention for HIV prevention: The Youthnet Trials. *AIDS and Behavior, 13*(3), 474–487.

Bull, S. S., McFarlane, M., & Reitmeijer, C. (2001). HIV and sexually transmitted infection risk behaviors among men seeking sex with men on-line. *American Journal of Public Health, 91*(6), 988–999.

Camacho-Gonzalez, A. F., Wallins, A., Toledo, L., Murray, A., Gaul, Z., Sutton, M. Y., … Chakraborty, R. (2016). Risk factors for HIV transmission and barriers to HIV disclosure: Metropolitan Atlanta youth perspectives. *AIDS Patient Care and STDs, 30*(1), 18–24. doi:10.1089/apc.2015.0163

Carballo-Dieguez, A., Miner, M., Dolezal, C., Rosser, B. R., & Jacoby, S. (2006). Sexual negotiation, HIV-status disclosure, and sexual risk behavior among Latino men who use the internet to seek sex with other men. *Archives of Sexual Behavior, 35*(4), 473–481.

Carey, J. W., Mejia, R., Bingham, T., Ciesielski, C., Gelaude, D., Herbst, J. H., … Stall, R. (2009). Drug use, high-risk sex behaviors, and increased risk for recent HIV infection among men who have sex with men in Chicago and Los Angeles. *AIDS and Behavior, 13*(6), 1084–1096.

Carpenter, K. M., Stoner, S. A., Mikko, A. N., Dhanak, L. P., & Parsons, J. T. (2009). Efficacy of a web-based intervention to reduce sexual risk in men who have sex with men. *AIDS and Behavior.* doi:10.1007/s10461-009-9578-2

Cashman, S. B., Adeky, S., Allen, A. J., 3rd, Corburn, J., Israel, B. A., Montano, J., … Eng, E. (2008). The power and the promise: Working with communities to analyze data, interpret findings, and get to outcomes. *American Journal of Public Health, 98*(8), 1407–1417. doi:10.2105/ajph.2007.113571

Casper, R. C., Redmond, D. E., Jr., Katz, M. M., Schaffer, C. B., Davis, J. M., & Koslow, S. H. (1985). Somatic symptoms in primary affective disorder. Presence and relationship to the classification of depression. *Archives of General Psychiatry, 42*(11), 1098–1104.

Centers for Disease Control and Prevention. (2003). Advancing HIV prevention: New strategies for a changing epidemic--United States, 2003. *Morbidity and Mortality Weekly Report, 52*(15), 329–332.

Centers for Disease Control and Prevention. (2016). *Compendium of evidence-based interventions and best practices for HIV prevention.* Retrieved from https://www.cdc.gov/hiv/research/interventionresearch/compendium/rr/index.html.

Chen, H. T., Grimley, D. M., Waithaka, Y., Aban, I. B., Hu, J., & Bachmann, L. H. (2008). A process evaluation of the implementation of a computer-based, health provider-delivered HIV-prevention intervention for HIV-positive men who have sex with men in the primary care setting. *AIDS Care, 20*(1), 51–60.

Chiasson, M., Hirshfield, S., Humberstone, M., DiFilippi, J., Koblin, B., & Remien, R. (2005). Increased high risk sexual behavior after September 11 in men who have sex with men: An internet survey. *Archives of Sexual Behavior, 34*(5), 527–535. doi:10.1007/s10508-005-6278-5

Chiasson, M., Hirshfield, S., Humberstone, M., Remien, R., Wolitski, R., & Wong, T. (2005). *A comparison of on-line and off-line risk among men who have sex with men.* Conference on Retroviruses and Opportunistic Infections.

Chiasson, M., Parsons, J., Tesoriero, J., Carballo-Dieguez, A., Hirshfield, S., & Remien, R. (2006). HIV behavioral research online. *Journal of Urban Health, 83*(1), 73–85.

Chiasson, M., Shuchat Shaw, F., Humberstone, M., Hirshfield, S., & Hartel, D. (2009). Increased HIV disclosure three months after an online video intervention for men who have sex with men (MSM). *AIDS Care, 21*, 1081–1089.

Chiasson, M. A., Hirshfield, S., Remien, R. H., Humberstone, M., Wong, T., & Wolitski, R. J. (2007). A comparison of on-line and off-line sexual risk in men who have sex with men: An event-based on-line survey. *Journal of Acquired Immune Deficiency Syndromes, 44*(2), 235–243.

Cochran, S., & Mays, V. (2000). Relation between psychiatric syndromes and behaviorally defined sexual orientation in a sample of the US population. *American Journal of Epidemiology, 151*, 516–523.

Cochran, S., Sullivan, J., & Mays, V. (2003). Prevalence of mental disorders, psychological distress, and mental health services use among lesbian, gay, and bisexual adults in the United States. *Journal of Consulting and Clinical Psychology, 71*(1), 53–61.

Cohen, M. S., Chen, Y. Q., McCauley, M., Gamble, T., Hosseinipour, M. C., Kumarasamy, N., ... Fleming, T. R. (2011). Prevention of HIV-1 infection with early antiretroviral therapy. *New England Journal of Medicine, 365*(6), 493–505.

Cohen, M. S., Chen, Y. Q., McCauley, M., Gamble, T., Hosseinipour, M. C., Kumarasamy, N., ... Godbole, S. V. (2016). Antiretroviral therapy for the prevention of HIV-1 transmission. *New England Journal of Medicine, 375*(9), 830–839.

Colfax, G., & Guzman, R. (2006). Club drugs and HIV infection: A review. *Clinical Infectious Diseases, 42*(10), 1463–1469.

Colfax, G., Shoptaw, S., Colfax, G., & Shoptaw, S. (2005). The methamphetamine epidemic: Implications for HIV prevention and treatment. [Review]. *Current HIV/AIDS Reports, 2*(4), 194–199.

Corbett, T. (2016). *New to Grindr profiles: HIV status and last test date fields*. Retrieved from http://www.grindr.com/blog/new-grindr-profiles-hiv-status-last-test date/.

Courtenay-Quirk, C., Horvath, K. J., Ding, H., Fisher, H., McFarlane, M., Kachur, R., ... Harwood, E. (2010). Perceptions of HIV-related websites among persons recently diagnosed with HIV. *AIDS Patient Care and STDs, 24*(2), 105–115.

Crepaz, N., & Marks, G. (2002). Towards an understanding of sexual risk behavior in people living with HIV: A review of social, psychological, and medical findings. *AIDS, 16*(2), 135–149.

Crepaz, N., Marks, G., Liau, A., Mullins, M. M., Aupont, L. W., Marshall, K. J., ... Wolitski, R. J. (2009). Prevalence of unprotected anal intercourse among HIV-diagnosed MSM in the United States: A meta-analysis. *AIDS, 23*(13), 1617–1629.

Denscombe, M. (2009). Item non-response rates: A comparison of online and paper questionnaires. *International Journal of Social Research Methodology, 12*, 281–291.

Dew, M., Becker, J., Sanchez, J., Caldararo, R., Lopez, O., Wess, J., ... Banks, G. (1997). Prevalence and predictors of depressive, anxiety and substance use disorders in HIV-infected and uninfected men: A longitudinal evaluation. *Psychological Medicine, 27*, 395–409.

Downing, M., Chiasson, M. A., & Hirshfield, S. (2016). Recent anxiety symptoms and drug use associated with STI diagnosis among an online U.S. sample of men who have sex with men. *Journal of Health Psychology, 21*(12), 2799–2812.

Duru, O. K., Collins, R. L., Ciccarone, D. H., Morton, S. C., Stall, R., Beckman, R., ... Kanouse, D. E. (2006). Correlates of sex without serostatus disclosure among a national probability sample of HIV patients. *AIDS and Behavior, 10*(5), 495–507.

Elford, J., Bolding, G., Davis, M., Sherr, L., & Hart, G. (2003). *Web-based behavioural surveillance among men who have sex with men: A comparison of online and offline samples in London, UK*. Paper presented at the STD/HIV prevention and the Internet 2003, Washington, DC.

Fortune, T., Wright, E., Juzang, I., & Bull, S. (2010). Recruitment, enrollment and retention of young black men for HIV prevention research: Experiences from the 411 for safe text project. *Contemporary Clinical Trials, 31*(2), 151–156.

Frosch, D., Shoptaw, S., Huber, A., Rawson, R. A., & Ling, W. (1996). Sexual HIV risk and gay and bisexual methamphetamine abusers. *Journal of Substance Abuse Treatment, 13*, 483–386.

Gamage, D. G., Sidat, M., Read, T., Cummings, R., Bradshaw, C. S., Howley, K., ... Fairley, C. K. (2011). Evaluation of health map: A patient-centred web-based service for supporting HIV-infected patients. *Sexual Health, 8*(2), 194–198.

Gilbert, P., Ciccarone, D., Gansky, S. A., Bangsberg, D. R., Clanon, K., McPhee, S. J., ... Gerbert, B. (2008). Interactive "video doctor" counseling reduces drug and sexual risk behaviors among HIV-positive patients in diverse outpatient settings. *PLoS One, 3*(4), e1988. doi:10.1371/journal.pone.0001988

Gilman, S., Cochran, S., Mays, V., Hughes, M., Ostrow, D., & Kessler, R. (2001). Risk of psychiatric disorders among individuals reporting same-sex sexual partners in the National Comorbidity Survey. *American Journal of Public Health, 91*(6), 933–939.

Goedel, W. C., & Duncan, D. T. (2015). Geosocial-Networking app usage patterns of gay, bisexual, and other men who have sex with men: Survey among users of Grindr, a mobile dating app. *JMIR Public Health and Surveillance, 1*(1), e4. doi:10.2196/publichealth.4353

Goedel, W. C., & Duncan, D. T. (2016). Contextual factors in geosocial-networking smartphone application use and engagement in condomless anal intercourse among gay, bisexual, and other men who have sex with men who use Grindr. *Sexual Health*. doi:10.1071/sh16008

Golden, M. R., Wood, R. W., Buskin, S. E., Fleming, M., & Harrington, R. D. (2007). Ongoing risk behavior among persons with HIV in medical care. *AIDS and Behavior, 11*(5), 726–735.

Gorbach, P. M., Drumright, L. N., Daar, E. S., & Little, S. J. (2006). Transmission behaviors of recently HIV-infected men who have sex with men. *Journal of Acquired Immune Deficiency Syndromes, 42*(1), 80–85.

Greenwood, G., White, E., Page-Shafer, K., Bein, E., Osmond, D., Paul, J., & Stall, R. (2001). Correlates of heavy substance use among young gay and bisexual men: The San Francisco Young Men's Health Study. *Drug and Alcohol Dependence, 61*(2), 105–112.

Grov, C. (2011). HIV risk and substance use in men who have sex with men surveyed in bathhouses, bars/clubs, and on Craigslist.org: Venue of recruitment matters. *AIDS and Behavior, 16*(4), 807–817.

Grov, C., Golub, S. A., & Parsons, J. T. (2010). HIV status differences in venues where highly sexually active gay and bisexual men meet sex partners: Results from a pilot study. *AIDS Education and Prevention, 22*(6), 496–508.

Grov, C., Hirshfield, S., Remien, R. H., Humberstone, M., & Chiasson, M. A. (2011). Exploring the venue's role in risky sexual behavior among gay and bisexual men: An event-level analysis from a National Online Survey in the U.S. *Archives of Sexual Behavior, 42*(2), 291–302.

Grov, C., Parsons, J. T., & Bimbi, D. S. (2007). Sexual risk behavior and venues for meeting sex partners: An intercept survey of gay and bisexual men in LA and NYC. *AIDS and Behavior, 11*(6), 915–926.

Groves, R. M., & Peytcheva, E. (2008). The impact of nonresponse rates on nonresponse bias. *Public Opinion Quarterly, 72*(2), 167–189.

Halkitis, P., Parsons, J., & Stirratt, M. (2001). A double epidemic: Crystal methamphetamine drug use in relation to HIV transmission among gay men. *Journal of Homosexuality, 41*(2), 17–35.

Halkitis, P., Parsons, J., & Wilton, L. (2003). Barebacking among gay and bisexual men in New York City: Explanations for the emergence of intentional unsafe behavior. *Archives of Sexual Behavior, 32*(4), 351–357.

Halkitis, P. N., & Parsons, J. T. (2003). Intentional unsafe sex (barebacking) among HIV-positive gay men who seek sexual partners on the Internet. *AIDS Care, 15*(3), 367–378.

Hall, H. I., Holtgrave, D. R., Tang, T., & Rhodes, P. (2013). HIV transmission in the United States: considerations of viral load, risk behavior, and health disparities. *AIDS and Behavior, 17*(5), 1632–1636. doi:10.1007/s10461-013-0426-z

Harawa, N. T., Williams, J. K., Ramamurthi, H. C., Manago, C., Avina, S., & Jones, M. (2008). Sexual behavior, sexual identity, and substance abuse among low-income bisexual and non-gay-identifying African American men who have sex with men. *Archives of Sexual Behavior, 37*(5), 748–762. doi:10.1007/s10508-008-9361-x

Harris, L. T., Lehavot, K., Huh, D., Yard, S., Andrasik, M. P., Dunbar, P. J., & Simoni, J. M. (2010). Two-way text messaging for health behavior change among human immunodeficiency virus-positive individuals. *Telemedicine Journal and E-Health, 16*(10), 1024–1029.

Hatfield, L. A., Horvath, K. J., Jacoby, S. M., Simon Rosser, B. R., Hatfield, L. A., Horvath, K. J., & Jacoby, S. M. (2009). Comparison of substance use and risky sexual behavior among a diverse sample of urban, HIV-positive men who have sex with men. *Journal of Addictive Diseases, 28*(3), 208–218.

Hightow-Weidman, L. B., Pike, E., Fowler, B., Matthews, D. M., Kibe, J., McCoy, R., & Adimora, A. A. (2012). HealthMpowerment.org: Feasibility and acceptability of delivering an internet intervention to young black men who have sex with men. *AIDS Care, 24*(7), 910–920.

Hirshfield, S., Chiasson, M. A., Joseph, H., Scheinmann, R., Johnson, W. D., Remien, R. H., ... Margolis, A. D. (2012). An online randomized controlled trial evaluating HIV prevention digital media interventions for men who have sex with men. *PLoS One, 7*(10), e46252.

Hirshfield, S., Downing, M. J., Parsons, J. T., Grov, C., Gordon, R. J., Houang, S. T., ... Chiasson, M. A. (2016). Developing a video-based randomized controlled trial for HIV-positive gay, bisexual and other men who have sex with men. *JMIR Research Protocols, 5*(2), e125.

Hirshfield, S., Grov, C., Parsons, J., Anderson, I., & Chiasson, M. A. (2015). Social media use and HIV transmission risk behavior among ethnically diverse HIV-positive men who have sex with men: Results of an online study in three U.S. States. *Archives of Sexual Behavior, 44*(7), 1969–1978.

Hirshfield, S., Remien, R., & Chiasson, M. (2006). Crystal methamphetamine use among men who have sex with men: Results from two National Online Studies. *Journal of Gay and Lesbian Psychotherapy, 10*, 85–93.

Hirshfield, S., Remien, R., Humberstone, M., Walavalkar, I., & Chiasson, M. (2004a). Substance use and high-risk sex among men who have sex with men: A national online study in the USA. *AIDS Care, 16*(8), 1036–1047.

Hirshfield, S., Remien, R. H., Walavalkar, I., & Chiasson, M. A. (2004b). Crystal methamphetamine use predicts incident STD infection among men who have sex with men recruited online: A nested case-control study. *Journal of Medical Internet Research, 6*, e41.

Hirshfield, S., Schrimshaw, E. W., Stall, R., Margolis, A. D., Downing, M. J., & Chiasson, M. A. (2015). Drug use, sexual risk, and syndemic production among MSM who engage in group sex encounters. *American Journal of Public Health*, e1–e10.

Hirshfield, S., Wolitski, R. J., Chiasson, M. A., Remien, R. H., Humberstone, M., & Wong, T. (2008). Screening for depressive symptoms in an online sample of men who have sex with men. *AIDS Care, 20*, 904–910.

Horvath, K. J., Carrico, A. W., Simoni, J., Boyer, E., Amico, K. R., & Petroll, A. E. (2013). Engagement in HIV medical care and technology use among stimulant-using and nonstimulant-using men who have sex with men. *AIDS Research & Treatment, 2013*, 121352. doi:10.1155/2013/121352

Horvath, K. J., Danilenko, G., Williams, M., Simoni, J., Amico, K. R., Oakes, J. M., & Simon Rosser, B. R. (2012). Technology use and reasons to participate in social networking health websites among people living with HIV in the US. *AIDS and Behavior, 16*(4), 900–910.

Horvath, K. J., Nygaard, K., Danilenko, G., Goknur, S., Michael Oakes, J., & Simon Rosser, B. (2012). Strategies to retain participants in a longterm HIV prevention randomized controlled trial: Lessons from the MINTS-II study. *AIDS and Behavior, 16*(2), 469–479.

Horvath, K. J., Alemu, D., Danh, T., Baker, J. V., & Carrico, A. W. (2016). Creating effective mobile phone apps to optimize antiretroviral therapy adherence: Perspectives from stimulant-using HIV-positive men who have sex with men. *JMIR Mhealth Uhealth, 4*(2), e48. doi:10.2196/mhealth.5287

Horvath, K. J., Michael Oakes, J., Simon Rosser, B. R., Danilenko, G., Vezina, H., Rivet Amico, K., ... Simoni, J. (2013). Feasibility, acceptability and preliminary efficacy of an online peer-to-peer social support ART adherence intervention. *AIDS and Behavior, 17*(6), 2031–2044.

Horvath, K. J., Oakes, J. M., & Rosser, B. R. S. (2008). Sexual negotiation and HIV serodisclosure among men who have sex with men with their online and offline partners. *Journal of Urban Health, 85*(5), 744–758.

Horvath, K. J., Rosser, B., & Remafedi, G. (2008). Sexual risk taking among young internet-using men who have sex with men. *American Journal of Public Health, 98*(6), 1059–1067.

Horvath, K. J., Smolenski, D., Iantaffi, A., Grey, J. A., & Rosser, B. R. (2012). Discussions of viral load in negotiating sexual episodes with primary and casual partners among men who have sex with men. *AIDS Care, 24*(8), 1052–1055.

Huang, E., Marlin, R. W., Young, S. D., Medline, A., & Klausner, J. D. (2016). Using Grindr, a smartphone social-networking application, to increase HIV self-testing among black and

Latino men who have sex with men in Los Angeles, 2014. *AIDS Education and Prevention*, *28*(4), 341–350. doi:10.1521/aeap.2016.28.4.341

Johnson, M. O., Dilworth, S. E., Neilands, T. B., Chesney, M. A., Rotheram-Borus, M. J., Remien, R. H., ... Morin, S. F. (2008). Predictors of attrition among high risk HIV-infected participants enrolled in a multi-site prevention trial. *AIDS and Behavior*, *12*(6), 974–977.

Kalichman, S. C., Cherry, C., Cain, D., Pope, H., & Kalichman, M. (2005). Psychosocial and behavioral correlates of seeking sex partners on the internet among HIV-positive men. *Annals of Behavioral Medicine*, *30*(3), 243–250.

Kalichman, S. C., Cherry, C., Cain, D., Pope, H., Kalichman, M., Eaton, L., ... Benotsch, E. G. (2006). Internet-based health information consumer skills intervention for people living with HIV/AIDS. *Journal of Consulting and Clinical Psychology*, *74*(3), 545–554.

Kalichman, S. C., & Hunter, T. L. (1992). The disclosure of celebrity HIV infection: Its effects on public attitudes. *American Journal of Public Health*, *82*(10), 1374–1376.

Kalichman, S. C., Rompa, D., & Cage, M. (2000). Sexually transmitted infections among HIV seropositive men and women. *Sexually Transmitted Infections*, *76*(5), 350–354.

Kelly, J. A., Murphy, D. A., Bahr, G. R., Koob, J. J., Morgan, M. G., Kalichman, S. C., ... St Lawrence, J. S. (1993). Factors associated with severity of depression and high-risk sexual behavior among persons diagnosed with human immunodeficiency virus (HIV) infection. *Health Psychology*, *12*(3), 215–219.

Kennedy, S., Dickens, S., Eisfeld, B., & Bagby, R. (1999). Sexual dysfunction before antidepressant therapy in major depression. *Journal of Affective Disorders*, *56*, 201–208.

Khosropour, C. M. (2011). *Retention and HIV testing of MSM enrolled in a 12-month online study*. Paper presented at the Sex Tech Conference, San Francisco, CA. Retrieved from http://www.slideshare.net/isisinc/retension-and-hivtestingkhosropour.

Kilmarx, P. H., & Mermin, J. (2012). Prevention with people with HIV in the United States: The nexus of HIV prevention and treatment. *Journal of Acquired Immune Deficiency Syndromes*, *60*(3), 219–220.

Kim, A., Kent, C., McFarland, W., & Klausner, J. (2001). Cruising on the Internet highway. *Journal of Acquired Immune Deficiency Syndrome*, *28*(1), 89–93.

Kipke, M., Kubicek, K., Weiss, G., Wong, C., Lopez, D., Iverson, E., & Ford, W. (2007). The health and health behaviors of young men who have sex with men. *Journal of Adolescent Health*, *40*, 342–350.

Klausner, J., Wolf, W., Fischer-Ponce, L., Zolt, I., & Katz, M. (2000). Tracing a syphilis outbreak through cyberspace. [see comment]. *JAMA*, *284*(4), 447–449.

Klitzman, R., Exner, T., Correale, J., Kirshenbaum, S. B., Remien, R., Ehrhardt, A. A., ... Charlebois, E. (2007). It's not just what you say: Relationships of HIV dislosure and risk reduction among MSM in the post-HAART era. *AIDS Care*, *19*(6), 749–756.

Kraut, R., Patterson, M., Lundmark, V., Kiesler, S., Mukopadhyay, T., & Scherlis, W. (1998). Internet paradox. A social technology that reduces social involvement and psychological well-being? *American Psychologist*, *53*(9), 1017–1031.

Kremer, H., & Ironson, G. (2007). People living with HIV: Sources of information on antiretroviral treatment and preferences for involvement in treatment decision-making. *European Journal of Medical Research*, *12*(1), 34–42.

Kurth, A. E., Spielberg, F., Cleland, C. M., Lambdin, B., Bangsberg, D. R., Frick, P. A., ... Holmes, K. K. (2014). Computerized counseling reduces HIV-1 viral load and sexual transmission risk: Findings from a randomized controlled trial. *Journal of Acquired Immune Deficiency Syndromes: JAIDS*, *65*(5), 611–620. doi:10.1097/qai.0000000000000100

Kwak, N., & Radler, B. (2002). A comparison between mail and web surveys: Response pattern, respondent profile, and data quality. *Journal of Official Statistics*, *18*(2), 257–273.

Landovitz, R. J., Tseng, C. H., Weissman, M., Haymer, M., Mendenhall, B., Rogers, K., ... Shoptaw, S. (2012). Epidemiology, sexual risk behavior, and HIV prevention practices of men who have sex with men using GRINDR in Los Angeles, California. *Journal of Urban Health*, *90*(4), 729–739.

Lasry, A., Sansom, S. L., Hicks, K. A., & Uzunangelov, V. (2012). Allocating HIV prevention funds in the United States: Recommendations from an optimization model. *PLoS One*, *7*(6), e37545.

Lau, J. T., Lau, M., Cheung, A., & Tsui, H. Y. (2008). A randomized controlled study to evaluate the efficacy of an Internet-based intervention in reducing HIV risk behaviors among men who have sex with men in Hong Kong. *AIDS Care*, *20*(7), 820–828.

Lelutiu-Weinberger, C., Pachankis, J. E., Gamarel, K. E., Surace, A., Golub, S. A., & Parsons, J. T. (2015). Feasibility, acceptability, and preliminary efficacy of a live-chat social media intervention to reduce HIV risk among young men who have sex with men. *AIDS and Behavior*, *19*(7), 1214–1227. doi:10.1007/s10461-014-0911-z

Lester, R. T., Ritvo, P., Mills, E. J., Kariri, A., Karanja, S., Chung, M. H., ... Plummer, F. A. (2010). Effects of a mobile phone short message service on antiretroviral treatment adherence in Kenya (WelTel Kenya1): A randomised trial. *The Lancet*, *376*(9755), 1838–1845.

Lewis, L., & Ross, M. (1995). *A select body: The gay dance party subculture and the HIV/AIDS pandemic*. New York: Cassell.

Lewis, M. A., Uhrig, J. D., Ayala, G., & Stryker, J. (2011). Reaching men who have sex with men for HIV prevention messaging with new media: Recommendations from an expert consultation. *Annals of the Forum for Collaborative HIV Research*, *13*(3), 11–18.

Lewnard, J. A., & Berrang-Ford, L. (2014). Internet-based partner selection and risk for unprotected anal intercourse in sexual encounters among men who have sex with men: A meta-analysis of observational studies. *Sexually Transmitted Infections*, *90*, 290–296.

Liau, A., Millett, G., & Marks, G. (2006). Meta-analytic examination of online sex-seeking and sexual risk behavior among men who have sex with men. *Sexually Transmitted Diseases*, *33*(9), 576–584.

Link, M. W., & Mokdad, A. H. (2005). Alternative modes for health surveillance surveys: An experiment with web, mail, and telephone. *Epidemiology*, *16*(5), 701–704.

Margolis, A. D., Joseph, H., Hirshfield, S., Chiasson, M. A., Belcher, L., & Purcell, D. W. (2014). Anal intercourse without condoms among HIV-positive men who have sex with men recruited from a sexual networking web site, United States. *Sexually Transmitted Diseases*, *41*, 749–755.

Marks, G., Bingman, C. R., & Duval, T. S. (1998). Negative affect and unsafe sex in HIV-positive men. *AIDS and Behavior*, *2*(2), 89–99.

Marks, G., & Crepaz, N. (2001). HIV-positive men's sexual practices in the context of self-disclosure of HIV status. *Journal of Acquired Immune Deficiency Syndromes*, *27*(1), 79–85.

Mathew, R. J., & Weinman, M. L. (1982). Sexual dysfunctions in depression. *Archives of Sexual Behavior*, *11*(4), 323–328.

Mays, V. M., Cochran, S. D., & Zamudio, A. (2004). HIV prevention research: Are we meeting the needs of African American men who have sex with men? *Journal of Black Psychology*, *30*(1), 78–105.

McFarlane, M., Bull, S., & Rietmeijer, C. (2000). The Internet as a newly emerging risk environment for sexually transmitted diseases. *JAMA*, *284*(4), 443–446.

McFarlane, M., Bull, S. S., & Reitmeijer, C. A. (2000). The Internet as a newly emerging risk environment for sexually transmitted diseases. *Journal of the American Medical Association*, *284*(4), 443–446.

Mckirnan, D., Ostrow, D., & Hope, B. (1996). Sex, drugs and escape: A psychological model of HIV-risk sexual behaviours. *AIDS Care*, *8*(6), 655–659.

McKirnan, D., Vanable, P., Ostrow, D., & Hope, B. (2001). Expectancies of sexual "escape" and sexual risk among drug and alcohol-involved gay and bisexual men. *Journal of Substance Abuse*, *13*(1–2), 137–154.

Mettey, A., Crosby, R., DiClemente, R., & Holtgrave, D. (2003). Associations between Internet sex seeking and STI associated risk behaviours among men who have sex with men. *Sexually Transmitted Infections*, *79*(6), 466–468.

Mills, T., Paul, J., Stall, R., Pollack, L., Canchola, J., Chang, Y., ... Catania, J. (2004). Distress and depression in men who have sex with men: The urban Men's health study. *American Journal of Psychiatry*, *161*, 278–285.

Mimiaga, M. J., Fair, A. D., Mayer, K. H., Koenen, K., Gortmaker, S., Tetu, A. M., ... Safren, S. A. (2008). Experiences and sexual behaviors of HIV-infected MSM who acquired HIV in the context of crystal methamphetamine use. *AIDS Education and Prevention*, *20*(1), 30–41.

Morgan, C., & Cotten, S. (2003). The relationship between Internet activities and depressive symptoms in a sample of college freshmen. *Cyberpsychology & Behavior*, *6*(2), 133–142.

Mustanski, B., Garofalo, R., Monahan, C., Gratzer, B., & Andrews, R. (2013). Feasibility, acceptability, and preliminary efficacy of an online HIV prevention program for diverse young men who have sex with men: The keep it up! Intervention. *AIDS and Behavior, 17*(9), 2999–3012. doi:10.1007/s10461-013-0507-z

Mustanski, B. S. (2007). Are sexual partners met online associated with HIV/STI risk behaviours? Retrospective and daily diary data in conflict. *AIDS Care, 19*(6), 822–827.

Newman, J., Des Jarlais, D., Turner, C., Gribble, J., Cooley, P., & Paone, D. (2002). The differential effects of face-to-face and computer interview modes. *American Journal of Public Health, 92*, 294–297.

Noar, S. M. (2011). Computer technology-based interventions in HIV prevention: State of the evidence and future directions for research. *AIDS Care, 23*(5), 525–533.

Noar, S. M., Black, H. G., & Pierce, L. B. (2009). Efficacy of computer technology-based HIV prevention interventions: A meta-analysis. *AIDS, 23*(1), 107–115.

Noar, S. M., & Willoughby, J. F. (2012). eHealth interventions for HIV prevention. *AIDS Care, 24*(8), 945–952.

Nodin, N., Valera, P., Ventuneac, A., Maynard, E., & Carballo-Diéguez, A. (2011). The Internet profiles of men who have sex with men within bareback websites. *Culture, Health & Sexuality, 13*(9), 1015–1029.

O'Leary, A., Horvath, K., & Simon Rosser, B. R. (2012). Associations between partner-venue specific personal responsibility beliefs and transmission risk behavior by HIV-positive men who have sex with men (MSM). *AIDS and Behavior, 1–7.*

O'Leary, A., & Wolitski, R. J. (2009). Moral agency and the sexual transmission of HIV. *Psychological Bulletin, 135*(3), 478–494.

Orellana, E. R., Picciano, J. F., Roffman, R. A., Swanson, F., & Kalichman, S. C. (2006). Correlates of nonparticipation in an HIV prevention program for MSM. *AIDS Education and Prevention, 18*(4), 348–361.

Ostergren, J. E., Rosser, B. R. S., & Horvath, K. J. (2010). Reasons for non-use of condoms among men who have sex with men: A comparison of receptive and insertive role in sex and online and offline meeting venue. *Culture, Health & Sexuality, 13*(2), 123–140.

Parsons, J. T., Halkitis, P. N., Wolitski, R. J., & Gomez, C. A. (2003). Correlates of sexual risk behaviors among HIV-positive men who have sex with men. *AIDS Education and Prevention, 15*(5), 383–400.

Parsons, J. T., Schrimshaw, E. W., Wolitski, R. J., Halkitis, P. N., Purcell, D. W., Hoff, C. C., & Gomez, C. A. (2005). Sexual harm reduction practices of HIV-seropositive gay and bisexual men: Serosorting, strategic positioning, and withdrawal before ejaculation. *AIDS, 19*(Suppl 1), S13–S25.

Parsons, J. T., Severino, J., Nanin, J., Punzalan, J. C., von Sternberg, K., Missildine, W., & Frost, D. (2006). Positive, negative, unknown: Assumptions of HIV status among HIV-positive men who have sex with men. *AIDS Education and Prevention, 18*(2), 139–149.

Pennise, M., Inscho, R., Herpin, K., Owens, J., Jr., Bedard, B. A., Weimer, A. C., & Kennedy, B. S. (2015). Using smartphone apps in STD interviews to find sexual partners. *Public Health Reports, 130*, 245–252.

Pequegnat, W., Rosser, B. R., Bowen, A. M., Bull, S. S., Diclemente, R. J., Bockting, W. O., … Zimmerman, R. (2007). Conducting Internet-based HIV/STD prevention survey research: Considerations in design and evaluation. *AIDS and Behavior, 11*(4), 505–521.

Perlis, T. E., Des Jarlais, D., Friedman, S., Arasteh, K., & Turner, C. (2004). Audio-computerized self-interviewing versus face-to-face interviewing for research data collection at drug abuse treatment programs. *Addiction, 99*, 885–896.

Pew Research Center. (2011). *Health topics: 80% of Internet users look for health information online.* Retrieved December 9, 2016 from http://www.pewinternet.org/files/old-media//Files/Reports/2011/PIP_Health_Topics.pdf.

Pew Research Center. (2014a). *Internet user demographics.* Retrieved from http://www.pewinternet.org/data-trend/internet-use/latest-stats/.

Pew Research Center. (2014b). *Cell phone and smartphone ownership demographics.* Retrieved from http://www.pewinternet.org/data-trend/mobile/cell-phone-and-smartphone-ownership-demographics/.

Phillips, G., Grov, C., & Mustanski, B. (2015). Engagement in group sex among geosocial networking mobile application-using men who have sex with men. *Sexual Health*, *12*(6), 495–500.

Plankey, M. W., Ostrow, D. G., Stall, R., Cox, C., Li, X., Peck, J. A., ... Jacobson, L. P. (2007). The relationship between methamphetamine and popper use and risk of HIV seroconversion in the multicenter AIDS cohort study. *Journal of Acquired Immune Deficiency Syndromes: JAIDS*, *45*(1), 85–92.

Poppen, P., Reisen, C., Zea, M., Bianchi, F., & Echeverry, J. (2004). Predictors of unprotected anal intercourse among HIV-positive Latino gay and bisexual men. *AIDS and Behavior*, *8*(4), 379–389.

Rabkin, J., McElhiney, M., & Ferrando, S. (2004). Mood and substance use disorders in older adults with HIV/AIDS: Methodological issues and preliminary evidence. *AIDS*, *18*(Suppl 1), S43–S48.

Radcliffe, J., Doty, N., Hawkins, L. A., Gaskins, C. S., Beidas, R., & Rudy, B. J. (2010). Stigma and sexual health risk in HIV-positive African American young men who have sex with men. *AIDS Patient Care and STDs*, *24*(8), 493–499.

Rajasingham, R., Mimiaga, M. J., White, J. M., Pinkston, M. M., Baden, R. P., & Mitty, J. A. (2012). A systematic review of behavioral and treatment outcome studies among HIV-infected men who have sex with men who abuse crystal methamphetamine. *AIDS Patient Care and STDs*, *26*(1), 36–52.

Rendina, H. J., Jimenez, R. H., Grov, C., Ventuneac, A., & Parsons, J. T. (2014). Patterns of lifetime and recent HIV testing among men who have sex with men in New York City who use Grindr. *AIDS and Behavior*, *18*(1), 41–49. doi:10.1007/s10461-013-0573-2

Rhodes, S. D., Hergenrather, K. C., Duncan, J., Ramsey, B., Yee, L. J., & Wilkin, A. M. (2007). Using community-based participatory research to develop a chat room based HIV prevention intervention for gay men. *Progress in Community Health Partnerships*, *1*(2), 175–184.

Rietmeijer, C., Bull, S., McFarlane, M., Patnaik, J., & Douglas, J., Jr. (2002). Risks and benefits of the Internet for populations at risk for sexually transmitted infections (STIs). *Sexually Transmitted Diseases*, *30*, 15–19.

Rietmeijer, C. A., Bull, S. S., & McFarlane, M. (2001). Sex and the Internet. *AIDS*, *15*, 1433–1434.

Roffman, R. A., Klepsch, R., Wertz, J. S., Simpson, E. E., & Stephens, R. S. (1993). Predictors of attrition from an outpatient marijuana-dependence counseling program. *Addictive Behaviors*, *18*(5), 553–566.

Rosenberg, E. S., Khosropour, C. M., & Sullivan, P. S. (2012). High prevalence of sexual concurrency and concurrent unprotected anal intercourse across racial/ethnic groups among a national, Web-based study of men who have sex with men in the United States. *Sexually Transmitted Diseases*, *39*(10), 741–746.

Ross, M. W., Rosser, B. R., & Stanton, J. (2004). Beliefs about cybersex and Internet-mediated sex of Latino men who have Internet sex with men: Relationships with sexual practices in cybersex and in real life. *AIDS Care*, *16*(8), 1002–1011.

Ross, M. W., Rosser, B. R., Stanton, J., & Konstan, J. (2004). Characteristics of Latino men who have sex with men on the Internet who complete and drop out of an Internet-based sexual behavior survey. *AIDS Education and Prevention*, *16*(6), 526–537.

Ross, M. W., Rosser, B. R. S., McCurdy, S., & Feldman, J. (2007). The advantages and limitations of seeking sex online: A comparison of reasons given for online and offline sexual liaisons by men who have sex with men. *Journal of Sex Research*, *44*(1), 59–71.

Rosser, B., Miner, M. H., Bockting, W. O., Ross, M. W., Konstan, J., Gurak, L., ... Coleman, E. (2009). HIV risk and the Internet: Results of the Men's INTernet Sex (MINTS) Study. *AIDS and Behavior*, *13*(4), 746–756.

Rosser, B., Oakes, J., Horvath, K., Konstan, J., Danilenko, G., & Peterson, J. (2009). HIV sexual risk behavior by men who use the Internet to seek sex with men: Results of the Men's INTernet Sex Study-II (MINTS-II). *AIDS and Behavior*, *13*(3), 488–498.

Rosser, B. R., Oakes, J. M., Konstan, J., Hooper, S., Horvath, K. J., Danilenko, G. P., ... Smolenski, D. J. (2010). Reducing HIV risk behavior of men who have sex with men through persuasive computing: Results of the Men's INTernet Study-II. *AIDS*, *24*(13), 2099–2107.

Rosser, B. R. S., Horvath, K. J., Hatfield, L. A., Peterson, J. L., Jacoby, S., Stately, A., & the Positive Connections. (2008). Predictors of HIV disclosure to secondary partners and sexual risk behavior among a high-risk sample of HIV-positive MSM: Results from six epicenters in the US. *AIDS Care, 20*(8), 925–930.

Rosser, B. R. S., West, W., & Weinmeyer, R. (2008). Are gay communities dying or just in transition? Results from an international consultation examining possible structural change in gay communities. *AIDS Care, 20*(5), 588–595.

Scheer, S., Chu, P., Klausner, J., Katz, M., & Schwarcz, S. (2001). Effect of highly active anti-retroviral therapy on diagnoses of sexually transmitted diseases in people with AIDS. *Lancet, 357*(9254), 432–435.

Schwarcz, S., Scheer, S., McFarland, W., Katz, M., Valleroy, L., Chen, S., & Catania, J. (2007). Prevalence of HIV infection and predictors of high-transmission sexual risk behaviors among men who have sex with men. *American Journal of Public Health, 97*(6), 1067–1075.

Semple, S. J., Zians, J., Strathdee, S. A., & Patterson, T. L. (2008). Sexual marathons and methamphetamine use among HIV-positive men who have sex with men. *Archives of Sexual Behavior, 38*(4), 583–590.

Shaw, L., & Gant, L. (2002). In defense of the Internet: The relationship between Internet communication and depression, loneliness, self-esteem, and perceived social support. *Cyberpsychology & Behavior, 5*(2), 157–171.

Shin, E., Johnson, T. P., & Rao, K. (2012). Survey mode effects on data quality: Comparison of web and mail modes in a U.S. National Panel Survey. *Social Science Computer Review, 30*(2), 212–228.

Simoni, J. M., Kutner, B. A., & Horvath, K. J. (2015). Opportunities and challenges of digital technology for HIV treatment and prevention. *Current HIV/AIDS Reports*, 1–4. doi:10.1007/s11904-015-0289-1

Simoni, J. M., & Pantalone, D. W. (2004). Secrets and safety in the age of AIDS: Does HIV disclosure lead to safer sex? *Topics in HIV Medicine, 12*(4), 109–118.

Smith, A. (2010a). Mobile Access 2010. *Pew Internet & American Life Project.* Retrieved November 8, 2011 from http://www.Pewinternet.Org/reports/2010/mobile-access-2010/part-2. Aspx – footnote3

Smith, A. (2010b). *Technology trends among people of color. Pew Internet & American life project.* Retrieved November 8, 2011 from http://www.pewinternet.org/Commentary/2010/September/Technology-Trends-Among-People-of-Color.aspx.

Stahlman, S., Lyons, C., Sullivan, P. S., Mayer, K. H., Hosein, S., Beyrer, C., & Baral, S. D. (2016). HIV incidence among gay men and other men who have sex with men in 2020: Where is the epidemic heading? *Sexual Health.* doi:10.1071/sh16070

Stein, M. D., Freedberg, K. A., Sullivan, L. M., Savetsky, J., Levenson, S. M., Hingson, R., & Samet, J. H. (1998). Sexual ethics. Disclosure of HIV-positive status to partners. *Archives of Internal Medicine, 158*(3), 253–257.

Sullivan, P. S., Hamouda, O., Delpech, V., Geduld, J. E., Prejean, J., Semaille, C., ... Fenton, K. A. (2009). Reemergence of the HIV epidemic among men who have sex with men in North America, Western Europe, and Australia, 1996–2005. *Annals of Epidemiology, 19*(6), 423–431.

Sullivan, P. S., Jones, J., Kishore, N., & Stephenson, R. (2015). The roles of Technology in Primary HIV prevention for men who have sex with men. *Current HIV/AIDS Reports, 12*(4), 481–488. doi:10.1007/s11904-015-0293-5

Tashima, K., Alt, E., Harwell, J., Fiebich-Perez, D., & Flanigan, T. (2003). Internet sex-seeking leads to acute HIV infection: A report of two cases. *International Journal of STD & AIDS, 14*(4), 285–286.

Taylor, M., Aynalem, G., Smith, L., Bemis, C., Kenney, K., & Kerndt, P. (2004). Correlates of Internet use to meet sex partners among men who have sex with men diagnosed with early syphilis in Los Angeles County. *Sexually Transmitted Diseases, 31*, 552–556.

Thiede, H., Jenkins, R. A., Carey, J. W., Hutcheson, R., Thomas, K. K., Stall, R. D., ... Golden, M. R. (2008). Determinants of recent HIV infection among Seattle-area men who have sex with men. *American Journal of Public Health, 99*(Suppl 1), S157–S164.

Tikkanen, R., & Ross, M. (2003). Technological tearoom trade: Characteristics of Swedish men visiting gay Internet chat rooms. *AIDS Education and Prevention, 15*(2), 122–132.

Topp, L., Hando, J., & Dillon, P. (1999). Sexual behaviour of ectasy users in Sydney, Australia. *Culture, Health, & Sexuality, 1*, 147–159.

Vanable, P. A., Carey, M. P., Carey, K. B., & Maisto, S. A. (2002). Predictors of participation and attrition in a health promotion study involving psychiatric outpatients. *Journal of Consulting and Clinical Psychology, 70*(2), 362–368.

Venkatesh, V., & Bala, H. (2008). Technology acceptance model 3 and a research agenda on interventions. *Decision Sciences, 39*(2), 273–315. doi:10.1111/j.1540-5915.2008.00192.x

Weiss, R., & Samenow, C. P. (2010). Smart phones, social networking, sexting and problematic sexual behaviors—A call for research. *Sexual Addiction & Compulsivity, 17*(4), 241–246.

White, J. M., Mimiaga, M. J., Reisner, S. L., & Mayer, K. H. (2012). HIV sexual risk behavior among black men who meet other men on the Internet for sex. *Journal of Urban Health, 90*(3), 464–481.

Wilson, P. A., Valera, P., Ventuneac, A., Balan, I., Rowe, M., & Carballo-Dieguez, A. (2009). Race-based sexual stereotyping and sexual partnering among men who use the Internet to identify other men for bareback sex. *Journal of Sex Research, 46*(5), 399–413.

Winter, A. K., Sullivan, P. S., Khosropour, C. M., & Rosenberg, E. S. (2012). Discussion of HIV status by Serostatus and partnership sexual risk among Internet-using MSM in the United States. *Journal of Acquired Immune Deficiency Syndromes: JAIDS, 60*(5), 525–529.

Wolitski, R., Vadiserri, R., Denning, P., & Levine, W. (2001). Are we headed for a resurgence of the HIV epidemic among men who have sex with men? *American Journal of Public Health, 91*(6), 883–888.

Wolitski, R. J., Flores, S. A., O'Leary, A., Bimbi, D. S., & Gomez, C. A. (2007). Beliefs about personal and partner responsibility among HIV-seropositive men who have sex with men: Measurement and association with transmission risk behavior. *AIDS and Behavior, 11*(5), 676–686.

Wong, N., Gullo, K., & Stafford, J. (2004). *Gays lead non-gays in cell phone use, cable TV and HDTV viewership.* Technology use and preferences of gay and non-gay consumers [News story]. Retrieved from http://www.prnewswire.com/.

Wright, E., Fortune, T., Juzang, I., & Bull, S. (2011). Text messaging for HIV prevention with young black men: Formative research and campaign development. *AIDS Care, 23*(5), 534–541.

Young, S. D., Holloway, I., Jaganath, D., Westmoreland, D., & Coates, T. (2014). Project HOPE: Online social network changes in an HIV prevention randomized controlled trial for African American and Latino men who have sex with men. *American Journal of Public Health, 104*, 1707–1712.

Yu, G., Wall, M. W., Chiasson, M. A., & Hirshfield, S. (2015). Complex drug use patterns and associated HIV transmission risk behaviors in an Internet sample of US men who have sex with men. *Archives of Sexual Behavior, 44*(2), 421–428.

Chapter 17
HIV Positive Gay Men, Health Care, Legal Rights, and Policy Issues

Sean Cahill

Introduction

Gay men living with HIV have complex health care needs involving physical and mental health, as well as side effects of long-term HIV infection and antiretroviral use and comorbidities with other health conditions. A life-course framework along with the constructs of minority stress and resiliency will be examined in understanding the social development of gay men. Aging and caregiving issues for HIV positive gay men will be explored. The concept of Treatment as Prevention will be examined, along with biomedical prevention technologies that can help HIV negative partners in serodiscordant couples remain negative. Legal issues such as criminalization and discrimination will be considered. The myriad changes in health policy will be addressed, including the expanded access to both private and public health insurance through the Affordable Care Act. The experiences of HIV positive gay men in the Veterans Administration system and in senior settings will also be examined, as well as policy changes that can better equip these systems to provide clinically competent care.

S. Cahill (✉)
The Fenway Institute, Fenway Health, Boston, MA, USA

Department of Health Sciences, Bouvé College of Health Sciences,
Northeastern University, Boston, MA, USA
e-mail: scahill@fenwayhealth.org

© Springer Science+Business Media LLC 2017
L. Wilton (ed.), *Understanding Prevention for HIV Positive Gay Men*,
DOI 10.1007/978-1-4419-0203-0_17

Health Issues Affecting Gay Men Living with HIV

Health Disparities and Intersectional Identities

Since the onset of the HIV epidemic in the USA, gay and bisexual men, and other men who have sex with men (MSM), have been disproportionately burdened by the virus, and continue to experience disproportionate rates of HIV infection. In 2010, the Centers for Disease Control and Prevention (CDC) reported that MSM are at least 44 times more likely to contract HIV than heterosexual men (Centers for Disease Control and Prevention (CDC), 2011a, 2011b, 2011c, 2011d, 2011e, 2011f). In 2014, MSM comprised 70% of all new HIV infections, and were the only risk category for which new infections increased (CDC, 2014). These findings are alarming given that MSM only make up about 2% of the US adult population (CDC, 2010a). For gay and bisexual men of color, the statistics are even more troubling; a startling 42% of new HIV diagnoses among MSM in the USA occur among Black MSM even though Black MSM represent only about 0.25% of the adult population (CDC, 2011a).

In addition to HIV, gay and bisexual men experience elevated rates of cigarette smoking; alcohol and recreational drug use; sexually transmitted infections (STIs), including viral hepatitis; eating disorders; cardiovascular disease; anal cancer and AIDS-related cancers; and violence and trauma stemming from hate crimes, domestic violence, and sexual assault (Fenway Institute, 2013).

The health disparities affecting gay and bisexual men must be understood in the context of widespread anti-gay discrimination, harassment, and social isolation, especially in adolescence and young adulthood. Despite the significant changes in US society in recent decades, most young people who are lesbian, gay, bisexual or transgender (LGBT) report discrimination and harassment in school (Kosciw, Diaz, & Greytak, 2008). Lesbian, gay, and bisexual (LGB) youth also report a range of health risk behaviors at higher rates than heterosexual youth (CDC, 2011b; Kann et al., 2016). These include carrying a weapon on school property, being injured in a fight or with a weapon on school property, use of tobacco and substances, having sexual intercourse before age 13, feeling depressed and hopeless, and using diet pills or laxatives (CDC, 2011b; Kann et al., 2016). According to the Massachusetts Youth Risk Behavior Survey, LGB students are two to three times as likely to have been pregnant or gotten someone pregnant (Massachusetts Department of Elementary and Secondary Education (DESE), 2010; Mass. DESE, 2012).[1] LGB youth of color in Massachusetts are at higher risk than White LGB youth for a number of conditions related to bullying and social isolation due to anti-gay prejudice. These include not attending or missing school due to feeling unsafe, suicide attempts, and having had four or more sexual partners in their lifetime. Asian LGB

---

[1] In 2009, 10.5% of LGB students reported having been pregnant or having gotten someone pregnant, compared with 5.2% of heterosexual students; in 2011, the rates were 13.0% versus 4.7%, respectively. Differences were significant at the $p < 0.05$ level.

youth are twice as likely as Black youth, and nearly three times as likely as White non-Hispanic youth, to skip school due to feeling unsafe (Goodenow, 2011).[2] Several other studies show that Black and Latino LGB youth may be more likely to attempt suicide than White non-Hispanic LGB youth (Meyer, Dietrich, & Schwartz, 2008; O'Donnell, Meyer, & Schwartz, 2011; Remafedi, 2002).

HIV-Related Comorbidities

As of 2015, about half of the HIV positive population in the USA is over age 50 (Effros et al., 2008). As people grow older with HIV and live decades with the virus, they are likely to develop comorbidities (Deeks & Philips, 2009). Common comorbid conditions among older adults living with HIV include liver, kidney, and cardiovascular disease, obesity, cognitive impairment, depression, neuropathy, osteoporosis, and a number of cancers (Cahill et al., 2010). A key research question is whether long-term use of antiretroviral medications or having HIV itself is the cause of the higher rates of comorbid conditions.

Other STIs (Syphilis, HPV, MRSA)

Like HIV, syphilis disproportionately affects gay and bisexual men in the USA. In 2010, 64% of syphilis cases occurred among men who have sex with men (MSM) (CDC, 2011c). Human papilloma virus (HPV) is one of the most common STIs in the USA. Every year six million people contract HPV, mostly through sexual contact. Currently, 20 million people in the USA have detectable infection with HPV (CDC, 2011d). Most cases of genital warts, found in about 1% of the US population (three million people), are caused by specific HPV types. MSM represent the majority of prevalent cases of genital warts. HPV also causes several forms of cancer, including anal cancer (estimated at 1600 cases per year in women and 900 cases per year in men) (CDC, 2011e). Anal cancer is emerging as among the most important non-AIDS-defining malignancies affecting people living with HIV, especially gay and bisexual men (Palefsky, 2009). MSM with HIV are at even greater risk for HPV and its related complications. Though rare among the general population, HPV-related anal cancer is 40–80 times more prevalent among HIV-infected MSM than among uninfected heterosexual men (Silverberg et al., 2012).

MRSA, or methicillin-resistant Staphylococcus aureus, is a strain of staph that is resistant to the broad spectrum of antibiotics commonly used to treat it. Over the past decade, a particularly virulent drug-resistant strain of MRSA, known as USA300, emerged in gay male communities in Boston, New York, and San

---

[2] All disparities are from pooled 1995 to 2009 data, except for percent of youth bullied at school, which are from 2003 to 2009 pooled data.

Francisco (Beck, 2012). A study in San Francisco found that this strain of MRSA could be transmitted not only through anal sex but also through skin-to-skin contact and touching contaminated surfaces. It also found that risk factors contributing to increased rates of HIV and syphilis among gay and bisexual men were also impli-cated in the spread of MRSA: crystal methamphetamine use, sex with multiple part-ners, participation in group sex parties, Internet-initiated sexual contacts, skin abrasions associated with sexual activity, and a history of STIs (Diep et al., 2008). While washing with soap and water immediately after sex can prevent against skin-to-skin transmission of MRSA, only safer sex practices—including condom and lubricant use and minimizing the number of sexual partners—can prevent sexual transmission of MRSA, as well as syphilis and HIV.

Mental Health and Substance Use

Some studies show higher rates of mental health burden among LGB populations compared to heterosexuals, including depression, anxiety, and suicidality (King et al., 2008). The Massachusetts Behavioral Risk Factor Surveillance Survey of adults and Youth Risk Behavior Surveys show higher rates of mental health burden among LGB individuals (Blosnich, Bossarte, & Silenzio, 2012a, 2012b; Goodenow, 2011).

Health risk surveys demonstrate higher rates of substance use among gay and bisexual men (CDC, 2008a). According to the Massachusetts YRBS, LGB adoles-cents smoke at four times the rate as heterosexual youth, and binge drink at nearly twice the rate. Sexual minority male youth report cocaine use at more than four times the rate of heterosexual male youth, and sexual minority females report cocaine use at more than five times the rate of heterosexual female youth. Nineteen percent of gay and bisexual male youth reported injected drug use, compared to 2% of heterosexual male youth; 4% of sexual minority female youth reported injected drug use, compared with 0% of heterosexual female youth (Goodenow, 2011). LGBT youth are more likely to be homeless than other youth (Institute of Medicine, 2011). This experience can also correlate with health risks and risk of victimization.

LGBT people experience barriers to accessing mental health services. One study found that experiences of discrimination among LGBT people made them less likely to seek needed mental health services: "Experiences of discrimination may engender negative expectations among stigmatized groups about how they will be treated within larger institutional systems, making them wary of entering those situations" (Burgess, Lee, Tran, & van Ryn, 2007). Compared with hetero-sexuals, LGBT people were more likely to report "that they did not receive mental health services, or that such services were delayed (Burgess et al., 2007)." One study of mental health and substance use services in rural areas found widespread experiences of discrimination among LGBT clients, at the hands of both providers and heterosexual clients. LGBT clients were frequently silenced and told not to raise issues of sexuality or gender identity in group settings. Counselors expressed disapproval of homosexuality and sought to convert clients to heterosexuality. LGBT clients were refused entry into programs to "protect" them from discrimination, or placed in isolation from other clients. Of 20 providers interviewed, only one had had formal training in LGBT mental health issues (Willging, Salvador, & Kano, 2006).

Resiliency Factors

School-Based Interventions

Anti-gay harassment and violence are widespread in schools across the nation (Bochenek & Brown, 2001). As a result, many feel unsafe and report higher rates of social isolation, depression, suicidal ideation, and unprotected sex (Cianciotto & Cahill, 2012). LGB youth who are harassed engage in health risk behaviors at higher rates than their heterosexual peers who are also harassed (Bontempo & D'Augelli, 2002). LGBT-affirming school-based interventions are key to combating anti-gay bias and promoting the psychological health and physical well-being of LGBT youth (Goodenow, 2007).

Among these LGBT-affirming interventions are Gay Straight Alliances (GSAs), nondiscrimination policies, anti-bullying curricula, and curricula designed to provide positive and inclusive examples of the contributions that LGBT people have made to US and world culture. Approximately 4000 Gay Straight Alliances are currently registered throughout the USA and GSAs bring together students, faculty, and school staff to end homophobia in their schools (Griffin & Ouellett, 2002).

School-based interventions such as GSAs can support young people to affirm and cultivate a healthy gay identity. One study involving students from a GSA in Salt Lake City found that following their involvement in the GSA, students reported an improved sense of physical safety and sense of belonging to the school community. They also reported improved relationships with their families, developing a higher comfort level with their own sexual orientation, learning strategies for dealing with others' presumptions about their sexuality, and felt better about their ability to contribute to society (Lee, 2002).

Family Acceptance of Gay and Bisexual Identities

Family rejection because of one's sexuality during adolescence correlates with poorer health outcomes for LGB young adults. One study indicates that in addition to higher rates of substance use, depression, and attempted suicide, LGB youth who were rejected by their families were 3.4 times more likely to report having engaged in unprotected sexual intercourse, compared with peers who reported little to no experiences of family rejection (Ryan, Heubner, Diaz, & Sanchez, 2009). For this reason, parental acceptance of gay and bisexual sons is central to reducing their risk of HIV infection. Social marketing campaigns should promote parental acceptance of gay sons as a public health strategy, as Gay Men's Health Crisis (GMHC) did with its 2008 "My son is my life" campaign. They can also promote positive images of older gay men and older people living with HIV to challenge stigma related to age, homosexuality, and HIV.

Resiliency in Community Connectedness

Connectedness to LGBT communities is an important coping resource for LGBT people that provides non-stigmatizing environments and affirms positive self-appraisals (Meyer, 2010). Community connectedness—including supportive social relationships—has also proven protective against HIV infection (Lauby et al., 2012). Greater community involvement counters the negative effects of anti-gay bias on safer sex practices among gay men by providing social support, enhancing feelings of self-efficacy and positive self-identity, and reinforcing peer norms supporting safer sex practices (Ramirez-Valles, 2002). Interventions are needed that support and nurture affirming social networks for older gay men living with HIV.

The Life-Course Framework

The Institute of Medicine, in its landmark report on *The Health of Lesbian, Gay, Bisexual and Transgender People*, uses the life-course framework as well as models of minority stress, intersectionality, and social ecology to understand LGBT health disparities (Institute of Medicine, 2011). The life-course perspective holds that cohort and age differences influence health needs. Differential experiences with "coming out" and social homophobia also influence gay men's willingness to be "out" to their health care providers (Mayer et al., 2008). Harassment and homelessness are especially salient issues for youth who may be kicked out of their homes for being gay, or who experience violence and social isolation in schools or other social institutions such as foster care. Cancer and cardiovascular disease can become greater threats among middle age and older gay men, while some issues scan the life course—such as body image and eating disorders, substance use, and mental health issues (Makadon, Mayer, Potter, & Goldhammer, 2008).

Prejudice, Stigma, and Minority Stress

Higher rates of mental health disorders among gay and bisexual men are often caused by the "hostile and stressful social environment" caused by anti-gay "stigma, prejudice, and discrimination" (Meyer, 2003). Gay-related stigma has been shown to diminish positive affect and increase depression among midlife and older gay men (Wight, LeBlanc, de Vries, & Detels, 2012). Minority stress is caused by external, objective events and conditions, expectations of such events, the internalization of societal attitudes, and concealment of one's sexual orientation (Meyer, 1995; Meyer, 2003). Internalized anti-gay stigma can correlate with higher rates of sexual risk behavior; this is related to being less "out" about one's same-sex behavior, to lower condom self-efficacy, and to lower sexual comfort (Ross, Rosser, Neumaier, & Positive Connections Team, 2008). Anxiety, often connected to experiences of anti-gay prejudice, correlates with sexual risk behavior, especially among older gay and bisexual men (Lelutiu-Weinberger et al., 2013).

A key structural driver of health disparities among gay and bisexual men is anti-gay stigma. Rejection and social isolation from family and community experienced by gay and bisexual men contribute to a multitude of negative health outcomes, including substance use and condomless anal sex, both of which increase vulnerability to HIV, syphilis, and other STIs (Ryan et al., 2009). Experiences of anti-gay violence correlate with risky sexual behavior among young MSM (Russell, Ryan, Toomey, Diaz, & Sanchez, 2011). The association of experiencing homophobia within the past year and unprotected anal sex has also been documented among Black and Latino MSM (Jeffries, Marks, Lauby, Murrill, & Millett, 2012; Mizuno et al., 2012). Thus, anti-gay stigma must be treated as a public health threat. To counter its pervasive and detrimental effects, community-based prevention interventions that reduce homophobia and affirm the healthy formation of gay identities are urgently needed. Such campaigns can take the form of social marketing, such as the "I Love My Boo" campaign by GMHC from 2008 through 2010 (GMHC, 2010). Posters were placed on phone kiosks, bus shelters, and subway trains. Youth-serving institutions should adopt nondiscrimination and anti-bullying policies, train staff and participants in the negative social and health effects of anti-gay prejudice and social isolation, and teach them how to intervene and stop such behavior.

Social Determinants of HIV Positive Gay Men's Health

A provider's knowledge of a patient's sexual orientation and gender identity is essential to providing appropriate prevention screening and care (Makadon, 2011). Patients who disclose their sexual orientation identity to health care providers may feel safer discussing their health and risk behaviors as well (Klitzman & Greenberg, 2002). A sample of New York City MSM from the 2004 to 2005 National HIV Behavioral Surveillance system (NHBS) found that 61% had not disclosed their same-sex orientation or behavior to their medical providers. White MSM and native born MSM were more likely to have disclosed than Black, Latino, Asian, and immigrant MSM. Disclosure correlated with having tested for HIV (Berstein et al., 2008).

Barriers to LGBT people's accessing culturally competent health care include: a reluctance of LGBT patients to disclose their sexual and gender identity; a lack of providers trained to address the specific health care needs of LGBT people; structural barriers preventing access to health insurance, such as the outlawing of domestic partner health benefits for public sector employees in Michigan, Ohio, Georgia, and other states (Cahill, 2007), and a lack of culturally appropriate prevention services (Mayer et al., 2008).

LGBT people also experience a shortage of primary medical care and mental health providers culturally competent to serve them. Many health care providers are uncomfortable providing care to LGBT people. Although anti-gay attitudes among providers appear to have declined significantly over the past two decades, a recent study found that 18% of doctors in California are "sometimes" or "often" uncomfortable caring for gay patients (Smith & Mathews, 2007). A recent survey of deans of medical education at medical schools in the USA and Canada found that the median time dedicated to teaching LGBT-related content in the entire medical school curriculum was 5 h. One-third of medical schools reported that zero hours of LGBT content were taught. Only 24% of the medical school deans considered their school's overall coverage of LGBT material as "good" or "very good" on a 5-category Likert scale (Obedin-Maliver et al., 2011).

Aging and Caregiving Issues

The health care infrastructure is ill-equipped to handle the unique treatment and care needs of older gay men living with HIV. In fact, the health care infrastructure is not ready to handle the influx of elder American baby boomers in general, who are hitting retirement age now; there are not enough geriatricians or other health care workers to care for them (Eldercare Workforce Alliance, 2011). There are even fewer providers with expertise treating elders with complex, chronic health conditions. Stigma presents challenges for those in need of services and health care, and can significantly affect mental health and HIV treatment adherence. The training of elder service providers and health care providers in meeting the needs HIV positive older adults, including gay men, is needed as the population ages. Aging with HIV/AIDS presents biomedical complexities only now beginning to reveal themselves. Higher rates of comorbidities are among the more severe biomedical issues facing older adults with HIV/AIDS (Deeks & Philips, 2009). Liver disease and cardiovascular disease, both associated with long-term use of ARVs, are leading causes of mortality among older people living with HIV (Deeks & Philips, 2009). Cognitive impairment is also widespread among people on treatment for a long time; this could be due to "chronic HIV-driven inflammation in an aging brain" (Portegies, 2010).

Social Support and Social Isolation

HIV positive individuals over 50 are more socially isolated than their younger counterparts (Emlet, 2006). Many experience barriers to receiving emotional and instrumental social support from friends and family, including concealment of HIV status and others' fear of casual transmission of HIV (Schrimshaw & Siegel, 2003). Opinion research indicates that older Americans are more likely than younger age cohorts to hold inaccurate beliefs about the casual transmission of HIV (Kaiser Family Foundation, 2009a, 2009b).

As the HIV positive population in the USA ages, greater emphasis on HIV prevention among older adults is necessary. Evidence suggests that, in addition to anti-gay bias, older gay men also experience issues related to aging and self-esteem. Some older gay men experience a phenomenon known as "accelerated aging," the concept of feeling older at an earlier age than one's chronological age (Rosario, Schrimshaw, Hunter, & Braun, 2006). This aging experience differs from that of their heterosexual counterparts, and may present issues of social isolation for older gay men who are single and equate physical attractiveness with youth. These men may put themselves at risk for HIV and/or other STIs by meeting anonymous partners on the Internet and coupling these experiences with alcohol and substance use.

Caring for Older Adults with HIV/AIDS

Many older adults living with HIV/AIDS are disconnected from traditional informal support networks, and rely heavily on formal care providers (Shippey & Karpiak, 2005). This is especially true of gay men with HIV, many of whom have been rejected by family members. However, many people living with HIV rely on informal caregivers. Informal caregivers in the USA report high rates of depression (Pirraglia et al., 2005) and emotional burden related to nondisclosure of the HIV status of the person for whom they care (Baker, Sudit, & Litwak, 1998). Informal caregivers often have less time to parent and to work, causing stress that can correlate with depression and an end to caregiving assistance (Mitchell & Knowlton, 2012).

With over half of HIV positive elders in the USA identifying as gay or bisexual men, cultural competency training of elder service staff is needed to provide clinically competent care to older HIV positive gay men (CDC, 2010b). Gay elders in nursing homes and assisted living facilities are often presumed heterosexual and feel it necessary to hide their sexual orientation from staff and other residents (Johnson, Arnette, & Koffman, 2005). This is problematic as evidence shows that long-term relationships with same-sex partners are often devalued, and those who are found to be gay often experience discrimination, abuse, and neglect by staff (Fairchild, Carrino, & Ramirez, 1996). Many gay and lesbian elders fear rejection or neglect by health care providers, including personal care aides, as well as other residents of long-term care facilities and nursing homes (Stein & Bonuck, 2001). Though research on HIV positive elders in congregate living facilities is limited, evidence suggests that stigma persists among other residents, as well as staff charged with the care and well-being of residents.

HIV-Related Health Issues

Treatment as Prevention (TasP) and the Need for Better Treatment Outcomes

Recent studies have demonstrated a dramatic decrease in HIV transmission when infected individuals initiate suppressive antiretroviral therapy at higher CD4 counts (Cohen M et al., 2011). HPTN 052, the study released in May 2011 that showed providing ARVs to HIV-infected partners lowers the risk of infection of HIV negative partners, has significant implications for HIV prevention. As Abdool Karim and Abdool Karim note, "[T]here is now no doubt that antiretroviral drugs prevent HIV infection" (Abdool Karim & Abdool Karim, 2011, p. e23). What is less clear is what the implications of Treatment as Prevention are for gay and bisexual men. Only 3% of the serodiscordant couples in HPTN 052 were gay male couples (about 50 out of 1763 couples). It was difficult to recruit serodiscordant gay male couples in which the positive partner was treatment naïve.

President Obama's 2010 National HIV/AIDS Strategy prioritizes "increase[ing] access to care and optimiz[ing] health outcomes for people living with HIV" in part by "establishing a seamless system to immediately link people to continuous and coordinated quality care when they are diagnosed with HIV" (White House Office of National AIDS Policy (ONAP), 2010, pp. viii–ix). This approach is also known as Test, Treat, and Link to Care (TLC+). It calls for improved treatment outcomes by expanded testing, diagnosis, and linkage to treatment and care (TLC+) to find the estimated 13% of people living with HIV who are undiagnosed, and to increase the percentage of people diagnosed with HIV who receive ongoing care (CDC, 2008b; Health Resources Services Administration, 2006; White House Office of National AIDS Policy, 2010; ONAP, 2016).[3] The need for better treatment outcomes among people living with HIV was underscored in late 2011, when the Centers for Disease Control and Prevention (CDC) reported that only 28% of people living with HIV in the USA are virally suppressed (Cohen SM et al., 2011).

Serodiscordant Couples, Pre-exposure Prophylaxis, and Rectal Microbicides

The recent scientific breakthroughs with Treatment as Prevention, as well as pre-exposure chemoprophylaxis (PrEP) and rectal microbicides for HIV prevention, are especially important to serodiscordant couples. Initial results from clinical prevention trials of PrEP, in oral pill form (oral PrEP), indicate that PrEP could

---

[3] The CDC estimates that only 51% of people in the US diagnosed with HIV are receiving ongoing care, and only 41% of people with HIV in the US "are both aware of their infection and receiving ongoing care" (Vital Signs, *MMWR*, 2011a, December 2).

significantly reduce HIV infections. PrEP involves taking antiretroviral medications to prevent HIV transmission through unprotected sex or sharing needles. The first PrEP trial to demonstrate efficacy among MSM was iPrEx, which enrolled 2499 MSM in Latin America, the USA, South Africa, and Thailand. The participants who took oral emtricitabine and tenofovir disoproxil fumarate (FTC-TDF) had a 44% lower rate of HIV infection than those who took the placebo. All were provided comprehensive HIV prevention services, including risk reduction counseling and HIV/STI testing. In a nested case-control study, among subjects with a detectable study-drug level (i.e., the most treatment adherent), there was a 92% lower rate of HIV infection than among those without a detectable level of FTC-TDF tested in the visit before seroconversion (Grant et al., 2010).

It is essential that PrEP be combined with behavioral interventions to maintain both PrEP adherence and continued fidelity to safer sex practices. A concurrent focus on TLC+ as well as behavioral interventions to support treatment adherence and safer sex practices would decrease community viral load and complement the effectiveness of PrEP. Implementing both PrEP and TLC+ together can be done efficiently through public health programs that maximize the effectiveness of both. Recent modeling of PrEP implementation coupled with scaled up treatment—focusing on MSM in San Francisco, the general adult population in Botswana, and sero-discordant couples in South Africa—predicts that PrEP could significantly reduce HIV incidence and prevalence (Hallett et al., 2011; Supervie, Garcia-Lerma, Heneine, & Blower, 2010; Supervie et al., 2011).

If targeted to the highest risk populations and if adherence and efficacy is high enough, PrEP can be cost effective. While clinical settings are the most feasible sites for PrEP implementation, alternative arrangements should be explored, such as substance use treatment sites. Training of health providers and non-clinicians in PrEP delivery is a key component of PrEP scale-up. Research shows widespread willingness to use PrEP among the most vulnerable populations, such as MSM in the USA and globally. However, concerns are widespread that PrEP may lead to risk compensation, which should be monitored and challenged through social marketing and behavioral interventions. Many gay men are unaware of PrEP, and many confuse PrEP and PEP (post-exposure prophylaxis, a technology that has been available for many years now). Many gay men and many providers are unaware of either. For example, a survey of more than 4500 MSM on social networking websites in 2011 found that only 36% had heard of PEP (Krakower et al., 2012). PrEP offers a teachable moment to increase knowledge of and access to PEP.

Among the greatest barriers to accessing PrEP is cost. The CDC estimates TDF-FTC would cost $8030 a year; generic TDF-FTC is available in the global south for $108 a year. Currently, private insurers and Medicaid are covering PrEP for patients. The Affordable Care Act mandates coverage of "Essential Health Benefits" by insurance offered in state Health Insurance Exchanges; these include prescription drugs and prevention and wellness programs, which could cover PrEP (Cahill, 2012a, 2012b). In July 2012, the US Food and Drug Administration approved FTC-TDF for use as PrEP by gay and bisexual men, high-risk heterosexual women and men, and serodiscordant couples. In August 2012, the CDC issued guidance for use of PrEP by serodiscordant couples and heterosexuals, building upon guidance for MSM issued in 2011. The World Health Organization also issued provider guidance about PrEP use in July 2012.

Rectal Microbicides

A related experimental technology is microbicides, topical gels that contain antiretroviral medications that are applied vaginally or rectally to prevent HIV transmission. Rectal microbicides, currently in development, involve an agent that can be included in topical gels, lubricants, douches, or enemas and applied to the rectum to prevent HIV transmission (International Rectal Microbicides Advocates, 2013). A tenofovir rectal gel was found effective in preventing simian immunodeficiency virus (SIV) transmission among macaques (International Rectal Microbicides Advocates, 2013). A number of safety and acceptability studies have been conducted with humans since 2004. For example, one study found UC781 (a gel that includes a thiocarboxanilide non-nucleoside reverse transcriptase inhibitor) to be safe and well tolerated when used rectally in humans (AIDSinfo.gov, 2013; LeBlanc, 2010). Another study looked at how much microbicide gel would be acceptable, and found that MSM generally tolerated up to 35 ml while having receptive anal intercourse (Carballo-Dieguez et al., 2007). Rectal microbicide trial results released in 2011 showed that a rectal gel could effectively deliver FTC-TDF to rectal tissue (Anton, Saunders, Adler, et al., 2011; Microbicide Trials Network, n.d.; Reuters, 2011). While rectal microbicides are still in development, at some point in the future they could provide another tool that serodiscordant gay male couples could use to protect the HIV negative partner.

Serosorting

Serosorting is the process by which an individual makes a choice about sexual partners based upon known or perceived HIV status. In recent years, many HIV positive people have advertised online for sexual partners who are also HIV positive. *Poz.com*, a social network dating site run by *Poz* magazine, is one example of HIV positive serosorting. While serosorting can lead to less HIV infection of HIV negative individuals, public health advocates are concerned that HIV positive serosorters who do not use protection may transmit other STIs. Dual infection or superinfection with new, possibly drug-resistant strains of HIV is another concern. This could further weaken the immune system, hasten disease progression, and potentially limit treatment options (Siconolfi & Moeller, 2007). If two individuals who think they are HIV negative engage in unprotected sex, STI infection and even HIV infection may occur due to the window period between HIV exposure and a positive HIV test. The body takes some time—as much as 3 months—between infection with HIV and the production of enough HIV antibodies to be detected by an HIV test (Butler & Smith, 2007).

HIV Prevention Using Social Media, the Internet, and Commercial Sex Venues

The Internet has become a central medium in the social lives of many adults, including among gay men searching for sexual partners (Bolding, Davis, Hart, Sherr, & Elford, 2005). Popular dating or cruising websites often allow an option for HIV status to be provided and can facilitate negotiation of sexual behavior, including serosorting and use of condoms (Bolding et al., 2005). Online outreach to gay and bisexual men is an effective way to disseminate safer sex messages, HIV/STI prevention information, and referrals to testing and services. Contact with individuals through online outreach takes place in public chat rooms and fora, as well as through other, more private Internet communication, such as instant messaging and via email.

For decades commercial sex venues (CSVs) have been important sites for HIV/STI prevention education. CSVs charge admission or request a donation for admission to a bathhouse, sex club, or private sex party, either in a fixed or roaming location. Gay men who frequent CSVs are at high risk of HIV and other STIs (Aynalem et al., 2006). A high percentage of MSM surveyed in New York City and Los Angeles recently met sexual partners at bathhouses (40%), through public cruising (30%), and at private sex parties (25%) (Grov, Parsons, & Bimbi, 2007). HIV positive men may be more likely than HIV negative men to participate in public sex venues and commercial sex venues (Parsons & Halkitis, 2002). Therefore, prevention education and HIV/STI testing at CSVs can be highly effective.

Legal Issues Affecting Gay Men Living with HIV

Criminalization

Laws criminalizing HIV and the nondisclosure of one's HIV status reinforce HIV-related stigma, prejudice, and discrimination in US society. Currently 34 states in the USA have laws punishing people for exposing another person to HIV, usually through nondisclosure of status. Hundreds of individuals have been prosecuted for nondisclosure of their HIV status (Strub, 2011). Such nondisclosure is criminal, even if the person's viral load is undetectable and even if HIV transmission does not occur. Those convicted often have to register as sex offenders for the rest of their lives. An especially egregious case is that of Willy Campbell, who was sentenced to 35 years for spitting on a police officer. Campbell was convicted of "assault with a deadly weapon," even though spit from an HIV positive person cannot infect someone, let alone kill him (Strub, 2011). A bill introduced by Congresswoman Barbara Lee (D-CA) in 2011, the REPEAL HIV Criminalization Act, would review and repeal such laws (Gonzalez, 2012).

HIV Discrimination in Employment, Housing, and Public Accommodations

Discrimination on the basis of HIV status is illegal in many contexts, but between fiscal year 2000 and fiscal year 2009 some 2175 complaints were filed with the US Equal Employment Opportunity Commission about HIV-related discrimination in employment (Lambda Legal, 2010). These include a man fired from his job at a Las Vegas sandwich shop in 2005 after he disclosed his HIV status on a workplace health insurance application. The man's employer said he believed that the employee posed a danger to customers (Lamda Legal, 2010).

Discrimination also occurs in health care, housing, public accommodations, federal employment, and prison. For example, in 2007, an Alabama RV campground refused to allow a two-year-old to use the swimming pool and showers because he had HIV. A 75-year-old former university provost was ejected from an Arkansas assisted living facility in 2009 due to his HIV status, in violation of the Americans with Disabilities Act, the Fair Housing Act, and analogous state nondiscrimination laws. In 2006, in Pennsylvania, paramedics refused medical care to a man experiencing chest pains because they learned he had HIV. The US military and US Public Health Service Commissioned Corps have policies against hiring people living with HIV, and until recently the US State Department had a similar ban on HIV positive employees. Prisoners in Alabama and South Carolina also experience discriminatory treatment, segregation, and violation of their privacy, being forced to wear armbands, badges, or uniforms that declare their HIV status to everyone, including visitors (Lambda Legal, 2010).

HIV-related discrimination is connected to stigma and misperceptions about how HIV is transmitted. A Kaiser Family Foundation survey found that more than one-third of Americans believed that HIV could be transmitted by sharing a drinking glass, touching a toilet seat, or sharing a swimming pool with an HIV positive person (Kaiser Family Foundation, 2009a, 2009b). Fear of HIV-related stigma and discrimination undermines public health. President Obama's National HIV/AIDS Strategy warns that it "causes some Americans to avoid learning their HIV status, disclosing their status, or accessing medical care" (ONAP, 2010).

Anti-gay Discrimination

Anti-gay discrimination, or discrimination based on real or perceived sexual orientation, was once widespread in both public sector and private sector employment (D'Emilio, 1998). As of 2016, 22 states and the District of Columbia outlawed discrimination on the basis of sexual orientation, as did hundreds of municipalities (American Civil Liberties Union, 2017). More than half the population lives in one of these states or municipalities. However, in much of the country, it is still legal to deny a person a job, promotion, housing, or access to a public accommodation due to real or perceived sexual orientation. A review of 50 studies of sexual orientation discrimination conducted from the 1980s through 2007 found that between 16 and 68% of LGB respondents reported experiencing workplace discrimination. Experiences included being fired, denied employment, denied a promotion, and getting a poor job rating or evaluation (Badgett, Lau, Sears, & Ho, 2007). A survey of LGBT residents of Topeka, Kansas, found widespread workplace discrimination as well as harassment and vandalism in the workplace, housing discrimination, and discrimination in receiving government services (Colvin, 2004). Another indicator of potential discrimination is earnings differentials. An analysis of nine studies using data from a range of sources including that National Health and Social Life Survey and General Social Survey found that gay men earn 10–32% less than heterosexual men (Badgett, 2001).

Policy Issues Affecting HIV Positive Gay Men

The Affordable Care Act and Expanded Health Care Access

The Patient Protection and Affordable Care Act (ACA) of 2010 expanded access to health insurance and seeks to improve outcomes and reduce costs. It requires insurance companies to cover all who apply for insurance and offer the same rates without regard to preexisting health conditions (United States Department of Health and Human Services (U.S. HHS), n.d.). Until 2015, roughly 40 states did not recognize same-sex relationships. Most of these states also banned domestic partner recognition and civil unions, including health insurance for same-sex partners of municipal or state government workers (National Gay and Lesbian Task Force, 2013). Because of the slew of anti-gay family laws and amendments that stripped thousands of same-sex partners of their employer-provided health insurance, as well as discrimination against gay families by private insurance companies, LGBT people were much less likely to have insurance coverage. For all these reasons, the ACA's expansion of health care access has disproportionately benefitted LGBT Americans.

The ACA also provides support for preventative care and HIV testing as well as treatment and prevention services. It prohibits insurance companies from denying coverage for preexisting medical conditions, such as HIV infection. Prior to implementation of the ACA, only 13% of the estimated 1.2 million Americans living with HIV have private insurance and 25% have no insurance (Cahill, 2012a). Only half of people with HIV in the USA were in regular medical care, and less than a one-third are being treated effectively, such that they are virally suppressed (Cohen et al., 2011). The preexisting condition provision means that thousands of people living with HIV can now access health insurance and healthcare, which will improve treatment outcomes, a key goal of President Obama's National HIV/AIDS Strategy. As of 2016, 20 million Americans have accessed private or public insurance through the ACA (U.S. Department of Health and Human Services, 2016).

Medicaid and Medicare

Medicare, Medicaid, and Social Security provide critical support to thousands of people living with HIV in the USA. At least 10% of all people living with HIV in the USA, or 120,000 people, are Medicare beneficiaries (Gilden, Kubisiak, & Gilden, 2007). Medicare is the federal government health insurance program for people who are 65 and over and for some younger people with disabilities. Thirty-four million Americans, including nearly all of the nation's elderly population, have health coverage through Medicare. People living with HIV qualify for Medicare based on age (most US seniors are on Medicare) or because they have received Social Security Disability Insurance for at least 2 years, after which 93% go on to qualify for Medicare (Kaiser Family Foundation, 2009a, 2009b).

Medicaid is a means-tested program proving health care for specific categories of eligible persons, mainly the disabled, low-income children and their parents, and the medically needy. In 2009, between 200,000 and 240,000 people living with HIV were covered by Medicaid (Kaiser Family Foundation, 2009a, 2009b). Medicaid is a key source of funding for antiretroviral therapy. However, with the expansion of Medicare into prescription drug coverage (Medicare Part D), Medicare spending on people with HIV now surpasses Medicaid spending on people with HIV (Kaiser Family Foundation, 2009a, 2009b).

The Medicaid Expansion

Many people with HIV receive Medicaid, a means-tested health insurance program for the poor and disabled. However, until the Affordable Care Act, childless adults could not qualify for Medicaid unless they were disabled. For people living with HIV, this required that they had an AIDS diagnosis. The Medicaid expansion to individuals who earn up to 138% of the poverty level, a key component of the Affordable Care Act, changed this in 2014. However, the June 2012 US Supreme Court ruling struck down the mandatory expansion of Medicaid (Supreme Court of the United States, 2012). The Supreme Court upheld the federal government's ability to promote expanded Medicaid coverage in the states through expanded federal funding (a carrot), but not the ACA's provision that would cut all federal Medicaid funding to states that do not comply (a stick). About half of the 30 million people newly able to access health coverage under the ACA as originally designed would have been covered under the Medicaid expansion, including low-income adults who are not disabled and who do not have dependent children (Washington Post Staff, 2010). This expansion would benefit many single gay people, many people living with HIV, as well as millions of other low-income Americans.

Health Insurance Exchanges, Essential Health Benefits, and Qualified Health Plans

State Health Insurance Exchanges (HIEs) are the mechanism whereby low- and moderate-income individuals and families eligible for federal subsidies, and employees of small businesses, are able to purchase affordable health insurance (Kaiser Family Foundation, 2013; Weil, Shafir, & Zemel, 2011). The exchanges became active in 2014. The US Affordable Care Act mandates that all insurers cover certain "essential health benefits" (EHB). An insurer's essential health benefits package must cover ten categories of benefits—including prescription drugs, outpatient health care, hospitalization, lab services, prevention and wellness programs, disease management, and mental health and substance abuse services. The law also indicates that the package should be equal to current typical employer plans, meet the needs of diverse populations, including those with disabilities, and not discriminate (Kaiser Family Foundation, 2011).

In December 2011, the US Department of Health and Human Services announced that "essential health benefits" would vary state to state, and could reflect varying needs and priorities from one state to the next. Instead of defining "a single uniform set" of essential health benefits, the Obama Administration "will allow each state to specify benefits within broad categories," including preventive care and prescription drugs (Pear, 2011). HHS Secretary Kathleen Sebelius said the Administration was undertaking this initiative to give states "the flexibility to design coverage options to meet their unique needs" (Pear, 2011). Such an action also undercuts conservative critiques of the Affordable Care Act as an imposition of federal mandates on states that usurps state authority. Under the approach announced by HHS in December 2011, each state will designate an existing health insurance plan as a benchmark. The benefits offered by the benchmark plan will be deemed essential and, in 2014, all insurers operating in the state were required to provide benefits of the same or greater value as those provided by the benchmark plan. This benchmark plan will be one of the following[4]:

1. One of the three largest small-group plans in the state
2. One of the three largest health plans for state employees

---

[4] The Fenway Institute commented January 31, 2012 on the US Health and Human Services proposal on Essential Health Benefits (EHBs) issued in December 2011. Fenway urged HHS to ensure nondiscriminatory treatment against people with disabilities, including HIV/AIDS, by establishing a strong national floor for coverage. In December, the Administration signaled it would allow states a great deal of flexibility to determine EHBs, which has raised concerns among AIDS advocates and others advocating for people with complex health care needs. Fenway also recommended that small-group plans and for-profit HMOs be eliminated as benchmark options for states, because such plans often have coverage restrictions and higher cost-sharing. The Fenway Institute also recommended that plans be prohibited from substituting benefits across and within categories, and that patients be able to access the care they need based on the standard of care, not cost concerns. Finally, Fenway asked HHS to ensure that prevention and mental health/substance use services—statutorily covered as EHBs—be clinically competent to serve LGBT people.

3. One of the three largest national health insurance options for federal employees
4. The largest health maintenance organization operating in the state's commercial insurance market

Among HIE and EHB concerns related to gay people and HIV are discrimination and lack of coverage of HIV medications and other medically necessary services. Rules promulgated by the US Department of Health and Human Services in 2012 required nondiscrimination in HIE activities on the basis of sexual orientation and gender identity, including in the activities of Qualified Health Plan (QHP) issuers. In 2014, when the HIEs began to operate, QHPs were required to be exchange-certified insurance plans that provide Essential Health Benefits, follow limits on cost-sharing (such as deductibles and co-payments), and meet other requirements (United States Department of Health and Human Services (U.S. HHS), n.d.). Efforts are also underway to ensure HIEs reach out to LGBT consumers, collect confidential patient data on sexual orientation and gender identity, ensure subsidies and enrollment systems include same-sex couples and children of same-sex couples, and prohibit exclusions of transgender people's health care needs.

It is also critical that people with HIV/AIDS and other vulnerable populations have access to essential care and treatment through the QHPs traded on the HIEs. People with HIV/AIDS must take at least three antiretroviral (ARV) drugs to effectively suppress HIV. Allowing plans to cover only one drug in each category covered by the benchmark, as proposed in the US Department of Health and Human Services' Informational Bulletin of December 2011, could mean that people with HIV are not able to access the life-saving ARVs that revolutionized HIV care in the mid-1990s. Utilization controls, such as requiring prior authorization to access ARVs, could also hinder access to treatment. Explicit language in EHB guidance and future HHS regulations is essential to ensure that people with complex health conditions such as HIV are able to access all medications necessary to treat their disease according to federal treatment guidelines. HHS should also issue guidance to ensure access to comprehensive mental health and substance use services, prevention services, chronic disease management, and other elements of the ten statutorily mandated EHB categories.

It is also important that people living with HIV be able to access the care they need based on the standard of care. HHS regulations should include patient protections to ensure that patients can access the care they need based on the standard of care, not cost. People with HIV/AIDS, cancer, and other chronic disease may require frequent medical visits and laboratory tests to ensure their health. Service or benefit limitations could hinder this goal. People should also be able to access specialists without paying excessive co-payments they cannot afford. HHS should ensure that these scenarios do not occur by writing patient protections into EHB guidance. If HHS fails to do this, state exchanges should take the initiative and thereby guarantee that the complex health care needs of people with HIV are met.

Ryan White

The Ryan White Program provides care and support services to half a million people living with HIV in the USA and their families. About a third of Ryan White's $2.3 billion in funds supports the AIDS Drug Assistance Program (ADAP), which helps people with HIV purchase antiretroviral medications. Most clients served by the Ryan White program are low-income, male, and people of color (Kaiser Family Foundation, 2011). Many are gay and bisexual men. Core medical services provided with Ryan White funds include outpatient and ambulatory health services, early intervention services, medical case management, treatment adherence services, medical nutrition therapy, legal services, and mental health and substance use treatment.

Social Security and Supplemental Security Income

Some people living with AIDS qualify for Social Security disability insurance or Supplemental Security Income (SSI). Eligibility is reserved for individuals who (1) cannot do the work they once did before, (2) the Social Security Administration decides that they cannot adjust to other work because of their medical condition(s), and (3) their disability has lasted or is expected to last for at least 1 year or to result in death. Only those who have worked long enough and paid into the program sufficiently can access Social Security disability insurance; SSI is available more broadly based on limited resources and income, not work history (United States Social Security Administration, n.d.).

Until the landmark changes brought about by the landmark Supreme Court ruling *U.S. v. Windsor* in 2013, striking down federal nonrecognition of same-sex marriages (Cahill & Vargas, 2015), Social Security regulations denied older gay men with partners or spouses access to funds from systems they pay into throughout their working lives, but could not access due to the unequal treatment of same-sex couples. Nearly two-thirds of US retirees rely on Social Security for more than half of their annual income and, for 15% of seniors, Social Security is their only source of income (Liu, 1999). Social Security survivor benefits allow widows, widowers, and dependent children to put food on the table and fairly compensate them when their spouse pays into the system his or her whole life but dies before being able to enjoy these retirement savings. But gay and lesbian survivors were not eligible for these benefits, even though they had paid taxes into the system for their entire lives. The 9/11 attacks illustrated the unfairness of this policy: same-sex survivors of victims were denied Social Security and worker's comp survivor benefits. They also had to struggle to access funds from the victims' compensation fund administered by the US Justice Department. Gay partners were also ineligible for spousal benefits, which allow a partner to earn about half his or her life partner's Social Security payment if that rate is higher. Following the *Windsor* ruling, the Social Security Administration moved to treat same-sex spouses the same as heterosexual spouses.

Veterans Affairs

The Department of Veterans Affairs (VA) is the largest single provider of medical care to people with HIV in the USA (US Department of Veterans Affairs, 2009). It has served 64,000 HIV positive veterans since 1981, and currently serves 23,000 HIV-infected veterans. With more than eight million individuals enrolled in the VA health care system, many gay and bisexual men receive health care there. Little is known about the experiences and needs of LGBT veterans. A few state Behavioral Risk Factor Surveillance Surveys ask about sexual orientation and all ask about veteran status. An analysis of Massachusetts BRFSS data from 2005 through 2010 found that LGB veterans reported higher rates of suicidal ideation compared with heterosexual veterans (Blosnich et al., 2012a). Other issues that may disproportionately affect gay veterans are "trauma from childhood adversity interacting with military trauma" (Blosnich et al., 2012b). Because so many gay veterans associate their military service with hiding their sexual orientation, and because some were dishonorably discharged under the prior policies banning homosexuals from serving, it is essential that the VA undertake affirmative outreach to LGBT veterans to ensure that they access the health care services and benefits to which they are entitled. It is also critical that VA staff be trained in LGBT issues so that they can provide clinically competent care. Such trainings have been conducted in New York, Massachusetts, and elsewhere, and there is a working group within the VA promoting training in LGBT health issues and advancing significant improvements in other areas.

Data Collection on Health Surveys and in Clinical Settings

Asking questions about sexual orientation and gender identity is important because there are significant documented health disparities affecting LGBT people (Healthy People, 2020; Mayer et al., 2008). While we know about some disparities, there remain wide gaps in research on LGBT health. Gathering sexual orientation and gender identity data in a standardized way will allow us to better understand LGBT health disparities, as well as to prevent, screen, and detect early conditions that disproportionately affect LGBT people (Bradford, Cahill, Grasso, & Makadon, 2012). Every state conducts the Youth Risk Behavior Survey and the Behavioral Risk Factor Surveillance Survey, yet until 2015 few states gathered data on sexual orientation, and even fewer on gender identity. In 2015, the CDC added sexual orientation questions (identity and behavior) to its core questionnaire, and now about half of states ask the questions (Kann et al., 2016). Few national surveys collect sexual orientation and gender identity data, although this improved significantly under President Barak Obama (Cahill, 2016). Gathering sexual orientation and gender identity data in health care settings allows providers to better understand and treat their patients, and to compare their patients' health outcomes with national samples of LGB or LGBT people from national health surveys. A number of federal agencies have taken steps to encourage or require the collection of sexual orientation and gender identity data in health care settings, such as in the Meaningful Use incentive program under the Centers for Medicare and Medicaid Services (Cahill, Baker, Deutsch, Keatley, & Makadon, 2016).

The Older Americans Act

The OAA funds social and nutritional services to people 60 and older and their caregivers. Services include a wide range of programs related to elder abuse and neglect, mental health, benefits counseling, civil engagement, nutritional services, healthy aging, evidence-based health promotion and disease prevention, adult day care, transportation, and caregiving (United States Administration on Aging, n.d.). The OAA also funds workforce training and research. The Older Americans Act (OAA), currently overdue for reauthorization, should broaden the definition of older adults with "greatest social need" to include older adults with HIV and LGBT elders. This would allow resources to be targeted to train elder service staff and conduct research to better understand the experiences of these populations in elder service settings. State units on aging can make such a designation: Massachusetts's Executive Office of Elder Affairs (EOEA) designated LGBT elders as such in 2012 (Krinsky & Cahill, 2017). The Massachusetts Special Legislative Commission on Lesbian, Gay, Bisexual and Transgender Aging has also called on EOEA to make a similar designation for older adults living with HIV (Krinsky & Cahill, 2017).

Conclusions

In conclusion, gay men living with HIV have complex health needs. These include disparities in physical and mental health, as well as side effects of long-term HIV infection and antiretroviral use and interactions with other health conditions. Older gay men living with HIV may experience social isolation and have often have significant caregiving and social support needs. Biomedical prevention research holds great promise for serodiscordant couples, and recent changes in federal health policy have enabled greater access to quality health care for gay men living with HIV.

References

Abdool Karim, S., & Abdool Karim, Q. (2011). Antiretroviral prophylaxis: A defining moment in HIV control. *The Lancet*, *378*, e23–e25.
AIDSinfo.gov. UC781. (2013). Retrieved from http://aidsinfo.nih.gov/DrugsNew/DrugDetailT. aspx?int_id=394#DescRef1384.

American Civil Liberties Union. (2017). *Non-discrimination laws: State-by-state information, map*. Retrieved from https://www.aclu.org/map/non-discrimination-laws-state-state-information-map.

Anton, P., Saunders, T., Adler, A., et al. (2011). *A phase 1 safety and acceptability study of the UC-781 microbicide gel applied rectally in HIV seronegative adults: RMP-01. UCLA U-19 Microbicide development program*. Presented at Conference on Retroviruses and Opportunistic Infections, Boston. Retrieved from http://rectalmicrobicides.org/teleconf.php.

Aynalem, G., Smith, L., Bemis, C., Taylor, M., Hawkins, K., & Kerndt, P. (2006). Commercial sex venues: A closer look at their impact on the syphilis and HIV epidemics among men who have sex with men. *Sexually Transmitted Infections, 82*(6), 439–444.

Badgett, L. (2001). *Money, myths, and change: The economic lives of lesbians and gay men*. Chicago: University of Chicago Press.

Badgett, L., Lau, H., Sears, B., & Ho, D. (2007). *Bias in the workplace: Consistent evidence of sexual orientation and gender identity discrimination*. Los Angeles: UCLA Williams Institute.

Baker, S., Sudit, M., & Litwak, E. (1998). Caregiver burden and coping strategies used by informal caregivers of minority women living with HIV/AIDS. *ABNF Journal, 9*(3), 56–60.

Beck A. (2012). *Drug resistant staph found to be passed in gay sex—Study*. Reuters. Retrieved from http://www.reuters.com/article/2008/01/14/us-staph-men-idUSN1337175820080114.

Berstein, K. T., Liu, K. L., Begier, E. M., Koblin, B., Karpati, A., & Murrill, C. (2008). Same-sex attraction disclosure to health care providers among New York City men who have sex with men. *Archives of Internal Medicine, 168*(13), 1458–1464.

Blosnich, J. R., Bossarte, R. M., & Silenzio, V. M. (2012a). Suicidal ideation among sexual minority veterans: Results from the 2005–2010 Massachusetts behavioral risk factor surveillance survey. *American Journal of Public Health, 102*(S1), 44–47.

Blosnich, J. R., Bossarte, R. M., & Silenzio, V. M. (2012b). Improved health care for sexual minority and transgender veterans. *American Journal of Public Health, 102*, e10–e11.

Bochenek, M., & Brown, A. W. (2001). *Hatred in the hallways: Violence and discrimination against lesbian, gay, bisexual, and transgender students in U.S. schools*. New York: Human Rights Watch. Retrieved from www.hrw.org/reports/2001/uslgbt/toc.htm

Bolding, G., Davis, M., Hart, G., Sherr, L., & Elford, J. (2005). Gay men who look for sex on the internet: Is there more HIV/STI risk with online partners? *AIDS, 19*, 961–968.

Bontempo, D. E., & D'Augelli, A. R. (2002). Effects of at-school victimization and sexual orientation on lesbian, gay, or bisexual youths' health risk behavior. *Journal of Adolescent Health, 30*(5), 364–374.

Bradford, J., Cahill, S., Grasso, C., & Makadon, H. (2012). *Why ask about sexual orientation and gender identity in clinical settings*. Boston: Fenway Institute. Retrieved from http://www.fenwayhealth.org/site/DocServer/Policy_Brief_WhyGather..._v6_01.09.12.pdf?docID=9141

Burgess, D., Lee, R., Tran, A., & van Ryn, M. (2007). Effects of perceived discrimination on mental health and mental health services utilization among gay, lesbian, bisexual and transgender persons. *Journal of LGBT Health Research, 3*, 1–14.

Butler, D., & Smith, D. (2007). Serosorting can potentially increase HIV transmissions. *AIDS, 21*(9), 1218–1220.

Cahill, S. (2007). The role of antigay family amendments in the 2004 election. In M. Strasser (Ed.), *Defending same-sex marriage, "Separate but equal" no more: A guide to the legal status of same-sex marriage, civil unions, and other partnerships* (vol. 1, pp. 119–140). Westport, Connecticut: Praeger.

Cahill, S. (2012a, June 28. *The Supreme Court's ruling upholding the ACA is especially important for LGBT people and those living with HIV/AIDS*. Huffington Post. Retrieved from http://www.huffingtonpost.com/sean-cahill/supreme-court-health-care-ruling-lgbt-people_b_1634742.html.

Cahill, S. (2012b, July). *Policy focus: Pre-exposure prophylaxis for HIV prevention: Moving toward implementation (2nd edn)*. Boston: The Fenway Institute. Retrieved from http://www.fenwayhealth.org/site/DocServer/PolicyFocus_PrEP_v7_02.21.12.pdf?docID=9321.

Cahill, S. (2016). Expanding capacity for the measurement of sexual orientation and gender identity in federal surveys: Discussion. In *Joint Statistical Meeting Proceedings, Social Statistics*. Alexandria, VA: American Statistical Association.

Cahill, S., Baker, K., Deutsch, M., Keatley, J., & Makadon, H. (2016). Inclusion of sexual orientation and gender identity in stage 3 meaningful use guidelines: A huge step forward for LGBT
health. *LGBT Health, 3*, 100–102.

Cahill, S., Darnell, B., Guidry, J., Krivo-Kaufman, A., Schaefer, N., Urbano, L., … Valadez, R.
(2010). *HIV and aging: Growing older with the epidemic*. New York: Gay Men's Health Crisis.
Retrieved from http://www.gmhc.org/files/editor/file/a_pa_aging10_emb3.pdf

Cahill, S., & Vargas, H. (2015). Policy and legal issues affecting LGBT health. In H. Makadon,
K. Mayer, J. Potter, & H. Goldhammer (Eds.), *The Fenway guide to lesbian, gay, bisexual,
and transgender health* (2nd ed.pp. 519–538). Philadelphia: American College of Physicians.

Carballo-Dieguez, A., Exner, T., Dolezal, C., Pickard, R., Lin, P., & Mayer, K. H. (2007). Rectal
microbicide acceptability: Results of a volume escalation trial. *Sexually Transmitted Diseases,
34*(4), 224–229.

CDC. (2008a). HIV risk, prevention, and testing behaviors among men who have sex with men—
National HIV Behavioral Surveillance System, 21 U.S. cities. *MMWR, 60*(14). Retrieved from
http://www.cdc.gov/mmwr/pdf/ss/ss6014.pdf.

CDC. (2008b). HIV prevention estimates—United States, 2006. *Morbidity and Mortality Weekly
Report (MMWR), 57*. Retrieved from http://www.cdc.gov/mmwr/preview/mmwrhtml/
mm5739a2.htm.

CDC. (2010a). *CDC analysis provides new look at disproportionate impact of HIV and syphilis
among U.S. gay and bisexual men*. Retrieved from http://www.cdc.gov/nchhstp/Newsroom/
msmpressrelease.html.

CDC. (2010b). *HIV among gay, bisexual, and other men who have sex with men (MSM)*. Atlanta,
GA: Author. Retrieved from http://www.cdc.gov/hiv/topics/msm/pdf/msm.pdf

CDC. (2011a). Vital signs: HIV prevention through care and treatment. *Morbidity and Mortality
Weekly Report (MMWR), 60*(47), 1618–1623.

CDC. (2011b). HIV surveillance in men who have sex with men (MSM). *HIV/AIDS Statistics
and Surveillance*. Retrieved from http://www.cdc.gov/hiv/topics/surveillance/resources/slides/
msm/index.htm?source=govdelivery.

CDC. (2011c). Sexual identity, sex of sexual contacts, and health-risk behaviors among students
in grades 9-12—Youth risk behavior surveillance, selected sites, United States, 2001–2009.
MMWR Early Release, 60, 1–133.

CDC. (2011d). *Sexually transmitted disease surveillance*. Syphilis. Retrieved from http://www.
cdc.gov/std/stats10/syphilis.htm.

CDC. (2011e). *Sexually transmitted disease surveillance 2010*. Retrieved from http://www.cdc.
gov/std/stats10/default.htm.

CDC. (2011f). *STD surveillance network—genital warts—prevalence among Sexually Transmitted
Disease (STD). Clinic patients by sex, sex of partners, and site, 2010*. Retrieved from http://
www.cdc.gov/std/stats10/figures/51.htm.

CDC. (2014). *HIV surveillance report, 26, 2015*. Retrieved from http://www.cdc.gov/hiv/library/
reports/surveillance/.

Cianciotto, J., & Cahill, S. (2012). *LGBT youth in America's schools*. Ann Arbor, MI: University
of Michigan Press.

Cohen, M., Chen, Y., McCauley, M. , Gamble T, Hosseinipour MC, Kumarasamy N … HPTN
052 Study Team. (2011). Prevention of HIV-1 infection with early antiretroviral therapy. *New
England Journal of Medicine, 365*(6), 493–505.

Cohen, S. M., Van Handel, M. M., Branson, B. M., Blair, J. M., Hall, I., Hu, X., … CDC, CDC.
(2011). Vital Signs: HIV prevention through care and treatment—United States. *Weekly,
60*(47), 1618–1623.

Colvin, R. (2004). *The extent of sexual orientation discrimination in Topeka, KS*. New York: National
Gay and Lesbian Task Force Policy Institute, Equal Justice Coalition of Kansas. Retrieved from
http://www.thetaskforce.org/downloads/reports/reports/TopekaDiscrimination.pdf

D'Emilio, J. (1998). *Sexual politics, sexual communities: The making of a homosexual minority in
the United States, 1940–1970*. Chicago: University of Chicago Press.

Deeks, S. G., & Philips, A. N. (2009). HIV infection, antiretroviral treatment, aging, and non-AIDS related morbidity. *BMJ, 338*(7689), 288–292.

Diep, B., Chambers, H., Graber, C., Szumowski, J. D., Miller, L. G., Han, L. L., ... Perdreau-Remington, F. (2008). Emergence of multidrug-resistant, community-associated, methicillin-resistant Staphylococcus aureus clone USA300 in men who have sex with men. *Annals of Internal Medicine, 148*(4), 249–257.

Effros, R. B., Fletcher, C. V., Gebo, K., Halter, J. B., Hazzard, W. R., Horne, F. M., ... High, K. P. (2008). Aging and infectious diseases: Workshop on HIV infection and aging: What is known and future research directions. *Clinical Infectious Disease, 47*(4), 542–553.

Eldercare Workforce Alliance. (2011). *Issue brief. Geriatric workforce shortfall: A looming crisis for our families*. Washington, DC: Author.

Emlet, C. A. (2006). An examination of the social networks and social isolation in older and younger adults living with HIV/AIDS. *Health and Social Work, 31*(4), 299–308.

Fairchild, S. K., Carrino, G. E., & Ramirez, M. (1996). Social workers' perceptions of staff attitudes toward resident sexuality in a random sample of New York state nursing homes: A pilot study. *Journal of Gerontological Social Work, 26*(1&2), 153–169.

Fenway Institute. (2013). *The Fenway guide to LGBT health, module 3: Health promotion and disease prevention*. Boston: The Fenway Institute. Retrieved from http://www.lgbthealtheducation.org/training/learning-modules/

Gilden, D. E., Kubisiak, J. M., & Gilden, D. M. (2007). Managing Medicare's caseload in the era of suppressive therapy. *American Journal of Public Health, 97*(6), 1053–1059.

GMHC. 2010. *I love my boo*. Retrieved from http://www.facebook.com/pages/I-Love-My-Boo/109154532462180.

Gonzalez C. (2012, April). Advocates seek an end to HIV criminalization. *Poz*.

Goodenow, C. (2007). *Protective and risk factors for HIV-related behavior among adolescent MSM: Analysis of Massachusetts youth behavior survey data. Speech to national HIV prevention conference*. GA: Atlanta.

Goodenow, C. (Mass. DESE). (2011). "Prevention needs of sexual minority youth, MYRBS 1995–2009." Powerpoint presentation. Massachusetts Department of Elementary and Secondary Education.

Grant, R., Lama, J., Anderson, P., McMahan, V., Liu, A. Y., Vargas, L., ... iPrEx Study Team, iPrEx Study Team. (2010). Preexposure chemoprophylaxis for HIV prevention in men who have sex with men. *New England Journal of Medicine, 27*, 2587–2599.

Griffin, P., & Ouellett, M. L. (2002). Going beyond gay-straight alliances to make schools safe for lesbian, gay, bisexual, and transgender students. *Angles, 6*(1), 1–8.

Grov, C., Parsons, J., & Bimbi, D. (2007). Sexual risk behavior and venues for meeting sex partners: An interceptive survey of gay and bisexual men in LA and NYC. *AIDS and Behavior, 11*, 915–926.

Hallett, T., Baeten, J., Heffron, R., Barnabas, R., de Bruyn, G., Cremin, Í., ... Celum, C. (2011). Optimal uses for antiretrovirals for prevention in HIV-1 serodiscordant heterosexual couples in South Africa; a modeling study. *PLoS Medicine, 8*(11), e1001123.

Health Resources Services Administration, HIV/AIDS Bureau. (2006). *Outreach: Engaging people in HIV care*. Retrieved from http://ftp.hrsa.gov/hab/HIVoutreach.pdf.

Healthy People. 2020. *Lesbian, gay, bisexual, and transgender health*. Retrieved from http://www.healthypeople.gov/2020/topicsobjectives2020/overview.aspx?topicid=25.

Institute of Medicine of the National Academies; Board on the Health of Select Populations; Committee on Lesbian, Gay, Bisexual, and Transgender Health Issues and Research Gaps and Opportunities. (2011). *The health of lesbian, gay, bisexual, and transgender people: Building a foundation for better understanding*. Washington, DC: The National Academies Press.

International Rectal Microbicides Advocates. (2013). *Rectal Microbicides 101*. Retrieved from http://rectalmicrobicides.org/docs/From%20Product%20to%20Promise%20FINAL%20English%20version/FINAL_eng_IRMA_2010_new%20lowres.pdf.

Jeffries, W. L., Marks, G., Lauby, J., Murrill, C. S., & Millett, G. A. (2012). Homophobia is associated with sexual behavior that increases risk of acquiring and transmitting HIV infection among black men who have sex with men. *AIDS and Behavior, 17*, 1442–1453.

Johnson, M. J., Arnette, J. K., & Koffman, S. D. (2005). Gay and lesbian perceptions of discrimi-
   nation in retirement care facilities. *Journal of Homosexuality, 49*(2), 83–102.
Kaiser Family Foundation. (2009a). *HIV/AIDS policy fact sheet: Medicare and HIV/AIDS*.
   Retrieved from http://www.kff.org/hivaids/7171.cfm.
Kaiser Family Foundation. (2009b). *Survey of Americans on HIV/AIDS*. Retrieved from http://
   www.kff.org/kaiserpolls/7890.cfm.
Kaiser Family Foundation. (2011). *Fact Sheet: The Ryan White Program*. Retrieved from http://
   www.kff.org/hivaids/upload/7582-06.pdf.
Kaiser Family Foundation. (2013). *Establishing Health Insurance Marketplaces: An overview of
   state effort*. Retrieved from http://www.kff.org/health-reform/issue-brief/establishing-health-
   insurance-exchanges-an-overview-of/.
Kann, L., O'Malley Olsen, E., McManus, T., Harris, W. A., Shanklin, S. L., Flint, K. H., … Zaza,
   S. (2016). Sexual identity, sex of sexual contacts, and health-related behaviors among students in grades 9–12 – United States and selected sites, 2015. *MMWR Surveillance Summaries,
   65*(9), 1–202.
King, M., Semlyen, J., Tai, S. S., Killaspy, H., Osborn, D., Popelyuk, D., & Nazareth, I. (2008).
   A systematic review of mental disorder, suicide, and deliberate self-harm in lesbian, gay and
   bisexual people. *BMC Psychiatry, 8*, 70. doi:10.1186/1471-244X-8-70
Klitzman, R. L., & Greenberg, J. D. (2002). Patterns of communication between gay and lesbian
   patients and their health care providers. *Journal of Homosexuality, 42*(4), 65–75.
Kosciw, J. G., Diaz, E. M., & Greytak, E. A. (2008). *2007 national school climate survey: The
   experiences of lesbian, gay, bisexual and transgender youth in our nation's schools*. New York:
   Gay, Lesbian and Straight Education Network.
Krakower, D., Mimiaga, M., Rosenberger, J., Novak, D. S., Mitty, J. A., White, J. M., & Mayer,
   K. H. (2012). Limited awareness and low immediate uptake of pre-exposure prophylaxis
   among men who have sex with men using an internet social networking site. *PLoS One, 7*(3),
   e33119. doi:10.1371/journal.pone.0033119
Krinsky, L., & Cahill, S. (2017). Advancing LGBT elder policy and support services: The
   Massachusetts model. *LGBT Health*. doi:10.1089/lgbt.2016.0184. [Epub ahead of print].
Lambda Legal HIV Project. (2010). *HIV stigma and discrimination in the U.S.: An evidence-based
   report*. Retrieved from http://data.lambdalegal.org/publications/downloads/fs_hiv-stigma-and-
   discrimination-in-the-us.pdf.
Lauby, J. L., Marks, G., Bingham, T., Liu, K. L., Liau, A., Stueve, A., & Millett, G. A. (2012).
   Having supportive social relationships is associated with reduced risk of unrecognized HIV
   infection among black and Latino men who have sex with men. *AIDS and Behavior, 16*,
   508–515.
LeBlanc, M. (2010). *From promise to product: Advancing rectal microbicides research and advo-
   cacy*. International rectal Microbicides advocates. Chicago. 27. Retrieved from http://rectalmi-
   crobicides.org/docs/From%20Product%20to%20Promise%20FINAL%20English%20version/
   FINAL_eng_IRMA_2010_new%20lowres.pdf.
Lee, C. (2002). The impact of belonging to a high school gay/straight alliance. *The High School
   Journal, 85*(3), 13–26.
Lelutiu-Weinberger, C., Pachankis, J. E., Golub, S. A., Walker, J. J., Bamonte, A. J., & Parsons,
   J. T. (2013). Age cohort differences in the effects of gay-related stigma, anxiety and identifi-
   cation with the gay community on sexual risk and substance use. *AIDS and Behavior, 17*(1),
   340–349.
Liu, G. (1999). Social security and the treatment of marriage; spousal benefits, earnings sharing
   and the challenge of reform. *Wisconsin Law Review, 1*, 1–64.
Makadon, H., Mayer, K., Potter, J., & Goldhammer, H. (Eds.). (2008). *The Fenway guide to lesbian, gay, bisexual, and transgender health*. Philadelphia: American College of Physicians.
Makadon, H. J. (2011). Ending LGBT invisibility in health care: The first step in ensuring equitable care. *Cleveland Clinic Journal of Medicine, 78*, 220–224.
Massachusetts Department of Elementary and Secondary Education (DESE). (2010). *Massachusetts
   high school students and sexual orientation; results of the 2009 youth risk behavior survey*.
   Malden, MA: Author.

Massachusetts DESE. (2012). *Massachusetts high school students and sexual orientation; results of the 2011 youth risk behavior survey.* Malden, MA: Author.

Mayer, K. H., Bradford, J. B., Makadon, H. J., Stall, R., Goldhammer, H., & Landers, S. (2008). Sexual and gender minority health: What we know and what needs to be done. *American Journal of Public Health, 98,* 989–995.

Meyer, I. (1995). Minority stress and mental health in gay men. *Journal of Health and Social Behavior, 36,* 38–56.

Meyer, I. (2003). Prejudice, social stress, and mental health in lesbian, gay, and bisexual populations: Conceptual issues and research evidence. *Psychological Bulletin, 129*(5), 674–697.

Meyer, I. (2010). Identity, stress, and resilience in lesbians, gay men, and bisexuals of color. *Counseling Psychology, 38*(3), 442–454.

Meyer, I., Dietrich, J., & Schwartz, S. (2008). Lifetime prevalence of mental disorders and suicide attempts in diverse lesbian, gay and bisexual populations. *American Journal of Public Health, 98*(6), 1004–1006.

Microbicide Trials Network. (n.d.). *Rectal microbicides fact sheet.* Retrieved from http://www.mtnstopshiv.org/node/2864.

Mitchell, M. M., & Knowlton, A. (2012). Caregiver role overload and network support in a sample of predominantly low-income, African-American caregivers in persons living with HIV/AIDS: A structural equation modeling analysis. *AIDS and Behavior, 16*(2), 278–287.

Mizuno, Y., Borkowf, C., Millett, G. A., Bingham, T., Ayala, G., & Stueve, A. (2012). Homophobia and racism experienced by Latino men who have sex with men in the United States: Correlates of exposure and associations with HIV risk behaviors. *AIDS and Behavior, 16,* 724–735.

NGLTF. (2013). *State laws prohibiting recognition of same-sex relationships.* Retrieved from http://www.thetaskforce.org/static_html/downloads/reports/issue_maps/samesex_relationships_5_15_13.pdf.

O'Donnell, S., Meyer, I., & Schwartz, S. (2011). Increased risk of suicide attempts among black and Latino lesbians, gay men, and bisexuals. *American Journal of Public Health, 101*(6), 1055–1059.

Obedin-Maliver, J., Goldsmith, E. S., Stewart, L., White, W., Tran, E., Brenman, S., … Lunn, M. R. (2011). Lesbian, gay, bisexual and transgender-related content in undergraduate medical education. *Journal of the American Medical Association, 306,* 971–977.

Palefsky, J. (2009). Human papillomavirus-related disease in people with HIV. *Current Opinions on HIV and AIDS, 4*(1), 52–56.

Parsons, J., & Halkitis, P. (2002). Sexual and drug-using practices of HIV-positive men who frequent public and commercial sex environments. *AIDS Care, 14,* 815–826.

Pear, R. (2011, December 16. *Health care law will let states tailor benefits.* New York Times. Retrieved from http://www.nytimes.com/2011/12/17/health/policy/health-care-law-to-allow-states-to-pick-benefits.html.

Pirraglia, P. A., Bishop, D., Herman, D. S., Trisvan, E., Lopez, R. A., Torgersen, C. S., … Stein, M. D. (2005). Caregiver burden and depression among informal caregivers of HIV-infected individuals. *Journal of General Internal Medicine, 20,* 510–514.

Portegies, P. (2010). HIV/HAART and the brain—what's going on? *Journal of International AIDS Society, 13*(Supp14), 035.

Ramirez-Valles, J. (2002). The protective effects of community involvement for HIV risk behavior: A conceptual framework. *Health, Education, and Research, 17*(4), 389–403.

Remafedi, G. (2002). Suicidality in a venue-based sample of young men who have sex with men. *Journal of Adolescent Health, 31*(4), 305–310.

Reuters. (2011). *AIDS drug shown to protect anal tissue from HIV.* Retrieved from http://us.mobile.reuters.com/article/idUSTRE71R3OX20110228?ca=rdt.

Rosario, M., Schrimshaw, E., Hunter, J., & Braun, L. (2006). Sexual identity development among lesbian, gay, and bisexual youths: Consistency and change over time. *Journal of Sex Research, 43*(1), 46–58.

Ross, M. W., Rosser, B. R., Neumaier, E. R., & Positive Connections Team. (2008). The relationship of internalized homonegativity to unsafe sexual behavior in HIV-seropositive men who have sex with men. *AIDS Education and Prevention, 20*(6), 547–557.

Russell, S., Ryan, C., Toomey, R., Diaz, R., & Sanchez, J. (2011). Lesbian, gay, bisexual, and transgender adolescent school victimization: Implications for young adult health and adjustment. *Journal of School Health, 81*(5), 223–230.

Ryan, C., Heubner, D., Diaz, R., & Sanchez, J. (2009). Family rejection as a predictor of negative health outcomes in white and Latino lesbian, gay, and bisexual young adults. *Pediatrics, 123*(1), 346–352.

Schrimshaw, E. W., & Siegel, K. (2003). Perceived barriers to social support from family and friends among older adults with HIV/AIDS. *Journal of Health Psychology, 8*(6), 738–752.

Shippey, R. A., & Karpiak, S. E. (2005). Perceptions of support among older adults with HIV. *Research on Aging, 27*(3), 290–306.

Siconolfi, D., & Moeller, R. (2007). Serosorting. *Bulletin of Experimental Treatments for AIDS, 9*(2), 45–49.

Silverberg, M. J., Lau, B., & Justice, A. C., Engels E, Gill MJ, Goedert JJ … North American AIDS Cohort Collaboration on Research and Design (NA-ACCORD) of IeDEA. (2012). Risk of anal cancer in HIV-infected and HIV-uninfected individuals in North America. *Clinical Infectious Disease, 54*(7), 1026–1034.

Smith, D. M., & Mathews, W. C. (2007). Physicians' attitudes toward homosexuality and HIV: Survey of a California medical society-revisited (PATHH-II). *Journal of Homosexuality, 52*, 1–9.

Stein, G. L., & Bonuck, K. A. (2001). Physician-patient relationships among the lesbian and gay community. *Journal of Gay & Lesbian Medical Association, 5*(3), 87–93.

Strub, S. (2011). *Prosecuting HIV: Take the test and risk arrest? Achieve.* New York: ACRIA and GMHC.

Supervie, V., Barrett, M., Kahn, J., Musuka, G., Moeti, T. L., Busang, L., & Blowera, S. (2011). Modeling dynamic interactions between pre-exposure prophylaxis interventions & treatment programs: Predicting HIV transmission & resistance. *Scientific Reports, 1*, 185.

Supervie, V., Garcia-Lerma, J., Heneine, W., & Blower, S. (2010). HIV, transmitted drug resistance, and the paradox of preexposure prophylaxis. *PNAS, 107*(27), 12381–12386.

Supreme Court of the United States. (2012). *National Federation of independent business et al. V. Sebelius,* Secretary of Health and Human Services. Retrieved from http://www.casebriefs.com/blog/law/health-law/health-law-keyed-to-furrow/health-care-cost-and-access-the-policy-context/national-federal-of-independent-business-et-al-v-sebelius/.

U.S. HHS. (2016, March 3). 20 million people have gained health insurance coverage because of the Affordable Care Act, new estimates show. Press release. Retrieved from https://www.hhs.gov/about/news/2016/03/03/20-million-people-have-gained-health-insurance-coverage-because-affordable-care-act-new-estimates.

United States Administration on Aging. (n.d.).*Older Americans Act.* Retrieved from http://www.aoa.gov/AoA_programs/OAA/index.aspx.

United States Department of Health and Human Services (U.S. HHS). (n.d.) *Key features of the law.* Retrieved from http://www.healthcare.gov/law/features/index.html.

United States Department of Veterans Affairs. (2009). *The state of care for veterans with HIV/AIDS.* Retrieved from http://www.hiv.va.gov/provider/state-of-care/summary.asp.

United States Social Security Administration. (n.d.). *Disability planner: Social security protection if you become disabled.* Retrieved from http://www.ssa.gov/dibplan/index.htm#a0=0.

Washington Post Staff. (2010). *Landmark: The inside story of America's new health-care law and what it means for us all.* New York: Public Affairs (Perseus).

Weil, A., Shafir, A., & Zemel, S. (2011). *Health insurance exchange basics.* State Health Policy Briefing. National Academy for State Health policy. Retrieved from http://nashp.org/sites/default/files/health.insurance.exchange.basics.pdf.

White House Office of National AIDS Policy. (2010). *National HIV/AIDS strategy.* Retrieved from https://www.whitehouse.gov/administration/eop/onap/nhas.

White House Office of National AIDS Policy. (2016). *National HIV/AIDS strategy for the United States; updated to 2020.* Indicator supplement. Retrieved from https://www.aids.gov/federal-resources/national-hiv-aids-strategy/nhas-2020-indicators.pdf.

Wight, R. G., LeBlanc, A. J., de Vries, B., & Detels, R. (2012). Stress and mental health among midlife and older gay-identified men. *American Journal of Public Health, 102*(3), 503–510.

Willging, C. E., Salvador, M., & Kano, M. (2006). Unequal treatment: Mental health care for sexual and gender minorities in a rural state. *Psychiatric Services, 57*, 867–870.

Index

© Springer Science+Business Media LLC 2017
L. Wilton (ed.), *Understanding Prevention for HIV Positive Gay Men*,
DOI 10.1007/978-1-4419-0203-0

Printed in the United States
By Bookmasters